DATE

EFFECTS OF NOISE ON HEARING

Effects of Noise on Hearing

Edited by

Donald Henderson, Ph.D
Associate Professor
Department of Otolaryngology
and Communication Sciences
State University of New York
Upstate Medical Center
Syracuse, New York

Roger P. Hamernik, Ph.D
Associate Professor
Department of Otolaryngology
and Communication Sciences
State University of New York
Upstate Medical Center
Syracuse, New York

Darshan S. Dosanjh, Ph.D
Professor
Department of Mechanical and
Aerospace Engineering
Syracuse University
Syracuse, New York

John H. Mills, Ph.D
Associate Professor
Department of Otolaryngology
Medical University of South Carolina
Charleston, South Carolina

Raven Press ▪ New York

Raven Press, 1140 Avenue of the Americas, New York, New York 10036

Made in the United States of America

International Standard Book Number 0–89004–012–5
Library of Congress Catalog Card Number 75–14576

Preface

We have been studying the effects of high-level impulse noise on the auditory system for the past six years. During the course of this research, it became evident that the answer to a seemingly straightforward question, that is, how much noise is too much, is highly complex and requires input from many disciplines. There are several excellent books (Kryter, *The Effects of Noise on Man,* Academic Press, 1970; Burns and Robinson, *Noise and Man,* 2nd edition, Lippincott, 1973), but these volumes are broad in scope and furthermore important advances have taken place since their publication.

The problems of noise pollution are increasingly becoming an environmental issue. Public interest groups are pressuring our legislature to develop comprehensive and protective guidelines for noise exposures. Our lawmakers are at a disadvantage because the information on the biological and psychological consequences of noise is both incomplete and contradictory. In 1975, the National Institute for Occupational Safety and Health supported a symposium on the Effects of Noise on Hearing, held at Cazanovia, New York. Forty experts from the fields of acoustics, anatomy, physiology, audiology, epidemiology, otolaryngology, and biochemistry were invited to write critical essays on the specific issues underlying the effects of noise on hearing. These essays should help form the scientific basis for the determination of noise standards, as well as point directions for future research.

The book is divided into six sections, the first of which puts the problem of noise pollution in perspective. The second and third sections outline the current understanding of the anatomical, biochemical, and physiological changes underlying noise-induced hearing loss. The fourth section shows the contribution that animal research can make. The fifth section integrates the information from demographic studies, and the final section deals with scientific, medical, and legal considerations for establishing a damage-risk criteria.

This book is useful as a text and source book for audiologists, otolaryngologists, engineers, sensory psychologists, and environmental scientists.

The editors would like to thank NIOSH, especially Dr. Alan Stevens, for their interest, encouragement, and support. We also appreciate the help from both the Department of Mechanical and Aerospace Engineering, Syracuse University and the Department of Otolaryngology and Communication Sciences, State University of New York Upstate Medical Center, for their support over the last two years. A number of individuals helped ensure the success of the symposium: Dr. R. Schmidt, President, State University of New York Upstate Medical Center, for his encouragement and advice on publication; Mr. Tom Vedder for the smooth operation of the audiovisual service; Mrs. H. Hayes and Mrs. G. Nortman for their patient and understanding secretarial help; Dick Salvi and Ken Hynson for helping to keep the symposium running smoothly. Finally, special thanks go to Mrs. Jeannette Levey for taking the responsibility of making the symposium actually work. Everyone associated with her benefited from her enthusiasm, and she made the whole experience much more enjoyable.

D.H.
R.P.H.

Introduction

The National Academy of Sciences, National Research Council Committee on Hearing and Bioacoustics (CHABA) has studied the existing research data and statistics on noise exposure up to 1965 and has created a set of public health guidelines. These guidelines are stated in the form of damage risk criteria (DRC), which specify that for a given combination of noise parameters, a predictable amount of hearing loss may develop in a certain percentage of the population. The DRC are based on several postulates concerning the relation between temporary loss of hearing (TTS) and the noise-induced permanent loss of hearing (NIPTS).

Postulate I. TTS_2 is a consistent measure of the effects of a single day's exposure to noise.

Postulate II. All exposures that produce a given TTS_2 will be equally hazardous.

Postulate III. The NIPTS eventually produced after 10 years of habitual exposure, 8 hours per day, is about numerically equal to the TTS_2 at 1 kHz produced in young normal-hearing ears by an 8-hour exposure to the same noise.

The primary sets of data for the CHABA report were either *ex post facto* correlations of hearing losses for people and their estimated noise exposure or experimental studies that predicted the NIPTS on the basis of how much TTS was produced by a limited exposure. Since the 1965 CHABA meeting, there have been major advances in the understanding and quantification of the effects of noise on hearing. These advances have an important and direct bearing on the problem of establishing a scientifically based DRC. Specifically: (1) Studies of asymptotic TTS, in humans and chinchilla, permit the development of a mathematical model that relates the physical parameters of a noise and the limits of both TTS and PTS that can be expected from a noise. (2) Studies of cellular ultrastructure have indicated such subtle changes as disruption of tight cell junctions, fractures in the reticular lamina and the ensuing mixing of cochlear fluids. These changes in the ultrastructure might be related to the hearing level of subjects. Preliminary analysis of cellular integrity has demonstrated that large losses of outer hair cells may not be manifested in the results of pure-tone audiometry; therefore, it appears that more powerful diagnostic procedures are necessary. (3) Several studies have shown traumatic interaction between safe noise and safe levels of ototoxic drugs as well as traumatic interactions between safe impulse and safe continuous noise. (4) Finally, neurophysiologists are now looking at the changes that take place in the single neurons of the auditory system when the system has been damaged by noise or ototoxic drugs. The results of these studies are useful in understanding the language of the auditory brain and have already given us new insights into possible central contributions to TTS.

Collectively, these experiments cast some doubt on the assumed TTS/NIPTS relation, question the efficacy of using pure-tone thresholds as an index of the status of the auditory system, and point out the deficiencies in the noise criteria.

The National Institute for Occupational Safety and Health (NIOSH) is committed to understanding the relation between noise and hearing loss. Therefore, considering the complexity of the problem and the new data available, NIOSH sponsored a symposium entitled Noise-Induced Hearing Loss: Critical Issues. The symposium was held at Cazenovia College, Cazenovia, New York on June 23–24, 1975. Scientists in the areas of anatomy, biochemistry, psychophysics, medicine and engineering were invited to write critical essays on the problems that are involved in establishing a scientific basis for DRC. Some of the questions that were posed to the experts were as follows:

1. What is the relationship between TTS and the transient cellular changes that occur in the cochlea? What processes are responsible for the different TTS recovery patterns? What is the relationship between TTS and NIPTS? Do the present CHABA postulates about TTS have to be modified?

2. What are the differential effects of low-level long-duration noise, high-level short-duration noise, impulse noise and continuous/impulse noise combinations? Is there a strategy for evaluating all types of noise on a common criterion?

3. How can results be extrapolated across species? This is particularly important because certain types of information can most efficiently be obtained from animal experiments; therefore, it is imperative to develop an algorithm for going from animal to human results.

4. What is the most appropriate measure of noise-induced damage to the auditory system? What are the optimum hearing conservation strategies for various noise environments? Are there any viable prophylactic procedures to prevent NIPTS? How does one separate the components of sociocusis, presbycusis, and noise-induced NIPTS for purposes of compensation?

Donald Henderson
Roger P. Hamernik
Darshan S. Dosanjh
John H. Mills

Contents

Part VI. Scientific, Medical, and Legal Considerations for Establishing a Damage Risk Criteria

Contributors

Harlow W. Ades
Loyola University of Chicago
Chicago, Illinois 60626
and
Bioacoustics Laboratory
University of Illinois
Chicago, Illinois 60612

Peter W. Alberti
University of Toronto
Toronto, Ontario, Canada

Robert C. Bilger
Bioacoustics Department
Department of Otolaryngology
Eye and Ear Hospital
University of Pittsburgh
Pittsburgh, Pennsylvania 15213

Barbara A. Bohne
Department of Otolaryngology
Washington University
School of Medicine
St. Louis, Missouri 63110

John F. Corso
State University of New York
Cortland, New York 13045

Terrence R. Dolan
Loyola University of Chicago
Chicago, Illinois 60626

Dennis G. Drescher
Laboratory of Neuro-otolaryngology
National Institute of Neurological
* and Communicative Disorders*
* and Stroke*
National Institutes of Health
Bethesda, Maryland 20014

John D. Durrant
Departments of Otorhinology
* and Physiology*
Temple University
School of Medicine
Philadelphia, Pennsylvania 19122

Kenneth McK. Eldred
Bolt, Beranek & Newman, Inc.
Cambridge, Massachusetts 02138

Donald H. Eldredge
Central Institute for the Deaf
St. Louis, Missouri 63110

E. F. Evans
University of Keele
Keele, England

Alan S. Feldman
Department of Otolaryngology
Communication Disorder Unit
State University of New York
Upstate Medical Center
Syracuse, New York 13210

Thomas J. Fria
University of Toronto
Toronto, Ontario, Canada

Roger P. Hamernik
State University of New York
Upstate Medical Center
and
Syracuse University
Syracuse, New York

Joseph E. Hawkins, Jr.
Kresge Hearing Research Institute
and
Department of Otorhinolaryngology
University of Michigan Medical School
Ann Arbor, Michigan 48104

Donald Henderson
State University of New York
Upstate Medical Center
and
Syracuse University
Syracuse, New York 13210

Terry Henderson
Physical Agents Branch
National Institute for Occupational
* Safety and Health*
Cincinnati, Ohio 45202

Lars-Goran Johnsson
Kresge Hearing Research Institute
and
Department of Otolaryngology

University of Michigan
  Medical School
Ann Arbor, Michigan 48104

Daniel Johnson
6570th Aerospace Medical
  Research Laboratory
Wright-Patterson Air Force Base, Ohio

John S. Keeler
University of Waterloo
Waterloo, Ontario, Canada

Karl D. Kryter
Stanford Research Institute
333 Ravenswood Avenue
Menlo Park, California 94025

John C. LeBlanc
University of Toronto
Toronto, Ontario, Canada

Alan Martin
Institute of Sound and
  Vibration Research
University of Southampton
Southampton, England

William Melnick
Ohio State University
Department of Otolaryngology
Columbus, Ohio 43210

John H. Mills
Department of Otolaryngology
Medical University of South
  Carolina
Charleston, South Carolina 29401

David B. Moody
Kresge Hearing Research Institute
University of Michigan
Ann Arbor, Michigan 48104

Peter Paul Morgan
University of Toronto
Toronto, Ontario, Canada

Robert J. Murphy
Loyola University of Chicago
Chicago, Illinois 60612

Douglas W. Robinson
National Physical Laboratory
Teddington, England

Richard J. Salvi
Department of Otolaryngology
  and Communication Sciences
Upstate Medical Center
Syracuse, New York 13210

Robert L. Smith
Institute for Sensory Research
Syracuse University
Syracuse, New York 13210

James B. Snow, Jr.
Department of Otolaryngology
  and Human Communication
University of Pennsylvania
  School of Medicine
Philadelphia, Pennsylvania 19104

Heinrich H. Spoendlin
Department of Otolaryngology
University of Zurich
Zurich, Switzerland

William C. Stebbins
Kresge Hearing Research Institute
University of Michigan
Ann Arbor, Michigan 48104

Ruediger R. Thalmann
Washington University
School of Medicine
St. Louis, Missouri 63110

Juergen Tonndorf
College of Physicians and Surgeons
Columbia University
New York, New York 10032

Constantine Trahiotis
Department of Psychology
University of Illinois
Champaign, Illinois 61820

Henning E. von Gierke
6570th Aerospace Medical
  Research Laboratory
Wright-Patterson Air Force
  Base, Ohio

W. Dixon Ward
Hearing Research Laboratory
University of Minnesota
Minneapolis, Minnesota 55455

Part I
Noise and Hearing: A Perspective on the Problem

Introduction

Terry Henderson

Physical Agents Branch National Institute for Occupational Safety and Health, Cincinnati, Ohio 45202

In my five years at the National Institute for Occupational Safety and Health I cannot recall any previous occasion on which so many distinguished experts were concentrated in one room to discuss the critical issues of noise and hearing loss. It is hard to imagine a conference program more directly aimed at our own concerns and research efforts than this one, and we are most grateful to be in the position of providing necessary sponsorship.

At this time, I would like to review a few ideas regarding occupational noise research that are of considerable concern to us.

First, I would urge you to seriously consider undertaking applied research projects dealing with noise-induced hearing loss in which actual industrial noise exposures are simulated. Particularly in the case of impact or impulsive noise, the need for further data is great. The technology now permits comprehensive animal-model research studies which would have been impossible a few years ago. It will require a great deal of routine, painstaking research to refine the dose-response formulas to the required level of accuracy, and some of that effort may not be as glamorous as we would like; but it is essential if we are going to establish and justify health criteria for our nation's workers.

Second, we must emphasize research efforts to relate noise-induced hearing loss to impairment of activities of daily life other than simply hearing speech in a noiseless environment. Most of the current controversies surrounding noise limits or "identified levels" really arise from uncertainty as to the actual handicap associated with a specific degradation in one's audiogram. This issue cannot be totally resolved until we have critically analyzed the variety of special functions that our ears actually perform in daily life, and have measured the effect of a noise-induced hearing loss upon each one of them.

Finally, I would like to suggest that we need more informal communication between the various laboratories that are engaged in hard-core noise-induced hearing loss research, particularly animal research. Some sort of informal newsletter might be helpful. At any rate, I would hope that everyone will make the most of this opportunity to establish or rekindle close friendships and professional contacts. Those of us from NIOSH would certainly like to get to know all of you.

Effects of Noise on Hearing, edited by Donald Henderson, Roger P. Hamernik, Darshan S. Dosanjh, and John H. Mills. Raven Press, New York © 1976

The Problems of Criteria for Noise Exposure

Donald H. Eldredge

Central Institute for the Deaf, St. Louis, Missouri 63110

How do we form a correct judgment with respect to the hazard to hearing inherent in exposures to noise? The process is complex because the answer depends on several correct judgments, or criteria, with respect to hearing, noise, and means for control of exposure to noise. Neither hearing nor exposure to noise is an all-or-none phenomenon. Hearing can be somewhat impaired without any practical disadvantage in everyday life. However, practical disadvantages grow fairly systematically with increasing degrees of hearing impairment. Similarly, noise is always with us and exposures differ only in degree in regard to level, frequency content, and duration. Given that neither universally perfect hearing nor universal absolute quiet is possible, where do we draw the line so as to reach an optimum compromise? Stated another way, the initial question was based on the false premise that there is a "correct" judgment regarding the hazard for hearing inherent in exposures to noise. The judgment must compromise values in a number of very different dimensions and, accordingly, can only be as good as the compromises. This chapter concerns the kinds of subsidiary questions and compromises that must be faced and made in the process of reaching one or more optimum or "best" judgments. Many of these questions have recently been discussed in considerable detail in the report compiled by Guignard (1) for the United States Air Force and the Environmental Protection Agency.

The first class of questions concerns the goals for hearing conservation. How do we use hearing and how much of this hearing should be protected? The second class of questions follows the first closely. How should we measure loss of hearing? Do the measurements that are possible truly reflect or match the decisions about the amount of hearing to be protected? The third class of questions is concerned with the physical measures that should be used to characterize exposures to noise. At a minimum these include dimensions related to level, frequency content, and duration of exposures. Various degrees of added complexity or simplicity are possible. The fourth class of questions concerns the causal relations between hearing loss and exposure to noise. Here the measures of exposure must be chosen to elicit these causal relations and are not necessarily identical to the measures chosen for the purposes of the second and third classes of questions. A fifth class asks: "How does one apply the available information to the writing of criteria, or standards for judgments, that will be used and not ignored?"

GOALS FOR CONSERVATION OF HEARING

In today's political and social climate there appear, in principle, to be only 2 acceptable goals for the conservation of hearing. The first is the prevention of any impairment at all. The second is the prevention of any material impairment, or handicap, for the hearing of everyday speech. However, some groups and many individuals find that the advantages of some activities that produce noise outweigh the minor disadvantages associated with somewhat greater degrees of hearing impairment. The concepts underlying these apparently simple statements require elaboration.

There are all degrees of loss of hearing short of total deafness and some loss of hearing with increased age appears to be the normal human condition. Medically, it is sometimes possible to restore normal hearing in diseased ears, but there is no way to improve on normal hearing. Accordingly, states of hearing are either normal or described in negative terms. Davis (2) has provided useful definitions for impairment, handicap, and disability of hearing. He defines impairment as a deviation or change for the worse in either structure or function, usually outside the range of normal. Handicap is defined as the disadvantage imposed by an impairment sufficient to affect one's personal efficiency in the activities of daily living. Finally, disability is defined as the actual or presumed inability to remain employed at full wages. These definitions represent a sequence such that there may be impairment without handicap; a handicap requires a greater impairment but may not be disabling in an economic or medicolegal sense, and a disability requires a handicap specifically related to employment. The definitions provided by Davis (2) are used in this chapter, but the reader is warned that these terms have been and still are often used in other ways or as loosely interchangeable equivalents. Furthermore, the nature of noise-induced hearing loss is such that impairments that are significant handicaps in everyday life rarely are handicaps when at work in the noise that produced the impairments. For this reason we consider goals only in terms of impairments and handicaps and eliminate disability from further consideration.

The most conservative goal for the conservation of hearing is the prevention of any impairment of hearing that could be attributed to exposure to noise. The Noise Control Act of 1972 (3) required the administrator of the Environmental Protection Agency to "publish information on the levels of environmental noise the attainment and maintenance of which in defined areas under various conditions are requisite to protect the public health and welfare with an adequate margin of safety." This goal requires that exposures to noise be limited in such a way that normal hearing does not become impaired hearing and so, in turn, requires that we be able to describe operationally the difference between normal and impaired hearing. This distinction is a standard statistical problem. For any measure of the ability to hear there are ranges of values that characterize a normal, young population. The measure of hearing for a single individual drawn randomly from another population must be tested against these ranges. The tests are in terms of the statistical probabilities that the individual measure could have belonged to the normal population. Any line drawn between normal and not-normal or impaired only characterizes a statistic of this kind. The problem and the statistic changes if, for a given individual, there are sets of measures appropriate to the usual or normal state for the individual and for a test state, such as the condition following a period of exposure to noise. Here the statistical tests are directed only at the reliability or repeatability of the individual measures. The distinction is operationally important to the definition of impairment because an individual with worse-than-average hearing may be considered normal, whereas another individual with average hearing can be considered to have impaired hearing if prior measures indicate a loss from better-than-average hearing. However, when the hearing of a test population is compared to that of a normal control population, statistically significant differences between the 2 populations may be detected when the differences are smaller than the range of normal values. These measures can be sensitive to, and accurately reflect, very small differences, provided the 2 populations are measured identically and are, in fact, equivalent, except for the independent variable, such as exposure to noise.

Impairment may be either structural or functional. Changes in the inner ear produced by exposures to noise cannot be examined in the intact individual; therefore, we are restricted to questions about the uses of hearing that can be impaired. The catalog of uses is potentially enormous, but, fortunately, it can be reduced to examples that are considered reasonably representative of the whole. One example is sensitivity to faint sounds over some range of frequencies. Another example is the ability to hear and to discriminate everyday speech and common environmental sounds.

The earliest function to become impaired by exposures to noise appears to be the sensitivity for the hearing of faint sounds in the frequency range 3–6 kHz. If one chooses a goal of no impairment to hearing, this function should be conserved.

The prevention of material impairment of health or functional capacity is another choice for a goal for the conservation of hearing. If we define "material impairment" as one that imposes a disadvantage in daily living, then we arrive at the equivalent to handicap. Many observers believe that the ability to hear faint sounds in the frequency range 3–6 kHz is not a material function in everyday life. Commonly, there is no handicap in everyday life, including the appreciation of music, in the presence of moderately large impairments of sensitivity for these frequencies.

The understanding of speech is such an important part of everyday life that the preservation of this ability is one logical goal for the conservation of hearing. An early expression of this goal was contained in a statement by the Council on Physical Medicine and Rehabilitation of the American Medical Association (4). Furthermore, the speech signal is complex enough in the acoustic dimensions of level, frequency, and time to be a rather good overall test of hearing function. In general, it has been assumed that, if there is no handicap for the hearing of speech, there is not likely to be any handicap for the hearing of other everyday sounds.

One reason that the ability to hear faint sounds was given so little value earlier is that they are commonly masked by the noise of everyday acoustic environments. For some, it follows that the goal of preservation of hearing for speech should imply the preservation of hearing for speech in everyday acoustic environments. As we shall see in the next section, it has not really been possible to devise and to standardize a satisfactory measure of the ability to hear speech for these purposes. The added difficulties required to specify the acoustic properties of everyday noise were so great that efforts to do so were abandoned, and both the AMA Committee on Medical Rating of Physical Impairment (5) and the American Academy of Ophthalmology and Otolaryngology (6) have advocated that material impairments, or handicaps, be calculated in terms of the hearing of everyday speech in the quiet.

The reader should note that the goals for these medical groups were different from the concerns of this chapter. These medical groups attempted to devise a method to calculate percent of impairment on a scale between no material impairment and total impairment. It is likely that these goals were adequately served even though the inquiry was limited to the hearing of everyday speech in the quiet, and, as we will see in the next section, indirect measures were applied as correlates of these abilities. When a major concern is the precise identification of the state of hearing that signals the onset of material impairment, it is possible that the same simplifications may be less appropriate and that the concept of the hearing for speech in environmental noise should be retained. Evidence supporting the necessity for this retention is, however, not compelling.

MEASUREMENT OF HEARING IMPAIRMENT AND HEARING HANDICAP

The measurement of hearing impairment has most commonly been tried in the form of a medicolegal scale encompassing the range from 0 to 100% impairment. The purposes for this scale commonly were related to compensation for accidental injury, occupational disease, or implied disability suffered as a consequence of military service. No completely satisfactory measures are available for these purposes, and opinions on the best measures vary. There are several reasons for this.

First, hearing function is inferred from the dimensions of acoustic signals that are heard correctly. The dimensions of these acoustic signals include level, frequency, complexity, and corresponding dimensions of accompanying noise. The key functions cited in the previous section included the detection of faint signals and discrimination of speech sounds in quiet and in noise. Beyond the fact that there is not agreement on the best way to measure hearing for speech lies the problem of abstracting a single score for impairment from sets of dissimilar measures. How do you add a speech recognition score in percent correct to a loss of sensitivity for faint sounds expressed in decibels? An early attempt at a Social Adequacy Index by Davis (7) that had been developed for clinical use on patients with mixed hearing loss did not survive the technical difficulties with standardization of speech tests because of problems such as those discussed by Silverman and Hirsh (8). This question has not been answered and present practice has retreated to schemes which infer impairment for hearing of everyday speech from measures of auditory sensitivity for pure tones as shown on the audiogram.

The pure-tone audiogram is a set of measures that compares the ability of an individual to detect the presence of faint pure tones in the quiet to the corresponding abilities in a normal population. Thus, the audiogram is a measure ideally suited to the goal of no impairment of hearing. If the audiograms of a population exposed to a noise do not differ significantly from those of a population that has not been exposed to noise, then we can infer no impairment of hearing that can be related to the exposure to noise. If the goal of no impairment of hearing is selected, then the criterion for the judgment of minimal hazard can be set for that exposure that just does or just does not produce some arbitrarily small, but statistically significant, difference between the audiograms of matched control and exposed populations.

In their retreat to the pure-tone audiogram the medical groups concerned chose to equate the onset of impairment for the hearing of everyday speech in the quiet with an average hearing threshold level for the frequencies 0.5, 1, and 2 kHz that was 15 dB less sensitive than the zero reference levels specified in 1951 by the American Standards Association (9). When new levels for reference zero recommended by the International Organization for Standardization (10) were widely adopted, and, in anticipation of their subsequent adoption in the United States, the Committee on Conservation of Hearing of the American Academy of Ophthalmology and Otolaryngology (2) recommended that the same thresholds for tones be retained as equivalent to the onset of handicap. Thus, the onset of handicapping impairment was now equated with an average hearing threshold for the frequencies 0.5, 1, and 2 kHz that was 26 dB less sensitive than the new reference zero. Above this level impairment was considered to increase 1.5% per dB up to 100% impairment for mean thresholds that were 82 and 93 dB less sensitive, respectively, than the 2 reference zeros.

In one sense our concerns with the details of this scale are limited because, for our purposes, we need to identify only the onset of handicap and, perhaps, to learn something about the slightly greater impairments that are risked if our judgments about the hazards of noise exposure are somewhat in error. Nevertheless, it is of additional interest to examine these choices more closely in order to identify some sources for differences of opinion.

The above scale for impairment was adopted because it was expedient, was workable, reflected clinical experience with speech tests in the hard-of-hearing at that time, and avoided many practical problems attending other choices. However, the scale can be criticized on several counts. First, clinical experience of those who have worked with the hard-of-hearing suggest that handicap with everyday speech in everyday life does not grow in simple proportion to the loss of sensitivity in decibels. Some form of a sigmoid relation with handicap increasing slowly, then more rapidly, and finally more slowly again appears to correspond better to the reports of patients. Such a relation was rejected because audiometric accuracy did not appear great enough to justify the differences from a simple 1.5% per dB relation. Thus, the scale was really one for the impairment of hearing sensitivity for pure tones and not for the more abstract concept of disadvantage with everyday speech.

Direct tests of the ability to discriminate speech for the purposes of a scale of impairment were seriously considered, but were rejected because of the complexities of speech perception. Some of these have been discussed by Hirsh (11), and important differences among tests include the nature of the speech material, the quality of the speech signal, the skill of the speaker, and the language skills of the listener. Some of these difficulties and some possibilities for solutions were discussed by Silverman and Hirsh (8), but solutions have not appeared. The concept of the articulation index introduced by French and Steinberg (12) included logical schemes for the evaluation of the effects of noise and of various forms of frequency distortion on the reception of speech. Although the intelligibility for nonsense syllables was easily reduced by either or both forms of interference, the redundancy and added clues in connected discourse, sentences, and polysyllabic words in the hard-of-hearing and in normals was enough to maintain intelligibility in the face of substantial interference.

The early studies that related pure-tone thresholds to hearing for speech used the threshold levels for correct recognition of 50% of spondaic words (13,14) or 50% of phonetically balanced monosyllabic (PB) words (15) by hard-of-hearing persons. This level in decibels of an arbitrary amount of speech reception was easily contrived and compared with pure tone thresholds, and, by inference from the more complete studies of speech intelligibility (see above), was a reasonable way to approximate difficulty with hearing for everyday speech. Although the highest correlation differed slightly, it appeared that the loss for speech as measured above was well approximated by the average loss of sensitivity at the 3 frequencies of 0.5, 1, and 2 kHz.

The intelligibility of speech is such that it remains high even in the presence of significant distortions (12,16). However, Harris (17) demonstrated that simultaneous, multiple distortions, no one of which, alone, significantly modified intelligibility, may greatly reduce intelligibility. Several studies (e.g., 18–20) have treated loss of sensitivity for pure tones at frequencies above 2 kHz as one form of distortion and demonstrated the intelligibility of speech to be significantly reduced when the speech signal was also filtered, speeded, or mixed with noise. One simple generalization from such studies is that the conditions for listening to speech can readily be made so difficult that auditory sensitivity for frequencies above 2 kHz becomes of major importance. A second generalization by these investigators (19,20) was that the average loss of sensitivity at 1, 2, and 3 kHz correlated better with loss of speech intelligibility in noise for the hard-of-hearing than did the average loss at 0.5, 1, and 2 kHz.

Both audiograms and speech-intelligibility tests are artificially contrived samples of listening tasks. What are the relations of hearing-threshold levels for pure tones or for speech-intelligibility scores to reports of difficulties or disadvantages in everyday life? Kell et al. (21) elicited responses to a social questionnaire from matched populations of older women with and without substantial hearing losses associated with years of exposure to industrial noise. As expected, reports of difficulty were more numerous with the greater losses of hearing. Pearson et al. (22) analyzed the relations among the reports of difficulty, measures of speech-reception thresholds (SRT) in noise, and pure-tone hearing threshold levels. The transition from little or no difficulty to difficulty with many everyday listening tasks was relatively abrupt and occurred as the SRT for phonetically balanced monosyllabic words in noise at 60 dBA changed from 65–69 dB to 80–84 dB. Their statistical analyses of the relations between difficulty in everyday life and hearing threshold levels led to a Dundee Index for Hearing Impairment. The hearing threshold level at 2 kHz plus one-half the quantity of the level at 6 kHz minus the level at 4 kHz sorted the noise-exposed population and the matched controls with respect to reported difficulty better than 6 other schemes including the 3-frequency averages 0.5, 1, and 2 kHz and at 1, 2, and 3 kHz. The first term of this index appeared to evaluate overall sensitivity for the so-called speech frequencies and the second term added a correction for the shape of the audiogram. Apparently a 4-kHz notch in an audiogram is not of practical importance until it has grown large enough to produce losses at 2 and 6 kHz.[1] Furthermore, quite normal hearing was associated with an index of 25 dB or less and an index of 25–35 dB was still in the lower range of normal hearing. This represents the class of observation that originally led to the concept of a low fence for the onset of impairment at 26-dB mean hearing threshold level.

We can conclude that the measurement of impairment of sensitivity for pure tones is relatively straightforward. When adequate precautions have been taken to assure quiet test environments, accurate audiometric calibrations, consistent audiometric techniques, and absence of temporary shifts of auditory thresholds, accuracy is limited only by the statistics of populations and of repeated measures. But a direct measure of material impairment or handicap has not been standardized. Furthermore, reasonable persons can easily adopt dif-

---

[1] Note that this index, which is specific to noise-exposed populations, is likely to be in error when hearing sensitivity is nearly normal for frequencies up through 4 kHz and then dips sharply at 6 kHz.

ferent criteria for the definition of a loss of hearing great enough to be a handicap in everyday life.

MEASURES OF EXPOSURES TO NOISE

Today measurements of noise are common, but the most useful and meaningful measures of exposures to noise are not really known, and, in any event, are likely to be different for different purposes. In the overall context for our original question, measures of noise are required (i) for determination of the relations between hearing loss and exposure to noise, (ii) for the specification of limits for safety (or hazard), and (iii) for the monitoring of exposure for compliance with safety limits.

How many physical measures of a habitual exposure to noise must we use to characterize the exposure with respect to the risk for hearing? In the total acoustic space above the quiet of the Brownian motion of molecules of the gases comprising air, there are 3 major categories of physical measures: sound level, sound frequency, and duration or temporal pattern of the sound. Since some sound is always present, duration alone does not determine hazard. The sound frequencies to which the human ear can respond are limited more or less to the range from 20 Hz to 20 kHz. Hearing is more sensitive in the range 0.5–5 kHz with diminishing sensitivity for progressively lower and higher frequencies. It follows that, to some extent, the frequency content of exposures must be important. Finally, since continuous noise at arbitrarily low levels is not a hazard, increasing sound level must eventually contribute to hazard.

In general, we will see in the next section that hazard to hearing is jointly determined by all 3 classes of measures and thus we basically require 3 entries in a table that will categorize hazard to hearing from an exposure to noise. As we will see in a subsequent section, consumers of safety standards rarely will tolerate complexity and a 3-entry table already seems too complex. Fortunately, one solution to the choice of specific measurements is not necessary. The only requirements are that the choice of measurements for each purpose be optimal and that scientists and consumers alike recall that the choice for one purpose need not have been optimal for other purposes.

The fundamental nature of energy for many physical relations suggests that measures of sound pressure that are related to energy may have equivalent lawful relations for the hazard to hearing. Thus, most commonly root-mean-square (rms) sound pressures or their approximations are measured and today there is a tendency to measure an exposure with fluctuations in sound pressure in terms of the level of a continuous noise that would have the same total energy as the fluctuating noise. The more sophisticated reader will have recognized that, as is commonly done, we have in our discussion of physical measurements passed over the acoustic pressure waveforms in time to reach their equivalents in the frequency domain. But the same acoustic energies in the frequency domain can be found combined in ways that produce either high or low ratios of peak pressures to rms pressures. If some portion of the hazard to hearing depends on peak pressures, then measures of peak pressures, of the ratio of peak-to-rms pressure, or the level exceeded n percent (e.g., 10 or 25%) of the time may be required.

The frequency content or spectrum of noise may be specified in relative detail by measures of sound pressure in the constant narrow bands of the wave analyzer, in one-third octave bands, or in octave bands. Less detailed measures can nearly always be inferred accurately from more detailed measures, but inferences in the opposite direction are not possible. In general, studies of *causal* relations between noise exposure and hearing loss require the spectrum to be specified at least as octave-band levels. This is true even though simpler measures prove to relate adequately to risk to hearing.

The simpler methods for treating frequency spectra are to sum the energy at all frequencies to arrive at a single overall level. For most sound-level meters the range of frequencies that are summed is limited to less than that of normal hearing by the response characteristics of the microphone. When the energy at all frequencies in the electrical signal from the microphone is summed equally, or essentially equally, the quantity measured is the overall linear sound pressure level or the C-weighted sound level. Various schemes have been used to weight the energy in the electrical signals unequally before summation to a single level. The most useful of these appears to be the A-weighted sound level. The frequency response of the A-weighting network is the reciprocal of an equal loudness curve at 40 phons and also roughly approximates the reciprocal of the auditory sensitivity for pure tones. Thus it tends to sum the acoustic energy in a manner potentially similar to the way the ear may. Alternatively, to the extent that the ear does not sum acoustic energy, but processes energy at different frequencies in a parallel fashion, the A-weighting network may serve to measure the overload to the inner ear equally for the different frequencies.

Rather less used is a B-weighting network with a response characteristic that is the reciprocal of an equal loudness function for pure tones at about 70 dB SPL. The D-weighting network is based in a similar way on the perceived-noisiness function, but is not presently used for purposes related to hazard.

The variety of temporal patterns and durations of exposures to noise is nearly infinite. Noise may be steady and continuous, fluctuating and continuous, intermittent and continuous, interrupted by periods of quiet, and so on. The noises that are most easily classified are those that are steady and continuous for discrete durations, commonly the working day. Noises that change levels frequently, fluctuate, or are interrupted are more difficult to classify. Either one must use many classes, each class differing in several dimensions, or else one must try to combine some of the inhomogeneous exposures into classes based on total energy or total A-weighted "energy" integrated over an appropriate period of time. Each approach has advantages and disadvantages.

RELATIONS BETWEEN HEARING LOSS AND EXPOSURE TO NOISE

Are the relations between hearing loss and exposure to noise sufficiently orderly and systematic to allow useful generalizations with respect to hazards, or are the relations so idiosyncratic as to defy useful generalizations? To some extent both propositions appear to be true and it is more profitable to begin with observations of the more systematic relations. To the extent that these do exist the quality of the relations observed will depend, among other things, on the choices of the correct measures of hearing loss and of exposures to noise. For measurements of large numbers of people the auditory thresholds for pure tones appear to be the only practical measures and, as noted earlier, reflect impairments of hearing with reasonable sensitivity. It has proven more difficult to find and to classify representative exposures that lead to systematic relations. At this time we must still use the quality of any relations that are observed between or among different measures to evaluate the relative correctness of such measures for these purposes.

Reports by Robinson (23,24), Robinson and Cook (25), Baughn (26), and Passchier-Vermeer (27,28) show reasonably systematic relations between loss of hearing and daily exposure to continuous, relatively steady noises throughout an 8-hour working day. When these noises with different spectral properties are converted to their A-weighted sound levels or to noise ratings (NR) based on curves with comparable spectral properties, hearing thresholds for tones increase systematically with level and with duration of exposure in terms of years. Individual differences, however, are great. Perhaps the most sophisticated analysis of the trends of these relations is that reported by Robinson (23). For the trends reflected by his data, interquartile ranges of 20 dB are common for age-corrected hearing levels and a range of more than 40 dB may be necessary to include the hearing levels of the exposed population falling between the 10th and 90th centiles.

Could this variability in loss among individuals have been reduced by the selections of other measures? We know a little more about the importance of individual variability than we do about the importance of spectral differences between noises with the same A-weighted sound levels. A few studies report the losses associated with a few relatively homogeneous exposures with durations extending to as long as 40 years (29,30). Hearing loss appears and grows differently for different frequencies. However, there is a tendency for the loss at each frequency to approach a limit that is systematically related to noise level. Further, these studies suggest that individuals differ more with respect to the rate at which they acquire a hearing loss than they do in the amount of hearing loss at the end of a working lifetime. Normal interquartile ranges begin relatively small, grow to be very large in the middle years of exposures to noise, and then become smaller again as a limiting shift is approached. When data from different kinds of exposures are combined, these trends may be partially obscured, and, in turn, they tend to obscure the practical consequences of some of the differences among exposures that have been equated by A-weighted sound levels.

The Environmental Protection Agency through the Aerospace Medical Research Laboratory has tried to face the problem of condensing as many data concerning the relations of hearing loss to noise exposure into the most useful form possible. Johnson (31) combined the trends from Robinson (23), Baughn (26), and the review by Passchier-Vermeer (27) to produce a table that summarizes the effects expected for continuous noise exposure at representative A-weighted sound levels. These relations, as amended for publication in the EPA "Levels Document" (32) are shown in Table 1. The average noise-induced permanent threshold shifts (NIPTS) for the frequencies 0.5, 1, and 2 kHz, for the frequencies 0.5, 1, 2, and 4 kHz and for the single fre-

TABLE 1. *Summary of the permanent hearing damage effects expected for continuous noise exposure at various values of the A-weighted average sound level[a]*

| | 75 dB for 8 hr | | |
	av. .5,1,2 kHz	av. .5,1,2,4 kHz	4 kHz
Max NIPTS 90th percentile	1 dB	2 dB	6 dB
NIPTS at 10 yr 90th percentile	0	1	5
Average NIPTS	0	0	
Max NIPTS 10th percentile	0	0	0
	80 dB for 8 hr		
	av. .5,1,2 kHz	av. .5,1,2,4 kHz	4 kHz
Max NIPTS 90th percentile	1 dB	4 dB	11 dB
NIPTS at 10 yr 90th percentile	1	3	9
Average NIPTS	0	1	4
Max NIPTS 10th percentile	0	0	2
	85 dB for 8 hr		
	av. .5,1,2 kHz	av. .5,1,2,4 kHz	4 kHz
Max NIPTS 90th percentile	4 dB	7 dB	19 dB
NIPTS at 10 yr 90th percentile	2	6	16
Average NIPTS	1	3	9
Max NIPTS 10th percentile	1	2	5
	90 dB for 8 hr		
	av. .5,1,2 kHz	av. .5,1,2,4 kHz	4 kHz
Max NIPTS 90th percentile	7 dB	12 dB	28 dB
NIPTS at 10 yr 90th percentile	4	9	24
Average NIPTS	3	6	15
Max NIPTS 10th percentile	2	4	11

Entries are the differences in decibels between pure-tone thresholds of noise-exposed and control populations matched for age. There are comparisons for three different measures of threshold, for four statistical indicators for the populations, and for four different levels of noise. See text for more detailed examples.
[a] From ref. 32.

quency 4 kHz that are produced by continuous noise exposures are shown for combinations of 4 A-weighted sound levels and for 4 statistical measures of populations so exposed.

The statistical measures were chosen to illustrate the ranges of changes observed as well as measures of central tendency. The statistic showing the greatest change across levels and across methods of measuring hearing loss was the maximum difference in decibels between the 90th percentiles of the noise-exposed and the control populations at any time throughout the period of 40 years of exposure. When these same 90th percentiles are compared after exposure for 10 years the differences were less, but also large enough to imply that the greater part of the change that will occur in 40 years occurs in the first 10 years. The entries listed as average NIPTS are gross average values obtained by averaging over a 40-year exposure and also over all the population percentiles, and differ no more than a couple of decibels from the median values after 20 years of exposure. The maximum NIPTS obtained by comparing the 10th percentiles in the exposed and control populations shows the least change attributable to noise exposure and, for this reason, helps to assure that the changes produced by noise are not concentrated in the 10% of the initially most sensitive ears. Rather the changes observed appear to apply to all the population with the greater changes appearing in the initially least sensitive ears. Thus measures directed at prevention of changes at the 90th percentile are almost certain to help the entire population.

Table 1 helps to clarify the importance of choice of goals for the conservation of hearing. Given daily exposures at 75 dB(A), 90% of a population should never show more than 6 dB difference in hearing level at 4 kHz from a normal control population, and the differences at lower frequencies are smaller yet. Although statistically significant, these changes are probably too small to measure with confidence on a single individual. Under EPA requirements for involuntary exposures the choice of a limit at 75 dB(A) for continuous exposure for 8 hr is adequately protective.

If a limit of 85 dB(A) for continuous exposures lasting 8 hr a day is chosen, Table 1 says 90% of the population will have 7 dB or less change in mean hearing levels for the 4 frequencies 0.5, 1, 2, and 4 kHz and 19 dB or less change at 4 kHz. It would be difficult to measure significant impairment of speech intelligibility in this group. If the limit is set at 90 dBA, the table says 90% of the population will show a change of 7 dB or less for the average hearing level for 0.5, 1, and 2 kHz, 12 dB or less when 4 kHz is included in the average and 28 dB or less at 4 kHz. Many argue that even these changes do not constitute impairments that are handicapping in everyday life. The more highly valued are operations that produce sound levels in excess of 85 dB(A), and the more difficult it is to reduce sound levels from 90 to 85 dB(A), the easier it is to accept 90 dB(A) continuously for 8 hr as a limit that is satisfactorily safe for 90% of persons so exposed.

The above presentation of Table 1 glosses over a number of practical audiometric problems. The data were combined from 3 reports to show the differences between exposed and control populations, each set of which had been matched as well as possible. There were differences among the hearing threshold levels measured in the different control populations and corresponding differences in exposed populations. Variously, some of these differences may be attributed to population selection, masking noises, temporary threshold shifts, and permanent threshold shifts from incidental, nonoccupational exposures to noise. Furthermore, some of the differences in audiometric techniques that led to the differences between the ASA-1951 (9) and the ANSI-1969 (33) references for audiometric zero persist in whole or in part in many surveys. Reports originating in the United States (34–36) continue to show normal thresholds more nearly like those of ASA-1951, whereas reports from Great Britain (37–39) show normal thresholds equal to or better than ANSI-1969. The report by Glorig et al. (40) implies that the pace of audiometry in U.S. surveys can be slowed enough to yield the more sensitive thresholds, but the reports cited suggest this does not often happen. Are the threshold audiograms collected in surveys of noise-exposed populations systematically less sensitive to the same degree as the matched control populations? If so, then the differences between the populations are the correct measures of the effects of the noise exposure. This author believes this to be more commonly true on the basis of the configurations of the normal audiograms. However, there is no unequivocal evidence either way and others, like Kryter (41), may continue to view measured hearing threshold levels in absolute terms and so find larger effects for the same exposures to noise.

When daily exposures to noise are shorter than 8 hr, are intermittent with rest periods in quiet, or fluctuate among several levels, periods at higher sound levels may be tolerated without an increase in risk to hearing. The simplest and most conservative scheme for evaluation of such exposures and the one recommended in the report compiled by Guignard (1) and repeated in the EPA "Levels Document" (32) assumes risks for hearing are no more than shown in Table 1 for any exposures to nonimpulsive noises for which the total energy in a 24-hr period is the same as for one of the continuous 8-hr exposures in the table. This equal-energy rule allows sound level to increase 3 dB each time the daily duration of exposure is halved.

Data show the equal-energy rule is actually best followed as a means of integrating the effects of continuous exposures over years, as in the concept of immission level proposed by Robinson (23) and Robinson and Cook (25). Data on temporary threshold shifts [e.g., Kryter et al. (42)] do not follow this rule. With practical industrial examples, the longer periods for the processes of recovery from a fatigued state more than offset the added effects of the higher levels for shorter periods. Under these circumstances experience suggests it is safe to allow sound pressures to increase by more than 3 dB when duration of exposure is halved. Available data do not, however, support the choice of any simple rule.

Passchier-Vermeer (43) has recently reviewed published reports of hearing loss associated with fluctuating and intermittent exposures to noise. She calculated the A-weighted sound levels for continuous 8-hr exposures that would have the same total energy as the shorter, time-varying exposures. Each measure of central tendency for hearing loss as a function of A-weighted equivalent level was plotted in relation to the trend curves for exposures to truly continuous noise. On the one hand, the relations from the different studies clustered about the trend curves in a manner that suggested underlying similar trends. But there were points that missed with hearing losses as much as 10 dB greater and others with hearing losses as much as 15 dB less. Since these misses are themselves measures of central tendency, they are probably significant, and suggest that we do not know and understand the relations between hearing loss and fluctuating or intermittent exposures to noise. Something more than total energy and possibly something more than A-weightings as a means of dealing with the differential frequency response of the ear are likely to be necessary.

PRACTICAL AND USEFUL STANDARDS

Some standard for exposure to noise that will in fact be used for the conservation of hearing is better than complete inaction for lack of a perfect standard. The problem is to find one that is acceptable and will be used. Standards can vary along one dimension between simplicity and complexity and along another dimension between low risk and high risk for impairment of hearing. The costs to society for different choices that can be made in this 2-dimensional space are not monotonically related to either dimension but depend in complex ways on the different costs of control of exposure to noise.

Engineering control of noise exposure includes steps that will reduce the level of noise at the source, or that will prevent the transmission of noise at high levels to the human environment. Either or both of these steps may be very costly and often truly satisfactory control of level is not possible. Administrative control of duration of scheduled exposures to noise is another method that can be used for the conservation of hearing. Here some degree of less efficient use of man-hours is likely to be the principal cost.

The range of degrees of risk to hearing that are socially acceptable are fairly well depicted in Table 1 and this can be used to illustrate the relations among other costs and values. If it is possible and reasonable to control exposures to noise to the low-risk equivalent of 75 dB(A) for 8 hr, then the costs of repeated measurements to monitor noise levels and repeated measurements of the hearing of exposed persons are not necessary. But if exposures are controlled only to the equivalent of 90 dB(A) for 8 hr, then other costs and measures are necessary to conserve hearing. First, the levels and durations of exposures should be monitored at reasonable intervals to assure that limits for exposures are not being exceeded. Second, the hearing thresholds of exposed persons should be monitored periodically to detect and to remove from further risk those 10–20% of persons showing the greater and more unacceptable losses of hearing. Thus, for an equivalent degree of conservation of hearing these costs for monitoring must be weighed against the costs necessary to reduce exposures to low-risk levels. Although it is always socially more desirable to reduce exposure to low-risk levels, practical and useful standards should preserve the options for alternative and sometimes less costly ways to reduce risk of hearing impairment.

Although standards can vary significantly along the dimension from simplicity to complexity, it has become clear that only simple standards are acceptable and therefore are the only ones that can become practical and useful. It is quite likely that the standards proposed by Kryter et al. (42) are more accurate than simpler standards being proposed today, but these have been used rarely. Both the concepts involved and the acoustic measurements required were impractical for everyday use. Current attempts at simple standards have been oriented toward specification of an A-weighted sound level, as in Table 1, that can be tolerated with some degree of safety for the usual 8 hr of the working day. The penchant for simplicity has been so strong that even Table 1 is too complex, and government agencies have been opting to draw the limit at a single A-weighted level. Now they are finding consumer resistance to these oversimplifications.

A rule that is somewhat lax, but strictly enforced, will have the merit that it reduces the risk to hearing from exposures that are likely to produce the greater and more handicapping impairments. It may permit substantial risks of lesser impairments and thus invite the negative attention of Ralph Nader and other crusaders. A rule based on a policy requiring a substantial margin of safety can too easily be demonstrated to be often overprotective and will be as easily ignored as the warning on a pack of cigarettes.

For industrial purposes the EPA currently recommends (32) a limit at 75 dB(A) for continuous exposures of 8 hr with other patterns of exposure restricted to the same total energy (3-dB rule). A corresponding limit of 90 dB(A) but with an allowable increase of 5 dB for each halving of the duration of exposure was proposed in 1969 by the American Conference of Governmental Industrial Hygienists (44) and is still used by the Occupational Safety and Health Administration (OSHA) (45). The EPA recommendation is considered by many to be overprotective and the OSHA rule is considered by as many others to be too lax.

Is it possible to draft a simple standard with reasonable margins for safety that can be accepted at a practical level? The answer is not clear. Some ingredients to be considered include:

1. An anchor for the standard at a level with a low risk for continuous exposures for 8 hr
2. A table of trading relations between level and duration that compensates

for the excesses in either direction that occur when using either the 3-dB or the 5-dB rule alone

3. A trading relation such that exposure limits are relaxed when exposure to noise and hearing sensitivities are monitored regularly

4. An explicit escape clause to allow for conditions of exposure that do not meet the standards but that are shown to be safe

Finally, if we are to increase our knowledge and understanding enough to be able to form better judgments with respect to the hazards to hearing inherent in exposures to noise, we must resist current trends toward the oversimplification necessary for useful standards and try to pursue new knowledge at the most sophisticated levels possible.

ACKNOWLEDGMENT

The preparation of this manuscript was supported in part by Grant No. NS 03856 from the National Institute for Neurological and Communicative Disorders and Stroke to the Central Institute for the Deaf.

REFERENCES

1. Guignard, J. C. (compiler and editor) (1973): *A Basis for Limiting Noise Exposure for Hearing Conservation.* Report Nos. AMRL-TR-73–90 and EPA-550/9–73–001-A, prepared for the Environmental Protection Agency by the Aerospace Medical Research Laboratory, Aerospace Medical Division, Air Force Systems Command, Wright-Patterson Air Force Base, Ohio.
2. Davis, H. (assisted by the Subcommittee on Hearing in Adults for the Committee on Conservation of Hearing of the American Academy of Ophthalmology and Otolaryngology) (1965): Guide for the classification and evaluation of hearing handicap in relation to the International Audiometric Zero. *Trans. Am. Acad. Ophthalmol. Otolaryngol.,* 69:740–751.
3. Noise Control Act of 1972. Public law 92–574, 92nd Congress, H.R. 11021, October 27, 1972.
4. AMA Council on Physical Medicine and Rehabilitation (1955): Principles for evaluating hearing loss. *Trans. Am. Acad. Ophthalmol. Otolaryngol.,* 59:550–552.
5. AMA Committee on Medical Rating of Physical Impairment (1961): Guide to the evaluation of permanent impairment; ear, nose, throat, and related structures. *JAMA,* 117:489–501.
6. AAOO Committee on Conservation of Hearing (Subcommittee on Noise in Industry) (1959): Guide for the evaluation of hearing impairment. *Trans. Am. Acad. Ophthalmol. Otolaryngol.,* 63:236–238.
7. Davis, H. (1948): The articulation area and the Social Adequacy Index for hearing. *Laryngoscope,* 58:761–778.
8. Silverman, S. R., and Hirsh, I. J. (1955): Problems related to the use of speech in clinical audiometry. *Ann. Otol. Rhinol. Laryngol.,* 64:1234–1248.
9. American Standard Specification for Audiometers for General Diagnostic Purposes, Z24.5–1951. American Standards Association, New York.
10. ISO Recommendation R 389 (1964): Standard Reference Zero for the calibration of pure-tone audiometers.
11. Hirsh, I. J. (1952): *The Measurement of Hearing,* Chap. 5. McGraw-Hill, New York.

12. French, N. R., and Steinberg, J. C. (1947): Factors governing the intelligibility of speech sounds. *J. Acoust. Soc. Am.*, 19:90–119.
13. Carhart, R. (1946): Speech reception in relation to pattern of pure tone loss. *J. Speech Disord.*, 11:97–108.
14. Quiggle, R. R., Glorig, A., Delk, J. H., and Summerfield, A. B. (1957): Predicting hearing loss for speech from pure tone audiograms. *Laryngoscope*, 67:1–15.
15. Harris, J. D., Haines, H. L., and Myers, C. K. (1956): A new formula for using the audiogram to predict speech hearing loss. *Arch. Otolaryngol.*, 63:158–176.
16. Hirsh, I. J., Reynolds, E. G., and Joseph, M. (1954): Intelligibility of different speech materials. *J. Acoust. Soc. Am.*, 26:530–538.
17. Harris, J. D. (1960): Combinations of distortion in speech. The 25 percent safety factor by multiple-cueing. *Arch. Otolaryngol.*, 72:227–232.
18. Harris, J. D., Haines, H. L., and Myers, C. K. (1960): The importance of hearing at 3 kc for understanding speeded speech. *Laryngoscope*, 70:131–146.
19. Kryter, K. D., Williams, C., and Green, D. M. (1962): Auditory acuity and the perception of speech. *J. Acoust. Soc. Am.*, 34:1217–1223.
20. Harris, J. D. (1965): Pure-tone acuity and the intelligibility of everyday speech. *J. Acoust. Soc. Am.*, 37:824–830.
21. Kell, R. L., Pearson, J. C. G., Acton, W. I., and Taylor, W. (1971): Social effects of hearing loss due to weaving noise. In: *Occupational Hearing Loss,* edited by D. W. Robinson, pp. 179–191. Academic Press, London and New York.
22. Pearson, J. C. G., Kell, R. L., and Taylor, W. (1973): An index of hearing impairment derived from the pure-tone audiogram. In: *Disorders of Auditory Function,* edited by W. Taylor, pp. 129–150. Academic Press, London and New York.
23. Robinson, D. W. (1970): Relations between hearing loss and noise exposure, analysis of results of retrospective study. In: *Hearing and Noise in Industry,* by W. Burns and D. W. Robinson, pp. 100–151. Her Majesty's Stationery Office, London.
24. Robinson, D. W. (1971): Estimating the risk of hearing loss due to exposure to continuous noise. In: *Occupational Hearing Loss,* edited by D. W. Robinson, pp. 43–62. Academic Press, London and New York.
25. Robinson, D. W., and Cook, J. P. (1970): Experimental basis for the concept of noise immission level. In: *Hearing and Noise in Industry,* by W. Burns and D. W. Robinson, pp. 152–161. Her Majesty's Stationery Office, London.
26. Baughn, W. L. (1973): *Relation Between Daily Noise Exposure and Hearing Loss Based on the Evaluation of 6,835 Industrial Noise Exposure Cases.* Report No. AMRL-TR-73–53, Aerospace Medical Research Laboratory, Aerospace Medical Division, Air Force Systems Command, Wright-Patterson Air Force Base, Ohio.
27. Passchier-Vermeer, W. (1968): *Hearing Loss Due to Exposure to Steady-State Broadband Noise.* Report No. 35, Research Institute for Public Health Engineering, TNO, Delft, The Netherlands.
28. Passchier-Vermeer, W. (1974): Hearing loss due to continuous exposure to steady-state broad-band noise. *J. Acoust. Soc. Am.*, 56:1585–1593.
29. Glorig, A., Ward, W. D., and Nixon, J. (1961): Damage risk criteria and noise-induced hearing loss. *Arch. Otolaryngol.*, 74:413–423.
30. Taylor, W., Pearson, J., Mair, A., and Burns, W. (1965): Study of noise and hearing in jute weaving. *J. Acoust. Soc. Am.*, 38:113–120.
31. Johnson, D. L. (1973): *Prediction of NIPTS Due to Continuous Noise Exposure.* Report Nos. AMRL-TR-73–91 and EPA-550/9–73–001-B, Aerospace Medical Research Laboratory, Aerospace Medical Division, Air Force Systems Command, Wright-Patterson Air Force Base, Ohio.
32. *Information on Levels of Environmental Noise Requisite to Protect Public Health and Welfare with an Adequate Margin of Safety* (1974): Report No. 550/9–74–004, U.S. Environmental Protection Agency, Washington, D.C.
33. *American National Standard Specifications for Audiometers—ANSI S3.6–1969* (1970): American National Standards Institute, Inc., New York.
34. Glorig, A., Wheeler, D., Quiggle, R., Grings, W., and Summerfield, A. (1957): *1954 Wisconsin State Fair Hearing Survey.* American Academy of Ophthalmology

and Otolaryngology, Research Center, Subcommittee on Noise in Industry, Los Angeles, California.

35. Riley, E. C., Sterner, J. H., Fassett, D. W., and Sutton, W. L. (1965): Re: Audiometric zero. *J. Acoust. Soc. Am.*, 37:924–926.

36. Lempert, B. L., and Henderson, T. L. (1973): *NIOSH Survey of Occupational Noise and Hearing: 1968 to 1972.* National Institute for Occupational Safety and Health, U.S. Department of Health, Education, and Welfare (Cincinnati, Ohio 45202).

37. Knight, J. J. (1966): Normal hearing threshold determined by manual and self-recording techniques. *J. Acoust. Soc. Am.*, 39:1184–1185.

38. Rice, C. G., and Coles, R. R. A. (1966): Normal threshold of hearing for pure tones by earphone listening with a self-recording audiometric technique. *J. Acoust. Soc. Am.*, 39:1185–1187.

39. Robinson, D. W. (1970): A note on the hearing level of the non-exposed controls. In: *Hearing and Noise in Industry,* by W. Burns and D. W. Robinson, pp. 235–241. Her Majesty's Stationery Office, London.

40. Glorig, A., Quiggle, R., Wheeler, D. E., and Grings, W. (1956): Determination of the normal hearing reference zero. *J. Acoust. Soc. Am.*, 28:1110–1113.

41. Kryter, K. D. (1973): Impairment to hearing from exposure to noise. *J. Acoust. Soc. Am.*, 53:1211–1234.

42. Kryter, K. D., Ward, W. D., Miller, J. D., and Eldredge, D. H. (1966): Hazardous exposure to intermittent and steady-state noise. *J. Acoust. Soc. Am.*, 39:451–464.

43. Passchier-Vermeer, W. (1973): Noise-induced hearing loss from exposure to intermittent and varying noise. In: *Proceedings of the International Congress on Noise as a Public Health Problem,* edited by W. D. Ward, pp. 169–200, Report No. 550/9–73–008. U.S. Environmental Protection Agency, Washington, D.C.

44. American Conference of Governmental Industrial Hygienists (1969): *Threshold Limit Values of Physical Agents Adopted by ACGIH for 1969.* Cincinnati, Ohio.

45. *Occupational Noise Exposure, Proposed Requirements and Procedures* (1974): United States Department of Labor, Occupational Safety and Health Administration (29 CFR Part 1910) (Docket No. OSH-11) Federal Register, Vol. 39, No. 207 (Thursday, Oct. 24), pp. 37773–37778.

Effects of Noise on Hearing, edited by Donald Henderson,
Roger P. Hamernik, Darshan S. Dosanjh, and John H. Mills.
Raven Press, New York © 1976

Demographics of Noise Pollution with Respect to Potential Hearing Loss

Kenneth McK. Eldred

Bolt Beranek and Newman Inc., Cambridge, Massachusetts 02138

This chapter briefly reviews 3 basic dimensions of potential noise-induced
hearing loss:

1. Individual exposure: What is an individual's noise exposure?
2. Exposed population: How many people are involved with potential risk
   to hearing?
3. Economics: What might it cost to control noise?

This review attempts to put the hearing-loss problem into perspective,
giving some insight into the range of current uncertainty on each of the dimensions, and to provide an overall context for the subsequent chapters.

QUANTIFICATION OF NOISE EXPOSURE

Lifetime Exposure

There is little need for sophisticated and precise measurement of the sound
exposure suffered by an individual standing by the muzzle of a large cannon,
which can produce major permanent hearing damage in 1 shot. For such
cases, when a single exposure is highly damaging, rather simple descriptions
of the event generally suffice.

However, the more general experience of an individual is a lifetime of exposure to a wide variety of milder sounds. For some people the magnitudes of
the sounds, together with their time patterns, are great enough to cause a
noise-induced permanent threshold shift.

The literature of hearing loss, as the result of noise exposure, has been concerned primarily with industrial noise exposure and its corresponding outcome
in terms of possible workmen's compensation. This interest has focused most
of the attention in defining noise exposure in terms of the "8-hr day; 5-day
week; 50-week year; 40-year working lifetime."

For the most part, this historical attention to industrial noise has been appropriate, except that it does not account for losses experienced through gunfire in military service or sport, or other accidental exposures. However, in
the second half of the 20th century, the general public may encounter rela-

tively high-level sound exposures. Such encounters can occur to them as passengers in transportation vehicles, as operators of recreational or home maintenance vehicles, etc. Consequently, it has become important to define an individual's total noise exposure, with reference to a "24-hr day, 7-day week, 52-week year, cradle-to-grave lifetime."

One of the greatest weaknesses in our current state of knowledge of noise-induced hearing loss is the lack of an accurate data base regarding total individual noise exposure. This lack extends also to noise exposure in the industrial workplace, because of the general change of sound levels over the years, and, during a given day, the change with individual position within a given workplace. To these gross uncertainties must be added the uncertainties associated with the definition of sound exposure for a single individual during a given day. The attempt to define the individual's daily exposure has created a need for sophistication and accuracy in our sound measurements, which still remains substantially unfulfilled.

Definition of a Specific Noise Exposure

Of the many problems that influence the reliability of measurement of sound exposure for a specific individual in a steady-state sound field, we will discuss only (i) accuracy of the sound level meter; and (ii) position of the microphone relative to the individual.

The sound level meter (SLM) generally required for measurement of individual exposure must meet the American National Standards Institute S1.4 1971 (1) standard, Type II tolerance with A-weighting. The random incidence frequency response and tolerances for a SLM meeting this standard are illustrated in Fig. 1.

The nominal tolerance of the instrument is ± 2 dB between the frequencies of 315 and 1,250 Hz, ± 3 dB between 50 and 2,000 Hz, and significantly greater at both lower and higher frequencies. The increased tolerance at lower frequencies (e.g., $+3$, -4.0 dB at 31.5 Hz) is not of great importance for most noises, since the A-weighting seriously attenuates low-frequency noise (e.g., 39.4 dB at 31.5 Hz). However, the increase in permitted tolerance at higher frequencies (particularly between 2,000 and 5,000 Hz, where the tolerance is $+6$, -5 dB) may be of major importance for the measurement of many sounds.

These tolerances apply to sound arriving at the ear with random incidence, a condition generally associated with a diffuse or reverberant sound field. Even greater tolerances apply to direct sounds at specific angles of incidence, particularly at frequencies above 2,000 Hz. Consequently, the A-weighted sound level for sounds dominated by energy at frequencies above 2,000 Hz may vary significantly (5–10 dB), depending on the characteristics of the particular sound field, the measuring instrument, and the operator's measurement technique.

The second major variable affecting a specific sound exposure measurement is the interaction of the individual with the sound field. In practice, measurements are often made without the presence of the individual. However, many noisy operations cannot occur at all without the presence of the operator, and the noise measurements are generally made "in the vicinity of the operator."

Figure 2 illustrates the variation in sound level at a position approximately ¼ in. from the entrance to the ear canal (2). For most frequencies between 250 and 8,000 Hz in a diffuse field, the sound level near the ear canal is about 3 dB greater than the level measured at the same point without the individual's presence. However, between 3,000 and 6,000 Hz, the ear-canal level is increased by as much as 11 dB because of diffraction of sound by the head.

Data (2) obtained in a plane wave in free field also indicate a high-frequency peak, for sound from the front or directly toward the ear. The latter also exhibits a 6-dB doubling over most of the frequency range. Conversely, over most of the frequency range, the level of sound arriving from the rear of the head is slightly below its value without the presence of the head.

Figure 3 gives similar comparison data (3) for chest and shoulder positions, showing the effect of variation in clothing. These data were obtained

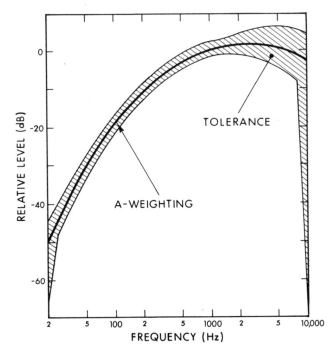

FIG. 1. Relative random incidence response level and tolerance for A-weighting for a type II sound level meter ANSI S1.4–1971.

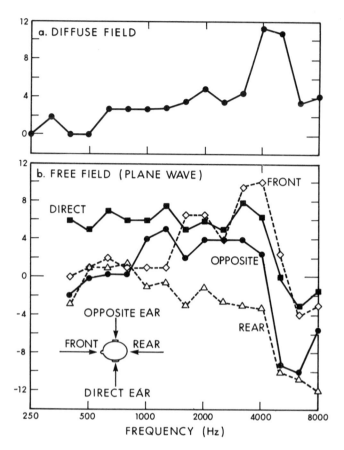

FIG. 2. Relative sound level at approximately ¼ inch from entrance to ear canal for diffuse and free fields with four angles of incidence.

in a semidiffuse room, averaged over a circular arc of 1-m radius. The data generally indicate a 2–3-dB increase at lower frequencies, with a marked decrease in level near the frequency for which the distance between the microphone and the individual is one-quarter of an acoustic wavelength.

Such data illustrate that the presence of an individual may have a significant effect on the sound measurement. Personal dosimeters worn by the individual will measure 2–3 dB higher for most frequencies than would a microphone placed in the same position without the presence of the individual.

Data obtained at other positions "in the vicinity of the individual" also may be expected to be affected by the individual's presence. Consequently, considerable variation in "measured" sound level may be expected among data obtained by different people utilizing different positioning techniques.

Additionally, in the 3,000–6,000-Hz region head diffraction may enhance the sound at the ear by as much as 11 dB. The pressure at the ear drum,

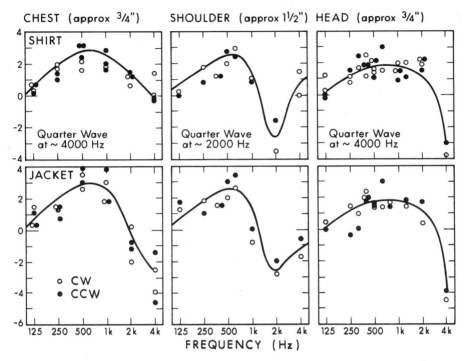

FIG. 3. Relative sound level at location on person for two positions with two types of clothing for semi-reverberant sound field.

relative to that on the head, is increased by the ear canal one-quarter wave resonance which occurs at ~3,000 Hz for the typical adult ear canal length. Consequently, for many sounds which are dominated by energy in the 2,500–6,000 Hz frequency range, the effective sound level at the eardrum is significantly higher than that measured in the field without the presence of an individual. This variation could be minimized by utilizing frequency weighting, such as D_2 (4) or E (5), which accounts better for these combined resonance and diffraction effects than does the A-weighting.

Combining Specific Exposures To Obtain a Total Exposure

A variety of rules of combination has been proposed to account for the time variation of sound magnitude in obtaining a measure of total exposure. One simplified set of rules is to integrate a function of the A-weighted sound level (L_A) over time (t) such that the exposure (E) is given by the following proportionality:

$$E \sim \int_{10}^{L_A(t)/10x} dt$$

Generally x is given a value between 1 and 2, leading to exchange rates for "equal exposure" ranging between 3 and 6 dB increase in noise level per halving of exposure duration.

The 2 exchange rates of most interest in current public discussion are 3 dB and 5 dB per halving of time. The 3-dB rate was utilized in the mid 1950s by the U.S. Air Force (6,7) and more recently was adopted by the Environmental Protection Agency (EPA) (8). The 5-dB rate (9) was adopted in 1969 by the Department of Labor (DOL) in the Walsh Healey Regulation (10) for protection of the hearing of workers.

Rules of combination may be used together with a standard noise level to define "allowable durations of exposure" at various noise levels relative to

TABLE 1. Comparison of "allowed durations" in 8-hr day for an A-weighted sound level standard of 90 dB

Sound level (dB)	5 dB/halving (hr)	3 dB/halving (hr)
105	1	0.25
100	2	0.8
95	4	2.5
90	8	8.0
85	16	25
80	32	80
75	64	253

the standard level. The standard level, usually referred to an 8-hr workday, is usually chosen to provide a stated probability of protection. The proposed standard levels of current interest range from 75 dB (EPA) (8) to 90 dB (DOL) (10). The effect of the 2 rules of combination on the allowed exposure durations for various levels may be observed in Table 1. As would be expected, the allowable durations for sound levels greater than the standard level are shorter for the 3-dB rule than for the 5-dB rule; the situation is reversed for noise levels below the standard level.

Figures 4 to 6 illustrate the time patterns and statistical distributions at 3 factory locations. They also give the fractional duration, defined as the summation of the actual duration at each noise level divided by the allowable duration at that level. The fractional durations were computed for all sound above 90 dB using both the 3- and 5-dB rules of combination. For these time patterns, the fractional duration for the 3-dB rule was approximately 2.3 times that found by using the 5-dB rule.

Figures 4–6 also give the equivalent level, defined here as the steady-state level, producing the same exposure as the time-varying sound, calculated in accordance with each rule. Whereas the ratios of fractional durations for these examples were essentially constant, the difference in equivalent level between the 3- and 5-dB rule varied from zero in Fig. 4 to 3.7 dB in Fig. 6. Such dif-

TIME HISTORY - DOFFING

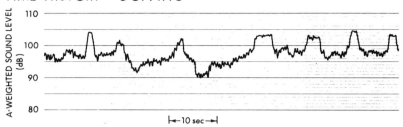

STATISTICAL DISTRIBUTION

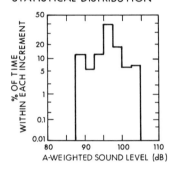

EFFECT OF COMBINATION RULE FOR
8 HOUR STANDARD LEVEL OF 90 dB

Combination Rule	Fract. Duration	Equiv. Level (dB)
5 dB/halving	3.45	99
3 dB/halving	7.87	99
Ratio	2.28	0

FIG. 4. Example of factory noise, doffing, illustrating the effect of combination rule.

TIME HISTORY - MORTISER

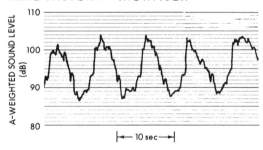

STATISTICAL DISTRIBUTION

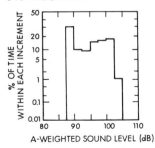

EFFECT OF COMBINATION RULE FOR
8 HOUR STANDARD LEVEL OF 90dB

Combination Rule	Fract. Duration	Equiv. Level (dB)
5 dB/halving	2.10	95.0
3 dB/halving	4.68	96.7
Ratio	2.23	1.7

FIG. 5. Example of factory noise, mortiser, illustrating the effect of combination rule.

TIME HISTORY - DEBUNGER

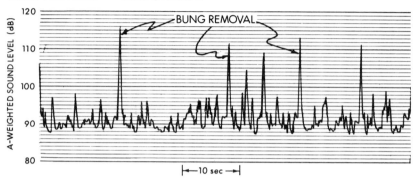

STATISTICAL DISTRIBUTION

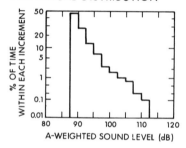

EFFECT OF COMBINATION RULE FOR
8 HOUR STANDARD LEVEL OF 90dB

Combination Rule	Fract. Duration	Equiv. Level (dB)
5 dB/halving	0.89	89.5
3 dB/halving	2.07	93.2
Ratio	2.33	3.7

Fig. 6. Example of factory noise, debunger, illustrating the effect of combination rule.

ferences in equivalent level, for relatively simple examples of time-varying factory noises, illustrate the difficulty in ascribing great accuracy to our existing data base, much of which has been obtained by eye averages of the SLM needle, using the "slow" dynamic characteristic.

Current data obtained with modern dosimeters can improve this situation for noise environments which are considerably in excess of the standard level. However, because the Walsh Healy regulation defined no allowable durations for levels below its standard of 90 dB, most available dosimeters ignore all of the sound exposure below 90 dB. Cutting off all energy below the standard level considerably distorts the noise data.

The effect of sound energy at levels below which noise exposure is not counted is illustrated in Figs. 7 to 9. Fractional durations and equivalent levels have been calculated for both the 3- and 5-dB combination rules with lower cutoffs of 90, 85, and 80 dB, in comparison to a 90 dB standard. The results illustrate that, for environments in which the noise level varies above and below the standard level, the fractional duration or equivalent level is considerably affected by the existence of a lower cutoff level. The most severe effect occurs when the lower cutoff coincides with the standard level. Also, these examples show that when all the sound levels are counted in the

TIME HISTORY - BOX FORMER MACHINE

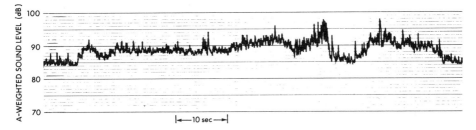

STATISTICAL DISTRIBUTION

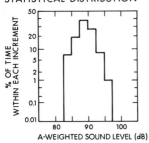

EFFECT OF COMBINATION RULE (3/5) AND LOWER CUTOFF FOR
INTEGRATION AND 8 HOUR STANDARD LEVEL OF 90 dB

	5 dB/Halving		3 dB/Halving	
Lower Cutoff	Fract. Dur.	Eq. Lev. (dB)	Fract. Dur.	Eq. Lev. (dB)
90	.48	84.5	.57	87.5
85	.89	89.0	.92	89.6
80	.92	89.3	.93	89.7
ΔdB		4.8		2.2

FIG. 7. Example of factory noise, box former machine, illustrating the effect of combination rule and lower cutoff for integration.

TIME HISTORY - DEPALLETIZER, POSITION B

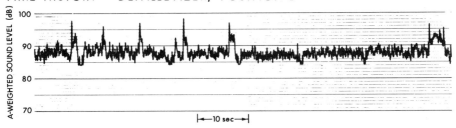

STATISTICAL DISTRIBUTION

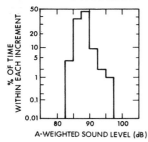

EFFECT OF COMBINATION RULE (3/5) AND LOWER CUTOFF FOR
INTEGRATION AND 8 HOUR STANDARD LEVEL OF 90 dB

	5 dB/Halving		3 dB/Halving	
Lower Cutoff	Fract. Dur.	Eq. Lev. (dB)	Fract. Dur.	Eq. Lev. (dB)
90	.16	77.0	.20	83.0
85	.72	87.5	.68	88.4
80	.73	87.5	.69	88.4
ΔdB		10.5		5.4

FIG. 8. Example of factory noise, depalletizer, position B, illustrating the effect of combination rule and lower cutoff for integration.

TIME HISTORY - DEPALLETIZER, POSITION C

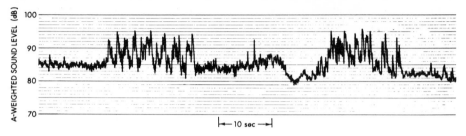

STATISTICAL DISTRIBUTION

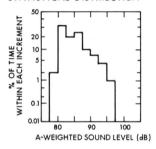

EFFECT OF COMBINATION RULE (3/5) AND LOWER CUTOFF FOR
INTEGRATION AND 8 HOUR STANDARD LEVEL OF 90 dB

Lower Cutoff	5 dB/Halving		3 dB/Halving	
	Fract. Dur.	Eq. Lev. (dB)	Fract. Dur.	Eq. Lev. (dB)
90	.18	74.8	.22	83.4
85	.41	83.5	.39	85.9
80	.58	86.3	.48	86.8
ΔdB		11.7		3.4

FIG. 9. Example of factory noise, depalletizer, position C, illustrating the effect of combination rule and lower cutoff for integration.

summation there is little difference between the 3- and 5-dB rules, because the 3-dB rule has greater allowable duration for levels below the standard than does the 5-dB rule, thus offsetting its lower allowable duration for levels in excess of the standard.

HOW MANY PEOPLE ARE EXPOSED TO NOISE
WHICH MIGHT PRODUCE HEARING LOSS?

There are several limitations to obtaining a reasonable estimate of the number of people exposed to noise that might produce hearing loss. The principle limitations are:

1. Lack of consistent data base identifying all segments of the population that might be exposed
2. Lack of agreement on the magnitude of exposure which should be utilized for screening (standard level and rule of combination)
3. Lack of a meaningful and accurate measured noise data base

Estimates are available for the number of exposed production workers from the DOL study (11), and, for the general public in nonoccupational situations, from the EPA Title IV report to Congress (12). These estimates, which will be summarized in the following paragraphs, do *not* include workers in many industries, including mining, transportation, construction, and agricultural industries, nor do they account for the military service and recreational activities involving firearms.

Production Workers

The DOL study (11) estimated that 26% of 14.3 million production workers were exposed to levels exceeding a 90-dB standard level, and that 59% were exposed to levels exceeding an 85-dB standard level. Details of the estimate by industry are summarized in Table 2. Most critical in terms of the 90-dB standard level are textile mill products, lumber and wood products, and food and kindred products. If the standard level were 85 dB, the most critical list would also include machinery products (electric and nonelectric), transportation equipment, and fabricated metal products, in addition to the 3 categories previously mentioned.

TABLE 2. *Estimate of production workers overexposed relative to 85 and 90 dB(A) standard levels*

Industry	SIC code	Thousands of workers exposed to over		Percentage of workers exposed to over	
		85 dB(A)	90 dB(A)	85 dB(A)	90 dB(A)
Food and kindred products	20	820	350	70	30
Tobacco manufacturers	21	48	40	76	63
Textile mill products	22	855	765	95	85
Apparel and related products	23	12	0	1	0
Lumber and wood products	24	542	390	100	72
Furniture and fixtures	25	236.6	67.6	55	15
Paper and allied products	26	395	206	71	37
Printing and publishing	27	132	99	20	15
Chemicals and allied products	28	137	66	23	11
Petroleum and coal products	29	58	23	50	20
Rubber and plastics products	30	266	106	50	20
Leather and leather products	31	3	0	1	0
Stone, clay, and glass products	32	416	139	75	25
Primary metals					
Primary steel	331	325	170	67	35
Foundries	332, 336	189	54	70	20
Primary nonferrous	333, 339, 335	63	35	27	15
Fabricated metal products	34	786	225	70	20
Machinery (except electric)	35	956	273	70	20
Electrical machinery	36	959	274	70	20
Transportation equipment	37	880	284	65	21
Utilities	49	445	188	71	30
		8,324	3,755	59.3	26.1

From ref. 11, with permission.

Nonoccupational Exposure

The EPA Title IV report to Congress (12) attempted to identify the non-occupational situations (except firearms) in which members of the general public could be exposed to risk of hearing damage. The principal identified sources are summarized in Table 3. This table also contains the 8-hr equivalent level estimated for both the 3- and 5-dB rules of combination, and for

TABLE 3. *Summary of estimated noise exposure for operators and passengers in nonoccupational situations*

Source	A-weighted sound level (dB)		Estimated annual duration (hr)[b]	8-hr Equivalent sound level (dB)[c]			
				3 dB/halving		5 dB/halving	
	Avg.[a]	Max.		Avg.	Max.	Avg.	Max.
Snowmobile	108	112	200	96	100	91	95
Motorcycle	95	110	250	84	99	80	95
Motorboat (>45 hp)	95	105	100	80	90	73	83
Chain saw	100	110	20	78	88	67	77
General aviation aircraft	90	103	100	75	88	68	81
Light utility helicopter	94	100	20	72	78	61	67
Trucks (personal use)	85	100	180	73	88	67	82
Subways	80	93	400	71	84	68	81
City buses	82	90	250	71	79	67	75
Commercial propeller aircraft	88	100	50	70	82	61	73
Lawn care (I.C. engine)	87	95	50	69	81	56	68
Home shop tools	85	98	30	65	78	55	68

[a] Average is median of group of available measures on various products.
[b] Year of 8-hr days has 2,920 hr.
[c] Equivalent level based on 2,000 hr/year (50 weeks at 40 hr/week) for 5-dB rule and 2,920 hr/year (52 weeks at 56 hr/week) for 3-dB rule.
Principal data source is EPA Title IV report to Congress (12).

the average and maximum source levels. It should be noted that the joint distribution of estimated usage and source levels is at present unknown; therefore, the actual *number* of people exposed at various levels and durations is also unknown.

The total number of "individual exposures" has been estimated for the average level and average annual duration as a function of the rule of combination and standard level. The results, summarized in Fig. 10, indicate that the nonoccupational individual exposures may range between 1.6 and 11.5 million, depending on the criteria employed in the evaluation.

Additional analysis of the Title IV data indicates that, for a given standard level, the 3-dB rule identifies approximately twice as many excesses as does the 5-dB rule.

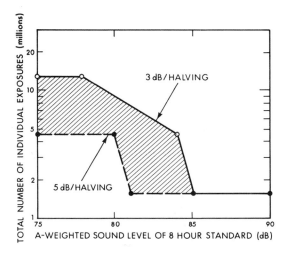

FIG. 10. Estimated number of operators and passengers potentially exposed to annual average equivalent sound levels in excess of stated 8-hr standard A-weighted sound level.

COST OF REDUCING NOISE

The cost of noise control is a function of 2 major variables:

1. Choice of the standard level and rule of combination that together determine how many things must be quieted and how much noise control is required

2. Time frame for compliance, which forces a choice between the amount of noise control accomplished by replacing old machines with new, quieter machines versus field quieting of old machines, and also affects the growth of cost-effective noise control technology

Despite the uncertainties previously mentioned in connection with the choice of a standard level and a rule of combination, the trend in overall cost can be assessed in terms of the time frame for compliance. If compliance is required only for new devices, the cost will be much less than if old devices must also be retrofitted for noise control. Additionally, if adequate lead time is given to compliance for new devices, the cost will be even less. This saving results from integrating the noise-control requirements with all the other requirements at the concept design stage for a new product.

An estimate of the cost for reducing the noise exposure for production workers was prepared in the 3-month DOL study (11). The results were based on an assumption of a 3–5-year program, utilizing existing retrofit technology and extrapolation of a small data base of unit cost and number of units to be retrofitted to entire industries.

It was estimated that a 3–5-year program to achieve a 90 dB–8 hr noise exposure for most production workers would cost $13.5 billion (approximately $3,600 per exposed worker), and that to achieve an 85 dB–8 hour noise exposure would cost $31.6 billion (approximately $3,700 per exposed worker). The large cost increase between achieving 90- and 85-dB goals was not the increase in cost to quiet an individual machine, but rather, a large increase in the number of machines to be quieted.

There is no way at present to obtain a statistically valid estimate of the accuracy of these estimates, but it is reasonable to assume at least ±3 dB uncertainty; this is only 1 dB greater than the tolerance of the Type 2 Sound Level Meter. With a ±3-dB tolerance, the range of costs for the 90-dB goal is $6.8 to $27 billion, and for the 85-dB goal, $15.8 to $63 billion.

If the compliance program were extended over a longer period of time, the costs could be expected to decrease significantly, because of the development of more cost-effective retrofit technology, and the replacement of old noisy machines with newly designed, quieter machines at minimal added cost.

SUMMARY

Our existing methodology for quantifying an individual's noise exposure needs significant improvement, specifically:

1. Accounting for an individual's total exposure
2. Improving frequency weightings to account better for the interaction of the individual and the sound field
3. Standardization of microphone placement relative to the individual

Without these improvements, we will continue to be plagued with an imprecise noise-exposure data base, both with respect to relating individual and public hearing loss to actual noise exposure, and defining the noise reduction requirements for control.

Determination of the number of individuals who have significant noise exposure is subject to the above uncertainties, in addition to the choice of a standard level and rule of combination appropriate for this task. The most

TABLE 4. *Estimated number of "individual exposures" to levels in excess of the stated A-weighted sound level 8-hr standard*

Type of exposure	8-hr Standard level (dB)		
	90	85	80
Production workers[a]	3.8	8.5	12.7
Nonindustrial operators/passengers (average levels)	1.6	1.6	9.0
Total[a]	5.4	10.1	21.7

[a] Total excludes people engaged in transportation, construction, agricultural, mining, military service, etc. and does not account for individuals who may be double counted.

current, though incomplete, estimate of the number of people affected is summarized in Table 4.

Estimating the cost of noise control is subject to all of the above uncertainties, together with those depending on the schedule for compliance. Short compliance schedules lead to higher costs than long time schedules, for the solution must be primarily that of retrofit with existing technology. Longer lead time can reduce costs by accomplishing much of the noise reduction by the replacement of old noisy machines with new, quieter machines, and by the development of more cost-effective noise control retrofit techniques.

REFERENCES

1. American National Standards Institute, Inc. (1971): Specification for Sound Level Meters. ANSI S1.4–1971.
2. Ollerhead, J. B. (1969): The Noisiness of Diffuse Sound Fields at High Intensities. FAA-No-70–3.
3. Young, R. W. (1974): Average Build-up of Sound Pressure Level on a Person in an Ordinary Room. Presented at *Acoust. Soc. Am.,* St. Louis, Mo.
4. Kryter, K. D. (1970): *Effects of Noise on Man.* Academic Press, New York.
5. Stevens, S. S. (1972): *Perceived level of noise by Mark VII in decibels (E). J. Acoust. Soc. Am.,* 51:575–601.
6. Eldred, K. M., Gannon, W., and von Gierke, H. E. (1955): Criteria for Short Time Exposure of Personnel to High Intensity Jet Aircraft Noise. WADC TN 55–355.
7. Department of Air Force, Washington, D.C. (1956): Air Force Regulation 160–3, Hazardous Noise Exposure.
8. EPA, 550.974–004 (1974): Information on Levels of Environmental Noise Requisite to Protect Public Health and Welfare with an Adequate Margin of Safety.
9. Radcliffe, J. C. et al. (1970): Guidelines for Noise Exposure Control. *S/V,* 4, #11, p. 21–24.
10. Occupational Safety and Health Standards, Part 1910.95, Federal Register 36FR 105–10466 (1971).
11. Bruce, R. D., Coelen, C., Fax, G. E., Fox, H. L., and Swanson, S. (1974): Impact of Noise Control at the Workplace, Bolt Beranek and Newman Inc. Report No. 2671. Submitted to U.S. Department of Labor.
12. Report To The President and Congress on Noise (1972): Report of the Administrator of the Environmental Protection Agency, Title IV Public Law 91–604, The Clean Air Act Amendments of 1970.

Discussion

J. Tonndorf: I'd like to make a comment to Ken Eldred's paper. Ken, I was very grateful to you for your last remark. Industry always tells us that noise abatement costs too many billions—they come up with these fantastic sums of money. I don't know the basis of these cost estimates, but they have them on paper. You made a very good point, that Industry writes off this equipment at a relatively fast rate, so if you give Industry a little time, say 5 years/5 dB, the cost of noise abatement becomes more reasonable.

D. Lipscomb: I've been trying for about the last 2 years to understand the audiogram, its role, and what it can tell us. What I've come up with is that it would appear that pure-tone tests give a good idea of the condition of the cochlear cells in the basal turn of the cochlea; for 2 kHz and above. For frequencies less than 2 kHz, it would appear that the pure-tone audiogram tells much more about what's going on in the conductive mechanism of the ear, including the conductive properties of the inner ear. I mention this for your consideration.

K. Kryter: I'd like to comment further on the use of pure-tone audiograms. The issue is not so much whether we should use pure-tone audiometry—I think that is perfectly acceptable. I think the real problem is in the interpretation, and conversion of these measures into something we define as hearing in everyday living. I also feel that Don Eldredge's presentation of AAOO definition is something that should be examined rather deeply.

H. von Gierke: I would like to emphasize the same point Karl Kryter just made. I was particularly shocked when hearing was defined with respect to normal limits. If I have 14 dB better than normal hearing to start with, I don't think my initial impairment should be measured with respect to the normal limit. I might get a 10-dB loss and still have an impairment with respect to normal. So it is time that we pay more attention to the individual person's capability to enjoy life, and to distinguish between the individual and impairment in the general sense with respect to the general population. I just cannot see the reason why, in this particular definition, the point is made only to the normal limits.

J. Miller: It is clear from the text of Dr. Eldredge's paper that we want to make sure that everyone understands the difference between two things: (a) how does the individual compare with the group and, (b) how does the individual compare with himself? In most of the text the point was not really to give an answer, but to make sure everyone understood the complexities involved.

J. Botsford: I've looked at this occupational hearing loss work on the industrial and application side over the years, and I'd like to comment on the AAOO formula. I think it is most vulnerable on the grounds that it allows an absorbable change for which there is no compensation. I don't believe there is any other kind of injury in workman's compensation where this is done. For example, if you cut off part of your arm, they don't say you can't be paid unless you lose at least 3 inches shorter than normal. The same applies to facial disfigurement. If there's any change or blemish as a result of injury, you are entitled to compensation.

J. Tonndorf: Historically, the only consideration was medico-legal. When you have the single individual and you don't have a preemployment audiogram, the best you can do is to determine his deviation from what you accept as normal. But we can do better now. First of all, we have more preemployment audiograms, and second, we can measure things a little bit better today. For the average population a 5-dB loss is a loss; for the individual it doesn't mean a thing.

R. Gannon: I should like to add a statement about the effects of age on the degree of handicap. I think that one must recognize the change that takes place, and the importance of hearing in the societal aspects of life with age. The older person, particularly in retirement, is much more dependent on communication with his friends, family, watching TV, etc., whereas the young person who is still working is mostly concerned with doing his 8 hours work during the day, and then trying to turn his wife on or off when he gets home at night.

Part II
Cochlear Anatomy and Biochemistry
Introduction

A succinct statement of the problem considered in this section is: what are the mechanisms of noise-induced cochlear pathologies? Within this context, it is necessary, but somewhat unfair, to consider the anatomy and the biochemistry of the cochlea together. The early descriptions of the conductive apparatus of the ear by Fallopius, coupled with the subsequent development of the microscope, provided the science of anatomy with a nearly 4-century jump on the biochemistry of the cochlea. It is only recently that the technology has become available for a quantitative study of the chemistry of the cochlea and the biochemical basis for sound transduction. Noise studies have led to a better understanding of the relationship between anatomy and hearing. Perhaps noise research where biochemical changes are charted can also lead to an understanding of the relationship between biochemistry and hearing. Data derived from such studies would thus serve a dual purpose of providing further guides for the prevention and possible treatment of cochlear disorders and basic science data on normal cochlear functions.

In comparison to cochlear biochemistry, the anatomy of the cochlea is, for the most part, well known and new advances are often in the area of a refinement of accepted principles. Many of the current problems in cochlear structure have arisen as a result of new and more detailed findings in electrophysiology and also as a consequence of new data from noise research. For example, the physiological response of the hair cells and the differential sensitivity of the outer and inner hair cells to otopathological agents requires the anatomist to ask, what are the morphological differences between OHC and IHC? Is there a morphological basis for an interaction between the IHC and OHC? What is the detailed quantitative neuroanatomy of the cochlea, i.e., the extent of single fiber OHC innervation, the anatomy of the type II neuron, etc.? Finally, what is the nature of the stereocilia attachments? Are there "filmy" and intricate connections within the subtectorial space between the OHC and IHC and the tectorial membrane as described and illustrated by Held and other early anatomists, or are these simply a turn of the century artifact? These are some of the questions to which the following authors will address themselves.

Effects of Noise on Hearing, edited by Donald Henderson,
Roger P. Hamernik, Darshan S. Dosanjh, and John H. Mills.
Raven Press, New York © 1976

Mechanisms of Noise Damage in the Inner Ear

Barbara A. Bohne

Department of Otolaryngology, Washington University School of Medicine, St. Louis, Missouri 63110

Although many investigators have observed the deleterious effects of noise
on inner ear structure, little conclusive evidence exists about the actual
mechanism(s) responsible for cellular injury and death. Most of the theories
that have been proposed are based on observations of noise-exposed ears.
Undeniably, this approach is necessary to provide a description of the events
which occur in the inner ear after exposure. However, since different investigators have exposed animals to various noises and then examined their
cochleae at different time intervals after exposure, reported findings have
been somewhat divergent, and this has resulted in the postulation of several
conflicting mechanisms of injury. Possibly, a more productive approach to
the study of mechanisms would involve a search for conditions that will
produce damage that mimics noise-induced changes. In this way, the proposed
mechanisms of injury could be studied individually.

Before discussing these hypothesized mechanisms, several general points
about exposure variables, timing of specimen collection, and histological
techniques must be reviewed.

PARAMETERS INFLUENCING EXPERIMENTAL RESULTS

Exposure Variables

There is a wide spectrum of exposures which will damage the inner ear
epithelium. For simplicity of discussion, these exposures will be grouped, on
the basis of their sound pressure level, into the following 3 categories: very
intense, intense, and moderate. The levels defining each category vary with
species and frequency of the exposure because of differences in the resonance
characteristics of the external canal and the transfer function of the middle
ear. However, the categories stand out relatively clearly when reviewing the
results of experiments on guinea pigs and chinchillas conducted at Central
Institute for the Deaf and Washington University in the past 25 years. The
anatomical appearance of the inner ear epithelium and the duration of exposure required to produce injury were used to identify the 3 categories.
This division appears valid because there is some evidence that cellular
damage and loss resulting from various exposures are mediated by different

mechanisms. For example, in ears examined shortly after exposure to very intense noise, a portion of the organ of Corti is often found to have been separated from the basilar membrane and to be floating free in the scala media (1–5). Cells in the detached portion of the organ of Corti have a relatively normal appearance. Since this type of lesion is found after brief exposures (on the order of minutes), it is most probable that it is the result of mechanical damage. That is, motion of the basilar membrane during exposure produces enough stress in the organ of Corti to cause its attachments to rupture (6–8).

The other classes of exposures must be presented for several hours or days in order to produce injury. In these cases, it is almost certain that one or more mechanisms other than mechanical are responsible for cellular damage and degeneration. The remainder of this chapter is concerned with damage produced by the lower intensity exposures and the mechanisms which may be responsible for this damage.

The locus of maximal injury in the organ of Corti is dependent on the frequency of the stimulus, with high-frequency sounds damaging the base and low-frequency sounds damaging the apex. However, damage can be more widespread than one would expect, based on the traveling-wave theory. Lesions can appear in the first turn of the cochlea in ears exposed for 9 days to an octave band of noise (OBN) centered at 500 Hz at 103 dB sound pressure level (SPL) (9). Conversely, it is possible to destroy 50–60% of the organ of Corti, leaving only the third turn uninjured, by a 3½-hr exposure to an OBN centered at 4 kHz at 108 dB SPL (10). These findings indicate that a complete picture of the damage caused by a particular exposure cannot be obtained unless the entire cochlea is examined.

Timing of Specimen Collection

The histological appearance changes and the amount of damage increases as the interval between exposure of an animal and fixation of its cochleae is lengthened (2,11,12). In order to determine the total amount of cochlear damage caused by a particular exposure, animals must be sacrificed after the ear has reached a static state, such that all degeneration and healing is completed. It has been shown that this stage is reached approximately 1 month following termination of the exposure (11,13). On the other hand, in order to obtain information on mechanisms of injury, cochleae must be fixed shortly after termination of the exposure. Cochleae examined between these 2 times will be in a dynamic stage of injury and repair. Some of the morphological changes seen in the ear at this stage may be the result of conditions which developed secondarily, after the initial effects of the noise exposure. For example, a change in the chemical environment of the organ of Corti may occur when a number of cells degenerate and release their cytoplasmic contents into the extracellular spaces. This change in environment could affect cells which were uninjured by the noise exposure.

In a study of mechanisms it is also important to examine ears after a static state has been reached so that one can determine what the initial changes mean as far as the health of the entire organ of Corti is concerned.

Histological Techniques

Several different histological techniques have been employed to study the noise-damaged inner ear. In many of the earlier studies, the entire cochlea was not examined but, rather, data were obtained from observations on representative samples (i.e., 1 out of every 5 cross sections of the cochlea) (14–16) or selected regions (i.e., one sample of the organ of Corti containing 100 inner hair cells from each turn of the cochlea) (17). These samples may not contain examples of all pathological changes present in the cochlea. Also, as mentioned previously, damage in 1 region of the cochlea may secondarily cause alterations in the cells in adjacent areas. These 2 points are particularly important to consider when attempting to study mechanisms of injury.

HYPOTHESIZED MECHANISMS OF INJURY

In addition to the mechanical theory mentioned earlier, the other frequently discussed mechanisms of noise injury are metabolic exhaustion of the stimulated cells and changes in vascular supply during exposure. Recently, the entrance of endolymph into the fluid spaces of the organ of Corti has been postulated as a mechanism to account for the progressive degeneration seen after noise exposure (11,18).

Metabolic Exhaustion

This theory attributes inner ear damage to a depletion of key enzymes and/or metabolites in the cells during prolonged noise exposure. Support for this theory comes primarily from observations of the ultrastructural appearance of cells in noise-exposed ears. Certain cytological alterations have been found consistently in the sensory cells shortly after termination of a variety of exposures. These changes include a distortion or swelling of the cells (19–23), an increase in osmiophilic bodies (lysosomes) in the outer hair cell apices (19,22,24,25), disarrangement or fusion of stereocilia (21–23,26), and an increase in size and number of whorls of smooth endoplasmic reticulum in the outer hair cells (19,20,23–25,27).

As time after exposure is lengthened, some of the damaged outer hair cells show definite necrotic changes, such as dilatation and eventual rupture of the cisternae of smooth endoplasmic reticulum (19–23,27) and karyolysis of the nuclei (23,27,28). Eventually, the plasma membranes of these severely damaged cells rupture (19–22,27,28). Little mention has been made of exactly which portion of the outer hair cell membrane ruptures first. Spoendlin (20,21) presented data that the surface of the hair cell which lacks cuticular plate material often ruptures so that cytoplasmic contents of the cell leak into the scala media. On the other hand, Engström et al. (27) found debris from degenerating cells within the fluid spaces of the organ of Corti. Lim and Melnick (22) found that the degenerating cells were sometimes pushed out into the scala media and sometimes pushed down into the fluid spaces of the organ of Corti.

Another relatively early finding after exposure has been described as extensive deformation (26) or softening (22) of the cuticular plates of damaged sensory cells. This change presumably precedes rupture of the cells.

Vascular Changes

The most frequently mentioned theory of noise damage is that of impaired circulation in the cochlear vessels during prolonged exposure, leading to a relative or absolute lack of oxygen and nutrients for cells in the inner ear (21,29,30). Evidence in support of this theory is based primarily on observations of capillary areas in the inner ear in histological preparations. Several investigators have noted a diminution or total lack of red blood cells in the vessels below the basilar membrane in noise-exposed ears (30,31). In some preparations, swollen endothelial cell nuclei were found to be partially occluding the capillary lumen and presumably impeding blood flow (7,31). Similar changes were also noted in spiral ligament above the attachment of Reissner's membrane, behind the stria, and in the spiral prominence (7), and also in the stria vascularis (30). In contrast to these findings, Kellerhals (12,32) found the strial vessels so densely packed with red blood cells that they appeared to form a homogeneous mass 24 hr after exposure to 200 gunshots. Aggregation of the red blood cells was thought to occur because of increased blood viscosity which, in turn, was presumably the result of decreased blood flow during exposure. All other vessels within the cochlea, including those below the basilar membrane, never showed this abnormality. Red blood cells were found packed in the strial vessels as long as several days after the exposure.

Although some histological studies indicate an impairment of cochlear blood flow during noise exposure, data of Perlman and Kimura (33) are not in agreement with this view. They observed blood flow in the capillaries of the stria and spiral ligament during exposure to a 277-Hz tone at different intensities. Moderate stimulation (90 dB) produced no visible change in flow rate. At slightly higher levels, flow rate increased, although dilatation of the vessels was rarely seen. Only when the tone was presented at 153 dB for 10 min did circulation cease in a few vessels. Narrowing or rupture of vessels was not observed and blood flow generally resumed when the exposure was terminated.

In addition to the sensory cell changes described in the preceding section, Spoendlin (20,21) has found tremendous swelling of the afferent nerve fibers to the inner hair cells and increased density in the efferent endings on the outer hair cells immediately after exposure (1 hr of white noise at 130 dB). The swelling of nerve fibers seen after noise exposure is identical to that seen by Spoendlin 1 hr after interruption of the blood circulation to the cochlea (20,34). However, Lim and Melnick (22) found minimal changes, consisting of swollen mitochondria, in the afferent nerve endings and no alterations in the efferent endings after exposure to an OBN at 117 dB for 4–24 hr. Finally, Beagley (19) found no evidence of ultrastructural changes in nerve endings or fibers after a 40-min exposure to a 500-Hz tone at 128 dB SPL.

Ionic Changes

In the inner ear, the presence of 2 fluids with very different ionic concentrations is well known. Endolymph, with its high concentration of potassium ions and low sodium, is found in the scala media, whereas perilymph, which is low in potassium and high in sodium, is found in the scala tympani and vestibuli. Studies by Tonndorf et al. (35), using vital dyes, and Ilberg (36), using thorotrast, have shown that the basilar membrane is rather freely permeable to the passage of small molecular weight substances. On the other hand, the reticular lamina of the organ of Corti was found to be impermeable to these same tracers. These studies provide good evidence that the fluid spaces of the organ of Corti are in communication with the scala tympani and, hence, must contain fluid which is quite similar to perilymph.

If noise exposure interrupts the continuity of the reticular lamina so that endolymph can gain access to the fluid spaces of the organ of Corti, cell membranes which are not normally in contact with fluid containing a high concentration of potassium ions may be damaged (11,18). This theory is based on findings in a number of cochleae which were prepared for phase-contrast microscopic examination shortly after termination of the noise exposure. In areas apical or basal to the maximally damaged portion of the organ of Corti, scattered outer pillars were found to have recently degenerated. Immediately adjacent to the missing outer pillars, outer hair cells were found to be grossly swollen or ruptured. Cells further away from the missing outer pillars had normal shapes (18). This finding tends to indicate that following loss of a few cells, endolymph enters the fluid spaces of the organ of Corti through the resulting hole in the reticular lamina. An additional number of cells surrounding the hole may then be damaged. The change in the concentration of ions within the fluid spaces of the organ of Corti may be 1 mechanism which can account for the continued degeneration seen in the inner ear at longer survival times (2,11,18,32).

There are 3 indirect lines of evidence which lend support to this theory. Goldstein and Mizukoshi (37) used pronase and a micromagnetic stirrer to separate individual outer hair cells from the organ of Corti. Cells undamaged by this procedure were suspended in either artificial perilymph or endolymph. Cells placed in perilymph retained their normal cylindrical shape, whereas those in endolymph swelled in the infranuclear region and assumed a pear-shaped appearance. Trump and Arstila (38) noted that it is possible to produce an isosmotic swelling in cells by substituting a penetrable ion, such as potassium, for extracellular sodium. Unless constrained by some external force which is equivalent to the internal hydrostatic pressure, the cells will continue to swell and eventually burst.

Also in support of this theory is a study by Duvall et al. (39) in which the endolymphatic surface of the organ of Corti was nicked with a microhook and pathological changes were observed in the inner ear at different times after surgery. Degeneration of sensory cells, supporting cells, and nerve fibers was observed to have spread beyond the initial site of injury at increased survival times. Based on these findings, it was hypothesized that mechanical rupture of the surface of the organ of Corti allows endolymph to enter the fluid spaces of the organ of Corti, perhaps resulting in degeneration of the supporting cells and neural elements.

At variance with the ionic theory of damage from noise exposure is the finding that early in the course of degeneration, supporting cells are joined together below the disintegrating sensory cell to form a tight seal between the endolymphatic space and the fluid spaces of the organ of Corti (20–22).

DYNAMIC CHANGES IN THE EAR AFTER NOISE DAMAGE

Cells and Nerve Fibers

Many of the conflicts in the literature just cited are probably attributable to the use of different noises for exposure and different techniques for both preserving and preparing the cochlea for microscopic examination. In an attempt to resolve some of these conflicts, a search was begun to find a noise exposure which would not cause a great deal of cell loss shortly after exposure, but which would consistently produce total degeneration of a segment of the organ of Corti after a month of recovery. In this way, the initial changes seen in the cells and nerve fibers would be free from contamination by any secondary events which may occur after noise exposure. Also, there would be no doubt as to the significance of the initial cellular changes.

It was found that, in chinchillas, exposure for 1 hr to an OBN centered at 4 kHz at 108 dB SPL fulfilled these preliminary requirements. After determining this, a large series of chinchillas were exposed to the noise and then sacrificed at different intervals so that all stages of cell degeneration and subsequent healing in the organ of Corti could be studied. All of the information obtained from this study will not be presented here; only those data which are relevant to the discussion of mechanisms of noise damage are discussed.

All cochleae were preserved by an *in vivo* perfusion of the perilymphatic spaces with a buffered solution of 1% osmium tetroxide. In order to determine the location and extent of damage in the noise-exposed ears, the cochleae were prepared as araldite-embedded, flat preparations (40). In each cochlea, the length of the organ of Corti was measured, counts of missing sensory cells were made, and the pathological changes present at each locus were noted. Selected regions within these specimens were then sectioned for more detailed study by light and electron microscopy.

Exposure to an OBN centered at 4 kHz produces maximal damage in the lower first turn ~4 mm from the basal end of the cochlea. Specimens perfused less than an hour after termination of the exposure were missing fewer than 10 outer hair cells in this area, whereas none of the inner hair cells and supporting cells were absent. Although most outer hair cells were present, they did not have entirely normal appearances. By phase-contrast microscopy, it was found that the outer hair cell bodies were slightly swollen and out of their normal positions. In addition, the cells contained accumulations of dense-staining material within their cytoplasm (Fig. 1B) which, by electron microscopy, turned out to be whorls of cisternae of smooth endoplasmic reticulum. The stereocilia pattern on these same outer hair cells was undisturbed (Fig. 1A). The rest of the cells and the nerve fibers within the organ of Corti, including fibers in the inner spiral bundle (Fig. 1C), had normal electron-microscopic appearances.

Ninety minutes after exposure, outer hair cells in the lower first turn showed more signs of damage. Phase-contrast microscopy showed that the stereocilia formed a dot pattern (Fig. 2A), rather than the smooth line seen earlier. By electron microscopy, this was found to be a fusion of several adjacent stereocilia to form a giant stereocilium (Fig. 2B). Outer hair cell bodies were more swollen, and there were areas where the plasma membrane of these cells appeared thinned (Fig. 2C). By electron microscopy, these areas were found to be regions in which the peripherally arranged cisternae of smooth endoplasmic reticulum had disappeared. Nerve fibers in the inner spiral bundles and within the tunnel space still had normal appearances at this time.

By 2 hr after exposure, no outer hair cell bodies were seen in a 1-mm-long segment of the organ of Corti in the lower first turn. All that remained below the reticular lamina were several enlarged nuclei which had lost most of their nucleoplasm and fragments of plasma membranes (Fig. 3B). From the arrangement of the fragments, it appeared that the cells were quite swollen

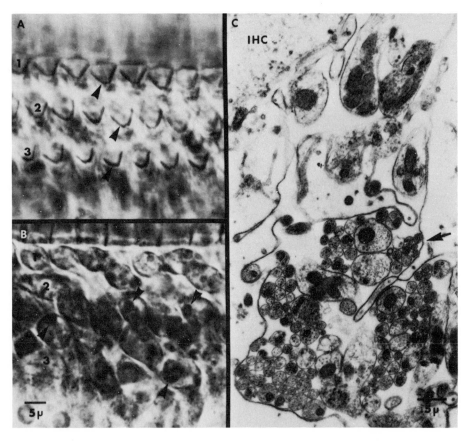

FIG. 1. Lower first turn of cochlea 23 min after termination of exposure (4 kHz OBN at 108 dB SPL for 1 hr). A. Phase-contrast photomicrograph of reticular lamina showing typical W-shaped pattern of stereocilia (*arrows*) on 3 rows of outer hair cells (OHC) (*1,2,3*). B. Focused below reticular lamina in A. Bodies of OHC are slightly swollen and out-of-position. There are accumulations of dense-staining material (*arrows*) in several of the cells. C. Electron micrograph of area below inner hair cells (*IHC*) shows normal appearance of nerve fibers in inner spiral bundle (*arrow*).

before the membranes ruptured. Study of the reticular lamina by phase-contrast microscopy indicated that apices of the 3 rows of outer hair cells were still present (Fig. 3A). However, sections cut tangential to the organ of Corti and examined by electron microscopy revealed that the surfaces of the outer hair cells had also disappeared. Small holes (Fig. 3C), the exact size of the missing hair cells, were left in the reticular lamina, since the phalangeal processes had not yet enlarged to form phalangeal scars. At the same time, the first signs of damage appeared in the radial tunnel fibers. This consisted of a clumping of axoplasm within the fibers, giving them the appearance of beads on a string (Fig. 3D). Electron microscopy showed some of the nerve fibers in the tunnel spiral bundle to be slightly swollen.

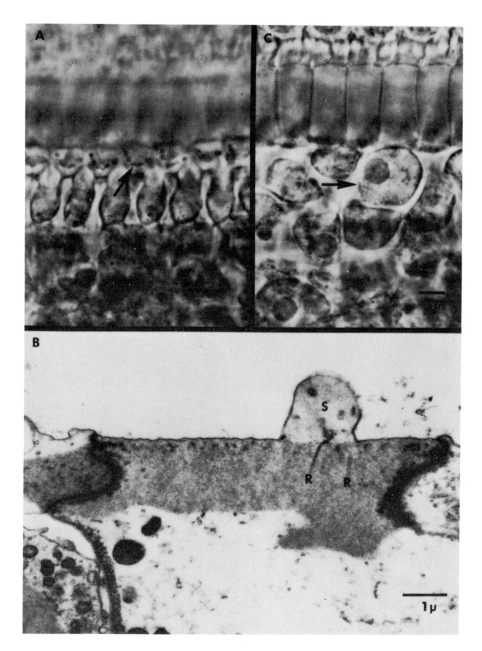

FIG. 2. Lower first turn of cochlea 1½ hr after termination of exposure (4 kHz OBN at 108 dB SPL for 1 hr). A. Phase-contrast photomicrograph of stereocilia (*arrows*) on first row outer hair cells (OHC). Note that stereocilia no longer form a smooth line but, instead, form a series of dots. B. Electron micrograph of cell in A shows that adjacent stereocilia (S) have fused and thus no longer form individual projections from cell surface. R, rootlets of 2 adjacent stereocilia. C. Focused below reticular lamina in A. OHC are quite swollen and distorted. At places, plasma membrane appears thinned (*arrow*).

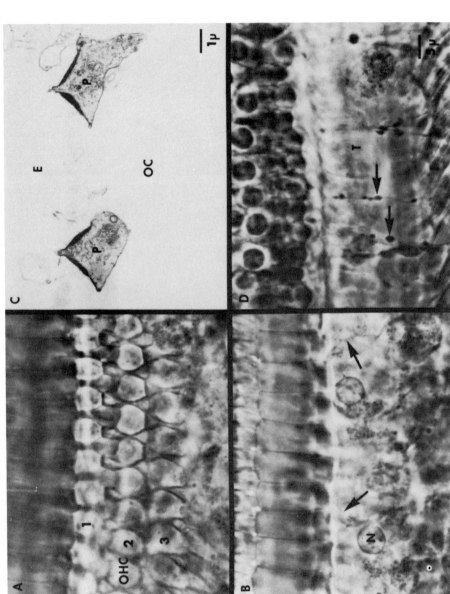

FIG. 3. Lower first turn of cochlea 2 hr after termination of exposure (4 kHz OBN at 108 dB SPL for 1 hr). A. Phase-contrast photomicrograph showing reticular lamina where it appears that 3 rows of outer hair cells (OHC) (1,2,3) are present. B. Focused below reticular lamina in A. All that remains of sensory cells is scattered degenerating nuclei (N) and fragments of plasma membranes (arrows). C. Electron micrograph of tangential section through second row OHC in A shows that surface membrane of sensory cell is gone. Hole remaining in reticular lamina provides route for communication between endolymphatic space (E) and fluid spaces of the organ of Corti (OC). Phalangeal processes (P) still have original shape at this time. D. Focused on tunnel space (T) in A. Axoplasm has formed clumps (arrows) in radial tunnel fibers.

As the time after exposure was lengthened beyond 2 hr, supporting cells and inner hair cells began to show signs of injury. These cells continued to undergo necrotic changes so that by the 14th day after exposure, an average of 1 mm of the organ of Corti was missing in the lower first turn.

Blood Vessels

The chinchillas used for the noise study reported here were exposed in the unanesthetized state. For this reason, it was not possible to perfuse the cochleae sooner than 20 min after termination of the exposure. Thus, some vascular alterations which may have been present during exposure could have resolved before the cochleae were perfused. With this limitation in mind, the condition of blood vessels below the basilar membrane was assessed.

Before describing the findings in noise-exposed ears, it is necessary to review the vascular anatomy of the adult chinchilla. Although present at birth, most of the vessel of the basilar membrane ceases functioning shortly thereafter. In chinchillas 8 days or older, the only functional portion of the vessel of the basilar membrane is found in the third turn (41). The vessel of the tympanic lip of the osseous spiral lamina, which has a small caliber when the vessel of the basilar membrane is still functioning (Fig. 4D), has a fairly large diameter in adults. Note that when the vessel is carrying a small amount of blood, the nuclei of the endothelial cells bulge into the lumen and appear to be impeding blood flow (Fig. 4D).

In chinchillas, the vessel of the tympanic lip forms a highly variable pattern. In some cases, the vessel forms a series of simple T junctions (Fig. 4A). In other areas, the vessel may be double (Fig. 4C), and elsewhere, the vessel may be entirely absent (Fig. 4B).

In order to enhance the possibility of finding vascular changes after noise exposure, chinchillas were exposed to noises which produced more damage than that described in the preceding section. In each case, the animals were sacrificed as soon as possible after termination of the exposure. Since the most likely location of vascular changes is in the vessels beneath the maximally damaged portion of the organ of Corti, only the condition of these vessels will be described.

Chinchillas exposed for 9 days to an OBN centered at 500 Hz at 95 dB SPL sustain considerable loss of outer hair cells in the lower third turn of the cochlea and also may have some loss in the lower first turn (9). The appearance of the organ of Corti in the lower third turn of the cochlea 55 min after exposure to this noise is shown in Fig. 5. The presence of cellular debris below the reticular lamina (Fig. 5B) indicates that many of the outer hair cells had recently degenerated. At this same locus, nerve fibers in the inner spiral bundle were of normal size and appearance (Fig. 5C). Despite the large amount of outer hair cell loss in this area, the vessel of the tympanic lip was well filled with red blood cells (Fig. 6A). In the same animal, there

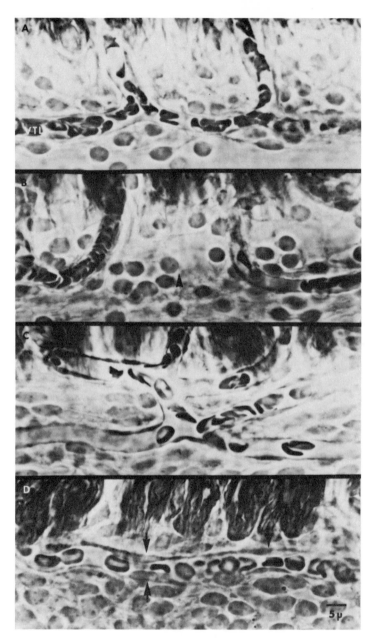

FIG. 4. Phase-contrast photomicrographs showing normal variation in pattern of vessel of tympanic lip (*VTL*) of osseous spiral lamina in chinchilla. A. VTL forming 2 typical T junctions in upper second turn. B. Avascular area (*arrow*) in upper second turn lying between 2 capillary beds. C. Complex arrangement in lower second turn with 3 vessels connected to VTL, which then becomes double. D. VTL in lower third turn of newborn animal. Scattered swollen endothelial cell nuclei (*arrows*) partially occlude lumen of vessel.

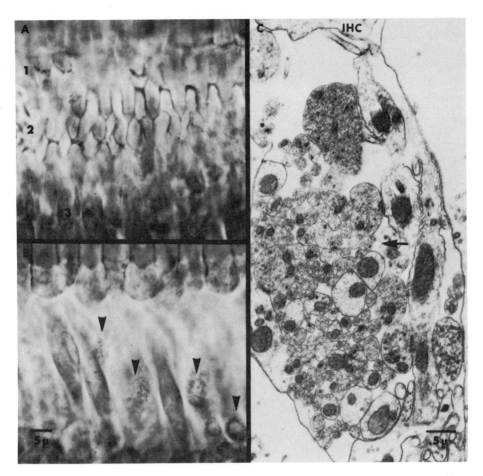

FIG. 5. Lower third turn of cochlea 55 min after termination of exposure (500 Hz OBN at 95 dB SPL for 9 days). A. Phase-contrast photomicrograph of reticular lamina shows extensive loss of OHC in first (1) and second (2) rows. Most cells in third row (3) are present. B. Focused below the reticular lamina in A. Few hair cell bodies are visible in first row. There is much cellular debris (arrows), indicating that the cells have recently degenerated. C. Electron micrograph of area below inner hair cells (IHC) shows nerve fibers in inner spiral bundle (arrow) have typical appearance.

was a region in the lower first turn in which several outer pillars had de-generated and a number of outer hair cells were quite swollen. The vessel of the tympanic lip at this locus was also found to be normal (Fig. 6B).

In animals exposed for 3½ hr to an OBN centered at 4 kHz at 108 dB SPL, more than one-half of the entire organ of Corti had degenerated by 1 month after exposure (10). Ears exposed to the same noise, but examined less than 1 hr after exposure were found to be missing all outer hair cells in a 2-mm-long segment of organ of Corti in the lower first turn. At this same locus, the vessel of the tympanic lip showed no abnormalities (Fig. 6C).

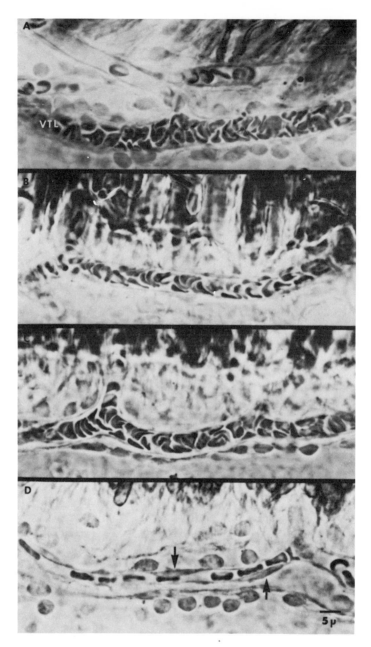

FIG. 6. Phase-contrast photomicrographs of vessel of tympanic lip (*VTL*) of osseous spiral lamina in chinchilla. A. Vessel in third turn of animal exposed for 9 days to a 500 Hz OBN at 95 dB SPL and perfused 55 min after termination of exposure. B. Vessel in first turn of animal described in A. C. Vessel in first turn of animal exposed for 3½ hr to 4 kHz OBN at 108 dB SPL and perfused 32 min after termination of exposure. D. Vessel in first turn of an ear which was ischemic for 1 hr prior to fixation. Swollen endothelial cell nuclei (*arrows*) partially occlude vessel lumen.

In all cochleae studied, including the nonexposed control ears, there were scattered short gaps in the column of red blood cells within the vessel of the tympanic lip. It is interesting to note that there were only 2 instances where swollen endothelial cell nuclei were observed in the vessel of the tympanic lip. One case was in the newborn chinchilla mentioned previously (Fig. 4D), and the other was in ears which were ischemic for a certain length of time prior to fixation (Fig. 6D). The ischemic ears are described in detail in the next section.

TESTING THE HYPOTHESES

Having obtained more precise details about the sequence of events which occur in the organ of Corti after excessive exposure to noise, it was decided that the time had come to test some of the theories on mechanisms of injury. The most readily testable hypotheses are those of ischemic and ionic damage.

Damage from Ischemia*

Anesthetized chinchillas were decapitated and their temporal bones were removed and opened widely to expose the cochleae.The specimens were then placed in a nitrogen atmosphere at 37°C for varying lengths of time prior to fixation. After perfusion, the cochleae were prepared exactly as described in the preceding section.

Signs of damage were present in both the stria vascularis and organ of Corti in specimens which were ischemic for 30 min prior to fixation. For the purposes of this chapter, only the changes seen in the organ of Corti are described.

In ears which were ischemic for 30 min, there were several clear signs of injury. Nerve fibers close to the base of the inner hair cells in the inner spiral bundle were swollen. By phase-contrast microscopy, small dots of extraneous material appeared to be attached to some of the radial tunnel fibers. Some of the inner and outer hair cells were slightly swollen. The supporting cells were essentially normal at this time.

After 1 hr of ischemia, the most peripheral portions of the myelinated nerve fibers in the osseous spiral lamina had begun to swell (Fig. 7A). There were more dots of extraneous material attached to the radial tunnel fibers (Fig. 7B), and nerve fibers in the inner spiral bundle were quite swollen (Fig. 7C). At this time, the inner and outer hair cells were no longer arranged in uniform rows, but, rather, were staggered in position, indicating that the cells were more swollen.

---

* The degenerative changes seen in cells after somatic death are often referred to as autolysis, to distinguish them from changes which occur in dead cells in a living body. However, this distinction is arbitrary because, in both cases, the same sequence of necrotic reactions takes place (38).

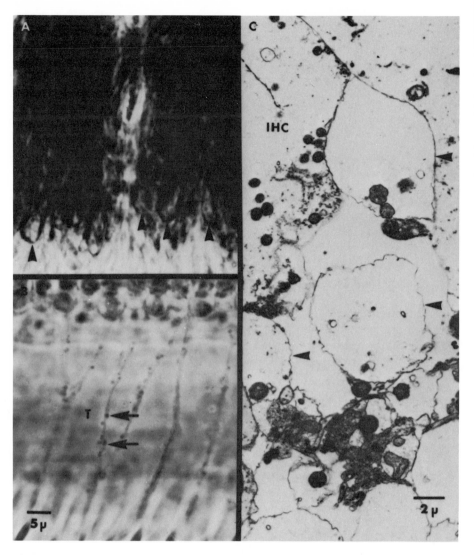

FIG. 7. Lower second turn of cochlea which was ischemic for 1 hr prior to fixation. A. Myelinated nerve fibers in osseous spiral lamina are slightly swollen (*arrows*) in region nearest organ of Corti. B. Small dots of extraneous material (*arrows*) appear to be attached to radial tunnel fibers as they cross the tunnel space (*T*). C. Electron micrograph of area below inner hair cells (*IHC*) shows swelling of fibers (*arrows*) in inner spiral bundle.

In ears which were ischemic for 2 hr, severe degenerative changes were present. Myelinated nerve fibers in the osseous spiral lamina were swollen throughout their lengths (Fig. 8A). All radial tunnel fibers were fragmented (Fig. 8B), and most of the nerve fibers in the inner spiral bundle had ruptured (Fig. 8C). Inner hair cells were quite swollen and contained

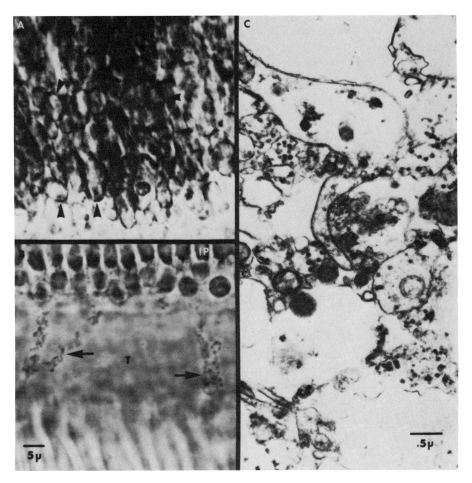

FIG. 8. Lower second turn of cochlea which was ischemic for 2 hr prior to fixation. A. Gross swelling (*arrows*) of nerve fibers in osseous spiral lamina is apparent along their entire extent. B. Radial tunnel fibers (*arrows*) within tunnel space (*T*) are fragmented. *IP*, inner pillar bases. C. Electron micrograph of area below inner hair cells shows that few identifiable nerve fibers remain in inner spiral bundle.

enlarged, pale-staining nuclei (Fig. 9A). The plasma membranes of some of these inner hair cells had actually ruptured. At the same locus, outer hair cells were also swollen (Fig. 9B), but had not yet reached the advanced stage of degeneration seen in the inner hair cells.

Damage from Ionic Changes

Since earlier studies have shown that the scala tympani communicates rather freely with the fluid spaces of the organ of Corti (35,36), solutions having different ionic compositions were perfused through the scala tympani

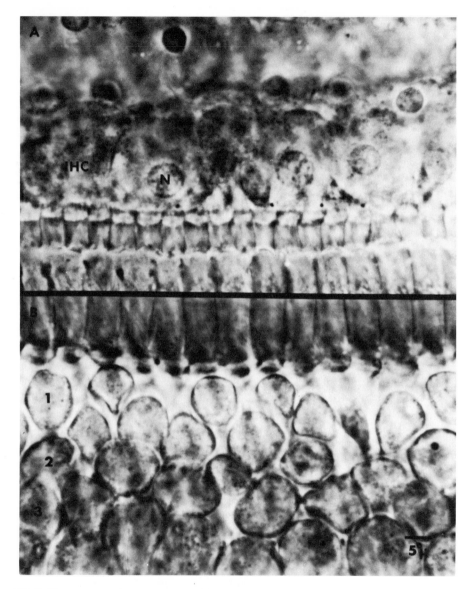

FIG. 9. Phase-contrast photomicrographs of lower second turn of cochlea which was ischemic for 2 hr prior to fixation. A. Inner hair cells (*IHC*) are quite swollen and have edematous cytoplasm and degenerating nuclei (*N*). B. Outer hair cells (*1,2,3*) at same locus are swollen but have not reached the advanced stage of degeneration seen in IHC.

in order to test their effect on the cells and nerve fibers of the organ of Corti.

For each perfusion, the chinchilla was anesthetized and one of its bullae surgically exposed and widely opened. A small hole was drilled in the scala tympani of the first turn near the round window and in the helicotrema at the apex. The animal's head was tightly clamped in a head holder to prevent

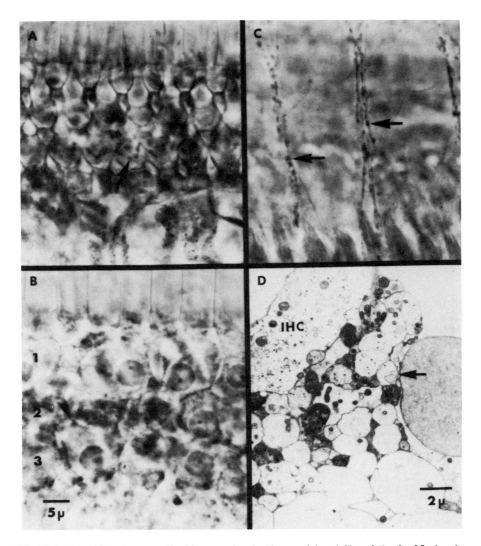

FIG. 10. Ear in which scala tympani had been perfused with an endolymph-like solution for 15 min prior to fixation. A. Phase-contrast photomicrograph of stereocilia on outer hair cells (OHC) in third row form a series of dots (arrow). B. Focused below reticular lamina in A. OHC bodies in all 3 rows (1,2,3) are quite swollen and have edematous cytoplasm. C. Axoplasm has formed clumps (arrows) in radial tunnel fibers. D. Electron micrograph of area below inner hair cells (IHC) shows swelling of nerve fibers in inner spiral bundle (arrow).

movement during perfusion. A micropipette (tip diameter 50–100 μm) connected to a Harvard infusion pump was positioned over the hole in the first turn with the aid of a micromanipulator. The perfusates were infused at a rate of 13.6 μl/min, with escape of fluid occurring from the apical hole.

In order to insure that the perfusion procedure did not cause any cytological alterations in the organ of Corti, the first experiments were conducted using various artificial perilymph solutions. It was found that an oxygen-saturated solution of Fex's artificial perilymph (42) could maintain the normal electron-microscopic appearance of cells and nerve fibers in the organ of Corti for perfusion durations of more than 1 hr. The pH of the perfusate was 7.3 and the osmolarity was 292 mOsm.

In the next set of experiments, cochleae were perfused with an oxygen-saturated, endolymph-like solution, which was prepared by reversing the potassium and sodium concentrations in Fex's artificial perilymph. The osmolarity and pH of this solution were the same as in the artificial perilymph.

A 15-min perfusion with artificial endolymph produced damage in the organ of Corti, which resembled that seen 1–2 hr after noise exposure (4 kHz OBN at 108 dB SPL for 1 hr). By phase-contrast microscopy, the stereocilia on the outer hair cells were seen to form a dot pattern (Fig. 10A). By electron microscopy, it was found that adjacent stereocilia had fused together. Outer hair cells in all 3 rows were quite swollen and had edematous cytoplasm (Fig. 10B), as did many of the supporting cells. Inner hair cells were distorted, but this appeared to be the result of indentation by swollen inner supporting cells. By phase-contrast microscopy, axoplasm in the radial tunnel fibers was seen to form a series of clumps (Fig. 10C). Nerve fibers near the basilar membrane in the inner spiral bundle were greatly enlarged, whereas those close to the base of the inner hair cells were less swollen (Fig. 10D).

After perfusion for 1 hr with artificial endolymph, the lateral part of the organ of Corti was found to be detached from the basilar membrane. Many inner and outer hair cells had ruptured and all of the radial tunnel fibers were gone.

In an attempt to determine whether or not the increased concentration of potassium in the perfusate was responsible for the cellular alterations, another endolymph-like solution was prepared. In this case, choline salts were substituted for the potassium salts in the artificial endolymph. Choline is a quaternary ammonium ion which does not cross intact biological membranes (43).

The use of choline maintained the osmolarity of the perfusate (291 mOsm) so that the effect of excess potassium ions could be determined. As can be seen in Fig. 11, the cells and nerve fibers within the organ of Corti had entirely normal appearances after a 15-min perfusion with the "choline–endolymph" solution.

DISCUSSION ANALYSIS

Metabolic Exhaustion

The early swelling of sensory cells after noise exposure is indicative of abnormal cell volume regulation, which may be the result of an increase in

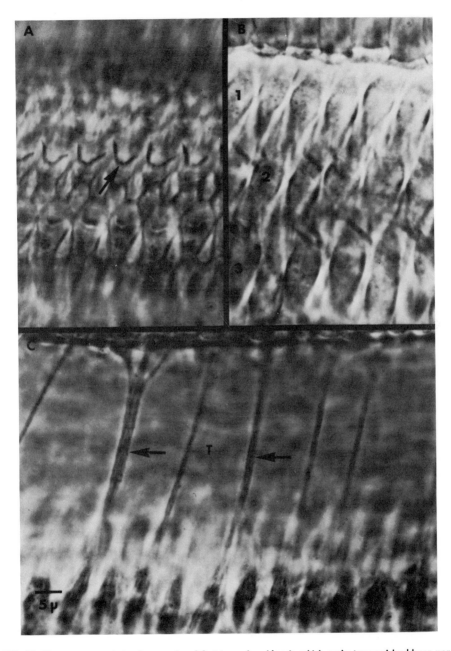

FIG. 11. Phase-contrast photomicrographs of first turn of cochlea in which scala tympani had been perfused for 15 min with an endolymph-like solution containing choline salts instead of potassium. A. Stereocilia on outer hair cells (OHC) form smooth W pattern (arrow). B. Bodies of OHC (1,2,3) have normal cylindrical shape. C. Radial tunnel fibers (arrows) crossing tunnel space (T) have normal appearance.

membrane permeability, a modification of ion-transport systems within the membrane, or a depletion of energy required for the transport systems (38). In turn, any of these alterations may be the result of the inability of the cell to maintain a normal rate of metabolism. Dilatation of the cisternae of smooth endoplasmic reticulum may also result from changes in ion and water movements across cell membranes (38).

As noted previously, an increased number of lysosomes (19,22,24,25) is often found in outer hair cells after noise exposure. It has been suggested that rupture of the lysosomes in a cell will cause it to enter a necrotic phase leading to death. However, Trump and Ginn (44) have found intact lysosomes in cells that were already in an advanced stage of degeneration. In many outer hair cells which appear severely damaged, intact lysosomes have also been observed (11). Thus, it seems unlikely that lysosomal rupture is responsible for sensory cell degeneration after noise exposure.

Vascular Changes and Ischemia

There are 2 questions to consider when discussing the relationship between cochlear microcirculation and noise-induced cochlear injuries. First, are there changes in blood supply to the cochlea during noise exposure? Second, if present, do these changes play any significant role in the production of cochlear injuries? The second question is raised because the source of oxygen supply for the organ of Corti is still in question.

At this time, the first question cannot be answered satisfactorily. Some histological studies have shown that vascular changes do result from noise exposure. However, in these studies, different changes were reported. In some cases, the vessels below the basilar membrane were reduced in number, or were totally devoid of red blood cells (7,30,31). In other cases, strial vessels were altered, being either packed with red blood cells (12,32) or completely empty (30).

The study of Perlman and Kimura (33) indicated that blood flow in the stria vascularis and spiral ligament was not impeded until the exposure was presented at a high-intensity level (153 dB SPL). This exposure is in the range of very intense and, hence, would probably have resulted in mechanical rupture of the organ of Corti. Cochlear damage has been found to occur at levels of exposure which were not found to produce any change in cochlear blood flow.

The observations in several physiological studies of normal cochlear circulation may help to explain some of these variations. Lawrence (45), using guinea pigs, has found that the diameter of the vessel of the basilar membrane is slightly larger than that of a red blood cell. Red blood cells generally travel single-file in this vessel. The occasional gaps seen in the column of red blood cells were thought to contain plasma. Costa and Brånemark (46) studied blood flow in the stria vascularis, spiral ligament, limbus, and vessels below the basilar membrane using a Leitz intravital microscope. Under optimal lighting conditions, all blood elements could be identified. The vascular networks were usually filled with blood at "various hematocrit." This implies that the number of red blood cells in any 1 vessel varied from moment to moment, depending on the amount of plasma present. Occasionally, a white blood cell was observed to block flow temporarily at the junction of 2 vessels. This resulted in a decrease in the number of red blood cells passing through 1 of the vessels.

The small gaps seen between red blood cells in histological preparations probably are the result of normal physiological variations in blood flow. In chinchillas exposed to noise, white blood cells have been found in increased numbers in the vessels of the tympanic lip of the osseous spiral lamina (41). The peak elevation in white blood cells was seen when there was a large amount of degenerating debris within the organ of Corti as a result of the recent rupture of a number of cells. Thus, it may be reasonable to expect some variation in vessel perfusion when the organ of Corti has been severely injured and there is an increased number of white blood cells in the vessels below the basilar membrane. In summary, it is quite possible that there are changes in cochlear blood flow during noise exposure. However, some of the changes may be indicative of physiological variations rather than pathological.

The question about the significance of vascular changes can be answered by comparing the relative susceptibility of various cells in the organ of Corti to noise exposure and ischemia. Almost all noise studies have shown that outer hair cells are the first to be injured, regardless of the exposure level. If damage is severe enough, many cells within the organ of Corti may degenerate, but the outer hair cells degenerate first. Inner hair cells generally do not disappear until a number of the pillars are gone. On the other hand, ischemic studies have indicated that inner hair cells are more susceptible to lack of oxygen than outer hair cells (47). In the present study, it was shown that inner hair cells were ruptured after 2 hr of ischemia, while the plasma membranes of the outer hair cells were still intact (Fig. 9). Thus, the picture of ischemia in the organ of Corti does not fit that of noise damage as far as hair cell susceptibility is concerned.

Data concerning damage to nerve fibers within the organ of Corti from noise exposure are conflicting. Spoendlin (20,21) has found swelling in the afferent nerve fibers to the inner hair cells shortly after a 1-hr exposure to white noise at 130 dB. In the present study, no changes were found in these fibers in ears exposed for 9 days to an OBN centered at 500 Hz at 95 dB SPL or in ears exposed for 1 hr to an OBN centered at 4 kHz at 108 dB SPL. In these cases, there were no areas in the organ of Corti in which the reticular lamina was found to be damaged shortly after termination of the exposure. However, swelling of the nerve fibers in the tunnel spiral bundle was observed shortly after termination of exposure to an OBN centered at 4 kHz at 108 dB SPL for 3½ hr (41). In this instance, all outer hair cells had degenerated in a 2-mm-long segment of the organ of Corti in the lower first turn of the cochlea. A corresponding number of holes remained in the reticular lamina as a result of the recent cell degeneration (11). It was at this locus that swelling of fibers in the tunnel spiral bundle was observed, and also where the radial tunnel fibers had the appearance of beads on a string (Fig. 3D).

Ionic Damage

The cellular changes seen in the organ of Corti following a 15-min perfusion of scala tympani with an oxygen-saturated solution of endolymph were described earlier (Fig. 10). It was noted that these changes were quite similar to those seen 1–2 hr after noise exposure (4 kHz OBN at 108 dB SPL for 1 hr; Figs. 2 and 3). The differences between these specimens can be explained by considering the route through which endolymph entered the organ of Corti. In the perfusion experiment, endolymph crossed the basilar membrane to enter the fluid spaces of the organ of Corti. Thus, outer hair cells (Fig. 10A,B) and nerve fibers crossing the tunnel space (Fig. 10C) and in the inner spiral bundle (Fig. 10D) all showed signs of damage after a short exposure to endolymph. On the other hand, in the noise experiment, endolymph could not enter the fluid spaces of the organ of Corti until the outer hair cells had degenerated and left holes in the reticular lamina (Fig. 3C). In this case, nerve fiber damage appeared after the outer hair cells had degenerated (Fig. 3D). It is interesting to note that in the endolymph-perfused ear, nerve fibers in the inner spiral bundle which were closest to the basilar membrane were more swollen than those near the inner hair cell base (Fig. 10D). Spoendlin (20,21) has found the afferent nerve fibers closest to the inner hair cell bases to be the first to swell after noise exposure. Perhaps in Spoendlin's studies (20,21) endolymph leakage was already present when the specimens were examined shortly after exposure. This, then, would account for the presence of swollen nerve fibers in the upper part of the inner spiral bundle.

SUMMARY

The mechanisms by which excessive exposure to noise can lead to degeneration of all the cells and nerve fibers in a segment of the organ of Corti are still unknown. However, based on a review of the literature and the data reported here, certain positive statements about mechanisms of noise injury can be made.

1. Exposure to noise at very high intensities often results in detachment of a portion of the organ of Corti from the basilar membrane. This lesion is probably a consequence of the stress which develops in the organ during exposure and, therefore, is purely mechanical in nature.

2. Outer hair cells are the first cells to be damaged by noise exposure, whereas inner hair cells are the first to degenerate from ischemia. Thus, it is unlikely that lack of oxygen during exposure is the cause of sensory cell degeneration.

3. Exposure to noise at high intensities may cause severe damage to a number of cells during the exposure. Although the mechanisms which are responsible for this initial damage have not been elucidated, it is likely that a change in membrane permeability is involved.

4. If, as a result of exposure to noise, a number of sensory cells degenerate simultaneously, small holes will be left in the reticular lamina for a finite length of time. These holes provide a pathway through which endolymph can enter the fluid spaces of the organ of Corti.

5. The presence of endolymph (or excessive potassium ions) in the fluid spaces of the organ of Corti causes uninjured cells and nerve fibers to undergo an isosmotic swelling and eventually to rupture. This may be the mechanism responsible for degeneration of many of the supporting cells and nerve fibers after noise exposure.

ACKNOWLEDGMENTS

This work was supported by NIH grants NS 01791 and NS 11417 to the Department of Otolaryngology, Washington University School of Medicine, and NIH grant NS 03856 to the Central Institute for the Deaf, St. Louis, Missouri.

The perfusion experiments were done by Mr. Thomas H. Comegys. Excellent technical assistance was provided by Ms. Rosie Saito, Ms. Virginia Schnettgoecke, and Ms. Diane Hasey.

REFERENCES

1. Lurie, M. H. (1940): Studies of acquired and inherited deafness in animals. *J. Acoust. Soc. Am.,* 11:420–426.
2. Lurie, M. H. (1942): The degeneration and absorption of the organ of Corti in animals. *Ann. Otol. Rhinol. Laryngol.,* 51:712–717.
3. Hawkins, J. E., Jr., Lurie, M. H., and Davis, H. (1943): Injury of the inner ear produced by exposure to loud tones. *Office of Scientific Research and Development, Committee on Medical Research, Suppl. Report,* Contract OEMcmr-194.
4. Covell, W. P., and Eldredge, D. H. (1951): Injury to animal ears by intense sound. *AF Technical Report No. 6561, Part I.* WADC, U.S. Air Force, Wright-Patterson AFB, Ohio.
5. Covell, W. P., and Eldredge, D. H. (1952): Injury to animal ears by intense sound. *AF Technical Report No. 6561, Part II.* WADC, U.S. Air Force, Wright-Patterson AFB, Ohio.
6. Schuknecht, H. F., and Tonndorf, J. (1960): Acoustic trauma of the cochlea from ear surgery. *Laryngoscope,* 70:479–505.
7. Hawkins, J. E., Jr. (1971): The role of vasoconstriction in noise-induced hearing loss. *Ann. Otol. Rhinol. Laryngol.,* 80:903–913.
8. Jordan, V. M., Pinheiro, M. L., Chiba, K., and Jimenez, A. (1973): Cochlear

pathology in monkeys exposed to impulsive noise. *Acta Otolaryngol.* [*Suppl.*] (*Stockh.*), 312:16–30.

9. Fried, M. P., Dudek, S. E., and Bohne, B. A. (1976): Basal turn cochlear lesions following exposure to low frequency noise. *Trans. Am. Acad. Ophthalmol. Otolaryngol.* (*in press*).

10. Bohne, B. A., and Eldredge, D. H. Unpublished data.

11. Bohne, B. A. (1971): *Scar Formation in the Inner Ear Following Acoustical Injury: Sequence of Changes From Early Signs of Damage to Healed Lesion.* Ph.D. dissertation, Washington University, St. Louis, Missouri.

12. Kellerhals, B. (1972): Pathogenesis of inner ear lesions in acute acoustic trauma. *Acta Otolaryngol.* (*Stockh.*), 73:249–253.

13. Stockwell, C. W., Ades, H. W., and Engström, H. (1969): Patterns of hair cell damage after intense auditory stimulation. *Ann. Otol. Rhinol. Laryngol.*, 78:1144–1168.

14. Alexander, I. E., and Githler, F. J. (1951): Histological examination of cochlear structure following exposure to jet engine noise. *J. Comp. Physiol. Psychol.*, 44:513–524.

15. Lawrence, M., and Yantis, P. A. (1957): Individual differences in functional recovery and structural repair following overstimulation of the guinea pig ear. *Ann. Otol. Rhinol. Laryngol.*, 66:595–621.

16. Eldredge, D. H., Covell, W. P., and Davis, H. (1957): Recovery from acoustic trauma in the guinea pig. *Laryngoscope,* 67:66–84.

17. Engström, H., Ades, H. W., and Andersson, A. (1966): *Structural Pattern of the Organ of Corti.* Almqvist and Wiksell, Stockholm.

18. Bohne, B. A. (1974): Mechanism for continuing degeneration in the organ of Corti. *J. Acoust. Soc. Am.*, 55:S77–S78.

19. Beagley, H. A. (1965): Acoustic trauma in the guinea pig. Part II. *Acta Otolaryngol.* (*Stockh.*), 60:479–495.

20. Spoendlin, H. H. (1970): Auditory, vestibular, olfactory and gustatory organs. In: *Ultrastructure of the Peripheral Nervous System and Sense Organs: An Atlas of Normal and Pathologic Anatomy,* edited by A. Bischoff, pp. 173–337. Mosby, St. Louis, Mo. (Thieme, Stuttgart).

21. Spoendlin, H. H. (1971): Primary structural changes in the organ of Corti after acoustic overstimulation. *Acta Otolaryngol.* (*Stockh.*), 71:166–176.

22. Lim, D. J., and Melnick, W. (1971): Acoustic damage of the cochlea. A scanning and transmission electron microscopic observation. *Arch. Otolaryngol.*, 94:294–305.

23. Ward, W. D., and Duvall, A. J. (1971): Behavioral and ultrastructural correlates of acoustic trauma. *Ann. Otol. Rhinol. Laryngol.*, 80:881–896.

24. Engström, H., and Ades, H. (1960): Effect of high intensity noise on inner ear sensory epithelia. *Acta Otolaryngol.* [*Suppl.*] (*Stockh.*), 158:219–229.

25. Spoendlin, H. H. (1962): Ultrastructural features of the organ of Corti in normal and acoustically stimulated animals. *Ann. Otol. Rhinol. Laryngol.*, 71:657–677.

26. Lindeman, H. H., and Bredberg, G. (1972): Scanning electron microscopy of the organ of Corti after intense auditory stimulation: Effects on stereocilia and cuticular surface of hair cells. *Arch. Klin. Exp. Ohr.-, Nas.-Kehlk. Heilk.*, 203:1–15.

27. Engström, H., Ades, H. W., and Bredberg, G. (1970): Normal structure of the organ of Corti and the effect of noise-induced cochlear damage. In: *Sensorineural Hearing Loss,* edited by G. E. W. Wolstenholme and J. Knight, pp. 127–156. Williams and Wilkins, Baltimore, Md.

28. Beagley, H. A. (1965): Acoustic trauma in the guinea pig. Part I. *Acta Otolaryngol.* (*Stockh.*), 60:437–451.

29. Lipscomb, D. M. (1972): Indicators of environmental noise. In: *Indicators of Environmental Quality,* edited by W. A. Thomas, pp. 211–241. Plenum Press, New York.

30. Lawrence, M., Gonzalez, G., and Hawkins, J. E., Jr. (1967): Some physiological factors in noise-induced hearing loss. *Am. Ind. Hyg. Assoc. J.,* 28:425–430.

31. Lipscomb, D. M., and Roettger, R. L. (1973): Capillary constriction in cochlear and vestibular tissues during intense noise stimulation. *Laryngoscope,* 83:259–263.

32. Kellerhals, B. (1972): Acoustic trauma and cochlear microcirculation. *Adv. Oto-rhinolaryngol.*, 18:91–168.
33. Perlman, H. B., and Kimura, R. (1962): Cochlear blood flow in acoustic trauma. *Acta Otolaryngol. (Stockh.)*, 54:99–110.
34. Spoendlin, H. H. (1969): Das ischämische Syndrom des Innenohres. *Pract. Oto-rhino-laryngol.*, 31:257–268.
35. Tonndorf, J., Duvall, A. J., and Reneau, J. P. (1962): Permeability of intracochlear membranes to various vital stains. *Ann. Otol. Rhinol. Laryngol.*, 71:801–841.
36. Ilberg. C. v. (1968): Elektronenmikroskopische Untersuchungen über Diffusion und Resorption von Thoriumdioxyd an der Meerschweinchenschnecke: 4. Mitteilung Basilarmembran und Cortisches Organ. *Arch. Otorhinolaryngol. (NY)*, 192:384–400.
37. Goldstein, A. J., and Mizukoshi, O. (1967): Separation of the organ of Corti into its component cells. *Ann. Otol. Rhinol. Laryngol.*, 76:414–426.
38. Trump, B. F., and Arstila, A. U. (1971): Cell injury and cell death. In: *Principles of Pathobiology*, edited by M. F. LaVia and R. B. Hill, Jr., pp. 9–95. Oxford University Press, New York, London, and Toronto.
39. Duvall, A. J., Sutherland, C. R., and Rhodes, V. T. (1969): Ultrastructural changes in the cochlear duct following mechanical disruption of the organ of Corti. *Ann. Otol. Rhinol. Laryngol.*, 78:342–357.
40. Bohne, B. A. (1972): Location of small cochlear lesions by phase contrast microscopy prior to thin sectioning. *Laryngoscope*, 82:1–16.
41. Bohne, B. A. Unpublished data.
42. Fex, J. (1967): Calcium action at an inhibitory synapse. *Nature*, 213:1233–1234.
43. Kuijpers, W. (1969): *Cation Transport and Cochlear Function*. Ph.D. thesis, Nijmegen University, The Netherlands.
44. Trump, B. F., and Ginn, F. L. (1969): The pathogenesis of subcellular reaction to lethal injury. In: *Methods and Achievements in Experimental Pathology*, Vol. 4, edited by E. Bajusz and G. Jasmin, pp. 1–29. Yearbook Medical Publishers, Chicago, Ill.
45. Lawrence, M. (1971): Blood flow through the basilar membrane capillaries. *Acta Otolaryngol. (Stockh.)*, 71:106–114.
46. Costa, O., and Brånemark, P.-I. (1970): Vital microscopic evaluation of the microvessels of the cochlea. *Adv. Microcirc.*, 3:96–107.
47. Jordan, V. M., Pinheiro, M. L., Chiba, K., and Jimenez, A. (1973): Postmortem changes in surface preparations of the cochlea. *Ann. Otol. Rhinol. Laryngol.*, 82:111–125.

DISCUSSION

J. Durrant: Have you observed any degradation to Reissner's membrane and/or the stria vascularis?

B. Bohne: No, neither with Reissner's membrane nor the stria vascularis, at least not at the levels I've generally used. However, we have seen in almost 100% of the animals exposed to one particular noise, an area of stria that was missing; it was not in a standard location and it had very little relation to the damage in the organ of Corti. This was an exposure that lasted for 9 days. It was almost uniform in its production of strial loss, and I mean total atrophy, such that there was a thin layer of epithelium separating spiral ligament from the endolymphatic space.

H. Spoendlin: For very high-intensity exposures, occasionally we find tears in Reissner's membrane, and in our experience it was only in those cases where Reissner's membrane was ruptured that we also found strial changes.

We were not able to find strial changes as described by Ward and Duvall (23).

K. Hynson: With regard to your comment about leakage of endolymph to the cells that apparently had not been directly affected by the noise exposure itself, would you expect the resultant cellular rupture and prolonged degeneration process to be extensive enough to eventually lead to a permanent increase in the threshold and, furthermore, how do you account for the presumed recovery of thresholds during this same time?

B. Bohne: First of all, there are exposures that produce only temporary threshold shift so you don't have that much cellular loss, but in areas where the damage is great enough to open up holes in the reticular lamina and to the organ of Corti, then the degeneration spreads, and that's why the longer you wait after exposure, the bigger the lesion is. Now, the part about recovery—you're right—is hard to explain. With compound threshold shift some of the cells that are affected only slightly by the noise become more affected by the ionic change, so that compounds the problem. If there were some way to stop the leak, perhaps the cells would recover, but since there is no way, they go on to degenerate.

R. Price: There is a parallel in the case of impulse noise: i.e., there is a growth of TTS over a period of several hours after exposure. During this time sensory cell lesions have been shown to be increasing in extent.

J. Hawkins: I do agree with Dr. Bohne about the proposition that endolymph is a poison to the organ of Corti, as it probably causes a serious upset in the microhomeostasis of the cochlea. It is absolutely essential that these 2 fluids, both important, be kept in their proper places.

Effects of Noise on Hearing, edited by Donald Henderson,
Roger P. Hamernik, Darshan S. Dosanjh, and John H. Mills.
Raven Press, New York © 1976

Anatomical Changes Following Various Noise Exposures

H. Spoendlin

Department of Otolaryngology, University of Zurich, Zurich, Switzerland

In order to study the structural alterations due to acoustic stimulation, an
easy and reliable technique is needed which allows a quantitative evaluation
of all parts of the cochlea, including the spiral ganglion and the stria vascularis at the light- and the electron-microscopic level in any animal. Preparation artifacts due to the dissection of the cochlea must be avoided if the
immediate effects of sound on the cochlear ultrastructure are to be studied.
Easy documentation at every step is essential.

Our block-surface technique meets all these requirements (Fig. 1) (1):
fixation and embedding is accomplished by a gentle perfusion of the whole
cochlea through carefully opened windows using a low-viscosity epoxy resin
(Spurr), which easily penetrates the cochlear tissues. After polymerization,
the block containing the whole cochlea is divided into halves by a mid-

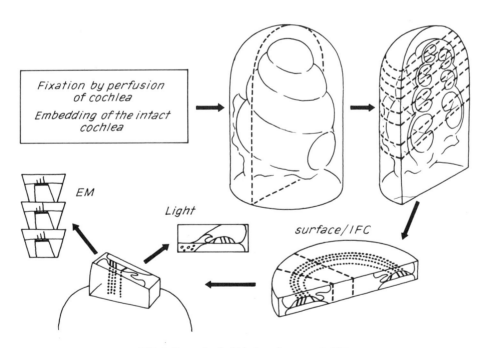

FIG. 1. The method of block-surface preparation.

modiolar cut, using a 0.1-mm-thick circular saw. Under the preparation microscope, the cochlear half-turns are cut out in the form of small disks, which are then arranged in the order of the cochlear turns (Fig. 2). In these small disks the organ of Corti and the osseous spiral lamina can be directly examined in a surface view, preferably with interference contrast of Nomarsky, which allows a recognition of all structural details throughout the entire thickness of the preparation. Thus, a quantitative assessment of practically the entire cochlea is possible. The findings can be represented schematically in a cochleogram that is the exact image of the original preparation (Fig. 2). The loss of sensory cells due to the preparation is less than 5% of the entire sensory cell population. Any selected area can now be further sectioned at any desired angle for light- and electron-microscopic examination.

In the present study, 240 guinea pigs and 5 cats were exposed to different types of wide- and narrow-band stimuli for exposure times of 30 sec to 1 week. The animals were sacrificed either immediately after the exposure, or after survival times of up to 1 year; their cochleae were prepared according to the block-surface technique. The spectrum of the wide-band noise had a fairly even frequency distribution between 500 and 8,000 Hz; the narrow-band noise had a bandwidth of one-third octave. For short sound exposures

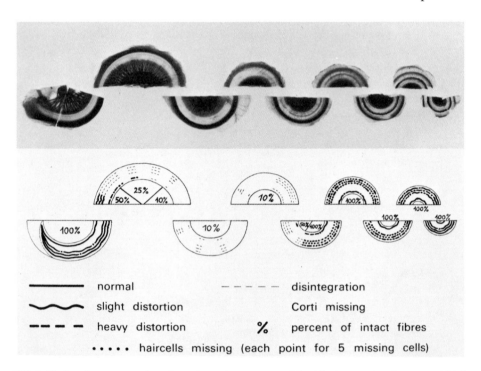

FIG. 2. Block-surface preparation of a guinea pig ear exposed for 10 min to an impulse noise of 12.5 msec 140 dB and a survival time of 3 months. Top: Original outlay. Bottom: Corresponding cochleogram with the different types of structural alterations.

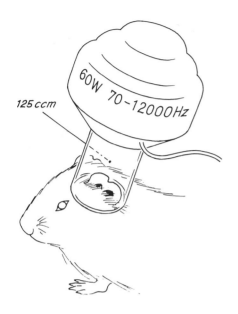

FIG. 3. Method of monaural acoustic overstimulation.

up to 1 hr, the guinea pigs were either kept awake in a small glass cylinder directly attached to the loudspeaker or, for better control of the exposure conditions, the animals were anesthetized with ketamine and the loudspeaker was adapted to 1 ear only by means of a small plastic tube (Fig. 3). For longer exposures of more than 1 hr, a larger metal container was used in which the animals were free to move around. The animal's hearing was roughly tested before and immediately after exposure and prior to sacrifice by means of the Preyer reflex.

MECHANISMS OF COCHLEAR DAMAGE

Primary structural damage, as seen immediately following relatively short acoustic overstimulation, gives valuable information on the mechanism of acoustic damage to the cochlea (2). Such immediate structural alterations are regularly found with exposure intensities above 125 dB; the severity of the damage increases with increasing sound intensity. The damage is most pronounced in the center of the main area of damage, and it decreases in the marginal zones.

The mildest changes which appear immediately after very short exposures of 30 sec are slight distortions of the outer hair cells, which take on an irregular shape instead of the normally regular cylindrical shape (Fig. 4). The next step is characterized by a regularly observed outward bending and occasional fusion of the sensory hairs of the inner hair cells (Fig. 5). The strict outward direction of the bending might reflect the stimulation mechanism of the inner hair cells, which, in fact, has been proposed to be a fluid flow out-

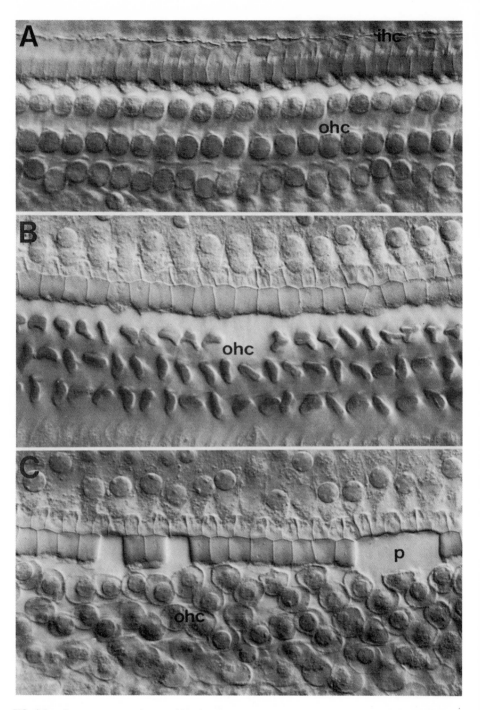

FIG. 4. Interference contrast pictures of block-surface preparations. A: a normal organ of Corti with regular cylindrical outer hair cells (ohc) and the normal sensory hairs of the inner hair cells (ihc). B: A light distortion of the outer hair cells (ohc) as the first degree of immediate acoustic traumatic alterations. C: Heavy distortion of the organ of Corti with swollen outer hair cells (ohc) and many missing pillar heads (p).

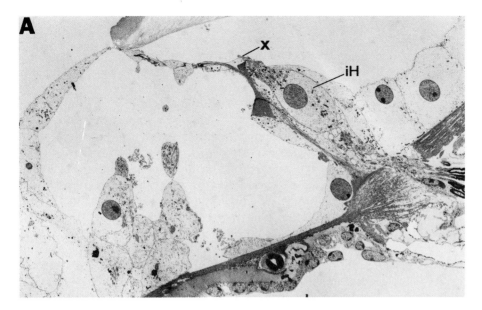

FIG. 5. Organ of Corti of the lower basal turn of a guinea pig 1 year after an overstimulation with 140 dB white noise for 20 min. Complete loss of outer hair cells. Supporting structures and inner hair cells (iH) essentially intact. Outward bending of the sensory hairs of the inner hair cell (x) as an irreversible damage. No appreciable retrograde degeneration.

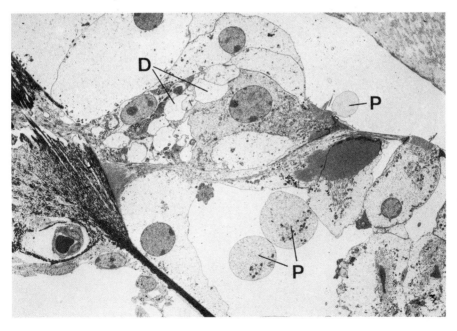

FIG. 6. Organ of Corti from the marginal damage zone of a guinea pig cochlea exposed to 1 hr 130 dB white noise. The great swelling of the afferent dendrites and endings (D) associated with the inner hair cells is clearly visible. Cytoplasmic protrusions at the surface and in the tunnel (P).

ward from the inner sulcus (4). Frequently, the afferent nerve fibers and their endings below the inner hair cells are greatly swollen and, occasionally, have even burst. Similar dendrite alterations are also found after ischemia of the inner ear. These dendrites appear to be a most sensitive structure to different kinds of influences (5). (Fig. 6). The efferent fibers and the afferent fibers to the outer hair cells remain essentially intact even when the outer hair cells are severely damaged and are degenerating. There is frequently an increased density of the synaptic vesicles in the efferent endings sometimes associated with the delayed appearance of some myelin figures, possibly as the structural manifestation of a functional activation (2) (Fig. 7).

Closer to the center of the main damage area, heavy distortion of the entire organ of Corti is found. The outer hair cells are swollen and their cytoplasmic contents are in great disorder. Many pillar heads are ruptured and cytoplasmic protrusions appear at the surface of the organ of Corti and in the tunnel. The tympanic lamina is shaken off the basilar membrane and accumulates in certain places as huge cell clusters (2,6,7).

In the area of maximal damage, the organ of Corti is frequently found in

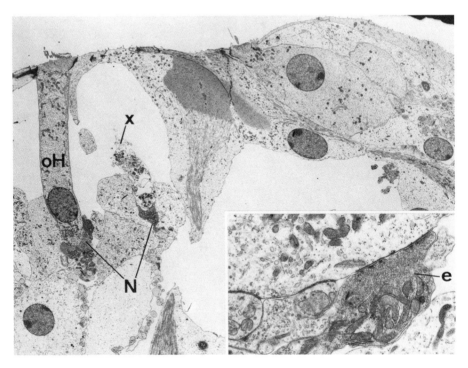

FIG. 7. Organ of Corti of the basal turn of a guinea pig after 1 week exposure to 110 dB white noise. Occasionally, scattered outer hair cells degenerate (x) among entirely normal-looking outer hair cells (oH). In spite of the degeneration of the hair cell the nerve endings remain essentially intact (N). *Inset:* Some of the efferent endings (e) have an increased density of synaptic vesicles.

complete disintegration with multiple ruptures of the reticular lamina and disconnection of the whole organ from the basilar membrane. Particularly weak points seem to exist along the lateral attachment of the reticular membrane at the Hensen cells, as described by Beagly (8), at the pillar heads and medial to the inner hair cell cuticule (2). Frequently, the whole organ of Corti is swept away from the basilar membrane, which eventually becomes completely bare with only the spiral vessel and the tectorial membrane remaining (Fig. 8). With exposure intensities of 140 dB and more, ruptures

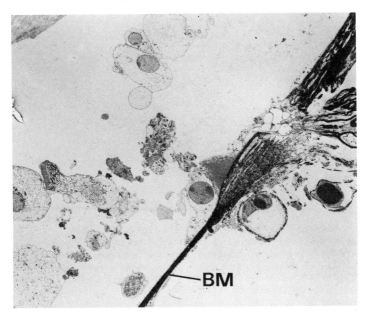

FIG. 8. Center of the damage area in the upper basal turn of a guinea pig cochlea immediately after a 5-min exposure to 140 dB white noise. All cellular elements of the organ of Corti are entirely disrupted and disconnected from the basilar membrane (BM).

of Reissner's membrane might occur, but we were never able to find perforations or tears in the basilar membrane as described by Voldrich (6).

In contrast to the findings of Duvall et al. (9), significant structural changes in the stria were never observed with any exposures, neither immediately after the exposure nor 1 day later, nor after any survival period up to 1 year (Fig. 9). Stria alterations were found only when the Reissner's membrane was ruptured.

A quite different type of alteration is found after longer exposure to sound pressure level (SPL) below 120 dB. There appears an increased number of swollen nuclei of outer hair cells mainly in the first row (3). After a certain delay, single outer hair cells degenerate amidst entirely normal cells, scat-

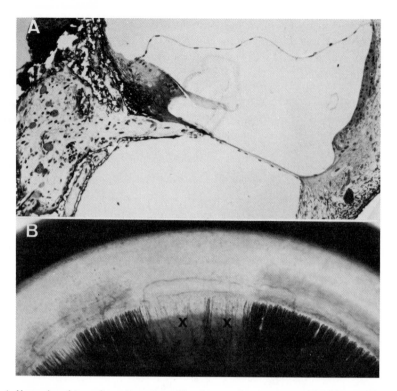

FIG. 9. A: Upper basal turn of a guinea pig cochlea 1 year after exposure of 2 × 20 min 140 dB white noise. Completely missing organ of Corti with a basilar membrane covered by 1 epithelial layer. The tectorial membrane remains. Retrograde degeneration of the cochlear neurons has greatly reduced the spiral ganglion cells, but about 10% of the neurons survive. The stria vascularis looks essentially normal. B: Spotty degeneration of the organ of Corti and the nerve fibers of the same animal in the lower basal turn. Substantial retrograde degeneration of the cochlear neurons occurs only in areas where the inner hair cells are missing (x).

tered over large distances. The primary changes are always confined to the sensory cells, which become swollen and show vacuolization of the cytoplasm and mitochondrial degeneration. Finally, the sensory cells degenerate completely, whereas the nerve endings still remain intact at this stage (Fig. 7). Such scattered degeneration also occurs spontaneously to a much smaller degree in normal animals. Therefore, a normally occurring process is merely enhanced by acoustic overstimulation.

The fact that we find, immediately after a 30-sec exposure, extensive membrane ruptures, or the organ of Corti entirely torn off the basilar membrane with the dislocation and loss of tympanic lamina cells, is clear evidence for a direct mechanical damaging effect of the acoustic overstimulation. On the other hand, swelling of dendrites and cytoplasmic changes in the outer hair cells, as a delayed phenomenon leading either to scattered degeneration of the hair cells or an accumulation of lysosomes, are probably the consequence of metabolic exhaustion or metabolic stress. Bending and fusion of sensory hairs is not necessarily the consequence of a mechanical effect, since such hairs are also found after intoxication (10) and genetic disturbances (11).

In conclusion, we must assume that, at high intensities above 125 dB, direct mechanical destructions and metabolic exhaustion are competing factors in acoustic damage to the cochlea. For lower intensities, metabolic effects are certainly predominant, and detectable structural alterations appear only as a secondary manifestation of the metabolic disturbance.

In all our animals exposed to intensities between 100 and 120 dB, the Preyer reflex was completely abolished after the exposure, but usually recovered within a few days. We were never able to find any significant ultrastructural changes as a morphological substrate of the temporary threshold shift (TTS). We must assume that the TTS is due to a reversible mild metabolic disturbance with no visible structural manifestations. The only delayed manifestation of chronically repeated TTS might, perhaps, be the accumulation of lysosomal inclusions in the hair cells as a visible but late unspecific sign of enhanced metabolic activity in the hair cells (12,13).

EVOLUTION OF STRUCTURAL CHANGES

The primary alterations evolve in the postexposure time to reach the final permanent status of damage only after a long period of time, probably about 2 months. In areas of disintegration of the organ of Corti, the whole organ disappears and only the bare basilar membrane remains covered by a single layer of flat epithelial cells, the spiral vessel and the tectorial membrane (Fig. 9). Areas of severe distortion finally appear as a collapsed group of supporting cells with entirely missing hair cells, or with only the inner hair cells left.

Slight distortion of the outer hair cells does not necessarily induce degeneration, but it seems to have a poor tendency to recover, since such distorted outer hair cells can still be found 3 months after the damaging exposure. The typical sensory hair distortions at the inner hair cells appear to be permanent with no chance to recover, but with no other effect on the sensory cell. One year after the exposure we can still find such distorted sensory hairs on otherwise entirely normal-looking inner hair cells (Fig. 5). Such permanent sensory hair alterations presumably have important functional bearings on the excitation mechanism of the hair cell.

The swelling of afferent dendrites at the inner hair cell level, the increased number of swollen outer hair cell nuclei, and the alteration in the efferent nerve endings at the outer hair cells are no longer found following postexposure times of 1 week or more, which indicates that these alterations are reversible (2).

Retrograde degeneration of the cochlear neurons is induced by the loss of inner hair cells or, more precisely, by irreversible damage to the afferent dendrites associated with the inner hair cells, which represent about 95% of all cochlear neurons (14). However, even in cases of total disappearance of the organ of Corti, throughout the cochlea retrograde degeneration is never complete, always leaving at least 10% of the neurons in an apparently healthy state (15) (Figs. 2 and 9). The loss of the outer hair cells has little effect on the retrograde degeneration of the afferent cochlear neurons, but they induce, contrary to the classical opinion (16), retrograde degeneration of the efferent fibers to a certain extent.

Quantitative evaluation of block-surface preparations was based on 2 parameters, believed to be the best indications of the degree of cochlear damage, and their extent on the basilar membrane measured: (i) the area of entirely missing and disintegrated organ of Corti associated with permanent total hair cell loss, and (ii) the total area of distortion, which usually leads only to a partial permanent hair cell loss of predominantly outer hair cells (Fig. 2).

DAMAGE LOCALIZATION

With white noise exposures, the main damage area is, as is well known, regularly situated in the upper basal and lower second turn (Fig. 10). With increasing exposures, the damage zones spread equally basalward and apicalward. It must be noted that this well-defined damage localization is also found immediately after very short exposures of 30 sec (Fig. 10), which cer-

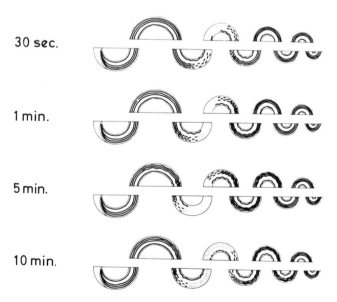

FIG. 10. Cochleograms of examples of cochleae exposed to 140 dB white noise with different exposure times.

tainly indicates that the determining factors for this localization are the mechanical properties of the cochlea, most probably the maximum volume displacement in this region. Other proposed causes, such as a poor vascular supply or a special mechanical susceptibility of this area, are very unlikely.

Occasionally, exceptions to this rule occur, for which, so far, no explanation can be given. In 2 out of 8 animals with a 1-week exposure to 110 dB of white noise, we found an isolated circumscribed lesion in the hook area with no, or only very weak, damage at the typical site in the upper basal turn (Fig. 7). Delayed permanent damage appears frequently to be less homogeneous than the primary alterations, with spotty defects and islands of preserved hair cells mainly in the marginal zones of the primary damage (Fig. 9B).

Narrow-band exposures with center frequencies from 250 to 8,000 Hz lead to tonotopical localization of the damage area (Fig. 11) (17). Surprisingly, however, the greatest damage was produced with bands in the lower and mid-frequency range when the same overall SPL was used for all frequency bands. More pronounced damage with higher frequency bands was observed only when the same intensity per hertz (dB/Hz) was given, i.e., 140 dB overall SPL at 250 Hz-thirdband corresponds to 152 dB at a 4,000 Hz-thirdband.

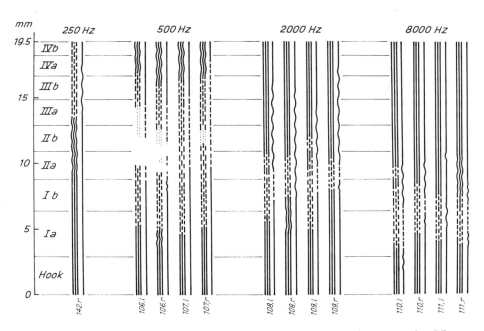

FIG. 11. Schematic representation of groups of cochleograms of guinea pig cochleae exposed to different narrow-band noises (140 dB, 5 min). The damaged areas are shown with the same signatures as in Fig. 2. The damage shows a clear tonotopical localization, more pronounced with a narrow-band noise, ~ 500 Hz, than with higher frequency bands.

INDIVIDUAL VARIABILITY OF DAMAGE

For continuous noise exposures with well-controlled parameters, the reproducibility of the extent of damage appeared to be satisfactory (Figs. 12 and 16). It is better for higher exposure intensities, especially if it is related to the area of heavy immediate mechanical damage such as a missing or disintegrated organ of Corti. The permanent delayed damage shows a greater spread of individual variations, probably because individual metabolic factors play an important role in the evolution of the primary alterations. A much greater variability of damage extent is found after impulse noise exposures, so that the damage for given exposure parameters is hardly predictable (Fig. 13).

After exposures in the free field with the animals awake, 1 ear was often much more damaged than the other, probably because the animal was able to protect 1 ear to a certain extent. This phenomenon of great differences in the damage of both ears was less pronounced with longer exposures to lower intensities, where the animal became adapted to the noise environment.

The susceptibility to acoustic traumatic inner ear damage probably varies among different species. Thus, we obtained, with the same exposures, clearly

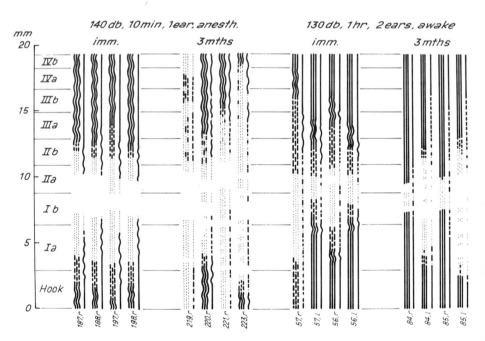

FIG. 12. Groups of cochleograms of guinea pig cochleae exposed to continuous white noise. The extent of immediate structural damage in monaural exposures and anesthesia is fairly constant. Delayed damage shows greater variations in extent. Binaural exposures of awake animals produce frequently great differences between both ears of the same animal.

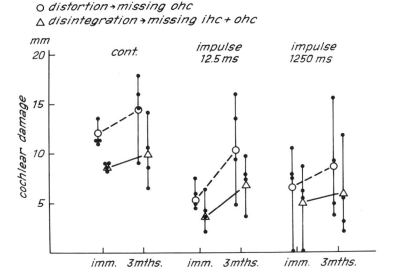

FIG. 13. Relation between immediate and late permanent damage in a guinea pig cochlea exposed to different types of white noise (140 dB, 10 min). There is a much greater variability in the late damage for the areas of distortion and for the areas of disintegration.

less damage in the cat than in the guinea pig. According to the findings of Ward and Duvall in 1971 (18), it would also appear that chinchillas are more susceptible than guinea pigs, as they obtained, with 123 dB, a similar damage we produced with only 130 dB in guinea pigs.

INTENSITY–TIME RELATIONS IN CONTINUOUS NOISE EXPOSURES

No simple relation seems to exist between exposure intensity levels and extent of structural damage. Short exposures up to 5 min produce very little damage at 130 dB, and very extensive damage at 140 dB (Fig. 14). At 120 dB, only mild immediate structural changes, predominantly of the metabolic type with consecutive hair cell loss, are found. One week of 110-dB continuous exposure is needed to produce very restricted, just-detectable changes. After relatively short exposures below 130 dB, no immediate structural changes of the mechanical type are found, whereas such changes occur regularly with rapidly increasing extent in intensities above 130 dB. It would appear that 130 dB is a critical intensity above which direct and immediate mechanical alterations occur with great regularity without much individual variation, and below which primary structural damage is exceptional. Below 130 dB metabolic delayed effects are predominant with great differences among individuals. Thus, with respect to the effects of acoustic trauma, 3 zones of intensity can be delineated (Fig. 15): up to about 90 dB, the critical intensity level, practically no damage is produced. From 90 to 130 dB,

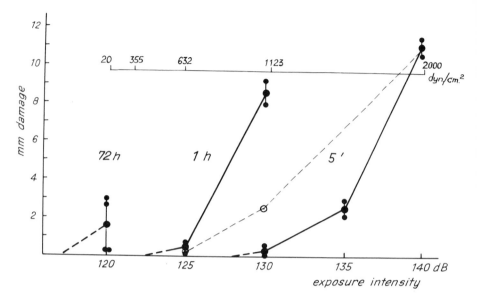

FIG. 14. Diagram representing the relationship between the extent of cochlear damage, total area of distortion and disintegration, to the exposure intensity at constant exposure times. Above a certain critical level the damage curves rise very steeply. Below the intensity of 130 dB practically no immediate damage is observed after relatively short exposure times. The interrupted line shows the damage extent of a 5-min exposure related to a linear SPL scale (upper inset scale, dyn/cm²).

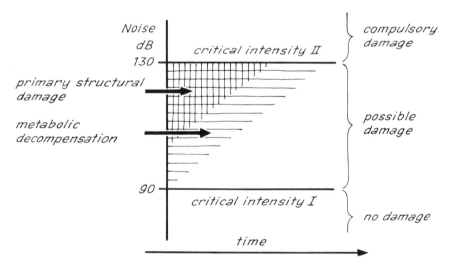

FIG. 15. Diagram representing the zones of sound intensity with respect to the acoustic traumatic effect. Up to 70–90 dB (critical intensity I) no damage is to be expected. Between 90 and 140 dB, metabolic de-compensation occurs increasingly and even primary structural damage might appear to a minor extent. In this intensity zone the organ of Corti may or may not be damaged and the exposure time is probably an important factor. Above the critical intensity of about 130 dB, there is always heavy structural irreversible damage of a direct mechanical type even after very short continuous exposures.

permanent acoustic traumatic damage, mainly of the metabolic type, may occur to a varying extent. Above 130 dB, severe irreversible structural damage is unavoidable. This critical level of 130 dB probably corresponds to an amplitude of basilar membrane movement on the order of 500 Å as extrapolated from Mössbauer measurements of basilar membrane amplitudes. It is, in fact, very surprising that such dramatic mechanical alterations are produced by such small amplitudes.

Damage of the metabolic type in the zone below 130 dB affects mainly the outer hair cells, whereas the inner hair cells frequently remain intact. According to the findings of Ward and Duvall (18) and Henderson et al. (19,20), the selective complete loss of outer hair cells does not seem to affect appreciably the threshold of hearing in experimental animals. This leaves us with the puzzling question about the functional role of the outer hair cells.

For intensities above 130 dB, very short exposure times are needed to produce heavy immediate damage. With longer exposure times, however, the damage extent does not increase in linear proportion to the exposure time. There seems to be a characteristic relation between the extent of immediate structural damage and different exposure times at a constant exposure intensity (Fig. 16). For 140 dB the curve flattens out to an almost

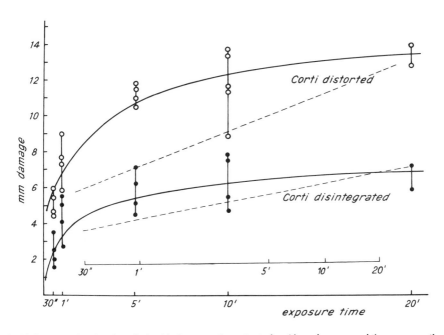

FIG. 16. Diagram showing the relationship between the extent of cochlear damage and the exposure time at constant intensity (140 dB). The upper curve relates to the entire area of distorted organ of Corti, whereas the lower curve relates to the area where the organ of Corti is entirely disintegrated or missing. After a very steep initial rising phase, the curve flattens out to become almost horizontal. If a logarithmic time scale is chosen (smaller inset scale), the curves become more or less straight (dashed lines).

horizontal course after a very short initial rising phase. Related to a logarithmic time scale, the curve becomes a straight line showing that structural damage increases as a linear function to the logarithm of time, as has been shown for asymptotic TTS. The lower the exposure intensity, the longer this initial rising phase becomes, where the time factor seems to be just as important as the intensity. For 140 dB, we found this rising phase to last about 10 min; for 130 dB, it extends over 1 hr; and for 120 dB, there was no tendency to level out for exposure times up to 72 hr. The principle of equal energy might be valid for this initial rising phase, very short for high intensities, and increasing to very long periods of time, probably on the order of years, for lower intensities. This phenomenon may clarify the reason why the hearing of workers who are exposed over years to the same noise does not deteriorate further after a certain number of years.

IMPULSE NOISE

Impulse noise certainly comes closest to the actual noise emissions to which we are exposed in modern life. The naturally occurring impulse noises are, however, very complex and difficult to define physically. Speech, for example, can be considered as a sequence of very short inhomogeneous impulses. The damage due to speech of the same average or peak intensity and duration as a continuous white noise is usually greater than the damage produced by the continuous noise. A complex stimulus such as speech, however, cannot be used to study the influences of different parameters of impulse noise as, for instance, impulse duration or rise time. For this purpose, we studied the effect of relatively long and simple wide-band impulses with well-defined and controlled parameters.

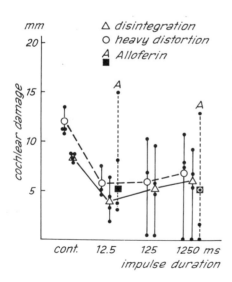

FIG. 17. Effect of different impulse durations on the extent of cochlear damage (140 dB, 10 min; impulse/interval = 1/1). The area of disintegration and the area of heavy distortion exhibit the same general pattern. Reproducibility is much better for continuous noise exposures, especially if the impulse durations are relatively long. The average damage and the great variability of damage is not changed very much by the elimination of the middle ear reflex with Alloferin.

In general, much greater variations of individual damage are found with impulse noise exposures. In some animals, no damage occurs, and in others, the damage is as extensive as that produced by a steady noise exposure, in spite of the much smaller total energy delivered (Fig. 17). The ratio of impulse level to interval has, as expected, an effect on the extent of damage; however, the many individual variations allow no precise prediction in the individual case (Fig. 18). Individual differences in the protective action of the middle ear muscle reflex do not seem to be responsible for the enormous damage variation, because the variability increases considerably after elimination of the middle ear reflex by a muscle relaxant (Alcuronium). If different impulse durations are delivered with an impulse–interval ratio of 1:1, the total delivered energy is always the same, but the average cochlear damage is less pronounced with very short impulse durations. In animals exposed to impulse noise under slight general anesthesia with ketamine, much greater damage was found than in animals exposed while awake. In the awake state, the whole animal would jerk with each impulse, which might considerably alter the exposure conditions and diminish the actual energy delivered to the ears. On the other hand, we cannot exclude an influence of the ketamine anesthesia on the acoustic middle ear reflex, which would help to explain the increased damage produced under general anesthesia. If measured under ketamine anesthesia, the protective action of the middle ear muscle reflex against acoustic trauma does not seem to be very significant. The average damage with or without middle ear reflex appears to be about the same (Fig. 17).

In a further series of experiments with impulse noise, we used rise times

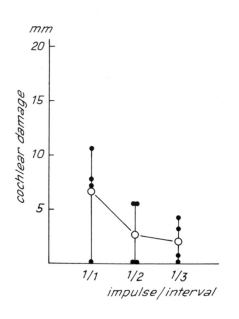

FIG. 18. The influence of the impulse–interval ratio on the extent of cochlear damage is difficult to estimate because of the great variability of the damage from impulse noise (140 dB).

varying from 25 to 250 msec. The most unexpected effect was a significant increase of damage with short rise times up to about 100 msec, as compared to the damage produced by square impulses (Fig. 19). This phenomenon can be observed with different impulse durations and impulse–interval ratios. Even with very slow rise times of 250 msec and very short peak SPL-duration damage is reduced only a little, although the total energy delivered is much smaller than with square impulses of equal peak level and duration. The structural alterations were highly diminished only when the peak level was not always reached in triangular-shaped impulses with slow rise times (Fig. 19).

It is difficult to explain the greater damaging effect of impulses with gradual rise times, in contrast to rectangular impulses. It is possible that more energy is lost in the middle ear conduction with rectangular impulses, which produce an abrupt intensification of sound energy, than with the gradual increments of energy created by trapezoidal impulses. The phenomenon is certainly related to the time constant of the ear.

The present quantitative structural analysis of acoustic traumatic cochlear damage allows the following conclusions: above a critical intensity of ~130 dB SPL, direct mechanical irreversible destructions occur regularly, whereas below 130 dB, partially reversible metabolic effects with delayed structural alterations seem to be predominant.

Exposure time and intensity do not seem to be equally responsible for structural damage. At high SPL exposure, intensity is more important for the

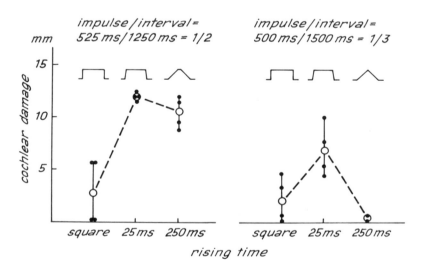

FIG. 19. Diagram showing the influence of the impulse rise time on the extent of cochlear damage. Short but gradual rise times clearly enhance the traumatic effect of the impulse noise as long as the peak level is reached, which probably is not always the case in triangular-shaped impulses (140 dB, 10 min).

determination of cochlear damage than exposure time, except for a short initial period where the time factor appears to be equally important. This initial period becomes increasingly longer with lower intensity levels.

Great variations of individual damage are found with impulse noise exposure. Gradual, but short, rise times of the impulses appear to enhance rather than reduce the damaging effect of impulse noise. Damage risks are difficult to predict for impulse noise, but they can be considerably higher when compared with the same total energy in steady noise.

REFERENCES

1. Spoendlin, H., and Brun, J. P. (1974): The block-surface technique for evaluation of cochlear pathology. *Arch. Otorhinolaryngol., 208*:137–145.
2. Spoendlin, H. (1971): Primary structural changes in the organ of Corti after acoustic overstimulation. *Acta Otolaryngol. (Stockh.), 71*:166.
3. Beck, Ch. (1956): Reaktionen der Kerne der äusseren Haarzellen beim Meerschweinchen auf adäquate Reize. *Arch. Otorhinolaryngol. (NY), 170*:81.
4. Dallos, P. (1973): Cochlear potentials and cochlear mechanics. In: *Basic Mechanisms in Hearing,* edited by Aage R. Møller, pp. 335–376. Academic Press, London.
5. Spoendlin, H. (1969): Das ischämische Syndrom des Innenohres. *ORL, 31*:257.
6. Voldrich, L. (1972): Experimental acoustic trauma. Part I. *Acta Otolaryngol. (Stockh.), 74*:392–397.
7. Werner, F. Cl. (1973): Experimentelle Schallwirkung und sekundäre Veränderungen in der Cochlea des Meerschweinchens. In: *Funktion und Therapie des Innenohres,* edited by Jakobi-Lotz, pp. 41–44. HNO-Heilkunde, Johann Ambrosius Barth, Leipzig.
8. Beagley, H. A. (1965): Acoustic trauma in the guinea pig. II. Electron microscopy. Including the morphology of cell junctions in the organ of Corti. *Acta Otolaryngol. (Stockh.), 60*:479.
9. Duvall, A. J., Ward, W. D., and Lauhala, K. E. (1974): Stria ultrastructure and vessel transport in acoustic trauma. *Ann. Otol. Rhinol. Laryngol., 83*:498–514.
10. Duvall, A. J., and Wersäll, J. (1964): Site of action of streptomycin upon inner ear sensory cells. *Acta Otolaryngol. (Stockh.), 57*:581.
11. Ernston, S. (1972): Cochlear morphology in a strain of the waltzing guinea pig. *Acta Otolaryngol. (Stockh.), 71*:469.
12. Spoendlin, H. (1970): Atlas of ultrastructure of the peripheral nervous system and sensory organs. In: *Normal and Pathological Anatomy,* edited by J. Babel, A. Bischoff, and H. Spoendlin, pp. 232–250. Thieme, Stuttgart.
13. Lim, D. J., and Melnick, W. (1971): Acoustic damage of the cochlea. *Arch. Otolaryngol., 94*:294–305.
14. Spoendlin, H. (1972): Innervation densities of the cochlea. *Acta Otolaryngol. (Stockh.), 73*:235.
15. Spoendlin, H., and Brun, J. P. (1973): Relation of structural damage to exposure time and intensity in acoustic trauma. *Acta Otolaryngol., 75*:220–226.
16. Fernandez, C. (1960): Innervation of the cochlea in relation to hearing loss. *Laryngoscope, 70*:363.
17. Stockwell, Ch. W., Ades, H. W., and Engström, H. (1969): Patterns of hair cell damage after intense auditory stimulation. *Ann. Otol. Rhinol. Laryngol., 78*:1144.
18. Ward, W. D., and Duvall, A. J. (1971): Behavioral and ultrastructural correlates of acoustic trauma. *Ann. Otol. Rhinol. Laryngol., 80*:1–16.
19. Henderson, D., Hamernik, R. P., and Sitler, R. (1974): Audiometric and anatomical correlates of impulse noise exposure. *Arch. Otolaryngol., 99*:62–66.
20. Hamernik, R. P., and Henderson, D. (1974): Impulse noise trauma. *Arch. Otolaryngol., 99*:118–121.

DISCUSSION

J. Tonndorf (to H. Spoendlin): I thoroughly agree with you, and I think almost everybody does, that there ought to be at least 2 mechanisms involved in the ultimate loss of sensory cells: 1 of a metabolic nature and 1 of a mechanically destructive nature. However, what looked odd to me was that you had these 2 mechanisms tied together by a continuous function of intensity. If you have 2 such mechanisms, you should have a discontinuity in the middle, which may be smoothed over, but nevertheless, there should be a discontinuity. Now, one way of smoothing over these functions is, if there are more than 2, perhaps 3 or 4 different components, I'd like to suggest that there may be destructive mechanisms that might be akin to metal fatigue or, perhaps something like the homogenation of the cell contents, which would be intermediate between the two extremes you have proposed, and this would tend to smooth out the curve.

H. Spoendlin: It is certainly possible that more than 2 mechanisms are involved.

R. Price: We have CM data which agree very well with what Dr. Tonndorf has said. We see a growth of loss in the CM which is linear in log time; this function changes rather suddenly at some intensity into a growth which is linear in time, which would imply a second mechanism of injury.

E. Evans: I would like clarification of your point where you claim that since 30 sec of noise exposure produces anatomical changes, these changes are, therefore, not of metabolic origin. How long was it between the noise exposure and the death of the animal and the preparation of the cochlea?

H. Spoendlin: The decapitation of the animal was done within a few seconds after the exposure and the cochleae were fixed within 2 min. You might still have some metabolic component of degeneration taking place in these 2 min, but, in practice, that's not at all what you see following the short-duration, high-level type of exposure. At least for the very severe destruction, essential metabolic factors probably can be excluded.

R. Smith: Dr. Spoendlin, you mention the bending of the inner hair cell stereocilia away from the tectorial membrane. Do you find that in the normal animals, the hairs do make contact with the tectorial membrane?

H. Spoendlin: I would say no; at least not in the way the stereocilia of the OHCs do. I've never seen the imprints of the IHC hairs on the lower surface of the tectorial membrane.

P. Stopp: In following on with Ted Evans' question, how much time do you allow before sacrificing the animal? Have you ever extended it a day or so?

H. Spoendlin: Our animals were sacrificed immediately, 1 day, 2 days, 3 days, etc. after exposure. I did show the time evolution that the sensory cell changes take; i.e., initial distortion of OHC leads eventually to degeneration of the cell in a few days.

J. Winslow: Dr. Spoendlin, did you find the characteristic radial bend of the stereocilia on outer hair cells also?

H. Spoendlin: Yes, but much rarer. Occasionally I found a fusion of the OHC stereocilia, as Bohne has shown, but not as consistently as with the hairs of the IHC. This is quite surprising.

W. Ward: I'm worried by Dr. Spoendlin's reviving the ghost of the critical intensity. I thought maybe we had gotten rid of that thing for all time. I say this because if there is a critical intensity, we are going to have even more problems trying to make a single damage risk standard that encompasses exposures from 75 or 80 dB up to impulse noises of 160 dB or so. As far as I can see from the present evidence that's published, although I think the equal energy hypothesis is conservative at low intensities, by the time you get up to the range of intensities that we're considering here (above 120–125 dB), a total energy assessment would be at least on the safe side. Now, a critical intensity would deny this; it implies that if you get to this intensity, then increasing above that level, even if you shorten the exposure time markedly so that you actually decrease the total energy, you will get more effect. Now, do you have any real definite evidence that you really have such a discontinuity?

H. Spoendlin: For continuous white noise, 130 dB clearly seems to be the critical intensity range above which immediate mechanical damage is produced in the guinea pig independently of exposure duration. This, however, does not seem to be applicable to impulse noise, the effect of which depends on additional factors.

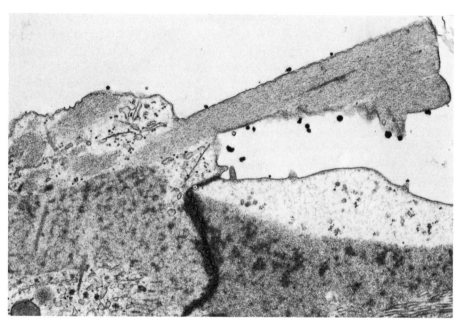

Editors' note: Figure shows outward bending fusion of sensory hairs of inner hair cell 4 days after 1-hr exposure to 130 dB white noise.

Effects of Noise on Hearing, edited by Donald Henderson, Roger P. Hamernik, Darshan S. Dosanjh, and John H. Mills. Raven Press, New York © 1976

Patterns of Sensorineural Degeneration in Human Ears Exposed to Noise

Joseph E. Hawkins, Jr. and Lars-Göran Johnsson

Kresge Hearing Research Institute and Department of Otorhinolaryngology, University of Michigan Medical School, Ann Arbor, Michigan 48104

Almost all of the human inner ears that we have examined, even those of teenagers, show some degree of degeneration of hair cells and nerve fibers in the lower basal turn of the cochlea. This loss of sensory and neural elements appears to be the result of a process that begins in childhood or even in infancy (1). As the degeneration ascends along the length of the basal turn, it produces the most common type of gradually progressive impairment of hearing with age, sensorineural presbycusis.

Many cochleae, particularly those of adult male patients, also show an area of degeneration that is confined largely to the second quadrant of the basal turn, i.e., the region between 9 and 13 mm. Such patients usually have a history of exposure to intense noise, whether in industrial employment, in hunting or other recreational pursuits, or in military service. Audiograms, when available, indicate a more or less severe permanent threshold shift for frequencies in the neighborhood of 4 kHz. Several cases of this type were reported in the early literature by Habermann (2,3), Brühl (4), Zange (5), and later by Crowe et al. (6), although the latter authors did not make specific mention of noise as a factor in causing the pathology that they described. A useful summary of those studies is given by Rüedi and Furrer (7). More recent descriptions of cochlear pathology caused by noise exposure are to be found in reports by Igarashi et al. (8) and Bredberg (9).

With the exception of Bredberg's material, all of the temporal bones of noise-exposed patients have been studied by the classical method of bright-field examination of stained serial sections from celloidin-embedded specimens. Unfortunately, even when precautions are taken to minimize post-mortem autolysis, that method has serious limitations for the evaluation of pathological changes in the organ of Corti and in the cochlear nerve fibers and minute blood vessels (10). The method of microdissection and phase-contrast examination of surface preparations (11,12), on the other hand, gives instructive views of the pattern of distribution of the hair cells and nerve fibers at low magnification, and permits a complete counting of the hair cells and mapping of any lesions in the form of a cytocochleogram.

CASE MATERIAL

The cases reported here were chosen from our collection of more than 200 pairs of human temporal bones, most of which were obtained at autopsy in the University of Michigan Hospital, the Ann Arbor Veterans Administration Hospital, or other associated institutions. In response to a questionnaire routinely sent to the next of kin, information indicating a history of vocational and/or recreational noise exposure was obtained in about 30 cases. In 20 pairs of bones from this group of patients the pattern of circumscribed degeneration in the basal turn of the cochlea was easily recognized. Cochleae from 8 other patients with characteristic dips in their audiograms and a history of noise exposure did not differ markedly from specimens obtained from patients in the same age group who had no such history. Another 5 pairs of bones were classified as representing patients who had probably been exposed to noise, because they showed the characteristic pattern of sensorineural degeneration, even though we were unsuccessful in eliciting information about their owners' history. For 10 cases good clinical audiograms were available, taken 1 to 3 years before death.

It is worth noting that all of these 33 pairs of bones were obtained from male patients. Taking affirmative action, we finally found, after diligent search, 1 pair of bones from a female patient with a circumscribed loss of nerve fibers in the basal turn of the left cochlea. The next of kin, however, denied that this patient had been exposed to noise. Thus, the group remains exclusively unregenerately male. Many of the patients had worked in the automotive or other noisy industries in the Detroit, Michigan area, and a number of them had also been exposed to the gunfire of hunting and target shooting. Four of the cases will be presented here.

METHOD

The temporal bones were prepared by our standard method (12), i.e., fixation with a 4% solution of buffered paraformaldehyde, and later staining for approximately 5 min by replacing the fixative with a 1% solution of osmium tetroxide (Millonig). In some instances, fixation and staining were carried out simultaneously by perfusing the perilymphatic space with Zetterqvist's buffered OsO_4 solution. The bones were then brought up to 70% alcohol, and the otic capsule was carefully removed after it had been thinned by means of mastoid and dental burrs. The cochlea was photographed under the dissecting microscope (Wild-Heerbrugg M-5), and, later, the entire length of the osseous and membranous spiral lamina was removed piecemeal (cf. Fig. 5). Cut into smaller fragments, it was mounted on glass slides in reagent-grade glycerol for microscopic examination with phase-contrast optics.

A complete count of missing hair cells was made, from one end of the basilar membrane to the other, on the basis of a yes-or-no decision as to the presence or absence of each cell, without attempting to make judgments about possible changes short of complete disappearance. Curves indicating the percentages of hair cells present in terms of an "ideal" pattern of 3 outer rows and a single inner row were then plotted, millimeter by millimeter, in the form of a cytocochleogram for the entire ear. Incomplete fourth and fifth rows were not taken into consideration. Because of the well-known irregularities of the outer hair cell pattern in the apical turn (10), the apparent reduction in the number of outer hair cells present, which was seen beyond the 30-mm point in all of the ears, should probably be regarded as normal.

OBSERVATIONS

The first case is that of GT, a 24-year-old man who died of a testicular carcinoma which had metastasized to the liver and lungs. He had worked for 6 months in noisy surroundings as a press operator, and had served in the U.S. Army for more than 5 years as a tank driver in Okinawa and Vietnam. The audiogram taken at bedside showed a typical 4-kHz dip of 70 dB in both ears. Three small, distinct areas of complete absence of the organ of Corti are seen in the second quadrant of the basal turn of the left cochlea (Fig. 1), giving the appearance of patchy degeneration similar to that described by Crowe et al. (6). The lesion appears to be relatively recent, since the areas of nerve degeneration are not sharply defined. They correspond, however, to the circumscribed portions of the basilar membrane where the organ of Corti has completely disappeared. The right ear does not display any similar area of nerve degeneration, except near the cecum vestibulare.

The second patient, EP, 72 years old, had not been exposed to industrial noise, but was described as an enthusiastic hunter. The asymmetry of the degeneration seen in his left and right ears (Figs. 2 and 3) gives a striking illustration of the protective effect of the acoustic shadow of the head for the right ear of a person shooting right-handed, i.e., from the right shoulder (13,14). The left ear shows an almost complete absence of organ of Corti and nerve fibers in the second quadrant. In the first quadrant the pattern of degeneration is more diffuse, and the presence of scattered nerve fibers is well correlated with the survival of supporting elements of the organ of Corti. At the beginning of the third quadrant there is a small island of supporting cells, also with a few remaining nerve fibers.

In the shadow-protected right ear the injury is much less. Only one small area of complete absence of sensory and neural elements is seen at the beginning of the third quadrant. There appears to be some thinning-out of the nerve pattern in the upper portion of the first quadrant.

Cytocochleograms for these 2 ears are shown in Fig. 4. The difference in the extent and severity of the lesions in the basal turn is striking. Hair cells are largely absent from the first 14 mm of the left cochlea, but only from the first 3 mm of the right. There is a second area, between 10 and 15 mm, of severe loss of outer hair cells from the right cochlea. Above the 15-mm

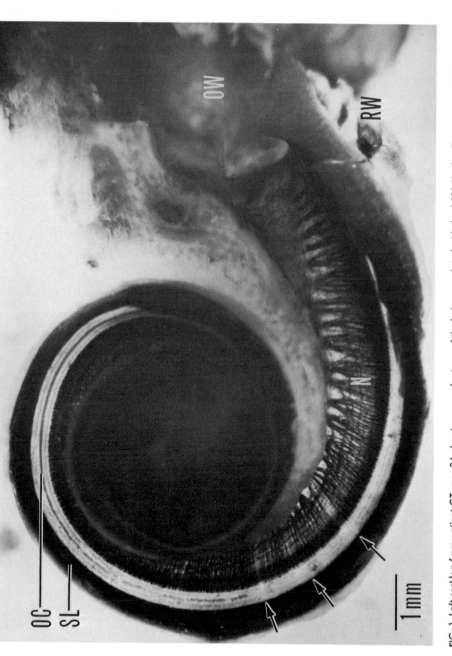

FIG. 1. Left cochlea from patient GT, age 24, showing an early stage of the lesion associated with the 4,000-Hz dip. The arrows at 9–11 mm indicate 3 narrow areas of complete degeneration of the organ of Corti (OC) and corresponding degeneration of nerve fibers (N) in the osseous lamina. SL, spiral ligament; OW, oval window; RW, site of round window.

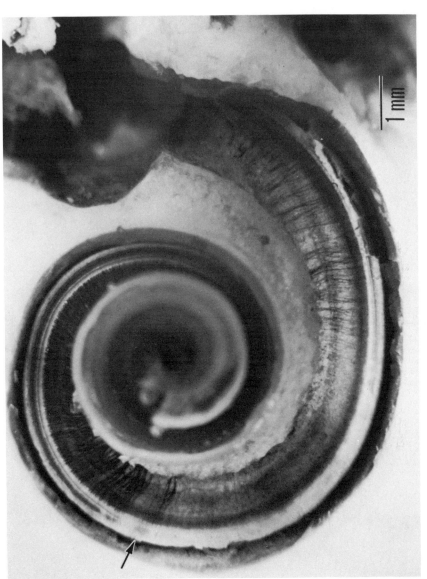

FIG. 2. Left cochlea from patient EP, a hunter, age 72, showing extensive loss of the organ of Corti and hair cells, especially in the second quadrant. The arrow (at 13 mm) shows a small surviving patch of supporting cells and nerve fibers. Similar sparsely innervated patches are seen in the first quadrant.

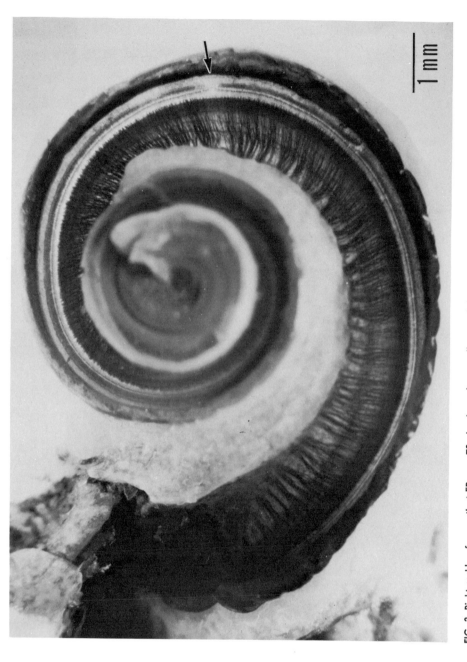

FIG. 3. Right cochlea from patient EP, age 72, showing only a small area of degeneration of organ of Corti and nerve fibers at about 13 mm (arrow). For a hunter shooting from the right shoulder, the right ear is partially protected by the sound shadow of the head.

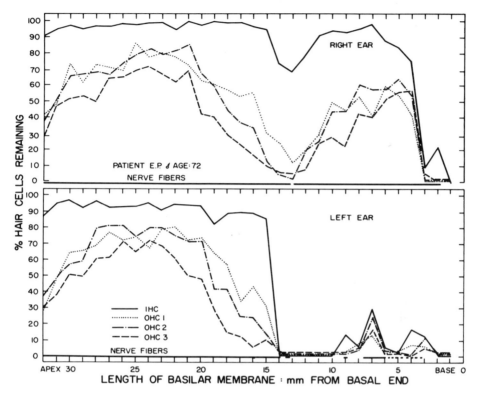

FIG. 4. Cytocochleograms for the 2 ears of patient EP, a hunter, showing the percentages of hair cells remaining per millimeter of length of the basilar membrane, measured from the cecum vestibulare. Separate curves represent the single row of inner hair cells and the 3 rows of outer hair cells. Incomplete fourth and fifth rows in the upper turns are disregarded. The falling-off of the outer hair cell curves near the apex probably represents the normal irregularity of the pattern in the apical turn (see Methods). The asymmetry of the loss below 15 mm reflects the protection, especially for higher frequencies, afforded the right ear by the sound shadow of the head. The black horizontal bar below each cytocochleogram indicates the presence of a population of nerve fibers in the osseous spiral lamina.

point the patterns of hair cell loss in the 2 ears are almost identical, indicating that the head shadow was effective only for the higher frequencies (15). To judge by the right cochlea, there appears to be surprisingly little hair cell loss, i.e., only 3 mm of the basal turn, that can be attributed to presbycusic changes, in spite of the patient's advanced age.

The third case is illustrated in Fig. 5, which shows the osseous and membranous spiral lamina after it had been dissected out of the left cochlea of a 25-year-old patient, RS. This man had not been exposed to industrial noise, but was reported to have used guns regularly, both 16-gauge shotgun and .22-caliber rifle, shooting right-handed. The pattern is obviously different from that of the first 2 cases, since the loss of hair cells and nerve fibers is confined almost entirely to the first 10 mm of the basal turn. The few bundles

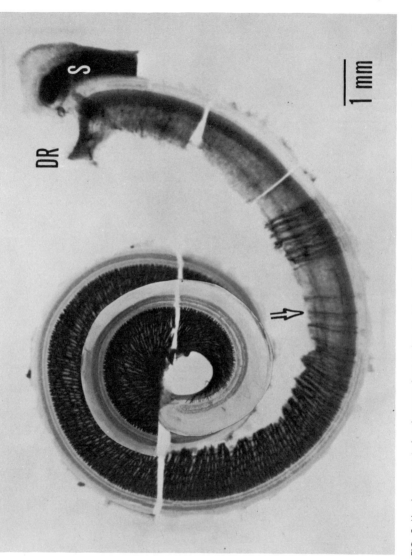

FIG. 5. Membranous spiral and osseous lamina dissected from the left cochlea of RS, age 25, a hunter, showing extensive loss of organ of Corti and myelinated nerve fibers from the first quadrant. Note the surviving nerve fibers at and below the arrow and even near the cecum vestibulare, wherever small patches of supporting cells and hair cells persist. DR, ductus reuniens; S, stria vascularis. (Reprinted with permission from *The Annals of Otology, Rhinology and Laryngology,* 83:294–303, 1974.)

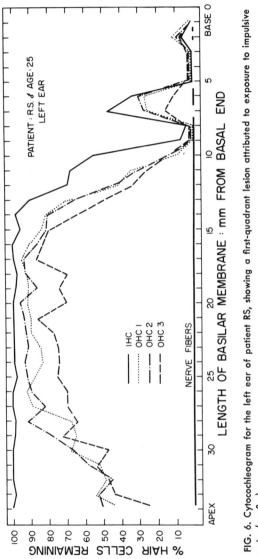

FIG. 6. Cytocochleogram for the left ear of patient RS, showing a first-quadrant lesion attributed to exposure to impulsive noise (gunfire).

of nerve fibers correspond to areas where the supporting structures of the organ of Corti and some of its hair cells remain. Again, the right ear, with the exception of the extreme basal portion, displayed a normal, dense nerve network. The cytocochleogram for the left ear is shown in Fig. 6.

The fourth case shows an almost complete loss of sensory and neural elements throughout the lower half of the basal turn (Fig. 7). The patient, GY, was 50 years old when he died. He had not been in military service, but we were told that he had worked on and off for 5 or 6 years in the pressroom of a factory making automobile bodies, and that he enjoyed hunting.

A knife-sharp transition is seen at 12 mm between the areas where neither nerve fibers nor organ of Corti can be seen and where both are present (Fig. 8). Figure 9 shows the appearance of the reticular lamina and hair cells in the fourth quadrant of the basal turn, well above the transition (at about 20 mm). In Fig. 9, the cytocochleograms for the 2 ears are remarkably symmetrical. An audiogram taken about a year before the patient's death indicates an abrupt hearing loss for frequencies above 2 kHz, with a maximum shift at 4 kHz of 80 and 90 dB in the respective ears (Fig. 10). The slight upturn at 8 kHz may have been the contribution of the tiny island of surviving organ of Corti and nerve fibers at 4 mm, although, by the time of the patient's death, no hair cells were to be seen there.

By way of contrast, a case of presbycusic degeneration is shown in Fig. 11. This female patient, CW, died of burns at the age of 92. The diffuse loss of organ of Corti and nerve fibers, especially from the first quadrant of the basal turn, is typical of sensorineural presbycusis in our series. There is also a small area of patchy degeneration at approximately 8 mm, apparently unrelated to noise exposure. With the thinning-out of the radial nerve-fiber bundles the pattern of the intralaminal spiral fibers (1) is nicely displayed. Unfortunately, no audiogram is available.

ANALYSIS

Although our series of cases of cochlear injury as a result of noise exposure includes only male patients, we would hardly be justified in inferring that female ears are somehow more resistant. It is reasonable to assume that economic, social, and cultural factors are involved, rather than a true sex difference in susceptibility. Women are somewhat less likely than men to have their ears exposed to intense occupational or recreational noise. When they are so exposed for many years, as in the Scottish jute-weaving industry, they can develop typical noise-induced permanent threshold shifts of respectable severity (16,17).

The four cases that we have presented illustrate the range of injury to the basal turn of the cochlea seen in patients known to have been exposed to industrial or impulsive noise. At one extreme we have the narrowly circumscribed areas of degeneration of sensory and neural elements in the left ear of

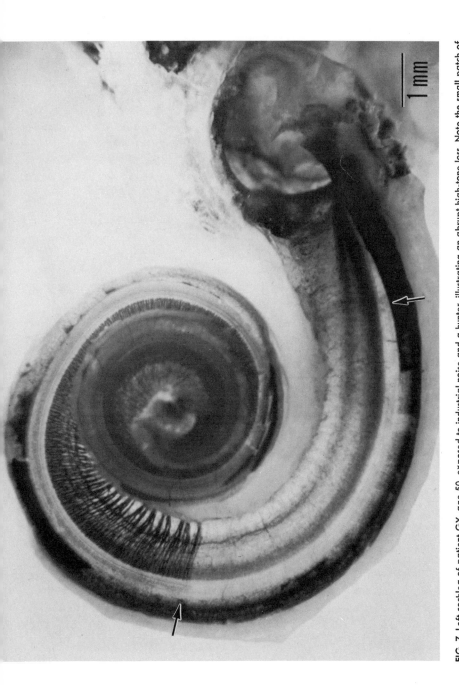

FIG. 7. Left cochlea of patient GY, age 50, exposed to industrial noise and a hunter, illustrating an abrupt high-tone loss. Note the small patch of surviving nerve fibers and supporting cells at 4 mm (lower arrow,) and the sharp transition (upper arrow) between complete degeneration and the normal-appearing pattern of nerve fibers and spiral organ. (Reprinted with permission from *The Annals of Otology, Rhinology and Laryngology,* 77:608–628, 1968.)

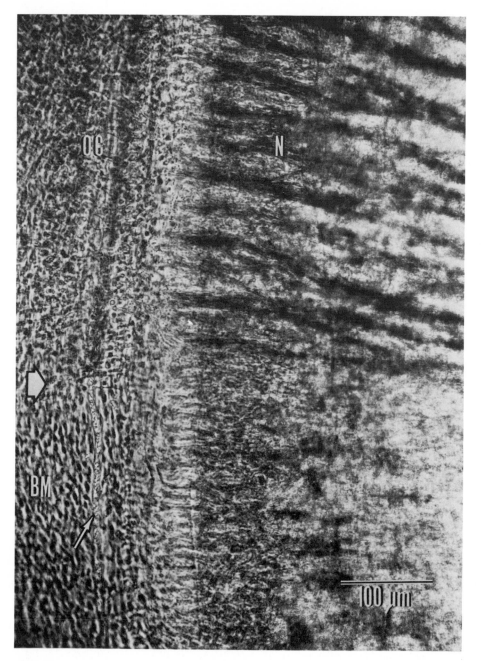

FIG. 8. Abrupt transition in the 12-mm region of the left cochlea of patient GY, age 50. The *broad arrow* marks the lower end of the surviving supporting structures of the organ of Corti (OC). Just above this point, the nerve fibers (N) are still present. Below it, the nerve channels of the osseous lamina are empty and the basilar membrane (BM) is covered by a simple epithelium, through which the outer spiral vessel (*lower arrow*) is visible.

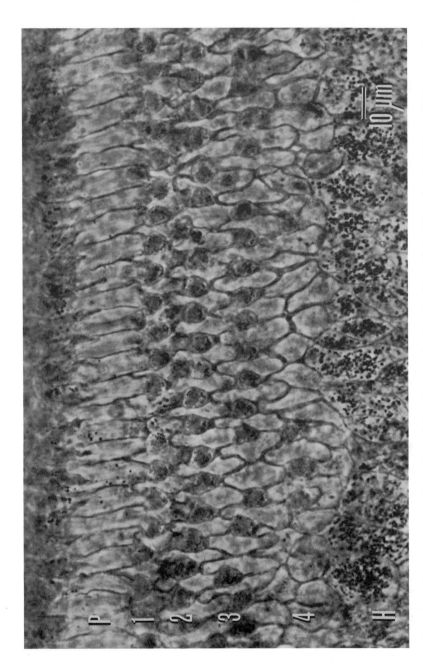

FIG. 9. Essentially normal pattern of outer hair cells from the upper basal turn (∼20 mm), left cochlea, of patient GY, age 50. Three outer hair cells are missing from the third row, and a few cells represent an incomplete fourth row. The inner hair cells are present, but not well displayed. P, pillar cells covering the tunnel; H, Hensen cells.

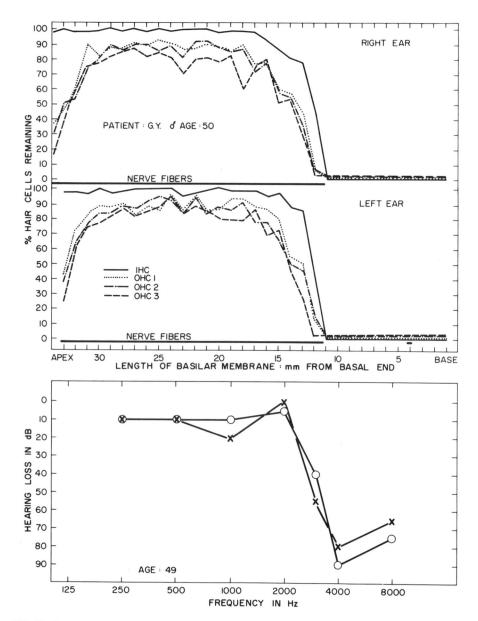

FIG. 10. Cytocochleograms for patient GY, with an audiogram taken 1 year earlier, showing the pattern of hair-cell and nerve-fiber degeneration and the symmetry of the abrupt high-tone loss. The placement of the logarithmic scale of frequencies for the audiogram with respect to the cytocochleograms is arbitrary, but agrees reasonably well with Guild's (6) diagram showing the localization of the upper frequencies along the basilar membrane.

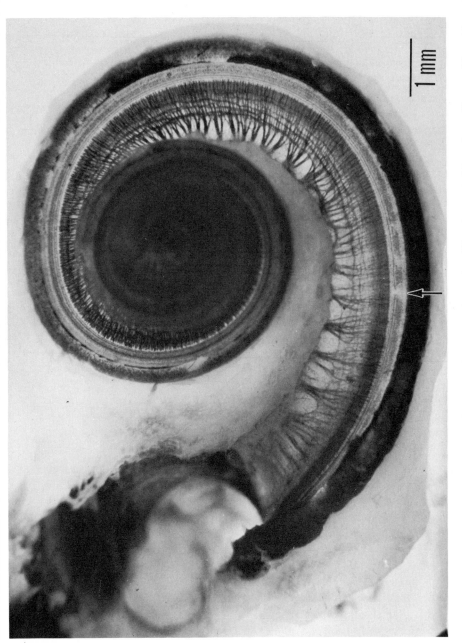

FIG. 11. Right cochlea of female patient CW, age 92, showing the pattern of somewhat diffuse, but graded, loss of nerve fibers, and the patchy degeneration of organ of Corti (arrow) that appears to be characteristic of sensorineural presbycusis.

GT (Fig. 1) and in the right ear of EP (Fig. 3); at the other, the widespread loss seen in the left ear of EP (Fig. 2), and the all but complete disappearance of the organ of Corti and its nerve fibers from the basal turn of both ears of GY (Figs. 7 and 10). When the findings in this group are contrasted with the diffuse sensorineural degeneration seen in the fifth case, CW (Fig. 11), it appears that the various patterns of degeneration caused by noise exposure can be differentiated from that of a typical sensorineural presbycusis.

The lesions seen in the left cochlea of GT, EP, and GY represent early and late stages in the development of the classic 4-kHz notch. For GT we have audiometric evidence of a narrow dip with a sharp maximum at 4 kHz. In GY, the upper limb of the curve has "broken away" (18), leaving an abrupt high-tone loss resembling that in several cases described by Crowe et al. (6).

The left ear of EP (Fig. 2) apparently represents a late transitional stage, with some supporting and neural elements remaining in the lower reaches of the basal turn, whence they have all but disappeared in the case of GY (Fig. 7). The pattern of degeneration in the left cochlea of EP resembles that in Bredberg's (9) case H107, a 71-year-old sawmill worker whose audiogram showed a broad noise-induced hearing loss for the higher frequencies, reaching a maximum of 70 dB at 2 kHz. Although it is regrettable that we have no audiogram for EP, we can surmise that the loss in his left ear would have followed the same curve as that of Bredberg's patient, despite the fact that its most likely cause was repeated exposure to the impulsive noise of gunfire, rather than the high-pitched scream of a power saw.

The chief difference between these 2 cases lies in the greater loss of nerve fibers from the first quadrant of EP's cochlea, seen also in the ear of RS (Fig. 5). In the latter, the lesion is largely confined to the first quadrant, and there is no loss of nerve fibers beyond 7 mm of the sort seen in GT, EP, and GY. Whether this type of first-quadrant loss is characteristic of the injury caused by gunfire remains to be established, but the sharp wave front of impulsive noise might be expected to set up a wave of high amplitude traveling for only a short distance and injuring hair cells and supporting structures in the first few millimeters of the spiral organ.

The early and late stages of the second-quadrant lesions associated with the 4,000-Hz dip are nicely illustrated in the ears of GT and EP, but they do little to further our understanding of the well-known susceptibility of this portion of the cochlea to injury by noise. We are inclined, however, to side with those who hold a "mechanistic" view of it as the locus of maximal acoustic stress along the length of the cochlear partition (19), possibly enhanced by the resonant properties of the external meatus (20). Nothing that we have observed in the density or arrangement of the microvasculature of the spiral ligament or stria vascularis of the 9–13 mm region would indicate that they are less generously supplied with blood than in other portions of the basal turn. It is true that the tributaries joining the outer spiral vessel at "T-junctions" become more and more widely spaced in the lower basal turn (21), but that fact seems hardly sufficient to characterize the area as a *locus minoris resistentiae* due to marginal or inadequate blood flow, as Crowe et al. (6) and other authors have postulated. Hinchcliffe (18) once seemed to imply that proximity to the oval and round windows might account for its vulnerability, since the basal portion of the cochlear partition is located between them in the direct path of vibratory motion from the stapes footplate to round-window membrane. This argument could apply to the *juxtafenestral lesion* so often seen in the so-called "hook" region, i.e., the first 2 mm of the basilar membrane (1,9), but we have regularly found that lesion even in patients who did not have a history of exposure to noise. It can hardly account for the *tonotopical lesion* of the 9–13 mm region corresponding to the 4,000-Hz dip, as should be clear from Fig. 1.

Crowe et al. (6) divided their 79 cases of impaired hearing for the higher frequencies into 2 groups, 1 with "gradual," the other with "abrupt" high-tone loss. Our cochlea from patient CW (Fig. 11) is not unlike their ear No. 12 from a 63-year-old woman, representing their group of patients with gradual high-tone loss. Their data for that cochlea indicate a gradually decreasing density of the nerve fiber pattern throughout the lower basal turn below ~15 mm. Such a pattern appears to be a common one in cases of sensorineural presbycusis. Our patient GY (Fig. 7), on the other hand, is a striking example of an abrupt high-tone loss, not unlike their case No. 69.

The remarkable symmetry of the audiograms and the patterns of degeneration of the 2 ears of GY (Fig. 10) may suggest to some readers the possibility of a genetically determined defect. The similarity to the left ear of EP, however, with the survival of the small patch of supporting cells and nerve fibers at 4 mm in the left cochlea, leads us to conclude that it was GY's known exposure to industrial noise and the sounds of gunfire rather than his heredity that was primarily responsible for his cochlear pathology and accompanying hearing loss. The sharp border of the lesion just above the 12-mm point underscores the dependence of the nerve fibers on the survival of the organ of Corti or its supporting structures. It also indicates that the radial nerve fibers, despite their multiple and seemingly irregular branching, must have a strict spatial arrangement.

A considerable period of time must be required for such complete degeneration of nerve fibers to occur throughout the basal turn. Abrupt transitions of this kind have not been seen in our monkeys kept for 1 month after noise exposure, even in those exposed to broadband noise (22). Some kanamycin- and neomycin-treated monkeys, however, have shown a transition from total absence of hair cells to a full complement within the space of 1 mm (23), thus meeting the criterion of Crowe et al. (6) for abrupt high-tone loss. By the time the animals were sacrificed, only a month or more after the end of treatment, the nerve fiber degeneration was far from complete in the area where all hair cells, inner as well as outer, had disappeared. Because the supporting structures remained intact, it appeared that they, in the absence of any inner hair cells, apparently determined the survival of the nerve fibers (24). How long those fibers might have continued to survive is an open question. On the other hand, in cats treated with gentamicin we have seen myelinated fibers persisting in the osseous lamina only where some of the inner hair cells were still present. Where the inner hair cells had disappeared, the nerve fibers also had degenerated, even though the outer hair cells and supporting cells were not affected (25). This observation is in accord with Spoendlin's findings in the cat and guinea pig (26), but it would appear that the retrograde degeneration of cochlear nerve fibers in primates may not follow precisely the same rules.

The method of microdissection and cytocochleographic evaluation reveals the patterns of sensorineural degeneration in noise-exposed ears with remarkable clarity. Our observations thus far suggest that there may be different patterns for impulsive and continuous noises, the former focused on the first quadrant of the basal turn, the latter on the second quadrant and characterized by the 4,000-Hz dip.

As Stacy Guild and his colleagues (6) insisted, the intelligent interpretation of audiological findings depends upon knowledge of the physiology and pathology of the cochlea. It follows that otopathological studies are most instructive when they can be correlated with the results of thorough audiological examinations. Bredberg's (9) and Schuknecht's (27) monographs show how every temporal bone for which such a correlation can be established acquires its own unique value. The difficulties and frustrations encountered in attempting to organize and carry out cooperative investigations of this kind, even on a modest scale, are hardly less than they must have been 40 years ago, but the need for the information to be gained from them is as great as ever.

SUMMARY

Patterns of degeneration of cochlear hair cells and myelinated nerve fibers are shown for 4 adult male patients known to have been exposed to either industrial noise or gunfire. In one young adult, a lesion restricted to the 9–13 mm region and showing relatively little nerve fiber degeneration was associated with a 4,000-Hz dip in the audiogram. An older hunter showed an extensive degeneration in the lower basal turn of the left cochlea, but little in the right, illustrating the effect of the acoustic shadow of the head in protecting the right ear against injury by the higher frequencies. In a second case exposure to gunfire had caused degeneration in the first quadrant of the left basal turn only. Thus the pattern of injury by impulsive noise may sometimes differ significantly from that produced in the second quadrant by continuous noise. In a case of industrial-noise exposure what apparently began as a 4,000-Hz lesion in the second quadrant had developed into a symmetrical abrupt high-tone loss when sensory and neural degeneration became almost complete throughout the lower basal turn in both ears. These findings are contrasted with those in a typical case of sensorineural presbycusis in an elderly female patient without a history of noise exposure, showing a somewhat diffuse, but graded, degeneration of nerve fibers in the basal turn.

ACKNOWLEDGMENT

This investigation was supported by grants from the Research Fund of the American Otological Society, Inc., and the John A. Hartford Foundation, and by USPHS Research Grant NS 05065 and Program Project Grant NS 05785.

REFERENCES

1. Johnsson, L-G., and Hawkins, J. E., Jr. (1972): Sensory and neural degeneration with aging, as seen in microdissections of the human inner ear. *Ann. Otol. Rhinol. Laryngol.*, 81:179–193.
2. Habermann, J. (1890): Über die Schwerhörigkeit der Kesselschmiede. *Arch. Ohrenheilkd.*, 30:1–25.
3. Habermann, J. (1906): Beitrag zur Lehre von der professionellen Schwerhörigkeit. *Arch. Ohrenheilkd.*, 69:106–130.
4. Brühl, G. (1906): Beiträge zur pathologischen Anatomie des Gehörorgans. *Z. Ohrenheilkd.*, 52:232–246.
5. Zange, J. (1911): Beitrag zur Pathologie der professionellen Schwerhörigkeit. *Arch. Ohrenheilkd.*, 86:167–174.
6. Crowe, S. J., Guild, S. R., and Polvogt, L. M. (1934): Observations on the pathology of high-tone deafness. *Johns Hopkins Med. J.*, 54:315–380.
7. Rüedi, L., and Furrer, W. (1947): *Das akustische Trauma*. Karger, Basel.
8. Igarashi, M., Schuknecht, H. F., and Myers, E. N. (1964): Cochlear pathology in humans with stimulation deafness. *J. Laryngol. Otol.*, 78:115–123.
9. Bredberg, G. (1968): Cellular pattern and nerve supply of the human organ of Corti. *Acta Otolaryngol. [Suppl.] (Stockh.)*, 236:1–135.
10. Johnsson, L-G., and Hawkins, J. E., Jr. (1967): A direct approach to cochlear anatomy and pathology in man. *Arch. Otolaryngol.*, 85:599–613.
11. Engström, H., Ades, H. W., and Andersson, A. (1966): *Structural Pattern of the Organ of Corti*. Almqvist and Wiksell, Stockholm.
12. Hawkins, J. E., Jr., and Johnsson, L-G. (1976): Microdissection and surface preparations of the inner ear. In: *Handbook of Auditory and Vestibular Research Methods*, edited by C. A. Smith and J. A. Vernon, pp. 5–52. Charles C Thomas, Springfield, Ill.
13. Kryter, K. D., and Garinther, G. R. (1965): Auditory effects of acoustic impulses from firearms. *Acta Otolaryngol. [Suppl.] (Stockh.)*, 211:1–22.
14. Taylor, G. D., and Williams, E. (1966): Acoustic trauma in the sports hunter. *Laryngoscope*, 76:863–879.
15. Keim, R. J. (1969): Sensorineural hearing loss associated with firearms. *Arch. Otolaryngol.*, 90:581–584.
16. Taylor, W., Pearson, J., Mair, A., and Burns, W. (1965): Study of noise and hearing in jute weaving. *J. Acoust. Soc. Am.*, 38:113–120.
17. Taylor, W., Pearson, J. C. G., Kell, R., and Mair, A. (1967): A pilot study of hearing loss and social handicap in female jute weavers. *Proc. R. Soc. Med.*, 60:1117–1121.
18. Hinchcliffe, R. (1967): Occupational noise-induced hearing loss. *Proc. R. Soc. Med.*, 60:1111–1117.
19. Schuknecht, H. F., and Tonndorf, J. (1960): Acoustic trauma of the cochlea from ear surgery. *Laryngoscope*, 70:479–505.
20. Wiener, F. M., and Ross, D. A. (1946): The pressure distribution in the auditory canal in a progressive sound field. *J. Acoust. Soc. Am.*, 18:401–408.

21. Johnsson, L-G., and Hawkins, J. E., Jr. (1972): Vascular changes in the human inner ear associated with aging. *Ann. Otol. Rhinol. Laryngol.*, 81:364–376.
22. Moody, D. B., Stebbins, W. C., Johnsson, L-G., and Hawkins, J. E., Jr. (1975): Noise-induced hearing loss in the monkey. (*this volume*).
23. Stebbins, W. C., Miller, J. M., Johnsson, L-G., and Hawkins, J. E., Jr. (1969): Ototoxic hearing loss and cochlear pathology in the monkey. *Ann. Otol. Rhinol. Laryngol.*, 78:1007–1025.
24. Johnsson, L-G. (1974): Sequence of degeneration of Corti's organ and its first-order neurons. *Ann. Otol. Rhinol. Laryngol.*, 83:294–303.
25. Hawkins, J. E., Jr., Johnsson, L-G., and Aran, J-M. (1969): Comparative tests of gentamicin ototoxicity. *J. Infect. Dis.*, 119:417–426.
26. Spoendlin, H. (1975): Retrograde degeneration of the cochlear nerve. *Acta Otolaryngol.*, 79:266–275.
27. Schuknecht, H. F. (1974): *Pathology of the Ear.* Harvard University Press, Cambridge, Mass.

DISCUSSION

W. Melnick: Dr. Hawkins, you showed, in one of your temporal bone slides, a complete absence of all nerves and sensory elements of the organ of Corti. The audiogram for that particular person showed a sharp 4-kHz notch with an improving slope to 8 kHz.

J. Hawkins, Jr.: That was an audiogram that had been taken a year before autopsy and, although there were not very many, there were some nerve fibers present in that region. Part of the problem was the person's noise exposure in that final year. I was trying to use that example to indicate that a certain amount of caution is necessary in interpreting such data, and the importance of trying to get a complete patient history from the next of kin as to noise exposure, both recreational and industrial.

As far as the connections to the inner hair cell stereocilia are concerned, I agree that the tympanic membrane connections are difficult to see, but we do occasionally see them in man, and Johnsson, in some of his preparations, sees inner hair cells clinging, not to the underside of the tympanic membrane, but to the fibers extending from Henson's stripe, and making contact with the cilia.

W. Melnick: Have you ever published those pictures?

J. Hawkins, Jr.: They have not been published yet. These connections are not very photogenic, but they ARE there.

Effects of Noise on Hearing, edited by Donald Henderson,
Roger P. Hamernik, Darshan S. Dosanjh, and John H. Mills.
Raven Press, New York © 1976

A Review of General Cochlear Biochemistry in Normal and Noise-Exposed Ears

Dennis G. Drescher

Laboratory of Neuro-otolaryngology, National Institute of Neurological and Communicative Disorders and Stroke, National Institutes of Health, Bethesda, Maryland 20014

The field of cochlear biochemistry is still in its infancy. However, micro-techniques are available (1–3) which allow quantitative biochemical investigations of cochlear function and dysfunction. It is the purpose of this review to examine selected studies in terms of the information they provide on possible biochemical mechanisms of the inner ear. The review material falls into 3 main categories: effects of noise on auditory behavior and on physiological parameters including cochlear potentials; biochemical studies on the cochlea, with some background biochemistry; and the possible effects of noise on cochlear biochemistry.

EFFECTS OF NOISE

Results of Behavioral Studies

Carder and Miller (4,5) and others (6–8) showed that when chinchillas and humans are exposed to continuous noise, their auditory thresholds reach an asymptote dependent on the level of exposure noise above some critical exposure level. If the noise is not too intense, normal auditory thresholds return after termination of the noise. In this chapter, the shift at asymptote is termed asymptotic temporary threshold shift (ATS). The ATS is, within a certain range of exposure levels, proportional to the level of the exposure noise (Fig. 1). Carder and Miller (5) showed by straight-line extrapolation that for chinchillas exposed to octave band noise with center frequency at 0.5 kHz, the expected maximum level for zero ATS is 65 dB SPL (sound pressure level) (Fig. 1). For exposure of chinchillas to octave band noise centered at 4 kHz, Mills (9) showed by extrapolation that the expected maximum level for zero ATS is 47 dB SPL. For high levels of noise, permanent threshold shifts (PTS) also occur (9) (Fig. 1). Thus, behavioral studies have suggested that, for noise of a specified band and for a given species, there is a range of "low" exposure levels for which there is little or no elevation of auditory thresholds, a range of "intermediate" levels for which com-

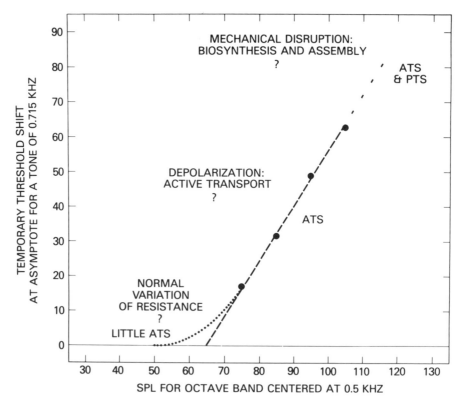

FIG. 1. Postulated molecular mechanisms for threshold shifts caused by continuous noise. The plot and data points are after H. M. Carder and J. D. Miller (5). Chinchillas were exposed to octave band noise with center frequency at 0.5 kHz for at least 2 days at levels designated by the abscissas. Thresholds at asymptote (ordinates) were determined for a test zone of 0.715 kHz. Dashed line shows one possible extrapolation of data points to zero asymptotic threshold shift (ATS), and dotted line shows another. "Low" exposure levels for this system are those producing little ATS below the dashed line intercept (65 dB SPL), "intermediate" levels are those causing ATS with complete recovery as observed by Carder and Miller, and "high" levels are those producing permanent threshold shift (PTS) as well as ATS (see text). Although no PTS was studied by Carder and Miller (thin dashed line), PTS occurs for sufficiently high exposure levels (9). The mechanisms listed for each range of levels are discussed in the text.

pletely reversible ATS occurs, and a range of "high" levels for which complete recovery to preexposure auditory thresholds does not occur.

Effects of Low Exposure Levels

What cochlear changes occur with exposure to sound at low levels resulting in little or no ATS? The mechanoelectrical theory of Davis (10) suggests that permeability changes occur when the resistance at the base of the cilia of the hair cells or in the cuticular membrane is varied by acoustic stimulation. Strelioff et al. (11) directly measured impedance changes between scala media and electrical ground in the guinea pig and found that the impedance followed the waveform of the acoustic stimulus, compatible with Davis' mechanoelectrical theory. Goldstein (12) studied the loss of fluorescein by hair cells as an indicator of changes in cellular permeability, and found that permeability increased for exposures to white noise at levels as low as 40 dB SPL. He concluded that permeability shifts are normal physiological functions of the hair cells. Changes in cochlear impedance and permeability may thus occur with low levels of sound (Fig. 1).

Effects of Intermediate Exposure Levels

Cochlear potentials are thought to reflect the functioning and state of the inner ear (13), and can be applied to the study of the reversible effects of noise at intermediate levels. Drescher (14,15) studied the change of cochlear microphonics (CM) with exposure of chinchillas to steady noise. The time course of noise-induced asymptotic reduction and recovery of CM is similar to the time course of change in behavioral auditory thresholds with noise (14–16). Noise-induced reduction of CM occurs only above a certain level of noise, as does ATS. Drescher and Eldredge (17) presented data supporting the idea that the minimum exposure level for reduction of CM can be estimated from the point of departure from linearity of the CM response. Reduction of CM by noise is hastened at high temperatures and retarded at low temperatures (14,15). Temperature-dependent biochemical or biophysical processes, such as division of cochlear energy reserves between active transport and general metabolism, or reversible alteration of cochlear membrane permeability, are suggested by these temperature studies. Even though intermediate levels of noise can cause minor hair cell loss (18), as well as changes of hair cell morphology (19), the reversible loss of auditory sensitivity in this range of levels must be caused by reversible processes, e.g., depolarization of hair cells during sound and active transport during the quiet (Fig. 1).

Effects of High Exposure Levels

At high levels of acoustic stimulation and with extended exposure, PTS becomes important (9) and cochlear potentials are lost irreversibly (20–22). Also at high levels, anatomical changes occur, including loss of cochlear elements (23–26). Biochemical repair processes may be important at levels of sound that cause disruption of cochlear structure (Fig. 1). Such biochemical processes include the biosynthesis of molecular components and assembly of membranes.

BIOCHEMISTRY: RELEASE OF ENERGY FROM CARBOHYDRATES

Chemical Energy

Cells of the cochlea obtain energy from carbohydrates such as glycogen and glucose, which they enzymically break down in steps, storing the energy

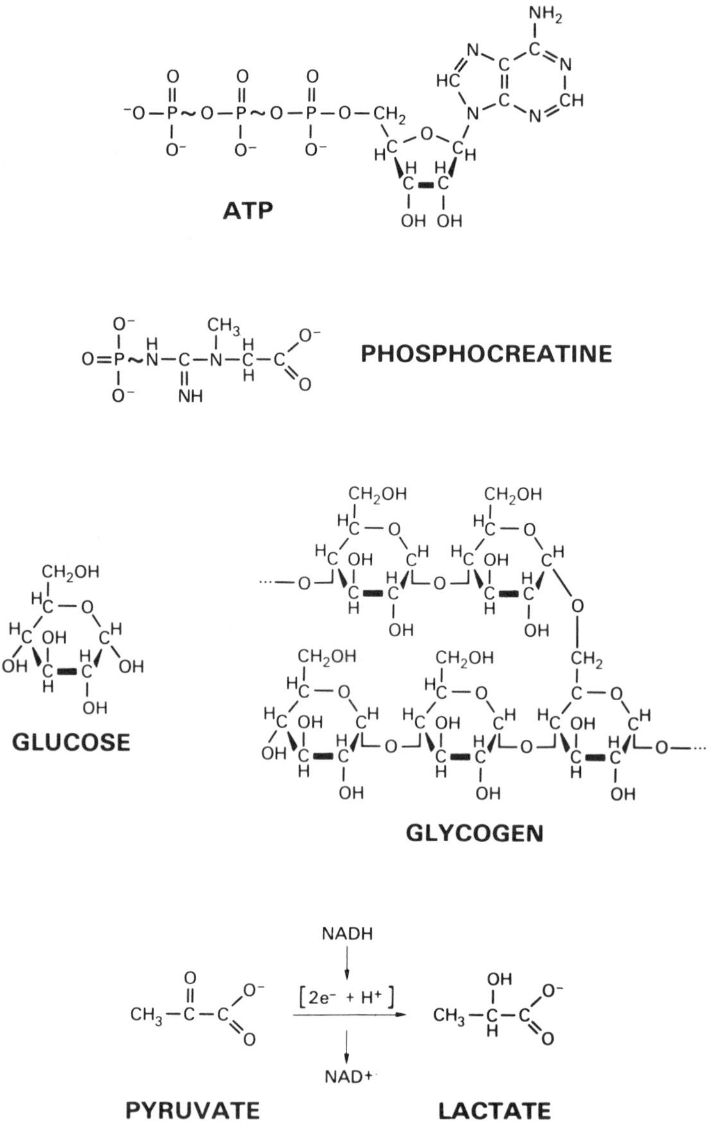

FIG. 2. Molecular structures relevant to cellular energy metabolism. Adenosine triphosphate (ATP) and phosphocreatine store chemical energy in high-energy phosphate bonds (∼). Glucose is degraded to smaller molecules, with transfer of energy in its chemical bonds to high-energy phosphate via glycolysis and the citrate cycle. Glucose can be stored as glycogen. The conversion of pyruvate to lactate is a reduction reaction of anaerobic glycolysis, producing the required oxidant NAD+.

released from the biochemical reactions in adenosine triphosphate (ATP) and phosphocreatine (Fig. 2). These molecules have been called high-energy phosphate compounds because the products of their hydrolysis are stabilized, and, owing to electrostatic repulsion, show little tendency to recombine.

Phosphocreatine serves as a reservoir of energy. The enzyme creatine phosphokinase catalyzes the reaction that interconverts phosphocreatine and ATP:

$$\text{phosphocreatine} + \text{ADP} \leftrightarrows \text{creatine} + \text{ATP}$$

Normally, the reaction favors the formation of ATP; therefore, if ATP supplies are exhausted, they are quickly replenished at the expense of phosphocreatine. The ATP molecule yields its energy as a reactant in a multitude of enzyme-catalyzed reactions. Such reactions include protein synthesis, lipid synthesis, synthesis of storage carbohydrates such as glycogen, and transport of ions against osmotic and electrical gradients.

Because chemical reactions that involve the participation of oxygen can yield large amounts of energy, oxygen is used by higher organisms in their metabolism. Any chemical reactant, including oxygen, that accepts electrons is called an oxidant. In the living cell, nicotinamide adenine dinucleotide in its reduced form (NADH; formerly, DPNH) provides electrons when it is oxidized, via several intervening reactions, by oxygen. In the oxidation of NADH to form oxidized NAD^+ and water, the released energy is stored in ATP. This process, called oxidative phosphorylation, takes place in the mitochondria, and yields 3 ATP molecules for every molecule of NADH oxidized. In the absence of oxygen, ATP can be produced from the sequence of reactions from glycogen through glucose to pyruvate, and on to lactate. This is termed glycolysis, and can occur in the cytoplasm of the living cell whether or not oxygen is available.

The reaction of pyruvate yielding lactate, catalyzed by the enzyme lactate dehydrogenase, results in oxidation of NADH to NAD^+ without formation of ATP (Fig. 2). The NAD^+ then provides more oxidant to maintain glycolysis. Lactate accumulates and is carried away by circulation. Without oxygen, 2 molecules of ATP are produced per molecule of glucose. Gluconeogenesis takes lactate back to glycogen by the reversal of most of the enzymic reactions that degrade glycogen in glycolysis. Thus, surplus carbohydrates can be stored in the cell. In the presence of oxygen, 38 ATP molecules can be produced per molecule of glucose (or 39 ATP per glucose unit from glycogen). Further details of carbohydrate metabolism and energy-yielding reactions can be found in several good texts (27–30).

Cochlear Metabolism

Most of the present knowledge about some of the intermediates of glycolysis and the citrate cycle, and activities of selected enzymes of carbohydrate metabolism in the cochlea is from the work of Matschinsky and Thalmann (31–35). These workers analyzed cochlear material using methods dependent upon the fluorescence of pyridine nucleotides (2,36). There was 3 times more glycogen and 10 times more glucose 6-phosphate in the organ of Corti than in the stria vascularis. From base to apex in the organ of Corti, glycogen increased (32) and phosphocreatine decreased (35). The activity of the glycolytic enzyme glycogen phosphorylase was 5 times higher in the organ of Corti than in the stria, and the citrate cycle enzymes, citrate synthase and malic dehydrogenase, were 2.5 times higher in the stria than in organ of Corti. The authors suggested that, although both organ of Corti and stria depend on aerobic metabolism, the organ of Corti appears to have more capacity for glycolysis than does the stria. However, enzymic activity alone cannot accurately reflect the quantities of enzymes present, since activity is dependent on the presence of activators and inhibitors, in an assay system and *in vivo*.

BIOCHEMISTRY: ENZYMES WITH SPECIAL FUNCTIONS

Adenosine Triphosphatase

Adenosine triphosphatase (ATPase), first described by Skou (37), is an enzyme that catalyzes the hydrolysis of adenosine triphosphate (ATP) to adenosine diphosphate (ADP) and inorganic phosphate. Activity of the isolated enzyme may depend on its association with membrane lipid (38). The ATPase is thought to be responsible for utilizing the energy released from ATP hydrolysis to transport ions against electrical or osmotic gradients or both (38). Such transport is called active transport, to distinguish it from passive transport, where ions are distributed according to their permeability through the membrane and the electrochemical gradient across the membrane (39).

There are 2 common kinds of ATPase activity, probably corresponding to 2 different enzymes (38), i.e., ATPase stimulated only by magnesium ions (Mg ATPase), and ATPase stimulated by sodium and potassium ions in the presence of magnesium ions (NaK ATPase). The NaK ATPase is inhibited by the cardiac glycoside ouabain, and activity due only to the NaK ATPase can be obtained by determining ATPase activity in the presence and absence of ouabain.

NaK ATPase activity has been found in the cochlea of the guinea pig by Iinuma (40) and Kuijpers et al. (41,42), and by Kuijpers et al. in the cochlea of both the rat (43) and chicken (41,42,44). There is ATPase activity in the mammalian stria vascularis and avian tegmentum vasculosum (41). Ouabain in the perilymph of scala vestibuli causes a depression of both the CM and the endocochlear potential (EP) (45). The CM and EP appear to depend on the high K^+/Na^+ ratio of endolymph (46). The NaK

ATPase of the cochlea may be important in maintaining the K^+ concentration in scala media. A reaction deposit ascribed to ATPase activity has been demonstrated histologically in the stria vascularis (47) and on the outer surface of the cells of the organ of Corti (48), where ATPase may maintain ion gradients. ATPase activity was not found along hair cell membranes in contact with the fluid of the tunnel of Corti.

Carbonic Anhydrase

Carbonic anhydrase catalyzes the hydration of carbon dioxide to form carbonic acid as follows:

$$CO_2 + H_2O \rightleftarrows H_2CO_3$$

Carbonic anhydrases are found in a wide variety of cells and tissues of the body (49,50), including K^+-secreting tissues such as the kidney, large intestine, and salivary glands (51). Erulkar and Maren (52) found carbonic anhydrase activity in the cochlear tissues of the cat. Tissues from the basal, middle, and apical turns had carbonic anhydrase of specific activity higher than that of whole blood, with the specific activity increasing apically. Acetazolamide, an inhibitor of carbonic anhydrase, caused endolymphatic K^+ to decrease to about one-fifth of control values. The authors concluded that cochlear carbonic anhydrase may play a part in the secretion of K^+ into the endolymph (52). In the kidney, carbonic anhydrase is thought to be important for the production of bicarbonate and H^+ ions, so that H^+ may be excreted into the urine and Na^+ may be reabsorbed by the kidney (53). Potassium ion competes with H^+ for the Na^+ exchange in the kidney. Acetazolamide produces a rise in carbon dioxide in the cells and metabolic acidosis, with increased loss of K^+ from cells into urine and diminished Na^+ resorption. In the cochlea, as stated previously, acetazolamide produces an increased loss of K^+ from endolymph.

Carbonic anhydrases have molecular weights of about 30,000 daltons; each molecule contains 1 atom of zinc, which is necessary for catalytic activity (49). Carbonic anhydrase exists in 2 isoenzyme forms in some tissues, 1 of high and 1 of low specific activity (51).

BIOCHEMISTRY: PROTEINS AND LIPIDS

Biological Membranes

Proteins and lipids are important to cochlear structure because they are the major components of biological membranes (54,55). Proteins are polymers of about 20 different L-α-amino acids, linked via their α-carboxyl and α-amino groups in the peptide bond (56,57). Lipids are molecules of biological origin, and are, as a rule, more soluble in organic solvents than in water. Polar lipids, such as phospholipids, and the sterol cholesterol, are found in biological membranes (27,55). Phospholipids alone can form bilayers consisting of 2 long rows of lipid molecules with nonpolar chains facing the inside of the bilayer and polar (phosphate) portions facing the outside (Fig. 3). The lipid bilayer is common to biological membranes (58),

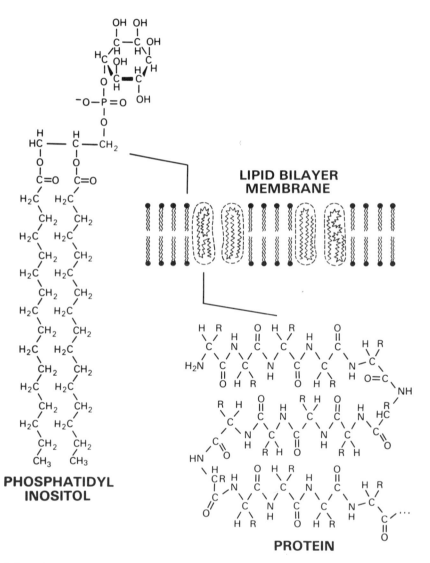

FIG. 3. Typical components of biological membranes. Polar lipids, such as the phospholipid phosphatidyl-inositol, can form lipid bilayers characteristic of membrane structure. Black dots represent polar head groups of the lipids, and pairs of wavy lines represent nonpolar "tails." Globular proteins, the zigzag traces bounded by dashed lines in the diagram, penetrate the lipid bilayer and may provide the membrane with pores and catalytic function. Part of the chain of amino acids constituting a globular protein is shown in the lower right-hand corner. Each R designates a side chain of a given amino acid.

with proteins partially or fully penetrating the bilayer (59). The biological membrane is probably not rigid, but fluid in the sense that proteins and lipids have rotational and translational freedom within the membrane (60).

Membrane Assembly

Membranes are formed from their component lipids and proteins without the aid of enzymes (61). This self-assembly is due to the attraction of the polar parts of the molecules to water and repulsion of the nonpolar parts from water and toward other nonpolar groups, causing the nonpolar portions to face the inside of the array. The component lipids and proteins are synthesized via enzymes.

Cochlear Proteins and Lipids

Little quantitative biochemistry has yet been applied to the isolation and characterization of proteins and lipids of the cochlea. The fractionation of some of the proteins of the whole cochlea of guinea pig is illustrated in the electrophoretic pattern in Fig. 4 (left). Here 30 to 40 bands are visible, resolved by discontinuous polyacrylamide gel electrophoresis (62). There are probably many more proteins present in concentrations too low to be visualized by staining, and still others with molecular weights too high to penetrate the gel.

Proteins are synthesized via messenger ribonucleic acid (mRNA). The synthesis of mRNA and other RNA species in the cochlea has been studied autoradiographically by Löbe (63), by injection of the labeled RNA precursor ^{3}H-uridine into the guinea pig. Löbe found that the stria vascularis, spiral limbus, tympanal lining cells, interdental cells, mesothelial cells of the scalae, and Reissner's membrane were intensely labeled. No labeling was detected in 35% of the outer hair cells and 24% of the inner hair cells. Localized labeling by ^{3}H-uridine may indicate regions of high protein turnover.

Glycoproteins, or mucopolysaccharides, are proteins bound to carbohydrates. Saito and Daly (64,65) studied mucopolysaccharides of the cochlea of the guinea pig. Using a turbidometric method for analysis of acid mucopolysaccharides and specific enzymes for cleaving the polysaccharide portions of the mucopolysaccharides, they determined the percentage of dry weight present as mucopolysaccharides to be about 0.1% for Reissner's membrane, 0.6% for stria vascularis, and 0.6% for the basilar membrane, organ of Corti, and spiral limbus combined. Lotz and Kuhl (66), employing column chromatographic techniques for purification, found the mucopolysaccharide content of cochlear tissue to be higher than that of muscle and connective tissue.

Scheibe et al. (67,68) separated cochlear lipids into major classes by thin-layer chromatography. Neutral lipids, phospholipids, and glycolipids of the

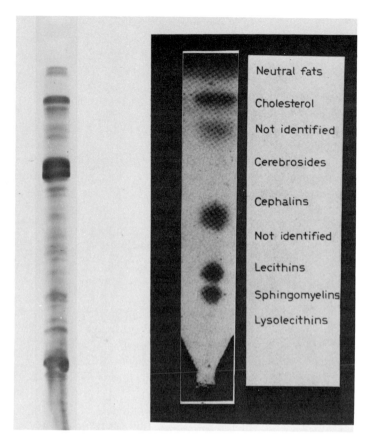

FIG. 4. Fractionation of cochlear proteins by disc electrophoresis (*left*) and cochlear lipids by thin-layer chromatography (*right*). Sample migration is from bottom to top. Electrophoresis of cochlear proteins from guinea pig was performed by the author. The thin-layer chromatogram is reproduced from ref. 68 (p. 99).

cochlear duct (see Fig. 4, right), Hensen's cells, and stria vascularis were investigated. The lipid classes were lysolecithins, sphingomyelins, lecithins, cephalins, cholesterol, and neutral fats, the latter of which included free fatty acids, triglycerides, and cholesterol esters. Hensen's cells contained a greater proportion of neutral fats than did the other cochlear fractions investigated, and neutral fats increased toward the apex. The authors suggested that lipids may be stored in the cochlea as neutral fats.

Schacht (69) labeled with radioactive phosphate the phospholipids of the organ of Corti and stria vascularis plus spiral ligament of the guinea pig. After 45 min, phosphatidylinositol phosphate and phosphatidylinositol diphosphate were labeled most. These results indicate that the phosphomonoester groups of the phosphatidylinositol phosphates exchange with inorganic phosphate. Phosphatidylcholine and phosphatidylinositol were not as highly labeled.

COCHLEAR BIOCHEMISTRY AND NOISE

Noise and Energy Metabolism

Konishi et al. (70) demonstrated that the cochlear potentials decrease with anoxia. Loud sounds may limit oxygen availability to the cochlea by decreasing cochlear blood flow in at least some of the cochlear vessels (71–73), but not necessarily in all (74). Schnieder (73) showed that the clearance rate for dye in the perilymph decreased during exposure to noise, which he ascribed to a decrease in cochlear blood flow. The endolymphatic oxygen concentration (75) and the EP (76) diminish with exposure to loud sound. The drop in cochlear potentials with higher levels of sound exposure may have a component due to insufficient oxygenation, caused by decreased oxygen supply or increased use of oxygen, or both. Tonndorf et al. (77) showed that the recovery of cochlear response (CM) after noise is slow during hypoxia. With anoxia, high ATP levels are maintained in the organ of Corti, whereas strial ATP, strial phosphocreatine, and phosphocreatine of the organ of Corti all decline rapidly (78).

Schnieder (73) found that lactate increased in the perilymph during noise exposure, suggesting that glycolysis may become more important to the cochlea during exposure to noise, or that noise causes decreased oxygen supply. Ishii et al. (79) found, by histochemical studies, that glycogen decreased in the outer hair cells of guinea pig cochlea after exposure to white noise for 30 min at 110 dB SPL. Changes in the size of glycogen granules after noise led these authors to suggest that during noise, glycolytic breakdown of glycogen occurred, and glycogen was synthesized in the quiet via gluconeogenesis. Stack and Webster (80) found a decrease in glycogen in the outer hair cells of the cochlea of the kangaroo rat, with some damage to the organ of Corti, for tones of up to 131 dB SPL for several hours duration. Tones at about 100 dB SPL for 12–13 hr produced little or no change in glycogen content of the hair cells. These histochemical approaches suffer from problems of degree of specificity of the stain as well as difficulty in quantification (81). Also, glycogen granules do not appear to be present in all species (79).

Noise and ATPase: Hypothesis

The hair cells possess a negative intracellular potential (82) that may be mainly a potassium diffusion potential. Exposure to intermediate levels of noise may result in a temporary increase in permeability somewhere in the reticular lamina. Leakage of K^+ down its electrochemical gradient from endolymph, through the reticular lamina, and along the sides of the hair cells could depolarize the cells, a hypothesis similar to that of Misrahy et al. (83). The depolarized cells might then be repolarized via NaK ATPase of the hair cell membranes. The influx of K^+ may be dependent on the noise level and the ATPase activity would be dependent on the supply of ATP and on the concentrations of Na^+ and K^+. During both exposure and recovery, active transport of ions requiring energy of ATP would be occurring. Interference with metabolic energy supply might be expected to alter the time course of these noise-induced changes.

Noise and Biochemical Repair

Proteins and lipids of living cells are constantly broken down and constantly replaced through enzyme-catalyzed biosynthesis. No significant study has yet been published on cochlear membrane turnover. Techniques are now available for such studies. We may expect that turnover and self-assembly of membranes play a part in resistance of cochlear membranes to noise damage and in their repair after traumatic exposures.

ACKNOWLEDGMENT

This work was supported by the Intramural Research Program, National Institute of Neurological and Communicative Disorders and Stroke, National Institutes of Health.

REFERENCES

1. Paparalla, M. M. (editor) (1970): *Biochemical Mechanisms in Hearing and Deafness*. Charles C Thomas, Springfield, Ill.
2. Lowry, O. H., and Passonneau, J. V. (1972): *A Flexible System of Enzymatic Analysis*. Academic Press, New York.
3. Neuhoff, V. (1973): *Micromethods in Molecular Biology*. Springer-Verlag, New York.
4. Carder, H. M., and Miller, J. D. (1971): Temporary threshold shifts produced by noise-exposure of long duration. *Am. Acad. Ophthalmol. Otolaryngol.*, 75:1346–1354.
5. Carder, H. M., and Miller, J. D. (1972): Temporary threshold shifts from prolonged exposure to noise. *J. Speech Hear. Res.*, 15:603–623.
6. Mills, J. H., Gengel, R. W., Watson, C. S., and Miller, J. D. (1970): Temporary changes of the auditory system due to exposure to noise for one or two days. *J. Acoust. Soc. Am.*, 48:524–530.
7. Mills, J. H., and Talo, S. A. (1972): Temporary threshold shifts produced by exposure to high-frequency noise. *J. Speech Hear. Res.*, 15:624–631.
8. Miller, J. D., Rothenberg, S. J., and Eldredge, D. H. (1971): Preliminary observations on the effects of exposure to noise for seven days on the hearing and inner ear of the chinchilla. *J. Acoust. Soc. Am.*, 50:1199–1203.
9. Mills, J. H. (1973): Temporary threshold shifts produced by nine-day exposures to noise. *J. Speech Hear. Res.*, 16:426–438.
10. Davis, H. (1965): A model for transducer action in the cochlea. *Cold Spring Harbor Symp. Quant. Biol.*, 30:181–190.

11. Strelioff, D., Haas, G., and Honrubia, V. (1972): Sound-induced electrical imped- ance changes in the guinea pig cochlea. *J. Acoust. Soc. Am.,* 51:617–620.
12. Goldstein, A. J. (1973): Permeability of the organ of Corti. *Ann. Otol. Rhinol. Laryngol.,* 82:166–174.
13. Wever, E. G. (1959): The cochlear potentials and their relation to hearing. *Ann. Otol. Rhinol. Laryngol.,* 68:975–989.
14. Drescher, D. G. (1974): Noise-induced reduction of inner-ear microphonic re- sponse: dependence on body temperature. *Science,* 185:273–274.
15. Drescher, D. G. (1974): Noise-induced reduction and recovery of chinchilla coch- lear microphonic response. *J. Acoust. Soc. Am.,* 56:S11(A).
16. Benitez, L. D., Eldredge, D. H., and Templer, J. D. (1972): Temporary threshold shifts in chinchilla: electrophysiological correlates. *J. Acoust. Soc. Am.,* 52:1115– 1123.
17. Drescher, D. G., and Eldredge, D. H. (1974): Species differences in cochlear fa- tigue related to acoustics of outer and middle ears of guinea pig and chinchilla. *J. Acoust. Soc. Am.,* 56:929–934.
18. Eldredge, D. H., Mills, J. H., and Bohne, B. A. (1973): Anatomical, behavioral, and electrophysiological observations on chinchillas after long exposures to noise. *Adv. Otorhinolaryngol.,* 20:64–81.
19. Bohne, B. A., Eldredge, D. H., and Mills, J. H. (1973): Cochlear potentials and electron microscopy applied to the study of small cochlear lesions. *Ann. Otol. Rhinol. Laryngol.,* 82:595–608.
20. Davis, H., and Associates (1953): Acoustic trauma in the guinea pig. *J. Acoust. Soc. Am.,* 25:1180–1189.
21. Eldredge, D. H., Covell, W. P., and Davis, H. (1957): Recovery from acoustic trauma in the guinea pig. *Laryngoscope,* 67:66–84.
22. Lawrence, M., and Yantis, P. A. (1957): Individual differences in functional re- covery and structural repair following overstimulation of the guinea pig ear. *Ann. Otol. Rhinol. Laryngol.,* 66:595–621.
23. Beagley, H. A. (1965): Acoustic trauma in the guinea pig. II. Electron microscopy including the morphology of cell junctions in the organ of Corti. *Acta Otolaryngol. (Stockh.),* 60:479–495.
24. Lim, D. J., and Melnick, W. (1971): Acoustic damage of the cochlea. *Arch. Otolaryngol.,* 94:294–305.
25. Spoendlin, H. (1971): Primary structural changes in the organ of Corti after acoustic overstimulation. *Acta Otolaryngol. (Stockh.),* 71:166–176.
26. Spoendlin, H., and Brun, J. P. (1973): Relation of structural damage to exposure time and intensity in acoustic trauma. *Acta Otolaryngol. (Stockh.),* 75:220–226.
27. Lehninger, A. L. (1970): *Biochemistry.* Worth, New York.
28. Mahler, H. R., and Cordes, E. H. (1971): *Biological Chemistry.* Harper and Row, New York.
29. White, A., Handler, P., and Smith, E. L. (1973): *Principles of Biochemistry.* McGraw-Hill, New York.
30. Watson, J. D. (1970): *Molecular Biology of the Gene.* Benjamin, New York.
31. Matschinsky, F. M., and Thalmann, R. (1967): Quantitative histochemistry of the organ of Corti, stria vascularis and macula sacculi of the guinea pig. I. Sampling procedures and analysis of pyridine nucleotides. *Laryngoscope,* 77:292–305.
32. Matschinsky, F. M., and Thalmann, R. (1967): Quantitative histochemistry of microscopic structures of the cochlea. II. Ischemic alterations of levels of glycolytic intermediates and cofactors in the organ of Corti and stria vascularis. *Ann. Otol. Rhinol. Laryngol.,* 76:638–646.
33. Thalmann, I., Matschinsky, F. M., and Thalmann, R. (1970): Quantitative study of selected enzymes involved in energy metabolism of the cochlear duct. *Ann. Otol. Rhinol. Laryngol.,* 79:12–29.
34. Matschinsky, F. M., and Thalmann, R. (1970): Energy metabolism of the cochlear duct. In: *Biochemical Mechanisms in Hearing and Deafness,* edited by M. M. Papa- rella, pp. 265–288. Charles C Thomas, Springfield, Ill.
35. Krzanowski, J. J., Jr., and Matschinsky, F. M. (1971): A phosphocreatine gradient opposite to that of glycogen in the organ of Corti and the effect of salicylate on

adenosine triphosphate and P-creatine in cochlear structures. *J. Histochem. Cytochem.,* 19:321–323.

36. Lowry, O. H., Passonneau, J. V., Schulz, D. W., and Rock, M. K. (1961): The measurement of pyridine nucleotides by enzymatic cycling. *J. Biol. Chem.,* 236:2746–2755.
37. Skou, J. C. (1957): The influence of some cations on an adenosine triphosphatase from peripheral nerves. *Biochim. Biophys. Acta,* 23:394–401.
38. Dahl, J. L., and Hokin, L. E. (1974): The sodium-potassium adenosinetriphosphatase. *Ann. Rev. Biochem.,* 43:327–356.
39. Katz, B. (1966): *Nerve, Muscle, and Synapse,* pp. 41–72. McGraw-Hill, New York.
40. Iinuma, T. (1967): Evaluation of adenosine triphosphatase activity in the stria vascularis and spiral ligament of normal guinea pigs. *Laryngoscope,* 77:141–158.
41. Kuijpers, W., Van der Vleuten, A. C., and Bonting, S. L. (1967): Cochlear function and sodium and potassium activated adenosine triphosphatase. *Science,* 157:949–950.
42. Kuijpers, W. (1969): Cation transport and cochlear function. *Acta Otolaryngol. (Stockh.),* 67:200–205.
43. Kuijpers, W. (1974): Na–K–ATPase activity in the cochlea of the rat during development. *Acta Otolaryngol. (Stockh.),* 78:314–344.
44. Kuijpers, W., Houben, N. M. D., and Bonting, S. L. (1970): Distribution and properties of ATPase activities in the cochlea of the chicken. *Comp. Biochem. Physiol.,* 36:669–676.
45. Kuijpers, W., and Bonting, S. L. (1970): The cochlear potentials. I. The effect of ouabain on the cochlear potentials of the guinea pig. *Pfluegers Arch.,* 320:348–358.
46. Konishi, T., Kelsey, E., and Singleton, G. T. (1966): Effects of chemical alteration in the endolymph on the cochlear potentials. *Acta Otolaryngol. (Stockh.),* 62:393–404.
47. Nakai, Y., and Hilding, D. A. (1966): Electron microscopic studies of adenosine triphosphatase activity in the stria vascularis and spiral ligament. *Acta Otolaryngol. (Stockh.),* 62:411–428.
48. Nakai, Y., and Hilding, D. (1967): Adenosine triphosphatase distribution in the organ of Corti. *Acta Otolaryngol. (Stockh.),* 64:477–491.
49. Edsall, J. T. (1968): The carbonic anhydrases of erythrocytes. *Harvey Lect.,* 62:191–230.
50. Maren, T. H. (1967): Carbonic anhydrase: Chemistry, physiology, and inhibition. *Physiol. Rev.,* 47:595–781.
51. Carter, M. J. (1972): Carbonic anhydrase: isoenzymes, properties, distribution, and functional significance. *Biol. Rev.,* 47:465–513.
52. Erulkar, S. D., and Maren, T. H. (1961): Carbonic anhydrase and the inner ear. *Nature,* 189:459–460.
53. White, A., Handler, P., and Smith, E. L. (1973): *Principles of Biochemistry,* pp. 932–935. McGraw-Hill, New York.
54. Guidotti, G. (1972): Membrane proteins. *Ann. Rev. Biochem.,* 41:731–752.
55. Tanford, C. (1973): *The Hydrophobic Effect: Formation of Micelles and Biological Membranes.* Wiley, New York.
56. Edsall, J. T., and Wyman, J. (1958): *Biophysical Chemistry,* Vol. 1. Academic Press, New York.
57. Schellman, J. A., and Schellman, C. (1964): The conformation of polypeptide chains in proteins. In: *The Proteins,* Vol. 2, edited by H. Neurath, pp. 1–137. Academic Press, New York.
58. Robertson, J. D. (1960): The molecular structure and contact relationships of cell membranes. *Prog. Biophys.* 10:344–418.
59. Singer, S. J. (1974): The molecular organization of membranes. *Ann. Rev. Biochem.,* 43:805–833.
60. Singer, S. J., and Nicolson, G. L. (1972): The fluid mosaic model of the structure of cell membranes. *Science,* 175:720–731.
61. Tanford, C. (1973): *The Hydrophobic Effect: Formation of Micelles and Biological Membranes,* pp. 1–11; 174–189. Wiley, New York.
62. Neville, D. M. (1967): Fractionation of cell membrane protein by disc electrophoresis. *Biochim. Biophys. Acta,* 133:168–170.

63. Löbe, P. (1974): Autoradiographic studies of the inner ear after cochlear perfusion of ³H-uridine. (in German). *Arch. Otorhinolaryngol.,* 208:61–70.
64. Saito, H., and Daly, J. F. (1970): Quantitative analysis of acid mucopolysaccharides in the normal guinea pig cochlea. *Acta Otolaryngol. (Stockh.),* 69:333–340.
65. Saito, H., and Daly, J. F. (1971): Quantitative analysis of acid mucopolysaccharides in the normal and kanamycin intoxicated cochlea. *Acta Otolaryngol. (Stockh.),* 71:22–26.
66. Lotz, P., and Kuhl, K.-D. (1970): Quantitative mucopolysaccharide-protein relation in the cochlea. (in German). *Arch. Otorhinolaryngol. (NY),* 197:122–128.
67. Scheibe, F., Gerhardt, H.-J., Esser, U., and Haupt, H. (1971): Dünnshicht-chromatographischer nachweis von Gewebelipiden aus der Meerschweinchenschnecke. *Acta Otolaryngol. (Stockh.),* 71:392–399.
68. Scheibe, F., Gerhardt, H.-J., Hache, U., and Haupt, H. (1973): Thin-layer chromatographic investigation of the lipids of inner ear tissues and perilymph of guinea pig. *ORL,* 35:96–103.
69. Schacht, J. (1974): Interaction of neomycin with phosinositide metabolism in guinea pig inner ear and brain tissues. *Ann. Otol. Rhinol. Laryngol.,* 83:613–618.
70. Konishi, T., Butler, R. A., and Fernández, C. (1961): Effect of anoxia on cochlear potentials. *J. Acoust. Soc. Am.,* 33:349–356.
71. Hawkins, J. E., Jr. (1971): The role of vasoconstriction in noise-induced hearing loss. *Ann. Otol. Rhinol. Laryngol.,* 80:903–913.
72. Misrahy, G. A., Arnold, J. E., Mundie, J. R., Shinabarger, E. W., and Garwood, V. P. (1958): Genesis of endolymphatic hypoxia following acoustic trauma. *J. Acoust. Soc. Am.,* 30:1082–1088.
73. Schnieder, E.-A. (1974): A contribution to the physiology of the perilymph. Part III: On the origin of noise-induced hearing loss. *Ann. Otol. Rhinol. Laryngol.,* 83:406–412.
74. Perlman, H. B., and Kimura, R. (1962): Cochlear blood flow in acoustic trauma. *Acta Otolaryngol. (Stockh.),* 54:99–110.
75. Misrahy, G. A., Hildreth, K. M., Shinabarger, E. W., Clark, L. C., and Rice, E. A. (1958): Endolymphatic oxygen tension in the cochlea of the guinea pig. *J. Acoust. Soc. Am.,* 30:247–250.
76. Rice, E. A., and Shinabarger, E. W. (1961): Studies on the endolymphatic dc potential of the guinea pig's cochlea. *J. Acoust. Soc. Am.,* 33:922–925.
77. Tonndorf, J., Hyde, R. W., and Brogan, F. A. (1955): Combined effect of sound and oxygen deprivation upon cochlear microphonics in guinea pigs. *Ann. Otol. Rhinol. Laryngol.,* 64:392–405.
78. Thalmann, R., Miyoshi, T., and Thalmann, I. (1972): The influence of ischemia upon the energy reserves of inner ear tissues. *Laryngoscope,* 82:2249–2272.
79. Ishii, D., Takahashi, T., and Balogh, K. (1969): Glycogen in the inner ear after acoustic stimulation. *Acta Otolaryngol. (Stockh.),* 67:573–582.
80. Stack, C. R., and Webster, D. B. (1971): Glycogen content in the outer hair cells of kangaroo rat (*D. spectabilis*) cochlea prior to and following auditory stimulation. *Acta Otolaryngol. (Stockh.),* 71:483–493.
81. Vosteen, K.-H. (1958): Die Erschöpfung der Phonoreceptoren nach funktioneller Belastung. *Arch. Otorhinolaryngol. (NY),* 172:489–512.
82. Weiss, T. F., Mulroy, M. J., and Altmann, D. W. (1974): Intracellular responses to acoustic clicks in the inner ear of the alligator lizard. *J. Acoust. Soc. Am.,* 55:606–619.
83. Misrahy, G. A., Hildreth, K. M., Shinabarger, E. W., and Gannon, W. J. (1958): Electrical properties of wall of endolymphatic space of the cochlea (guinea pig). *Am. J. Physiol.,* 194:396–402.

DISCUSSION

C. Trahiotis: I'd like to know, at least in gross terms, the biochemical effects that might be occurring in the cochlear nerve fibers; what seems sort of startling in the work of Benitez, Eldredge, and Templer (1) is that, at roughly

24–48 hr after an exposure that produces an ATS, the CM and the behavioral thresholds have recovered, while there was a tremendous loss in the AP; in fact, they stated that 5 hr after recovery they could not get AP from 90-dB clicks and, even 24 and 48 hr after recovery, there was still a severe AP depression. Do you think biochemical changes could have affected the nerve fibers and not the hair cells?

D. Drescher: That's a very difficult question to answer, but I think that in the study there was a higher response; i.e., an AER. This would indicate, as you imply, that the hair cells and higher neural centers were working or recovering in parallel, but the first-order neurons were not functioning properly; now, your question was, what caused this? The reason of Benitez et al. was that there was a desynchronization between the individual hair cells. There are a number of possibilities: e.g., it could have something to do with lactate; this is an acidic material, if it increases to the extent that Schnieder (2) has measured, it could be having some sort of effect on the naked nerve fibers, which would cause the desynchronization, but as to the actual mechanism of desynchronization, it is impossible, without more data, to say anything more definite. We could go into possible ionate mechanisms, but that would not be getting nearer to the truth.

J. Hawkins, Jr.: There is a paper by Schnieder which denies the possible role of lactate in producing fatigue effects in the cochlea. They maintain that the lactate would be washed away by the perilymph stream. On the other hand, that was written before they showed changes in the clearance rate of the cochlear fluids as a result of the noise exposure, so I think that the possibility is open again.

D. Drescher: To augment that point, you have 16 μm liters of perilymph in the guinea pig with a half-life turnover of about 10 min. It seems reasonable, even with that kind of flow rate, to think that there could be some sort of trapping in, say, the tunnel of Corti area, which would lead to a buildup of lactate. However, that flow rate by itself is impressively high and perilymph must be just coursing through the scala.

J. Hawkins, Jr.: Perhaps after noise exposure, the flow rates are also altered.

D. Drescher: Let's say it decreases by one-half, that might give you some buildup, but it's still a relatively high clearance rate.

P. Stopp: We have observed that under ouabain the N_1 response is lost and then later the CM; however, the CM recovers well before you get any N_1 response.

D. Drescher: Perhaps ouabain is being very specific.

P. Stopp: No. Ouabain will affect all cochlear responses, but in a different order.

D. Drescher: That could have to do partially with the binding of the ouabain, or the permeability of the ouabain to various structures it encountered. I would expect that there is a considerable difference in permeability between a hair cell and, say, the sort of very lipid type membrane of the nerve. And such permeability effects could definitely be differential when you consider both the start and the recovery processes.

G. Price: I presume these reactions must be temperature-sensitive. How much of a temperature change do you estimate would make a difference? Is it possible that minute temperature changes can take place in the cochlea as a result of sound stimulation?

R. Thalmann: We have shown that 2° has a tremendous effect on CM changes, while the EP is virtually insensitive to temperature. This is very strange, because the EP demonstrates a threshold; i.e., it's an all-or-none phenomenon.

J. Hawkins, Jr.: I was happy that Dr. Drescher brought up the matter of carbonic anhydrase in the cochlea. This has been rather neglected. I must confess to a slight concern as to what happened to the H^+ ions in this case; are they sopped up by the spiral ligament, or are they spirited away by the blood vessels behind the stria vascularis? It is certainly something that needs careful consideration.

REFERENCES

1. Benitez, L. D., Eldredge, D. H., and Templer, J. D. (1972): Temporary threshold shifts in chinchilla: Electrophysiological correlates. *J. Acoust. Soc. Am.*, 52:1115–1123.
2. Schnieder, E. (1974): A contribution to the physiology of the perilymph. Part III: On the origin of noise-induced hearing loss. *Ann. Otol. Rhinol. Laryngol.*, 83:406–412.

Effects of Noise on Hearing, edited by Donald Henderson, Roger P. Hamernik, Darshan S. Dosanjh, and John H. Mills. Raven Press, New York © 1976

Quantitative Biochemical Techniques for Studying Normal and Noise-Damaged Ears

Ruediger R. Thalmann

Department of Otolaryngology, Washington University School of Medicine, St. Louis, Missouri 63110

One of the most important open questions concerning inner ear function is: "What are the biochemical mechanisms involved in the response of the cochlear transducer to adequate stimulation at physiological levels?" The answer to this question would seem to be a prerequisite for the understanding of potential biochemical alterations induced by exposure to unphysiologically high levels of sound; however, under practical conditions it may be more realistic to reverse the strategy and to attempt detection of changes in the biochemical state induced by more intense, unphysiological sound exposure. The observed biochemical response patterns may then signify simply an exaggeration of normal processes, which could help elucidate the basic mechanisms; alternatively, of course, they may constitute patterns characteristic only in specific kinds of sound exposure.

In the preceding chapter Dr. Drescher presented various schemes that could represent biochemical correlates of functional changes induced by noise. It is my task to describe feasible and meaningful approaches that could lead to technical realization of the schemes discussed and provide experimental tools to test some of the hypotheses forwarded. My presentation falls into 3 sections:

1. Description and discussion of biochemical techniques that might be of use in noise studies, with emphasis upon quantitative approaches

2. Selection of promising animal models to which these techniques can be applied in a meaningful way

3. Brief presentation of preliminary quantitative biochemical results on noise-exposed ears (and discussion of these results in the context of known biochemical characteristics of the organ of Corti)

Before discussing in more detail the quantitative analytical techniques emphasized in this chapter, it may be appropriate to review briefly some other available biochemical approaches to the noise problem. Broadly speaking, these can be categorized as direct and indirect approaches.

INDIRECT APPROACHES

Most important in this category is the study of electrophysiological correlates of noise in combination with deliberate experimental interferences,

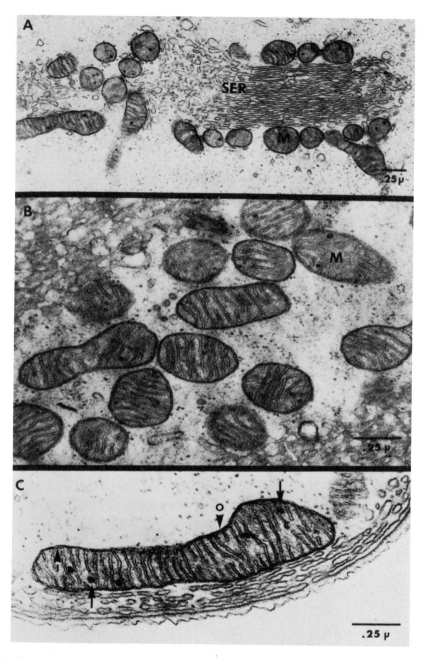

FIG. 1. Electron micrographs of outer hair cells from chinchillas with asymptotic threshold shifts of about 50 dB. A. Cell in lower third turn in animal exposed to an octave band of noise centered at 500 Hz. In central cytoplasm is an accumulation of smooth endoplasmic reticulum (SER). Note close association of mitochondria (M) to excess membranes. B. Tangential section of cell in middle of first turn in animal exposed to octave band of noise centered at 4 kHz. Peripherally arranged mitochondria (M) have entirely normal structures. C. Peripheral mitochondrion in cell from lower third turn of animal described in A. Outer (O) and inner (I) limiting membranes, cristae (C) and intramatrical granules (arrows) are clearly demonstrated. The outer mitochondrial compartment, located between the inner and outer limiting membranes, and the inner compartment into which the cristae project are both of normal size. Enlargement of the outer compartment at the expense of the inner compartment would be indicative of a reduction of the ATP/ADP ratio. (Courtesy B. A. Bohne.)

which are intended to alter chemical processes in a controlled way. From ensuing changes in electrophysiological response patterns biochemical mechanisms can be inferred. This approach was exemplified by Dr. Drescher in the preceding chapter when he described his most interesting experiments on the influence of temperature upon the rate of development of asymptotic threshold shift (ATS) and recovery therefrom. Another potentially profitable approach using electrophysiological responses as functional (and thereby biochemical) monitors is alteration of the chemical environment of the inner ear by omission or addition of metabolic substrates, application of enzyme inhibitors, etc. An example of the latter is the effect of iodoacetate, a powerful inhibitor of glycolysis, upon the sensitivity of the cochlear microphonics (CM) to sound (1). When the CM are predamaged by iodoacetate, short-term exposure to sound of a sound pressure level (SPL) of about 100 dB re 0.0002 μbar produces a drastic and irreversible further reduction of the potential.

Another important indirect approach is transmission electron microscopy, which can give certain indications about biochemical changes (state of the mitochondria [Fig. 1], ribosomes, lysosomes, membrane systems, etc.).

DIRECT APPROACHES

In this case the biochemical state of tissues and fluids of the inner ear are determined directly, either qualitatively or quantitatively.

Qualitative Techniques[1]

Qualitative histochemistry is also frequently referred to as slide or staining histochemistry. The outstanding advantage of this technique is its high resolution, which can in no way be matched by current quantitative techniques (2). Of particular interest are the more recent techniques at the electron-microscopic level. Disadvantages are that the data obtained are at best semiquantitative and that there are limitations in the types of substances that can be studied. The methods are in general restricted to the study of enzymes and other high molecular weight substances (e.g., glycogen). This, of course, limits the value of the entire approach, since enzyme activities (whether measured by qualitative or quantitative methods) do not usually reflect the rate at which a particular reaction is taking place, but rather indicate the capacity of a given enzymic step or sequence of steps. It is generally known that most enzymes perform at a much lesser rate *in vivo* than the activity measured *in vitro* under optimal conditions (maximal *in vitro* rates) would

---

[1] Since the majority of methods in this category are concerned with the determination of enzymes, some comments on *quantitative* enzyme histochemistry have been included under this heading for the purpose of comparison with and evaluation of qualitative approaches.

indicate. Nevertheless, relative enzyme patterns do give clues about preferred pathways, bottlenecks, primary sites of metabolic activity, etc. In the case of the organ of Corti (OC) and stria vascularis (SV), the prevailing type of energy generation has been identified by both qualitative and quantitative techniques, although certain patterns were exaggerated in the qualitative technique: For instance, a very high activity of lactic dehydrogenase was found in the OC, particularly in the outer hair cells, suggesting strong reliance upon glycolytic processes (3). This was confirmed by quantitative studies (4). However, virtually no lactic dehydrogenase was detectable in the SV by qualitative methods. This was later identified as an artifact due to poor penetration of the incubation medium into the dense strial tissue. Quantitative measurements indicated that lactic dehydrogenase activity in the SV is almost as high as in the OC (4). A high activity of malic dehydrogenase and other respiratory enzymes in the SV has been shown by both qualitative and quantitative techniques, in line with the high mitochondrial density and the high respiratory and metabolic rate (use rate of high energy phosphate) of this tissue (2–6).

The enzymes discussed above provide information about energy-releasing

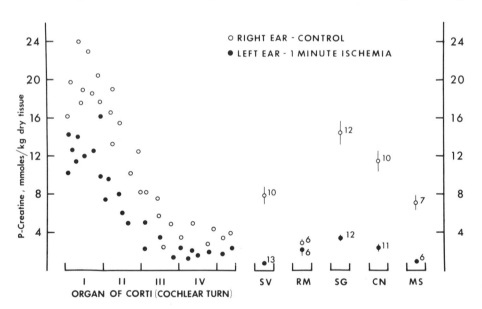

FIG. 2. Concentration of phosphocreatine in the organ of Corti and in other inner ear structures at control conditions and following ischemia of 1-min duration. All values are from the same guinea pig. Both bullae were widely opened, and on the left side the labyrinthine artery was exposed. Following electrocauterization of the artery the cochlear microphonics started to decline and both temporal bones were frozen in situ 1 min later. In the case of the organ of Corti the position of the symbols relative to the abscissa indicates the approximate location of each sample within the cochlea. For the remaining inner ear structures, only the means for the indicated number of individual values are recorded. The vertical bars indicate the standard error of the mean. RM, Reissner's membrane. SG, spiral ganglion. CN, cochlear nerve. MS, macula sacculi. (From ref. 40.)

processes; on the other hand, energy-consuming processes are reflected by the activity of ATPases. The distribution of Na⁺K⁺–ATPase, for instance, gives clues about the capacity of the corresponding $Na^+:K^+$ exchange systems. By quantitative methods it was shown that the SV has an exceedingly high activity of this enzyme (7,8). By contrast, the activity of Na⁺K⁺–ATPase is low in the OC and in Reissner's membrane, indicating a lesser capacity of these tissues for active transport. By qualitative histochemical techniques at the ultrastructural level, ATPase has been demonstrated in membranes and organelles of various cells of the inner ear (9), but the distribution of Na⁺K⁺–ATPase has not yet been determined.

With respect to noise experiments, alterations of enzyme activities due to long-term exposure may indicate true variations in the amount of enzymes present, i.e., enzyme induction or repression, and in this way may also provide indirect information about protein metabolism. On the other hand, a reduc-

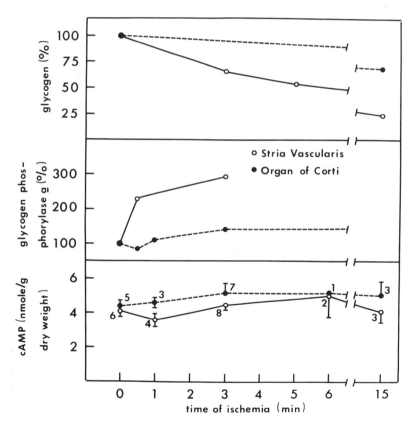

FIG. 3. Influence of ischemia upon cyclic AMP (*lower panel*), state of activation of glycogen phosphorylase (*middle panel*), and rate of degradation of glycogen (*upper panel*) in the organ of Corti and the stria vascularis. In the case of cyclic AMP the mean ± SEM for the indicated number of ears are given (2 determinations per ear). (From ref. 21.)

tion of activity may simply mean that membrane permeability is impaired and that the enzyme has leaked out of the cell.

Although enzymes are chemically labile substances, most of them are biologically stable. That is, they do not at all reflect the rapid metabolic adjustments taking place during short-term experimental interference, whereas steady-state levels of certain labile low molecular weight substances may be drastically altered (Fig. 2). One of the exceptions to this rule is glycogen phosphorylase, which interconverts rapidly from the inactive to the active form during metabolic impairment (Fig. 3) (8).

A number of qualitative studies have been performed concerning the influence of various types of noise upon the cochlea, but the results obtained so far do not allow firm conclusions to be made (2,3). A study by Ishii et al. (10) indicates that the distribution and amount of glycogen in the outer hair cells is changed by exposure to white noise of comparatively high intensity. This, of course, could signify alterations in glycogenolysis and glycolysis and consequent changes in energy generation. An acceleration of glycolysis during noise exposure is suggested also by the observation of Schnieder (11) that lactate levels in perilymph increase significantly.

Quantitative Biochemical Techniques

In the following, a brief review of potentially profitable techniques for the quantitative study of the biochemical basis of noise damage is given. Two important quantitative tools of neurochemistry—arteriovenous difference studies and tissue slice techniques—are not applicable to the inner ear in a meaningful way; however, in spite of a variety of complicating factors (microscopic size and fragility of the tissues, comparatively large interlocking fluid spaces with steep chemical and electrical gradients between compartments, close association of the soft tissues with bone), it is possible to adapt quantitative histochemical techniques to inner ear tissues (8,12).[2]

Although various approaches can be chosen for specific purposes, the following basic requirements must be satisfied by any quantitative histochemical technique:

1. The chemical profile of the tissues in question must be maintained faithfully. This poses particular problems when biologically labile substances are to be studied.

2. It must be possible to separate tissue units at a sufficient degree of resolution, e.g., whole OC at different points along the extent of the cochlea, cell layers containing populations of individual cell types, etc.

---

[2] In this context the term "quantitative histochemistry" is used only in the sense of quantitative *in vitro* analysis of nonviable tissue elements and does not apply to (semi)-quantitative optical or electron-probe techniques of tissues *in situ* or tissue sections.

3. It must be possible to determine the size of the sample, e.g., by measuring its weight, protein content, etc.

4. Because of the small size of inner ear tissues and because of the low concentration of most substances, highly sensitive analytical methods must be available.

Quantitative histochemical techniques of Lowry and Passonneau (13): The technique that we have stressed in the past and which appears to be optimally suited to the study of many biologically labile substances is an adaptation of Lowry's quantitative histochemical method, and consists of the following steps (8,12).

1. Rapid freezing of the cochlea with Freon 12 cooled to its melting point with liquid nitrogen
2. Freeze-drying of the cochlea *in toto* at low temperature ($-40°C$)
3. Microdissection of freeze-dried cochlear tissue units and populations of cell types of the OC in the three-dimensional state at room temperature at low relative humidity
4. Determination of the dry weight on a quartz fiber balance
5. Ultramicrochemical analysis by catalytic fluorometric techniques, including "enzymic cycling"

Regarding points 1 and 2: Rapid freezing arrests chemical processes with minimal delay and prevents formation of large ice crystals which would cause major tissue disruption. Freezing can be carried out *in situ* at any stage of a physiological experiment including, of course, experiments concerned with noise exposure. Once frozen, tissues are chemically stable when maintained at sufficiently low temperature and, in principle, analysis could follow at this stage; however, in the case of the cochlea, it is virtually impossible to distinguish and dissect the tissues of interest in the frozen state (in contrast to cochlear fluids, which can be sampled with a certain degree of accuracy while frozen) (14). This problem is eliminated by freeze-drying of the temporal bone *in toto,* which not only maintains (in most instances) the chemical state existing at the time of freezing, but also preserves the three-dimensional structure of cochlear tissues surprisingly well.

Regarding point 3: Because of the highly regular and organized arrangement of cochlear structures, they can be easily identified in the stereomicroscope and dissected out by techniques similar to those used for conventional surface preparations of fixed or fresh material. The OC can be further broken down into layers representing reasonably pure populations of component cell types (Fig. 4); in the case of the outer hair cells and Hensen cells further subdivision into single cells is possible (Fig. 5) (15). When working with the OC, particularly when it has been exposed to potentially harmful influences, evaluation of the quality of morphologic preservation is of great importance. Preliminary examinations can be carried out using the higher powers

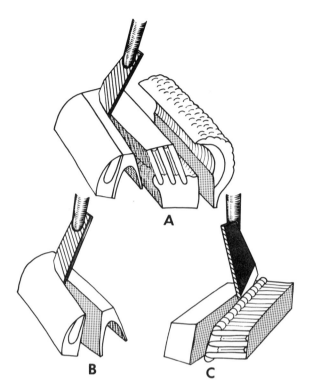

FIG. 4. Schematic diagram of the method for the separation of the organ of Corti into cell layers by dissection from the surface. A. The sample is positioned with the reticular lamina facing upward. With a razor-blade knife, longitudinal incisions are made as shown, dividing the specimen into 3 portions. B. The inner hair cell layer is separated from the tunnel layer by means of a longitudinal incision with the knife. C. The portion containing the outer hair cells and the Deiters cells is laid on its side, and an incision is made at the base of the hair cells transsecting the Deiters cups. These can be removed in part by cautious wiping with a hairpoint. (From ref. 41.)

of a stereomicroscope (50–100×) in transmitted illumination. More precise evaluations are possible by (i) phase-contrast or Nomarski differential interference-contrast microscopy from the surface, after the freeze-dried opaque samples have been rendered translucent; (ii) imbedding the samples in plastic and thin sectioning; or most conveniently (iii) using scanning electron microscopy; for the latter technique, the dissected structures need merely be affixed to a stub and coated with a thin metal film (12).

Regarding point 4: Definition of the size of the sample by its dry weight represents a convenient standard. It must be understood, of course, that dry weight varies greatly with the relative content of water and solids of the cell types in question. When such differences are disregarded, concentration gradients which are artifactual and not representative of the actual *in vivo* situation may become apparent between cell types, or else existing gradients may be obscured. Using the protein content of the tissues in question will, in general,

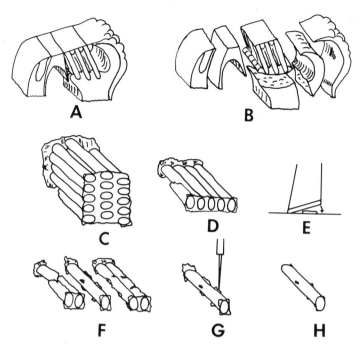

FIG. 5. Schematic diagram of the method for separating single outer hair cells from free-hand "cross section" of freeze-dried organ of Corti. Sequence of steps is left to right, top to bottom. By means of appropriate incisions and fractures, single outer hair cells can be isolated; debris, consisting of remnants of the Deiters cups, phalangeal processes, and precipitate from extracellular fluids, can be removed in part with fine quartz fiber "hairpoints" or electrically etched tungsten needles. (From ref. 15.)

constitute a more meaningful standard. We are presently in the process of determining the protein versus dry weight ratio of different cell types of the OC, which should allow establishment of appropriate correction factors for dry weight.[3]

Regarding point 5: The method of Lowry and Passonneau (13) undoubtedly is the most sensitive and most widely applicable microanalytical technique. Any substance that can be linked directly or via intermediate enzymic steps to a DPN- or TPN-dependent reaction can be assayed. A high sensitivity is achieved by using inherently sensitive fluorometric techniques. An almost unlimited further increase of sensitivity is possible by enzymic cyling, which is illustrated in Fig. 6. Since all reactions are enzymically controlled, the method provides also a high degree of specificity.

The Lowry technique alone provides many of the tools for a potentially profitable attack of the chemical aspects of the noise problem at various levels. The great advantage is that the steady-state levels of nearly any metabolic

---

[3] In neural structures, which exhibit pronounced variations in lipid content, the lipid-free dry weight represents a suitable index of sample size.

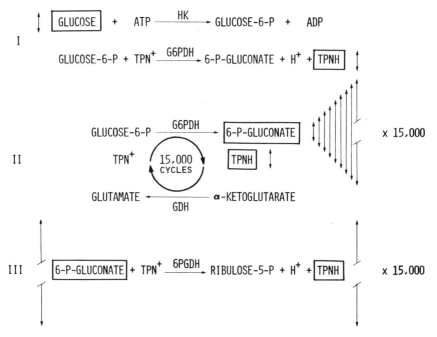

FIG. 6. Principle of enzymic cycling after Lowry and Passonneau (13) exemplified in the analysis of glucose. By means of auxiliary enzymes and cofactors, glucose is converted to glucose-6-P which in turn is converted to 6-P-gluconate, producing equimolar amounts of TPNH. TPNH exhibits native fluorescence; the amounts obtained in submicrogram samples, however, are too low for direct fluorometry; therefore, the TPNH produced in reaction (I) is introduced into the cycling system (II), where each pyridine nucleotide molecule is alternately oxidized and reduced in rapid succession; 6-P-gluconate and glutamate accumulate accordingly. The amount of 6-P-gluconate is finally determined in the indicator reaction (III). The TPNH formed in reaction III is a multiple of the TPNH formed in reaction I and is now measurable by direct fluorometry. (From ref. 41.)

substrate, intermediate, and cofactor can be measured, and in the case of certain substances, changes occurring within a matter of seconds following experimental interference can be detected. A limitation, of course, is that steady-state levels do not reflect actual reaction rates; however, these can be inferred to some extent from changes due to controlled experimental interference (16,17).

What are some of the biochemical processes that may be affected by exposure to noise and that could be attacked by the technique presented? It is reasonable to assume that the workload of the OC is increased during noise exposure, and the first possibility that comes to mind is an inability of the tissue to generate the excess energy required. This could be due to exhaustion of the primary energy sources, as suggested by the qualitative results of Ishii et al. (10), which indicate changes in glycogen levels of the outer hair cells; alternatively, it could be due to a failure of glycolytic and respiratory processes to keep up with the increased energy demands. Up to a certain point an acceleration of glycolysis (with or without concomitant increase of respiration) should be able to compensate for the increased demands of energy. If energy expenditure exceeds the amounts provided, this would be reflected by a reduction of the steady-state level of ATP; however, subtle reductions of ATP cannot be detected readily because of the relatively high base levels of this substance and because of biologic and experimental variability. By contrast, the corresponding small *absolute* increase of AMP may be readily detected, because of the low base level of this substance, and the consequent large percentage change. AMP is a positive modulator of several enzymic reactions leading to increased ATP production, and because of its disproportionate relative changes, can be considered as part of a biochemical amplification system (17). Another indication of incipient failure of energy generation may be a reduction of the level of P-creatine, the immediate reserve form of biochemical energy. A lowered level of P-creatine in the presence of normal or near-normal ATP levels could, therefore, signify that, due to increased demands, energy generation is on the verge of decompensation. In the OC, P-creatine levels indeed decline relatively fast in total ischemia, whereas ATP is maintained at a comparatively high level for appreciable periods of time (6,8).

Various mechanisms may be at fault with amino acid metabolism during noise exposure. Of particular interest are the putative amino acid transmitters γ-aminobutyric acid (GABA), glycine, glutamate, and aspartate. The first 2 substances are considered potential inhibitory transmitter substances; the latter 2 have been shown to be excitatory transmitters in certain neural systems. GABA is virtually absent in the OC; however, the other amino acids are present at substantial levels (18). It would seem plausible that at least the afferent amino acid transmitters could be compromised by excessive exposure to noise. However, because of the double function of these compounds in transmission and metabolism, reduction of their steady-state levels would not necessarily imply an impairment of auditory transmission or transduction. At this point there exists no hard evidence that amino acids play any role in transmission in the inner ear. Since these molecules are small, reduction of their steady-state levels could, of course, simply be due to leakage through damaged cell membranes.

Alternate micropreparatory and microanalytical procedures: The basic analytical technique of Lowry described above can be applied directly to the determination of substances such as glucose, lactate, amino acids, and enzymes in nanoliter samples of cochlear fluids.

For microrespirometric studies (see later) it is, of course, necessary to use freshly dissected OC or SV. The use of fresh material in combination with suitable microhomogenization techniques may also be advantageous in certain enzyme studies. Although the SV can be readily dissected in the native state, micropreparation of the OC is not very satisfactory, because separation from the basilar membrane invariably results in mechanical damage. Cell layers of the OC cannot be prepared in the native state, but digestion of the OC by

Pronase results in separation of single viable outer hair cells (15); however, chemical analyses of cells separated in this way have not as yet been technically realized. In some instances, for example, for the measurement of phospholipid turnover, cochlear tissues may be chemically fixed and dissected by means of routine surface preparation methods (19).

New microanalytical methods are increasingly becoming available. Microradioimmunochemistry, for instance, offers a powerful approach for the quantification of substances present at very low concentrations, such as cyclic AMP. This substance is of universal importance in cellular regulatory processes and, *inter alia,* is known to control and/or mediate a variety of permeability and transport phenomena. Cyclic AMP is known to play a key role in the reaction of the sensory cells of the retina to light. It is quite conceivable that cyclic AMP is involved in auditory transduction or transmission and could be compromised by the effects of noise.

A highly specific microradioimmunoassay developed by Steiner (20) can be scaled down sufficiently to measure steady-state levels of cyclic AMP in microgram samples of inner ear tissues (21) (Fig. 3; and Paloheimo and Thalmann, *unpublished*). Although the fluorometric method of Lowry possesses the requisite sensitivity to detect the small amounts of cyclic nucleotides present in inner ear tissues, the necessity for destroying other interfering nucleotides (some of which are present at levels 3 orders of magnitude higher), by enzymic degradation or by chromatography, poses serious limitations.

Analogous changes in permeability and transport phenomena due to noise could well be caused by an impairment of phospholipid metabolism. Phospholipids are important constituents of cell membranes. Schacht and associates (19) have already demonstrated marked changes in phospholipid metabolism due to the action of neomycin. When perfusing the perilymphatic space with ^{32}P-inorganic phosphate in artificial perilymph, they found that the most highly labeled lipids in cochlear structures were phosphatidylinositol phosphate and -diphosphate. Following treatment with neomycin, labeling of these polyphosphoinositides (but not of other lipids) decreased. Through *in vitro* studies on inner ear tissues and on cerebral cortex subcellular fractions these investigators found that this effect is mediated by inhibition of polyphosphoinositide turnover. In addition, they demonstrated that neomycin is a competitive inhibitor of calcium binding *in vitro* and, therefore, interferes with calcium homeostasis at the membrane level. Since the tissues may be chemically fixed there is no need for freezing and freeze-drying. The method as presently used (250 μCi/ml) is sensitive enough for analysis of samples of OC or SV pooled from 1 single ear; further increase of sensitivity is possible (Schacht, *personal communication*).

As alluded to during the discussion of potential changes of enzyme levels, it is conceivable that long-term noise exposure may lead to an inhibition of protein metabolism. The activity of protein metabolism can be estimated from the rate of incorporation of radioactively labeled amino acids administered *in vivo* via perilymphatic perfusion. Following application of ^{3}H-leucine of high specific activity in artificial perilymph (final activity 100–300 μCi/ml), incorporation rates can be determined for pooled freeze-dried samples of the OC with a combined dry weight of 2–4 μg. The sensitivity of the assay can be increased considerably by applying a suitable mixture of labeled amino acids. Higher sensitivity is necessary if it is desired to study incorporation rates for different cell layers of the OC, or if incorporation rates are to be determined for protein fractions separated by microdisc electrophoresis (12,22).

Another quantitative biochemical approach of potential value in noise studies is microrespirometry. Microdiver techniques have been successfully used for the determination of respiratory rates of inner ear structures by Chou and Hughes (5). Considerable technical improvements have been made in this field since these early studies. The presently available magnetic diver microgasometers are excellent tools for the quantitative study of a variety of physiological and biochemical parameters in minute tissue elements (23). This includes oxygen uptake, carbon dioxide evolution, and substrate utilization of separated live tissue, as well as determinations of enzyme activities in live or freeze-dried material.

A major disadvantage in respect to noise studies is the fact that none of these gasometric measurements can be carried out during noise exposure, but only upon its termination and following micropreparation and loading of the tissue in question. There is no meaningful way for noise stimulation *in vitro*. However, in certain types of noise-induced dysfunctions, such as ATS, long-term biochemical changes could be present in the OC, and might be detectable for prolonged periods in separated live tissue *in vitro*. Potential changes in the respiratory rate may then be compared to the rate of utilization of high-energy phosphate as determined by the "closed system" method of Lowry et al. (16) and as applied to the inner ear by Thalmann et al. (6).

Certain enzymes are most readily measured at the microscale by gasometric techniques. One typical example is carbonic anhydrase, an enzyme which may be of great importance in cochlear function, as pointed out by Dr. Drescher in the preceding chapter. The original measurements carried out by Erulkar and Maren (24) indicated an extremely high activity of carbonic anhydrase in cochlear duct tissue; however, the distribution between different structures of the cochlear duct has not yet been determined. The colorimetric microtechnique used by these investigators is not very sensitive and suffers from the disadvantage that the enzyme activity is measured under conditions which result in marked changes of the pH. A gasometric method based on the evolvement of CO_2, which was scaled down by Giacobini (25) to the ultramicrolevel, avoids artifacts produced by major changes in pH and can be used for the measurement of carbonic anhydrase in minute tissue elements; however, meaningful kinetic studies appear hardly feasible with presently available microtechniques.

With respect to quantitative determinations of cations in cochlear fluids, both integrating-flame photometry and helium-glow photometry offer the sensitivity necessary for the determination of exact concentrations of sodium (and, of course, potassium) in nanoliter samples of endolymph. Helium-glow photometry can also be used to measure calcium and magnesium concentrations in minute endolymph samples. However, fluid sampling techniques are in the process of being supplanted by ion-specific electrode techniques. Most spectacular in this respect is the sodium electrode used by Bosher (26), which is linear down to an activity of 1 mEq/liter or less. Simultaneous measurements of the endolymphatic potential and of sodium, potassium, and chloride activities are currently being conducted in Bosher's laboratory (*personal communication*). It is hoped that this elaborate technique will be applied to the study of noise-induced changes of ion activities in endolymph, suggested by the pertinent studies of Nakashima et al. (27).

ANIMAL MODELS FOR THE STUDY OF BIOCHEMICAL CORRELATES OF NOISE

In order to take advantage of the available quantitative techniques at our disposal, it is necessary to select a type, degree, and duration of sound exposure which has a high probability of producing significant biochemical changes, but does not produce morphological changes of an extent which would make quantitative analyses meaningless. A preparation that demonstrates marked and well-reproducible functional changes with minimal morphologic alteration—asymptotic threshold shift (ATS)—has been developed over the years by Staff Members of the Central Institute for the Deaf. A large amount of information from different disciplines has already been collected on this particular animal model and quantitative studies of potential biochemical correlates of ATS are in progress in collaboration with Dr. D. H. Eldredge and associates.

Carder and Miller (28) first observed this phenomenon in the chinchilla by behavioral methods. They demonstrated that continuous exposure to moderately intense noise (above 65 dB and below 100 dB re 0.0002 μbar) produced a progressive threshold shift until a steady-state level was attained within 24 to 48 hr. Complete behavioral recovery occurred within 3 to 6 days after cessation of exposure. Benitez et al. (29) established the electrophysiological counterparts of these behavioral data and found changes in the CM and the whole nerve action potential essentially paralleling those of the behavioral data. However, alterations in the action potential (poor synchronization) persisted at a time when behavioral responses and the CM had almost recovered to normal. It is noteworthy that no significant changes of the endolymphatic potential were noticeable at a time when the CM and the action potentials were maximally depressed. For this reason, we have not yet explored potential biochemical changes occurring in the SV.

As an anatomical correlate of ATS, Bohne found conspicuous ultrastructural changes confined to the outer hair cells in the form of proliferations of the cisternae of the smooth endoplasmic reticulum which forms the peripheral membrane system (Fig. 7). It should be noted, however, that a small percentage of outer hair cells are completely destroyed following exposure to narrow band noise of 95 dB SPL for a duration of 48 hr, although the majority of hair cells are entirely normal except for the mentioned intracellular ultrastructural changes (29,30).

Drescher (31) demonstrated that the time course of the changes of the CM during development of ATS and recovery therefrom is markedly influenced by temperature. This, of course, is strong evidence for a biochemical nature of ATS.

The marked functional changes in the absence of gross morphologic disturbances and the establishment of a new functional steady state made this model very attractive for the study of potential biochemical correlates of noise exposure. Since most existing quantitative (and qualitative) biochemical data

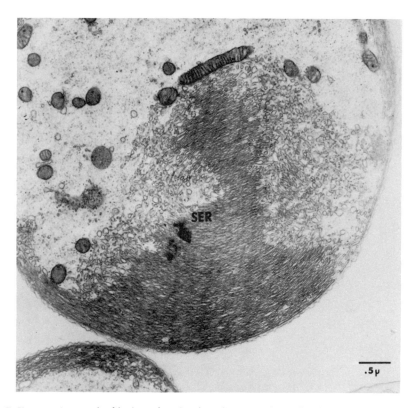

FIG. 7. Electron micrograph of horizontal section through an outer hair cell in lower third turn of a chinchilla cochlea with an asymptotic threshold shift of about 50 dB. There has been a tremendous proliferation of cisternae of smooth endoplasmic reticulum (SER) in response to noise exposure. Membranes fill about one-half of the cells at this point. (Courtesy B. A. Bohne.)

about the OC have been obtained in the guinea pig, it was originally planned to carry out the ATS studies in this species. However, marked differences in several acoustic parameters of the middle and inner ears of chinchillas and guinea pigs were demonstrated by Drescher and Eldredge (32), the net effect being a considerably lesser susceptibility of the guinea pig to the same free-field noise. Because the establishment of a complete new set of electrophysiological and anatomical correlates of ATS (not to speak of behavioral data, which are far less reliable in the guinea pig) would have been necessary, it was deemed preferable to carry out the planned biochemical studies on ATS in the chinchilla. This, of course, made necessary establishment of biochemical baseline data in this species. However, most substances investigated to date do not exhibit major species differences [lactic dehydrogenase, glucose 6-phosphate dehydrogenase, ATP, GABA, glutamate, and glycogen, with glycogen exhibiting a gradient rising in apical direction, similar to that in the guinea pig (8)]. The only substance which is markedly different is aspartate; the average steady-state level is about 3 times higher than in the guinea pig and there is a gradient decreasing in apical direction (opposite to that of glycogen) (33).

Since the outer hair cells seem to be the cells most likely to exhibit early biochemical changes due to noise (see ultrastructural changes described above) and since these cells make up a much larger proportion of the OC in the apical regions (where, in addition, the outer hair cell layer can be dissected more readily) we selected the lower of the 2 noise bands that have been studied extensively by other disciplines. This is an octave band centered at 500 Hz, which was presented free-field at an SPL of 95 dB re 0.0002 μbar for 48 hr. This stimulation is known to result in an average threshold shift of 48 to 50 dB at a test frequency of 715 Hz and produces maximum morphological changes in the upper second and lower third turn.

Under the assumption that there is much less variability due to unspecific causes between 2 ears of the same animal than there is between ears of different animals, it appeared advantageous to use 1 ear from each noise-exposed animal as a normal control, since we expected that if any biochemical changes did occur, they would be subtle changes. Therefore, the ossicular chain of the left middle ear was interrupted by removing the malleus and incus in a preliminary operation.[4] This afforded sufficient attenuation (34) to reduce the level of exposure to the control ear to less than 65 dB SPL, which theoretically, by extrapolation, is the lowest level at which ATS occurs.

Although behavioral data suggested that the threshold does not depart significantly from the asymptotic level within the first hour following cessation of stimulation (28), Drescher's (31) recent data, which demonstrate that significant early recovery of the CM does occur, dictate that the biochemical state

---

[4] All noise exposures and preliminary operations in the chinchilla were carried out by Dr. D. H. Eldredge and associates at the Central Institute for the Deaf, St. Louis, Mo.

existing during ATS should be fixed as soon as possible. We have found that the shortest practicable interval from removal of the animal from the noise environment to freezing of the cochleae is about 30 min. If shorter intervals should be required it would become necessary to use a closed sound system analogous to that employed by Drescher (31) in his temperature studies.

Evaluation of potential noise-induced changes becomes more complicated when the substances under study exhibit gradients along the extent of the cochlea. For instance, as mentioned earlier, glycogen would seem to be a promising candidate for quantitative study (10); however, since it exhibits a marked longitudinal gradient in both chinchilla and guinea pig (Fig. 8), and since the longitudinal extent of significant functional and morphological changes produced by the 500 Hz octave noise band at 95 dB SPL is rather narrow (upper second and lower third turn) (29,30) it may be difficult to differentiate subtle changes due to noise from artifacts due to overlap with the preexisting natural gradient. Therefore, we plan to use a broader noise band in the future. This would also be advantageous in the absence of gradients, since more samples per ear would be available for comparative study.

During the course of our studies it became evident that it would be useful to have an animal model available in which pronounced functional changes could be produced within shorter periods of time by exposure to high-intensity noise via a closed system in the anesthetized animals. For practical reasons,

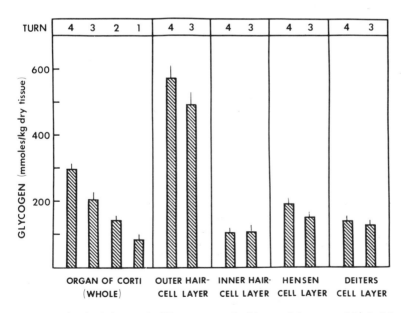

FIG. 8. Steady-state levels of glycogen in different turns and cell layers of the organ of Corti of the guinea pig. For whole organ of Corti the mean ± SEM is given for seven animals (6 to 8 samples per turn). For substructures 2 ears were used with 10 to 12 samples of each layer per turn and per ear. The whole number of subsamples was used in the calculation of the SEM. (Adapted from ref. 35.)

the guinea pig was selected and an exposure of 6 hr was chosen, since an exposure of this duration, including ancillary procedures, can be handled in an average workday. For initial experiments we used essentially the same noise band as in the ATS experiments in the chinchilla. In pilot experiments it was established that the maximum amount of noise to which the ears could be exposed for 6 hr without producing morphological changes of the OC at the light-microscopic level was 115 dB SPL (re 0.0002 μbar) measured at the tympanic membrane with the bulla open. Obvious advantages of this preparation are that various experimental variables can be introduced during exposure (such as temperature changes, hypoxia, application of enzyme inhibitors), if desired in combination with electrophysiological monitoring. In addition, the chemical state can be fixed while the ear is still being exposed to sound.

RESULTS AND DISCUSSION

The biochemical results obtained so far in ATS are disappointing. Preliminary experiments indicate that no significant changes in the maximum *in vitro* activity of lactic dehydrogenase and glucose 6-phosphate dehydrogenase (Table 1) occur in the outer layer[5] of the OC in chinchillas that have undergone an ATS of 48–50 dB. According to the localization of ultrastructural

TABLE 1. *Activity of glucose 6-phosphate dehydrogenase in the outer layer* of the organ of Corti in a chinchilla with asymptotic threshold shift*

Cochlear turn	Control	Exposed
Lower third	1.3	1.6
	1.7	1.6
	1.8	1.7
	1.7	1.7
		1.8
Upper second	1.6	1.9
	1.5	1.4
	1.6	1.8
	1.6	1.7
		1.5
Mean ± SD	1.60 ± 0.14	1.67 ± 0.14

The animal was exposed to an octave band noise centered at 500 Hz at an SPL of 95 dB for 48 hr. The ossicular chain of the "control" ear had been interrupted in a preliminary operation, thereby reducing the effective level of exposure to this ear below 65 dB, considered to be the lowest level at which asymptotic threshold shift occurs. The enzyme activity is expressed in moles per kilogram dry weight per hour.

 * The outer layer of the organ of Corti consists of the outer hair cells, Hensen cells, and Deiters cells.

---

[5] The outer layer of the OC consists of the outer hair cells, Deiters cells, and Hensen cells.

changes the regions investigated were the upper second and lower third turn.

We next analyzed ATP in the outer layer of the OC in a series of experiments, but did not find significant differences between exposed and control ears. Determinations of ATP were initiated also in the outer hair cell layer[6] to eliminate the possibility that subtle changes in the hair cells may be masked when the whole outer layer of the OC was investigated; again, there do not seem to be major differences in ATP levels between exposed and control ears. No data are as yet available on the inner hair cell layer, but, judging from the absence of morphological alterations of the inner hair cells in ATS, the likelihood of detectable biochemical changes is not very high.

It should be remembered that in the ATS experiments an interval of 30 min elapsed from cessation of noise exposure until the chemical state of the cochlea was fixed by rapid freezing. It is conceivable that some recovery of ATP levels may have occurred during this rest period. However, it has been mentioned before that behavioral thresholds do not change and that recovery of the CM is not too significant during a 30-min rest period (31). It therefore seems safe to assume that potential long-term changes in the chemical state of the OC due to ATS would persist to a large extent during such a comparatively short recovery period.

Since these data suggest that any possible alterations of energy generation are not severe enough to cause decompensation with a significant reduction of the steady-state levels of ATP,[7] we next explored the potential effects of ATS upon the putative afferent amino acid transmitters, glutamate and aspartate. Again no significant differences were detectable in the outer layer of the OC in corresponding areas of exposed and unexposed ears; we have not yet explored potential subtle effects at the level of individual cell layers.

The parallel experiments in the guinea pig using high-intensity noise for 6 hr also appear to be negative. Initial data indicate that the steady-state levels of ATP, glutamate, and aspartate overlap in the experimental and the opposite "control" ears (Figs. 9 and 10). The noise level reaching the opposite ear is attenuated by at least 40 dB and, according to pilot experiments, the attenuation may be as high as 60 dB in the frequency band used (D. H. Eldredge, *personal communication*). In order to avoid leakage of sound via air conduction, the ossicular chain of the opposite ear was interrupted. Nevertheless, it is possible that the effective noise level reaching the opposite ear may be above 65 dB SPL, considered to be the lowest level at which ATS occurs. It will therefore be necessary to validate the obtained preliminary results by comparing groups of exposed animals with animals whose ears were not exposed to any potentially damaging noise.

---

[6] The outer hair cell layer consists of the outer hair cells, the phalangeal processes and parts of the Deiters cups.

[7] An unchanged steady state level of ATP could, of course, exist in the presence of a pronounced deficiency of energy generation, if the cells are unable to utilize energy, for instance, for active ion transport.

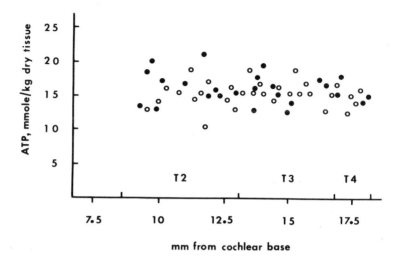

FIG. 9. Steady-state levels of ATP in the outer layer* of the organ of Corti in a guinea pig exposed for 6 hr to an octave band noise centered at 500 Hz in a closed system at 115 dB SPL (*filled circles*). The temporal bone was frozen immediately upon termination of noise stimulation and processed for dissection and chemical analysis as described (12). At this exposure no morphological changes are visible at the light-microscopic level. Exposure at 120 dB SPL results in morphological changes in the lower three-quarters of the third turn and in the upper third of the second turn. The *open circles* refer to the opposite "control" ear. See text for discussion of the validity of this "control."

* The outer layer of the organ of Corti contains the outer hair cells, Hensen cells and Deiters cells.

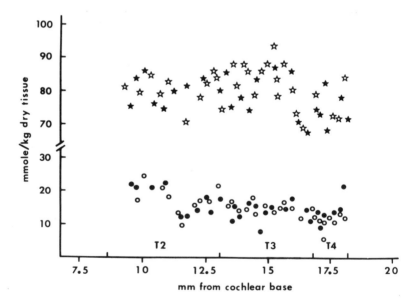

FIG. 10. Steady-state levels of aspartate (*circles*) and glutamate (*stars*) in the outer layer of the organ of Corti in a guinea pig exposed to noise in the same manner as described in Fig. 9 (*filled symbols*). The *open symbols* refer to the opposite "control" ear.

The absence of changes in ATP levels in the OC of ears that have undergone pronounced ATS or short-term exposure to intense noise levels is surprising, although it is known from previous experimentation with total ischemia and application of sodium cyanide that ATP levels are maintained in the OC for considerable periods during metabolic stress (6,8). Recent experiments in the guinea pig indicate that ATP levels in the outer hair cells of the third and fourth cochlear turn are hardly changed during 5 min of ischemia. This is the location where glycogen levels are extremely high (up to 600 mmoles/kg; Fig. 8) (35) and where the mitochondrial density is comparatively low (B. A. Bohne, *personal communication;* Fig. 11). This suggests that the outer hair cells of the upper turns rely strongly upon glycolysis. This is further supported by recent experiments with iodoacetic acid. When the cochlea was perfused with a 5×10^{-3} M solution of this compound in artificial perilymph the initial effects upon ATP levels in the outer layer of the OC were most pronounced in the apical portions of the cochlea (15 min). Only following longer exposure to this agent (30 min) was ATP depleted also in the lower turns.

As mentioned before, we intentionally, and for purely practical reasons, selected for our initial experiments a low-frequency noise band, because the outer hair cells make up a considerably larger portion of the OC in the upper turns, and because it is possible to dissect purer populations of hair cells. It is dangerous, however, to extrapolate from the results obtained in higher turns of the cochlea to the situation in the cochlear base, where the vast majority of available advanced electrophysiological data, in general, and in regard to noise, have been collected. Apart from the well-known morphologic differences of the OC along the extent of the cochlea (Fig. 11), marked biochemical gradients (Figs. 2 and 8) and electrophysiological gradients (endolymphatic potential) (7) do exist. Therefore, in the future it will be important to include biochemical studies on the effects of high-frequency noise. It is understood that low-frequency noise does not stimulate only the apical regions, but that, according to the traveling wave law, the cochlear base is stimulated as well. In fact, according to recent morphologic studies, it appears that the basal parts of the cochlea may be as heavily damaged as the apex by low-frequency, high-intensity noise (Fried et al.) (34).

Quantitative results of the reaction of inner hair cells to ischemia are not yet known for comparison. The inner hair cells contain much smaller amounts of glycogen (Fig. 8) (35) and, judging from morphologic criteria, they are more sensitive to anoxia than the outer hair cells (B. A. Bohne, *personal communication*). This, of course, is in contrast to the situation with respect to noise and most ototoxic agents, which usually injure the outer hair cells first.

Considering the absence of changes in ATP levels in the outer layer of the OC, and the apparent lack of change in the outer hair cells, what should be our future strategy in approaching the noise problem? First, of course, we must confirm the preliminary data on the outer hair cell layer. Next, it would be of interest to investigate whether the rate of glycogenolysis and glycolysis

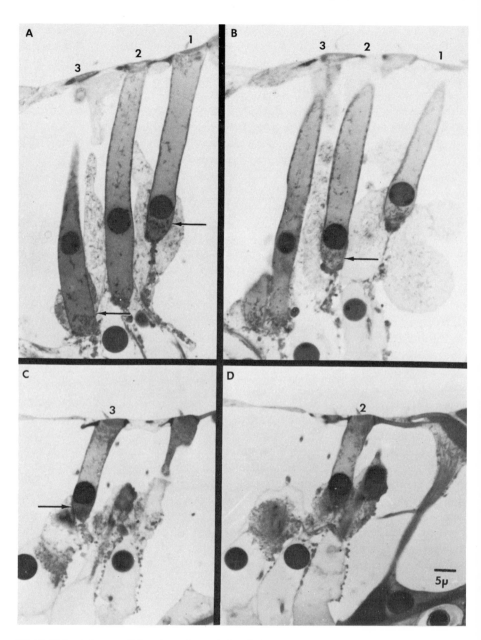

FIG. 11. Stained, 1-μm, radial sections of outer hair cells from a normal guinea pig. Note nuclear position and size of infranuclear group of mitochondria (*arrows*) in cells from different cochlear turns. (A) Lower fourth turn; (B) lower third turn; (C) and (D) lower first turn; (*1*) first row OHC; (*2*) second row OHC; (*3*) third row OHC. (Courtesy B. A. Bohne.)

is indeed increased; this would be reflected by changes in glycogen and lactate levels, in the state of activation of phosphorylase, and in the ratio glucose 6-phosphate/fructose-1,6-diphosphate, which would give indirect evidence about changes in flux at the P-fructokinase step, one of the most important metabolic control points. We should perhaps also pay closer attention to the energy state of the OC, by determining AMP, and in addition, ADP, which would make possible the calculation of the energy charge of the adenylate pool generally considered to be the most representative quantitative measure of the energy state of a given tissue (Atkinson) (36).

$$\text{Energy charge} = \frac{1}{2}\left(\frac{[\text{ADP}] + 2[\text{ATP}]}{[\text{AMP}] + [\text{ADP}] + [\text{ATP}]}\right)$$

The energy charge has not as yet been determined in normal OC; however, no matter what the exact value of the energy charge may be, the constancy of ATP observed in the OC in our preliminary experiments would seem to preclude a *major* reduction of the energy charge due to the types of noise exposures used. This would also follow from the observations of the state of mitochondria of the outer hair cells in ATS, which suggest that the energy charge is high (B. A. Bohne, *personal communication;* Fig. 1).

Of perhaps greater importance will be the determination of P-creatine. P-creatine is the only substance investigated so far in the OC which exhibits significant changes in short-term ischemia or other metabolic interference (Fig. 2). As mentioned earlier, we have not yet analyzed this substance in noise experiments because of its pronounced longitudinal gradient. If P-creatine should exhibit a significant reduction in noise-exposed ears, this would undoubtedly signify a strain upon energy-generating mechanisms, but the question arises whether a potential loss of P-creatine in the presence of near-normal levels of ATP could cause serious functional changes. Jongkind (37) has demonstrated, in the forebrain of the chick embryo, a rapid ischemic loss of electrophysiological activity in close correlation with the decline pattern of P-creatine. By contrast, ATP levels were largely unchanged at a time when electrophysiological responses were completely abolished. In order to account for this apparent paradox, Jongkind proposed a bicompartmental model in which 1 compartment, with a large P-creatine pool, acts as the primary energy source for the maintenance of electrical activity via a negligible "shuttle" pool of ATP, while the large ATP pool in the other compartment is relatively static and not directly involved in the generation of electrical potentials. Under any circumstances, in spite of unchanged overall levels of ATP, subtle changes may exist at discrete locations in the cells, which would not be amenable to quantitative study by the most sensitive available techniques. In fact, there is no reason why alterations of energy *generation* should necessarily be the pathophysiological mechanism of noise action; it is quite possible that energy is made unavailable through interference with energy *utilization,* for instance, by inhibition of active transport processes. In the SV this type of dysfunction has been shown to occur in intoxication with ouabain and salidiuretic drugs, and is reflected by pronounced changes in the endolymphatic potential (38). It is conceivable that similar dysfunctions may prevail in the OC due to aural overload. In fact, if biochemical alterations are at all the basis of the functional effects of noise it could be more profitable to concentrate upon membrane permeability, and transport phenomena mediated, for instance, by cyclic AMP or reflected by changes in phospholipid turnover and calcium homeostasis at the membranes (as discussed in the description of available quantitative biochemical techniques). Again, the presently available resolving power of these techniques may not be sufficient to detect subtle changes.

Several investigators have noticed marked effects of noise upon the SV and even upon the spiral vessel and the vessel of the tympanic lip. As mentioned before, we did not believe it worthwhile to study potential biochemical changes in the SV in our ATS experiments, as, in these preparations, the endolymphatic potential is not impaired. In addition, Duvall et al. (39) demonstrated in a recent article that the changes in the SV due to exposure to high levels of noise were always preceded by changes in the OC. This makes unlikely the proposition that (acute) noise damage to the OC may be due to alterations of the SV and subsequent interference with cochlear homeostasis. However, biochemical investigations of the effects of noise upon the SV may be of great interest in their own right, and because of the extremely active metabolism of this structure, biochemical changes may more readily be detectable by analytical methods presently available.

ACKNOWLEDGMENTS

The author thanks Dr. B. A. Bohne for providing the light and electron-micrographs and Dr. D. H. Eldredge for performing sound exposures and preliminary surgical procedures.

This work was supported by NIH grants RO1 NS 06575 and PO1 NS 11417.

REFERENCES

1. Bornschein, H., and Thalmann, R. (1963): Die Beeinflussung der Cochlearpotentiale durch endocochleare Applikation von Jodazetat. *Experientia,* 19:413–416.
2. Schätzle, W. (1972): *Histochemie des Innenohres.* Urban and Schwarzenberg, Munich, Berlin, Vienna.
3. Vosteen, K. H. (1961): Neue Aspekte zur Biologie und Pathologie des Innenohres. *Arch. Ohren-Nasen-Kehlkopfheilk.,* 178:1–104.
4. Thalmann, I., Matschinsky, F. M., and Thalmann, R. (1970): Quantitative study of selected enzymes involved in energy metabolism of the cochlear duct. *Ann. Otol. Rhinol. Laryngol.,* 79:12–29.
5. Chou, J. T. Y., and Hughes, D. E. (1964): Respirometrie. In: *Biochemie des Hörorgans,* edited by S. S. Rauch, pp. 446–453. Thieme, Stuttgart.
6. Thalmann, R., Miyoshi, T., and Thalmann, I. (1972): The influence of ischemia upon the energy reserves of inner ear tissues. *Laryngoscope,* 82:2249–2272.

7. Kuijpers, W. (1969): Cation transport and cochlear function. Thesis, University of Nijmegen, The Netherlands.
8. Matschinsky, F. M., and Thalmann, R. (1970): Energy metabolism of the cochlear duct. In: *Biochemical Mechanisms in Hearing and Deafness,* edited by M. M. Paparella, pp. 265–288. Charles C Thomas, Springfield. Ill.
9. Hilding, D. A., and Sugiura, A. (1970): Electronmicroscopic histochemistry of the cochlea. In: *Biochemical Mechanisms in Hearing and Deafness,* edited by M. M. Paparella, pp. 137–147. Charles C Thomas, Springfield, Ill.
10. Ishii, D., Takahashi, T., and Balogh, K. (1969): Glycogen in the inner ear after acoustic stimulation. *Acta Otolaryngol.,* 67:573–582.
11. Schnieder, E. A. (1970): Die Entstehung des Schalltraumas. Ein Beitrag über die Physiologie der Perilymphe. Thesis, Würzburg, Germany.
12. Thalmann, R. (1975): Quantitative histochemistry and cytochemistry of the ear. In: *The Handbook of Auditory and Vestibular Research Methods,* edited by C. A. Smith and J. Vernon. Charles C Thomas, Springfield, Illinois. (*in press*).
13. Lowry, O. H., and Passonneau, J. V. (1972): *A Flexible System of Enzymatic Analysis.* Academic Press, New York, and London.
14. Rauch, S. S. (1964): *Biochemie des Hörorgans,* pp. 144–154. Thieme, Stuttgart.
15. Thalmann, R., Thalmann, I., and Comegys, T. H. (1972): Quantitative cytochemistry of the organ of Corti. Dissection, weight determination and analysis of single outer hair cells. *Laryngoscope,* 82:2059–2078.
16. Lowry, O. H., Passonneau, J. V., Hasselberger, F. X., and Schulz, D. (1964): Effect of ischemia on known substrates and cofactors of the glycolytic pathway in the brain. *J. Biol. Chem.,* 239:18–30.
17. Lowry, O. H., and Passonneau, J. V. (1964): The relationships between substrates and enzymes of glycolysis in brain. *J. Biol. Chem.,* 239:31–41.
18. Godfrey, D. A., Carter, J. A., Lowry, O. H., and Matschinsky, F. M. (1975): Levels of putative transmitter amino acids in guinea pig cochlea. (*in preparation*).
19. Orsulakova, A., Stockhorst, E., and Schacht, J. (1975): Effect of neomycin on phosphoinositide labeling and calcium binding in guinea pig inner ear tissues *in vivo* and *in vitro. J. Neurochem.* (*in press*).
20. Steiner, A. L. (1973): Radioimmunoassay for cyclic nucleotides. *Pharmacol. Rev.,* 25:309–313.
21. Ahlström, P., Thalmann, I., Thalmann, R., and Ise, I. (1975): Cyclic AMP and adenylate cyclase in the inner ear. *Laryngoscope,* 85:1241–1258.
22. Neuhoff, V. (1973): *Micromethods in Molecular Biology.* Springer, New York.
23. Oman, S., and Brzin, M. (1972): The magnetic diver microgasometer. *Anal. Biochem.,* 45:112–127.
24. Erulkar, S. D., and Maren, T. H. (1961): Carbonic anhydrase and the inner ear. *Nature,* 189:459–460.
25. Giacobini, E. (1962): A cytochemical study of the localization of carbonic anhydrase in the nervous system. *J. Neurochem.,* 9:169–177.
26. Bosher, S. K. (1974): The significance of the ethacrynate induced changes in endolymph sodium. 11th International Workshop on Inner Ear Biology. Würzburg, Germany.
27. Nakashima, T., Sullivan, M. J., Snow, J. B., and Suga, F. (1970): Sodium and potassium changes in inner ear fluids. *Arch. Otolaryngol.,* 92:1–6.
28. Carder, H. M., and Miller, J. D. (1971): Temporary threshold shifts produced by noise exposure of long duration. *Trans. Am. Acad. Opthalmol. Otolaryngol.,* 75:1346–1354.
29. Benitez, L. D., Eldredge, D. H., and Templer, J. W. (1972): Temporary threshold shifts in chinchilla: Electrophysiological correlates. *J. Acoust. Soc. Am.,* 52:1115–1123.
30. Bohne, B. A. (1973): Anatomical correlates of a temporary shift in the threshold of hearing. *J. Acoust. Soc. Am.,* 53:292.
31. Drescher, D. G. (1974): Noise-induced reduction and recovery of chinchilla cochlear microphonic response. *J. Acoust. Soc. Am.,* 56:S 11.
32. Drescher, D. G., and Eldredge, D. H. (1974): Species differences in cochlear fatigue

related to acoustics of outer and middle ears of guinea pig and chinchilla. *J. Acoust. Soc. Am.,* 56:929–934.

33. Thalmann, R. (1975): Biochemical studies of the auditory system. In: *Human Communication and its Disorders.* Raven Press, New York. (*in press*).
34. Fried, M. P., Dudek, S. E., and Bohne, B. A. (1975): Basal turn cochlear lesions following exposure to low-frequency noise. *Trans. Am. Acad. Opthalmol. Otolaryngol.* (*in press*).
35. Thalmann, R., Thalmann, I., and Comegys, T. H. (1970): Dissection and chemical analysis of substructures of the organ of Corti. *Laryngoscope,* 80:1619–1645.
36. Atkinson, D. E. (1968): The energy charge of the adenylate pool as a regulatory parameter. Interaction with feedback modifiers. *Biochemistry,* 7:4030–4034.
37. Jongkind, J. F. (1971): Biochemical correlates of neural activity. In: *Recent Advances in Quantitative Histochemistry and Cytochemistry,* edited by U. C. Dubach and U. Schmidt, pp. 213–230. H. Huber, Bern, Stuttgart, Vienna.
38. Thalmann, R., Kusakari, J., and Miyoshi, T. (1973): Dysfunctions of energy releasing and consuming processes of the cochlea. *Laryngoscope,* 83:1690–1712.
39. Duvall, A. J., Ward, W. D., and Lauhala, K. E. (1974): Stria ultrastructure and vessel transport in acoustic trauma. *Ann. Otol. Rhinol. Laryngol.,* 83:498–514.
40. Thalmann, R., Miyoshi, T., Kusakari, J., and Thalmann, I. (1973): Quantitative approaches to the ototoxicity problem. *Audiology,* 12:364–382.
41. Thalmann, R. (1971): Metabolic features of auditory and vestibular systems. *Laryngoscope,* 81:1245–1260.

DISCUSSION

D. Henderson: Rudi, you mentioned striking negative results for ATP in hair cells. Have you looked for changes of ATP levels in the stria vascularis?

R. Thalmann: No, not in the stria vascularis. The reason we have not done much in the stria vascularis is because of the absence of changes in the EP in ATS. But I have heard so much from your group and other groups about morphological and vascular changes in the stria, that I think it would perhaps be quite profitable to look at potential biochemical alterations in this tissue. I would think that if there are vascular changes in the stria due to noise, that they would be accompanied by biochemical changes because of the extremely active metabolism of the stria. Any such changes, for instance, a decrease of ATP or P-creatine levels, should be readily detectable in this tissue.

J. Hawkins, Jr.: There is no question as to the importance of biochemical changes. Ours is probably the last of the physiological specialties to apply biochemistry to solving its problems. It was pointed out by Vinnikov and Titova (1), in their well-taken criticisms of the mechanoelectrical theory of cochlear action; not that their substitute for it was particularly good, but it very obviously pointed out that the physical–chemical process involved in transduction in the cells of the organ of Corti must depend upon or be regulated by biochemical changes. Thanks to Drs. Drescher and Thalmann, we are beginning to just scratch the surface of those important events.

I'd like to say that Dr. Thalmann's application of the Lowry biochemical techniques to the problem of cochlear biochemistry is a tremendous contribution to our field. The study of cyclic AMP which is of universal importance in relation to membrane permeability, is a very important aspect of this whole problem.

Finally, I'd like to say that in the guinea pig, even at 90 dB SPL (8 kHz band), after 1 week of exposure that does not alter the CM recorded from the round window, we find scattered hair cell losses in the second turn, or upper basal turn, so that I suspect that over a long period of time that sort of minimal change might be cumulative. Thus changes that don't immediately lead to PTS may gradually add up to one. As for stria vascularis changes, it is only after very long exposure that we see any real evidence of strial atrophy. On the other hand, we do see, after relatively short exposures, especially in the chinchilla, a sort of loosening of stria vascularis, and not the edema of the sort that Ward and Duvall (2) have talked about. Although much of these stria vascularis changes seem to be reversible, they may set off changes in cochlear microhomeostasis that could lead to hair cell loss.

REFERENCES

1. Vinnikov, Ya. A., and Titova, L. K. (1964): *The Organ of Corti: Its Histophysiology and Histochemistry.* Consultants Bureau, New York.
2. Ward, W. D., and Duvall, A. J. (1971): Behavioral and ultrastructural correlates of acoustic trauma. *Ann. Otol. Rhinol. Laryngol.,* 80:881–897.

Part III

Mechanical and Electrophysiological Characteristics of the Ear

Introduction

This section systematically delineates the contribution of the mechanical trans-duction system, the cochlear potentials, and the central auditory nuclei to the profile of symptoms accompanying noise-induced hearing loss.

The electrical response of the cochlea was first reported by Wever and Brey in 1930. Although there is still debate on the exact nature of the endolymphatic potential, the cochlear microphonic, the whole nerve action potential, and the summating potential, it is useful to study their changes following acoustic trauma. Theories have been proposed to explain the development of cochlear lesions; a possible strategy to evaluate these theories is to correlate the developing cochlear lesion and hearing loss with the systematic changes in the cochlear potentials. Conversely, perhaps we can learn more about the role of the cochlear potentials in normal hearing by noting their changes in cochleas with well-defined lesions.

Some of the symptoms associated with noise-induced hearing loss include recruitment, tinnitus, and a truncated temporal integration function. It is now possible to record, from single neurons in the eighth nerve and higher nuclei when the auditory system has been damaged by noise. The chapters by Smith and Evans review the changes in the eighth nerve firing patterns when the cochlea is in a state of either TTS or PTS from drugs or noise. The implications of the single unit studies extend beyond acoustic trauma to other issues in hearing. For example, one basic issue is the difference between the broad mechanical tuning of the basilar membrane and the sharply tuned response of eighth nerve fibers. Why is tuning of the eighth nerve fibers broader following noise and ototoxic drug treatment?

A more practical issue is the problem of implanting hearing aids in patients with large sensorineural hearing losses. Presumably, these patients would have only a fraction of their afferent supply to the cochlea intact and, in order to interface the aid with the patient, it is necessary to learn the limits of performance of the remaining neurons. The final chapter in this section develops the case for a central component to TTS. This is an intriguing idea, because most of the theories about normal phenomena in audition are typically based on cochlear processes. A prac-tical consequence of central TTS relates to the scientific basis for the current DRC. The original CHABA DRC proposal drew heavily on TTS data, despite the fact that there appears to be a low correlation between TTS and PTS. One possible reason for this poor correlation is that TTS involves central as well as peripheral processes.

Effects of Noise on Hearing, edited by Donald Henderson,
Roger P. Hamernik, Darshan S. Dosanjh, and John H. Mills.
Raven Press, New York © 1976

Relationship Between the Transmission Characteristics of the Conductive System and Noise-Induced Hearing Loss

Juergen Tonndorf

College of Physicians and Surgeons, Columbia University, New York, New York 10032

It is customary to list the protection of the inner ear among the various functions of the outer and middle ears. We should therefore examine the question if the 2 latter portions of the ear are able to provide such protection against the effects of intense and sustained noises as they typically occur in industrial environments.

For the purpose of this discussion, I would like to differentiate between passive protection and active protection. *Passive* protection is provided by the nonlinearities of the transmitting systems, both in the frequency domain (i.e., bandpass limitation) and in the amplitude domain (i.e., amplitude limitation, with its corollary, nonlinear distortion). The latter is potentially interesting from the standpoint of the cochlea in which energy is concentrated upon a limited region along the cochlear partition due to the traveling-wave event. If nonlinear distortion would indeed occur in the middle ear, energy would be distributed over wider frequency bands and hence also spread over a wider region along the cochlear partion. *Active* protection refers to any means by which outer and middle ears might actively interfere with the transmission of energy. The middle-ear reflex is the prime example.

PASSIVE PROTECTION

External Ear

First, we shall discuss 2 passive effects that have to do with the external ear and are due (i) to the diffraction of sound by the head and the pinna, and (ii) to the resonance of the ear canal. These phenomena were first described by Wiener and Ross (1) and have since been largely confirmed by Shaw (2,3) who elaborated on their underlying mechanisms in great detail.

Diffractional Effects

We note from Fig. 1 that the sound pressure in front of the tympanic membrane (TM), in reference to that in the free field, depends upon the azimuthal

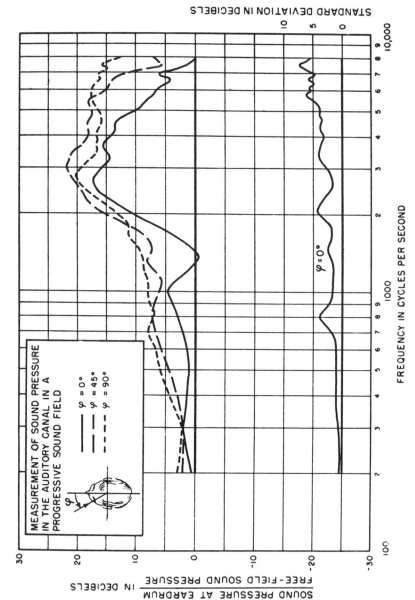

FIG. 1. The ratio between sound pressure at the TM and that in the free-field for 3 azimuthal angles. The phase relation is given for only 1 angle, i.e., $\phi = 0°$. (From ref. 1, with permission.)

angle. This sound pressure ratio is smallest when the sound source is in front of the observer (grazing incidence to the ear) and highest when the sound source faces the ear directly (perpendicular incidence). With frequency, differences vary between 5 and 10 dB (Fig. 1). As a consequence of this finding, CHABA (4) recommended that, for grazing incidence, noise levels might be 10 dB higher than for perpendicular incidence. Experimental animals, when being exposed to noise, are usually quick in learning which head position results in minimal sound pressure at their TMs, and they often maintain that position rigidly throughout the exposure period (5). However, it should be noted that in a hard-walled room the sound pressure is practically uniform, and there is no dependence on the angle of incidence. Consequently, there is no advantage in one head position over the other.

Canal Resonance

Figure 1 shows the resonance of the ear canal which occurs around 3 kHz and slightly below it, the exact frequency depending on the angle of incidence. As a consequence of this resonance, for frequencies around 3 kHz, the sound pressure in front of the TM increases by a whole order of magnitude over that existing in the free field. Threshold shifts induced by pure tones are well known to be maximal in the frequency region about ½ octave higher than the stimulating frequency. After exposure to industrial noises, audiometric curves show a characteristic notch at around 4 kHz (Fig. 2). The ½ octave point below that frequency is 2.84 kHz. It is quite conceivable, therefore, that the 4-kHz notch is causally linked to the elevation of sound pressure around 3 kHz in front of the TM, due to canal resonances. Other explanations for this notch given in the past include the following:

1. According to Guild and coworkers (7), there might be an insufficient blood supply at the boundary between the supply regions of the 2 cochlear arteries, i.e., in the middle of the first cochlear turn; this happens to be the place of reception of 4 kHz.

2. According to Hilding (8), there might be mechanical effects due to fluid streaming produced by AC stapedial displacements; because of the cochlear coiling, such streaming was thought to impinge upon the organ, once more in the middle of the first turn.

3. According to Schuknecht and Tonndorf (9), the accelerations the cochlear duct is undergoing might be maximalized in the same region, i.e., where the speed of propagation of the traveling wave is still sufficiently high and the amplitude of displacement is beginning to build up.

The present explanation is attractively simple and logical and thus may be superior to the 3 others just mentioned.

The basal-turn hair cells, mainly the outer ones, are known to be especially susceptible to a variety of other agents, e.g., some antibiotics. Although it may

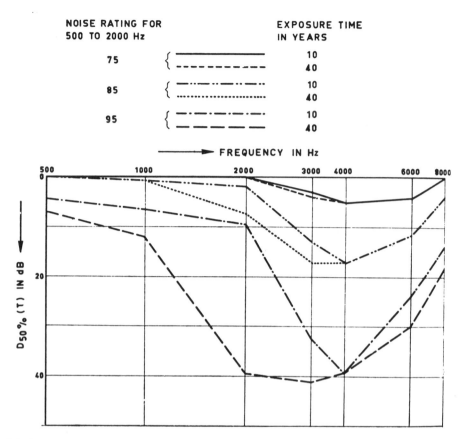

FIG. 2. The noise-induced part of the change in the median hearing level (D$_{50\%}$) for exposure to durations (T) of 10 and 40 years *versus* frequency. Note that the noise rating (NR) closely corresponds to the dB(A) level. (From ref. 6, with permission.)

well be a contributing factor, this increased, possibly metabolic, susceptibility cannot be the sole cause of the noise-induced 4-kHz notch, for it would not account for the relatively greater resistance of 6 and 8 kHz to noise exposure (Fig. 2).

Conclusions

With respect to the effects of the external canal we may thus state that, except for the decrease in sound pressure at the TM by 10 dB for grazing incidence, it does not afford any tangible protection against noise at levels encountered in industrial situations. On the contrary, by elevating the sound pressure at the TM around 3 kHz, it may well be the main cause of the noise-induced 4-kHz notch.

Middle Ears

Amplitude-Dependent Nonlinearities

The next question we shall discuss concerns the potential role of amplitude-dependent nonlinearities of the middle ear in the protection of the inner ear. If you would have broached this question to Helmholtz, his answer would have been strongly in the affirmative, for he did not believe that a purely mechanical system, like the middle ear, would possess a wide dynamic range. Helmholtz considered the middle ear to be the source of all the amplitude-dependent nonlinearities displayed by the ear. However, as was first demonstrated by Lewis and Reger (10), and since then confirmed by many others, using a variety of different approaches, it is really the cochlea which is the place of origin of most aural distortion products. [For a recent discussion, see Pfeiffer and Kim (11).]

The generation of subharmonics by the TM (12,13) occurs over very limited amplitude and frequency regions. It is therefore of no practical significance from the present standpoint.

Contrary to Helmholtz's expectations, the middle ear turned out to be a system with an amazingly wide linear range. In the midfrequencies, it reaches up to 140 dB SPL (sound pressure level), or even higher (14,15). By contrast, cochlear distortion manifests itself at about 75 dB SPL (16,17).

Curiously enough, it was Helmholtz (18) who first recognized one of the reasons why the middle ear should not be prone to nonlinear distortions. He pointed out that the TM, with its exponential cone shape, ought to resist mechanical membrane "breakup," the usual source of distortion in vibrating membranes. He also argued that the displacement amplitudes could never become large enough to reverse the direction of curvature of the TM. Recent quantitative studies have confirmed these notions (15,19).

Stapediovestibular joint

Békésy (20) pointed to another potential protective mechanism which must be mentioned in this connection. At amplitudes "below the threshold of feeling," i.e., at about 130 dB SPL, he found the displacement of the stapes footplate to occur around an axis running *vertically* near its posterior edge (Fig. 3a). That is to say, the footplate was being displaced like a door around a vertical hinge. [Observations by Guinan and Peake (14) in cats, which seemed to contradict Békésy's findings, may have their explanation in the fact that the stapediovestibular joint is differently structured in the 2 species (21).]

At higher amplitudes—apparently when the incudal displacements were large enough to include a sizable vertical component—there was an additional, rotational mode of displacement, this time around a *horizontal* axis that ran through the middle of the footplate. Such seesawlike motions should tend to minimize the resultant volume displacement of the cochlear fluids, and thus

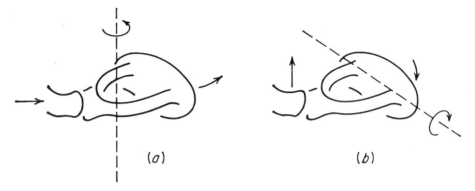

FIG. 3. Modes of stapedial vibrations. a: At SPLs of approximately 130 dB. b: At SPLs of approximately 140 dB. (From ref. 20, with permission.)

"protect" the inner ear. They would also introduce even-harmonic distortion.

If this secondary mode appeared above 130 dB SPL, as Békésy stated, i.e., perhaps at 140 dB, it is clear that it is of little, if any, significance for the protection of the inner ear at noise levels encountered in industrial situations.

Conclusions

Taken as a whole, we must conclude that middle-ear distortion in the amplitude domain does not provide any appreciable protection for the inner ear at industrial noise levels.

Frequency-Dependent Nonlinearities

Let us now take a look at nonlinearities in the frequency domain. Customarily, middle-ear function is given in terms of its displacement transfer function, which is the only practical way it can be assessed. This function is frequency-independent at low frequencies, dropping off with 12 dB/octave above ~1.5 kHz. It stands to reason, however, that displacement (charge in electrical terms!) is not the best way to indicate the power admitted to a given system or that transmitted through it. One can either use mallar displacement data, or those of middle-ear impedance, to calculate, under some simplifying assumptions, the *power* admitted to the middle ear (22).

The mechanoacoustic power (P_{ac}) entering a given system is the product of the complex sound pressure (p) acting upon that system, and the resultant complex volume velocity (v), times the cosine of the phase angle (ϕ) between them:

$$P_{ac} = pv \cos \phi \qquad (1)$$

The sound pressure can be measured directly. The volume velocity can only be assessed indirectly. If one obtained acoustic impedance data (Z_{ac}), the volume velocity for any pressure value is given as

$$v = pZ_{ac} \qquad (2)$$

If one obtained displacement data (d) and measured also the area, A (of the TM in the present case), the volume velocity for a given frequency (f) is given as

$$v = dA(2\pi f) \qquad (3)$$

provided the displacement is that of a rigid piston or at least a reasonable approximation thereof (22).

Figure 4a presents the results of 2 such calculations for the cat, and Fig. 4b for man, using displacement data and impedance data. Admittedly, the fit between the power admission data and the auditory threshold curve is not perfect. The reasons for these shortcomings are partly in measurement errors and partly in the underlying assumptions: (i) in live animals, phase measurements cannot be obtained with sufficient accuracy; especially when the angle is around 90°, i.e., when cos ϕ approaches zero, even small errors in phase angle have profound effects upon the results; (ii) it is recalled that the power calculated is that admitted *to* the ear, not that transmitted *through* it; there are insertion losses, especially in the TM, since it is not displaced like a piston (19), and also in both ossicular joints (24,25). However, crude as these calculations probably are, they suggest that the shape of the sensitivity curve, both at the low-frequency and at the high-frequency ends, is primarily determined by the admission of energy to the middle ear.

The reason for the low-frequency limitation in the middle ear lies mainly in the fact that the oval window/stapes footplate mechanism is capacitative in nature. In the cat, for example, the impedance was found to decrease with frequency at -12 dB/octave for $f < 630$ Hz (26).

Incudomallar joint

If results obtained in cats are valid for man, there may be some added protection at very low frequencies (25). As was just mentioned, the impedance of the oval window/stapes footplate mechanism increases with inverse frequency at 12 dB/octave for $f < 630$ Hz. At $f < 100$ Hz it thus becomes more than 100 times higher than it is at 1 kHz. Impedance must then be so high that, as shown in Fig. 5, the incudomallar joint begins slipping, suggesting that the latter may represent a friction-coupled joint.

This slippage at very low frequencies may, to some extent, attenuate the low-frequency effects upon the auditory system, but also upon the vestibular system (27); this should include protection against the slow-acting (low-frequency) pressure fluctuation caused by explosions. We must note in this regard that, as the power of rocket engines is increased, their maximal acoustic output is shifted to lower and lower frequencies. Typical figures for current space propulsion rockets are in the range of 10 Hz and less (27).

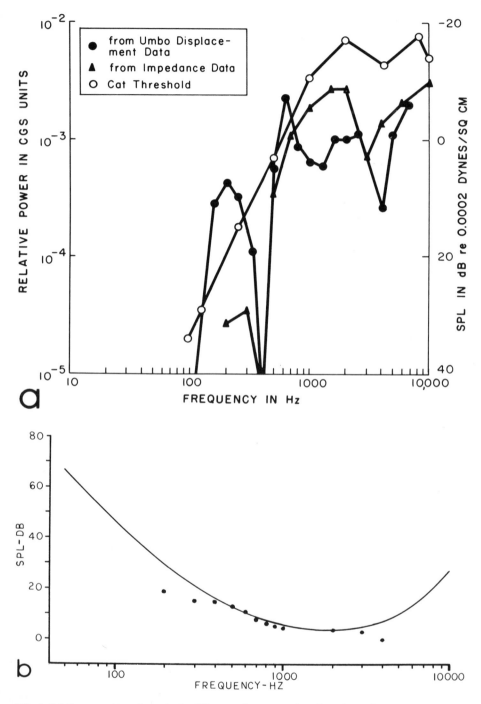

FIG. 4. Relative power transfer onto the TM versus frequency plotted on the auditory threshold curve. a: Calculated from umbo displacement data and impedance data obtained in cats (from ref. 22). b: Same as a, but calculated from human impedance data (from ref. 23).

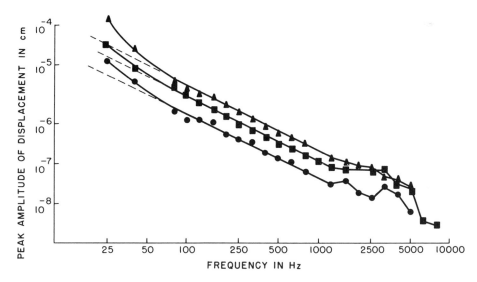

FIG. 5. Displacements of the manubrium mallei mechanically driven at the umbo for a constant CM output versus frequency. Results from 3 different cats. There was also a phase lag cumulating with inverse frequency at f < 100 Hz. When the stapes was driven in the same manner, the curves remained straight at the low-frequency end. These results were only obtained in young animals. (From ref. 25, with permission.)

Conclusions

The middle ear, due to its frequency limitation, must provide *some* protection to the inner ear at the low-frequency end and also at the high-frequency end. This protection finds its tangible expression in the use of the dB(A) scale of sound level meters, instead of the dB(C) scale, for the estimation of noise-exposure magnitudes.

ACTIVE PROTECTION

Many mammals (e.g., horses and dogs) can turn their pinnae to reduce the admission of sound into the ear canal. Some other mammals (e.g., seals) are able to close their ear canals tightly. These faculties are obviously lost in man.

Stapediovestibular Joint

The oval window/stapes footplate mechanism is part of the conductive system of the ear. Using time-averaged holography, Khanna and Tonndorf (28) have found evidence in cats for a *dynamic* increase in impedance at this point, especially at low frequencies, when very high-sound pressure levels, i.e., SPLs > 140 dB, were acting directly on the footplate. The middle ear had been amputated beforehand. This increase in impedance was only observed in *live* animals, never in cadavers. The increase occurred in inverse relation to frequency. Although the effect appeared to outlast the signal for some time, no time courses can so far be given, since the method, time-averaged holography, does not lend itself to the obtaining of such information. Therefore, these findings are still tentative.

Middle Ear Muscles Reflex

There is no question that contractions of the 2 muscles of the middle ear, the *tensor tympani* and the *stapedius,* are capable of attenuating middle-ear transmission, especially for brief periods of time. Much of the available information stems from experimental animals, notably cats and bats, which are capable of producing more powerful contractions of these muscles than those found in man. In cats and in some other animals, the tensor tympani is a thick broad-based muscle, and in man, where it is housed in a bony canal, it is a fusiform muscle. Fusiform muscles are known to execute large contractions, which, however, are not very powerful. Also, the distributions of thin and thick fibers differ significantly in the 2 types (29).

Experimental Animals

Short-term effects

In bats (30) optimal attenuations concomitant with their own voicing averaged around 18 dB, with the contractions becoming quickly less even over brief time spans of 3–4 msec. (In these animals, the middle-ear muscles contract synchronously with the laryngeal muscles. This arrangement serves to protect the ear while the cry is being issued which echo the ear must receive some 10 msec later: animal sonar.)

The mechanism underlying the attenuation effect, at least for the stapedius, was revealed in observations on humans by Zwislocki (24). On activation of the stapedius, the middle-ear impedance decreased, indicating the occurrence of a partial decoupling in the incudostapedial joint when the head of the stapes is being pulled sideways upon muscular action. Whether or not the resultant tilting of the footplate in the oval window may itself lead to functional stapes fixation cannot be decided with certainty (31). The fact that there is attenuation not only for air-conducted sounds, but also for bone-conducted sounds, could be solely accounted for by the elimination of the middle-ear bone conduction component on decoupling of the incudostapedial joint. The occurrence of a Carhart notch is not limited to stapedial fixation. It is observed whenever the middle ear is functionally separated from the inner ear (32).

Figure 6 shows the efficiency of the reflexes of both muscles in the cat. It is seen that, while, at a level of 85 dB SPL, the tensor tympani has practically no effect at any frequency, the stapedius provides 10–20 dB attenuation at low frequencies to reach near zero at high frequencies. In the cat, the threshold of the reflex of both muscles acting together is at 45 dB SPL (33); in man, it varies between 70 and 100 dB SPL with a mean around 85 dB (34).

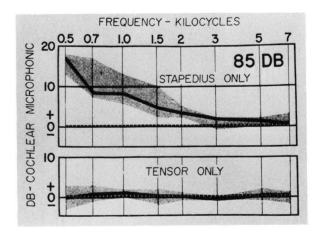

FIG. 6. Attenuation of middle-ear transmission versus frequency observed at an approximate SPL of 85 dB. Results were obtained by comparing the CM output in awake cats with that obtained in the same animals in deep general anesthesia. Median values and interquartile ranges are given. (From ref. 33, with permission.)

Long-term effects

The effects of relatively long-lasting, high-intensity stimulation upon the reflexes in feline ears were studied by Simmons (35,5). Attenuation values were assessed by comparing the round window cochlear microphonic or the N_1 (click) responses, measured in awake animals, with those obtained after putting the same animals into deep general anesthesia and thus eliminating the reflexes. After an initial and rather powerful contraction, lasting for a mere fraction of a second, the muscles relaxed rapidly during the first 30 sec to reach finally a steady-state contraction, although some fluctuations were going on all the time, apparently due to chewing and/or swallowing on the part of the animals. Figure 7 shows both the initial and terminal values and their between-animal variations for SPLs between 45 and 115 dB. At 75 dB, for example, the initial attenuation was as high as 20 dB, but the terminal one was a mere 5 dB.

The same group of animals, whose results are shown in Fig. 7, were then exposed to 1 kHz and 135 dB SPL for 2 hr. Also included in this second experiment was a number of animals in which either muscle, or both, had been surgically severed beforehand.

Temporary threshold shift (TTS) and its recovery were measured in terms of the cochlear microphonic (CM) responses to 2-kHz test tones and clicks (Fig. 8A), and of the N_1 (click) responses (Fig. 8B). As regards the CM responses, the unoperated animals showed an initial TTS on the order of 25–30 dB which recovered fully, usually within 1 or 2 days, although individual variations were considerable. For the N_1 (click) responses, variations were still wider, the initial TTSs were larger, but the recovery progressed more

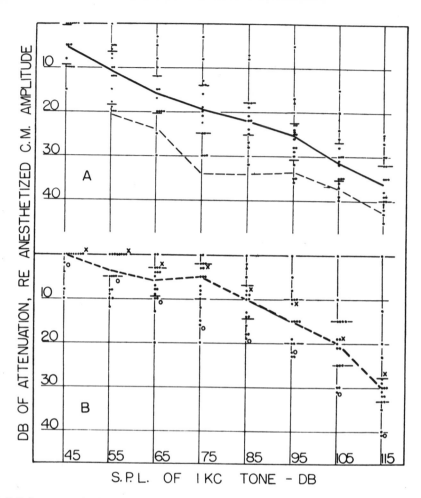

FIG. 7. Reflex attenuation in response to a 1 kHz stimulus versus signal level. A: Initial value. B: Terminal value after 30 sec. An animal with poorly maintained contractions (✕) showed a CM loss of 45 dB and a N_1 loss of more than 70 dB measured 45 min postexposure (1 kHz, 135 dB SPL for 2 hr). Conversely, an animal with good contractions (○) showed only a CM loss of 15 dB and a N_1 loss of 35 dB, 20 min postexposure. (From ref. 5, with permission.)

quickly. There were good correlations between the results of Figs. 7 and 8. That is to say, animals that had shown good attenuation values (Fig. 7), as a rule, displayed minimal TS (Fig. 8) and vice versa. All animals in which one of the muscles had been severed grouped with those most severely affected among the nonoperated animals. Their initial TTSs were larger, ~40–44 dB, and recoveries were delayed up to 40 days. In the 2 animals in which both muscles had been severed, the initial TTS was most severe, beyond the range of the testing equipment, i.e., larger than 80 dB, with little or no recovery up to the limit of 40 days.

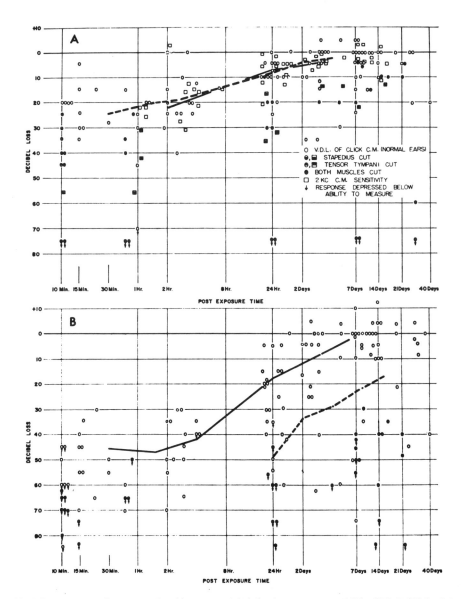

FIG. 8. Depression and recovery of cochlear potentials following exposure to 1 kHz, 135 dB SPL for 2 hr. A (*solid line*): mean changes of the CM responses to 2 kHz; (*dashed line*): mean changes of the click response (VDL, visual detection level); B: mean changes of the N_1 response (VDL); (*solid line*): mean changes for 16 normally muscled ears; (*dashed line*): mean changes for 5 ears with more severe losses. (From ref. 5, with permission.)

Short-Term Protection in Man

Fletcher and Riopelle (36) found a practical application for the short-term protection provided by the middle-ear muscle reflex, i.e., for the protection of the ears of riflemen on the rifle range. Since the latency of the reflex in man is on the order of 10 msec, and thus too slow for signals with fast rise times, Fletcher and Riopelle employed a preactivating signal. A brief tone of 1 kHz and 100 dB SPL was switched on, 200 msec prior to each firing of 1 round from a machine gun, and it was kept on until the gun had been fired. The resulting TTS after 100 rounds turned out to be significantly smaller than it had been without the preactivation of the reflex.

Long-Term Protection in Man

The question as to how these results can be extrapolated for exposures of 8 hr/day, 5 days/week, and for extended time periods should be approached with some caution. In some of his cats, Simmons (5) found the reflex quite stable with time. In others, it varied considerably from day to day. In still others, there was clear evidence for habituation, i.e., the attenuation became less with time. An example of the latter group is shown in Fig. 9.

One promising approach to this problem seemed to be to look at the effects of noise exposure in persons after unilateral stapedectomy and the concomitant loss of the stapedius muscle. Kos (37) reported 2 cases in which rifle firing or tractor driving seemed to have contributed to a fast-developing, high-frequency hearing loss in the operated ear. Later studies were unable to confirm Kos' findings. Steffen et al. (38) saw *some* large variations in TTS, but these are also found in normal ears. Likewise, Ferris (39,40) and Smith (41) found no evidence that stapedectomized ears would be more sensitive to the effects of noise exposure than are normal ears.

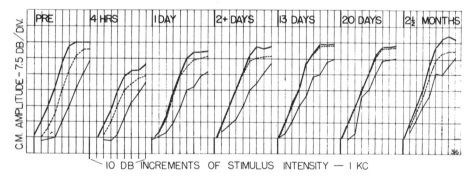

FIG. 9. CM input/output curves taken at the days indicated, following sound exposure (1 kHz, 135 dB SPL for 2 hr). At each level, 10 dB apart, responses were obtained to 1 kHz tones of 60 sec duration. (*Solid lines*): animal deeply anesthetized; (*dashed lines*): animal awake; (*thin solid lines*): responses immediately following each 1 min exposure. Note the habituation with time. (From ref. 5, with permission.)

Conclusions

Taken as a whole, it does not appear that reflex contractions of the middle-ear muscles during exposure to noise of long duration, e.g., for 8 hr/day, afford a substantial protection of the inner ear. Habituation, fatigability over long periods of time, and the long latency of the reflex may all be contributing to this failure.

MIDDLE EAR LESIONS—PROTECTION

One should also mention the attempts that have been repeatedly made during the past 50 years, i.e., to allow people with chronic middle-ear disorders to work in noise. This was based upon the belief that their inner ears would be well protected against the effects of noise exposure.

Although not directly related to the problem at hand, there is one obvious advantage: Willis' paracusis. In persons with conductive losses, both the noise and the signal are attenuated. Since everybody else speaks louder in the presence of noise, the signal to noise (S/N) ratio is then improved for such people. I have repeatedly observed this phenomenon in persons with a degree of conductive loss that ordinarily required them to use a hearing aid. In noise, they were able to carry on a conversation unaided and without apparent difficulty.

The only large-scale study in regard to the above problem that I know of was made by Temkin (42) in Russia. An appreciable number of workmen in a large industrial population had chronic middle-ear infections. Temkin found that the onset of sensorineural hearing losses was delayed and its extent made smaller, but only in those subjects in whom the infection was completely quiescent. When the infection was still active, sensorineural hearing losses developed at a rate that was often faster than was seen in normal-hearing workmen. In other words, not only was there no protection of the inner ear, but cochlear lesions were aggravated.

The explanation for the latter observation could be in a recent finding by Arnold and von Ilberg (43). According to these authors, the lymphatic vessels of the middle-ear mucosa are in direct communication with the perilymph of scala tympani via the round-window membrane. Vibrations could conceivably aid in letting toxic material pass from the middle ear into the perilymph, leading to a circumscribed labyrinthitis.

MIDDLE EAR—COMPLEX NETWORK

The fact that the middle ear is simultaneously capable of transmitting a maximum of the incident energy at low levels, while reducing transmission at higher levels, is, in last analysis, due to its complex structure. The middle ear does not only act as an impedance-matching transformer, but it represents a complex network (44,24,45). Decoupling and/or mismatching may occur at various places when the input sound pressure becomes too large.

SUMMARY

1. Protection of the inner ear against exposure to industrial noise levels was examined separately for passive and active effects.

2. Passive protection

a. Diffraction around head and pinna and the resulting directivity account for a reduction in sound pressure at the TM of up to 10 dB for grazing incidence as compared to perpendicular incidence, but only in a free field.

b. The resonance of the ear canal elevates the sound pressure at the TM by as much as 20 dB in the region of 3 kHz. This elevation is suggested to be the main cause of the audiometric 4-kHz notch, typically found after noise exposure.

c. Middle-ear amplitude distortion does not occur until SPLs of approximately 140 dB are reached.

d. Distortions in the frequency domain produce some limitations both at the low- and high-frequency ends, justifying the use of the dB(A) scale of sound level meters for the estimation of the incidence of noise-induced threshold shifts and their magnitude.

e. The mode change in stapedial displacement, which might conceivably limit the resulting volume displacement of the cochlear fluids, does not occur until SPLs of 140 dB are exceeded.

3. Active protection

a. A dynamic dependence of inner-ear impedance, especially for low frequencies, on SPL might, if confirmed, have a marginal effect. So far, it has only been observed in cats after amputation of the middle ear.

b. Reflex contractions of the middle ear, although affording short-term protection, do not appear to be effective with respect to long-duration exposures due to habituation, fatigability, and the long latency of the reflex.*

4. Allowing persons with conductive lesions to work in noise was advocated in the past because of the built-in "protection." An older survey indicated that, with chronic middle-ear infections, this is permissible only if the

---

* During the conference, Dr. A. R. Møller drew my attention to several recent studies done under his direction on the function of the middle-ear muscles. Of particular interest to the present problem is a paper by J. E. Zakrisson (*Acta Otolaryngol.,* 79:1–10, 1975). The author examined the TTS produced by 2 different, one-third octave band noises, one centered around 0.5 kHz, the other around 2.0 kHz, in patients with unilateral stapedius muscle paralysis caused by Bell's palsy. Results were compared to the TTS produced in normal ears and/or that in the same ears after recovery. Zakrisson found that the stapedius muscle reflex reduces the TTS in the low frequencies, but does not affect that occurring at higher frequencies, the implication being that the stapedial muscle reflex does protect the ear against damage caused by *low*-frequency noise exposure.

disease is completely quiescent. If it is still active, noise exposure may aggravate the occurrence of hearing loss.

5. From all available evidence, one is forced to conclude that the outer and middle ear were not designed as protective devices for the inner ear with present industrial noise exposure in mind.

REFERENCES

1. Wiener, F. M., and Ross, D. A. (1946): The pressure distribution in the auditory canal in a progressive sound field. *J. Acoust. Soc. Am.,* 18:401–408.
2. Shaw, E. A. G. (1973): Sound pressure transformation from the free field to the eardrum. *J. Acoust. Soc. Am.,* 53:291.
3. Shaw, E. A. G. (1974): The external ear. In: *Handbook of Sensory Physiology,* Vol. 7, edited by W. D. Keidel and W. D. Neff, pp. 455–490. Springer-Verlag, Berlin.
4. Kryter, K. D., Daniels, R., Fair, P., Fletcher, J. L., Garinther, G., Hodge, D. C., Kraul, C. W., Loeb, M., Harris, D., Parrack, H. O., Donley, R., Eldredge, D., Miller, J. D., and Ward, W. D. (1965): *Hazardous Exposure to Intermittent and Steady-state Noise.* Report of working group 46, NAS–NRC Committee on Hearing, Bioacoustics, and Biomechanics (CHABA), ORN Contract NONR 2300 (05).
5. Simmons, F. B. (1963): Individual sound damage susceptibility: role of the middle ear muscles. *Ann. Otol. Rhinol. Laryngol.,* 72:528–548.
6. Passchier-Vermeer, W. (1971): Steady-state and fluctuating noise: its effect on the hearing of people. In: *Occupational Hearing Loss,* edited by D. W. Robinson, pp. 15–33. Academic Press, London.
7. Crow, S. J., Guild, S. R., and Polvogt, L. M. (1934): Observations on pathology of high-tone deafness. *Johns Hopkins Med. J.,* 54:315–379.
8. Hilding, A. C. (1953): Studies on otic labyrinth: anatomic explanation for hearing dip at 4,096 Hz characteristic of acoustic trauma and presbycusis. *Ann. Otol. Rhinol. Laryngol.,* 62:950–956.
9. Schuknecht, H. F., and Tonndorf, J. (1960): Acoustic trauma of the cochlea from ear surgery. *Laryngoscope,* 70:479–505.
10. Lewis, D., and Reger, S. N. (1933): An experimental study of the role of the tympanic membrane and the ossicles in the hearing of certain subjective tones. *J. Acoust. Soc. Am.,* 5:153–158.
11. Pfeiffer, R. R., and Kim, D. O. (1973): Considerations of nonlinear response properties of single cochlear nerve fibers. In: *Basic Mechanism in Hearing,* edited by A. Møller, pp. 555–592, Academic Press, New York.
12. von Gierke, H. E. (1950): Subharmonics generated in human and animal ears. *J. Acoust. Soc. Am.,* 22:675.
13. Dallos, P., and Linnell, C. O. (1966): Subharmonic components in cochlear microphonic potentials. *J. Acoust. Soc. Am.,* 40:4–11.
14. Guinan, J., and Peake, W. T. (1967): Middle-ear characteristics of anesthetized cats. *J. Acoust. Soc. Am.,* 41:1237–1261.
15. Tonndorf, J., and Khanna, S. M. (1972): Tympanic-membrane vibrations in human cadaver ears studied by time-averaged holography. *J. Acoust. Soc. Am.,* 52:1221–1233.
16. Fletcher, H. (1929): *Speech and Hearing.* Van Nostrand, New York.
17. Lawrence, M., and Yantis, P. A. (1956): Onset and growth of aural harmonics in the overloaded ear. *J. Acoust. Soc. Am.,* 28:852–858.
18. Helmholtz, H. (1868): Die Mechanik der Gehörknöchelchen und des Trommelfells. *Pfluegers Arch.,* 1:1–60.
19. Khanna, S. M., and Tonndorf, J. (1972): Tympanic membrane vibrations in cats studied by time-averaged holography. *J. Acoust. Soc. Am.,* 51:1904–1920.
20. Békésy, G. von (1936): Zur Physik des Mittelohres und über das Hören bei fehlerhaftem Trommelfell. *Akust. Beih.,* 1:13–23 [quoted from: *Experiments in Hearing,* McGraw-Hill, 1960].

21. Bolz, A., and Lim, D. J. (1972): Morphology of the stapediovestibular joint. *Acta Otolaryngol.* (*Stockh.*), 73:10–17.
22. Khanna, S. M., and Tonndorf, J. (1969): Middle ear power transfer. *Arch. Hals Heilkd.* 193:78–88.
23. Khanna, S. M.: Unpublished data.
24. Zwislocki, J. J. (1962): Analysis of the middle-ear function: Part I: input impedance. *J. Acoust. Soc. Am.,* 34:1514–1523.
25. Tonndorf, J., and Khanna, S. M. (1967): Some properties of sound transmission in the middle and outer ears of cats. *J. Acoust. Soc. Am.,* 41:513–521.
26. Tonndorf, J., Khanna, S. M., and Fingerhood, B. J. (1966): The input impedance of the inner ear in cats. *Ann. Otol. Rhinol. Laryngol.,* 75:752–763.
27. Alford, B. R., Jerger, J. F., Coats, A. C., Billingham, V., French, B. O., and McBrayer, R. O. (1966): *Trans. Am. Acad. Ophthalmol. Otolaryngol.,* 71:40–47.
28. Khanna, S. M., and Tonndorf, J. (1972): The vibratory pattern of the round window in cats. *J. Acoust. Soc. Am.,* 50:1475–1483.
29. Candiollo, L. (1965). Ricerche anatomo-comparativo sul musculo tensore, con riferimento alla innervazione propriocettiva. *Z. Zellforsch.,* 67:34–56.
30. Henson, O. Jr. (1966): The activity and function of the middle-ear muscles in echo-locating bats. *J. Physiol.* (*Lond.*), 180:871–887.
31. Simmons, F. B. (1975): Personal communication.
32. Tonndorf, J. (1970): Cochlear mechanics and hydrodynamics. In: *Foundations of Modern Auditory Theory,* edited by J. V. Tobias, Vol. I, pp. 203–259. Academic Press, New York.
33. Simmons, F. B. (1959): Middle ear muscles activity at moderate sound levels. *Ann. Otol. Rhinol. Laryngol.,* 58:1126–1143.
34. Jerger, J., Jerger, S., and Mauldin, L. (1972): Studies in impedance audiometry, I: normal and sensorineural ears. *Arch. Otolaryngol.,* 96:513–523.
35. Simmons, F. B. (1960): Middle ear muscle protection from the acoustic trauma of loud continuous sound. *Ann. Otol. Rhinol. Laryngol.,* 59:1063–1071.
36. Fletcher, J. L., and Riopelle, A. J. (1959): Effect of a loud pre-exposure tone on TTS resulting from impulsive noise. *J. Acoust. Soc. Am.,* 31:831.
37. Kos, C. M. (1962): Experience with vein plug stapedioplasty in otosclerotic hearing loss. In: *Otosclerosis,* edited by H. F. Schuknecht, pp. 496–508. Little, Brown, Boston, Mass.
38. Steffen, T. N., Nixon, J. C., and Glorig, A. (1963): Stapedectomy and noise. *Laryngoscope,* 73:1044–1060.
39. Ferris, K. (1965): On the temporary effect of industrial noise on the hearing at 4000 c/s of stapedectomized ears. *J. Laryngol. Otol.,* 79:881–887.
40. Ferris, K. (1966): The temporary effects of 125 c/s octave-band noise on stapedectomized ears. *J. Laryngol. Otol.,* 80:579–582.
41. Smith, M. F. W. (1975): personal communication.
42. Temkin, J. (1933): Die Schädigung des Ohres durch Lärm und Erschütterung. *Monatsschr. Ohrenheilk. Laryngo-Rhinol.,* 67:257–299; 450–479; 527–553; 705–736; 823–834. [English translation in Transl. of the *Belt. Inst. Hear. Res.,* No. 27, July, 1973.]
43. Arnold, W., and von Ilberg, Ch. (1972): Neue Aspekte zur Morphologie und Funktion des runden Fensters. *Laryngol. Rhinol. Otol* (*Stuttg.*), 51:390–399.
44. Onchi, Y. (1949): A study of the mechanism of the middle ear. *J. Acoust. Soc. Am.,* 21:404–410.
45. Møller, A. (1961): Network model of the middle ear. *J. Acoust. Soc. Am.,* 33:168–176.

DISCUSSION

D. Lipscomb: In testing about 7,000 people, we find many, many more with a maximum hearing loss at 6,000 Hz, rather than at 4,000 Hz, and I wonder if you would apply the same reasoning to a 6 kHz dip.

J. Tonndorf: It's the length of the ear canal which determines the resonant frequency. Some people have longer ear canals than others.

H. von Gierke: Do cats contract the auditory canals?

J. Tonndorf: Yes, they do.

H. von Gierke: Is that excluded or included in your discussion of protective mechanisms?

J. Tonndorf: The animals are rather smart and find the point where the sound pressure in the field is minimal. Many animals can close their ear canal very effectively, and that is, of course, part of the picture which complicates the story a little.

H. von Gierke: Was the sound pressure measured at the tympanic membrane or in the field?

J. Tonndorf: Sound pressure was measured in the field.

H. von Gierke: Second question—discussing the protective mechanism of the middle ear, you did not say anything about the protective mechanism of pressure changes. Our recent experiments with low-frequency noise (infrasound) suggest that if you have such low frequencies, they protect against high-frequency transmission in the same way static pressure changes do. I think that's an important additional protective mechanism.

Editors Note: Drs. Trahiotis, Tonndorf, and Price discussed the transfer function of the middle ear and its possible influence on the production of noise-induced hearing losses, especially the 4-kHz notch. A major point of agreement was that stapes displacement is probably not the most appropriate dimension and that energy or power would be a more meaningful measure of the input to the cochlea. In other words, one of the issues in noise-induced hearing loss is the specification of the stimulus (noise) at the stapes footplate. What is the most appropriate dimension, i.e., the volume and velocity of the stapes, the acceleration of the stapes, energy per cycle, etc.?

G. Smoorenburg: With impulse noises we have found that TTS and PTS had maxima at different test frequencies. I think data such as these are difficult to explain solely by resonances of the ear canal.

J. Tonndorf: There are other reasons as well, including, as Stacy Guild [et al. *Acta Otolaryng.,* 1931, 15:269] has pointed out, vasculature of the cochlea. Indeed, there are many factors which could be operating here.

W. Ward: If the blood supply was involved, one might expect TTS to grow faster and to recover more slowly at 4.0 kHz than at other frequencies. Of course, this does not happen, and thereby, in my opinion, dispatches the notion of the blood supply as a significant mechanism.

Effects of Noise on Hearing, edited by Donald Henderson,
Roger P. Hamernik, Darshan S. Dosanjh, and John H. Mills.
Raven Press, New York © 1976

Effects of Noise on Cochlear Potentials

John D. Durrant

*Departments of Otorhinology and Physiology, Temple University School of Medicine,
Philadelphia, Pennsylvania 19140*

In 1930 Wever and Bray (1) reported their historical observation of
electrical responses recorded from the 8th nerve, which were later found
to consist of electrical potentials from the cochlea as well as the auditory
nerve. Within the next 4 years, Wever and his coworkers (2) and Hughson
and Witting (3) published reports on the effects of traumatic sound exposures
on the cochlear potentials, and by the late 1940s a fairly steady flow of
similar reports began to appear in the literature (4–6). The progress in research in this area since the middle 1940s has been painstaking but substantial; still, after 4 decades of study of the cochlear electrophysiological
manifestations of acoustic trauma, much has yet to be learned. The purpose
of this chapter is to present what appears to be the salient characteristics of
the changes observed in the cochlear potentials following exposure to intense
sound. The majority of studies in the literature concern the effects of pure-
tone exposures rather than noise per se. Also, there has been little distinction
between temporary and permanent impairment of the cochlear function.
Consequently, the term *acoustic trauma* will be used here and it will be applied in the broadest sense. Most of the cochlear electrophysiological studies
of acoustic trauma have centered around the cochlear microphonics (CM),
therefore, this potential will be the primary subject of discussion.

EFFECTS OF TRAUMATIC SOUND EXPOSURES
ON COCHLEAR MICROPHONICS

Influence of Exposure Parameters

The reduction in sensitivity which can be observed in the microphonic
recording following exposure to intense sound appears to be directly related
to the sound pressure level (SPL) and the common logarithm of the duration
of the exposure. Eldredge and his associates (7,8) have presented data
suggesting that exposures of different intensities and durations will bring
about comparable reductions in the CM as long as they contain 'the same
energy. However, the equal energy relationship has not been clearly demonstrated over a wide range of exposure conditions, and some exceptions are

evident in the literature. The data of Gerhardt and Wagner (9), Wagner and Gerhardt (10), and Jankowski et al. (11) reflect a linear relationship between the change in CM and the intensity and duration of the exposure, when replotted in log–log coordinates. (This is true except near the lowest levels at which some change in the CM can be induced.) Price's data (12,13) suggest a similar relationship for exposure levels ranging from 0 to 20 dB above the SPL at which the maximum CM output is observed. Higher levels of exposure appear to cause a dramatic increase in the loss of CM sensitivity which deviates from the (essentially) straight-line relationship established at lower levels. Thus, no simple function relating loss of CM sensitivity to intensity of the exposure may exist which holds for all intensities. This may also be true for duration. Findings of Burgeat and Burgeat-Menguy (14; also in Aubry et al., 15) suggest that, for very brief exposures, e.g., 3 sec), the function relating the reduction in CM to intensity is linear on a semilog plot, that is, percent CM vs dB SPL. Eldredge et al. (7,8) also observed that the equal energy relationship does not hold for intense exposures of short duration (i.e., 133 dB SPL for 1 min), but rather, the shift in CM sensitivity tends to be determined primarily by the sound pressure and little by duration.

Another test of the equal energy concept is provided by the observations of the effects of intermittent tonal exposures. Intermittent stimuli have been demonstrated to have comparable effects on CM as that seen under continuous pure tones of equivalent durations, that is, equal total on-times (16,17). However, the influence of duty cycle has not been extensively studied, particularly under conditions in which significant recovery might be expected during the off-times. Only Wagner et al. (18) appear to have examined a very wide range of duty cycles, although they did not obtain their data under constant total on-times. It is also noteworthy that Eldredge and Covell (7) found less narrow-band noise to be required to cause the same depression of CM sensitivity as a pure tone presented at a level equal to the overall SPL of the noise—the opposite of what might be expected.

Ultimately, it would be desirable for a damage risk criterion (DRC) based on the CM (19,20), to determine the critical parameters which lead to permanent versus temporary depression of the microphonics. Such factors have yet to be firmly established. There is a consensus that the microphonic is vulnerable to acoustic trauma of some form whenever the SPL of the sound stimulus exceeds that at which the input–output function of the CM deviates from linearity (21). Thus, the bendover of the input–output function does, in fact, appear to represent the level of sound which can overload the cochlea.

Most investigators have not found the frequency of the exposure stimulus very critical. Data from studies incorporating either round-window or differential recording techniques suggest that one frequency of exposure does not appear to be substantially more detrimental than another (6,22–24). Of course, in the case of differential recording, the maximum reduction in

CM sensitivity is observed following exposure at frequencies which tonotopically correspond to the site of recording (8,23,25,26).

Influence of Parameters of the Test Stimulus

Various researchers have examined the so-called "electrical audiogram," that is, the graph of the decibel difference in the isopotentials recorded from the round window before and after exposure. Comparable reductions in CM sensitivity are seen regardless of frequency. In other words, the electrical audiogram is frequently found to have a somewhat flat configuration (4–6, 12,13,21,22,24,27–31). However, when some systematic difference in the effects of a given sound exposure are observed at different test frequencies, the frequency of maximum depression in the CM tends to occur below the exposure frequency (5,12,19,22).

Following exposure, it is typically observed that change in the maximum CM output (ΔCM_{max}) is proportionately less than the change in the sensitivity of the CM (ΔCM_{sens}) or, in more general terms, the CM evoked at levels below the SPL at which the input–output functions deviate from linearity (8,23–26,32–34). This phenomenon is illustrated in Fig. 1. In this case ΔCM_{max} is seen to be 5 dB, whereas ΔCM_{sens} is 15 dB. The actual reduction in

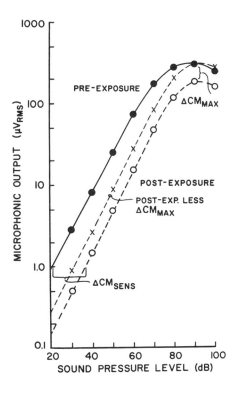

FIG. 1. Microphonic input–output functions obtained in the first turn of the guinea pig utilizing differential electrodes and monitored at 10 kHz before and after 15 min exposure to a 10-kHz tone presented at 100 dB SPL (re 2×10^{-5} N/m²). The change in sensitivity (ΔCM_{sens}) was 15 dB, whereas the change in maximum output (ΔCM_{max}) was 5 dB following exposure. The middle graph (x—x) was derived by shifting the postexposure curve upward to correct for loss in maximum output (see "Discussion and Conclusions").

either ΔCM_{sens} or ΔCM_{max} output is such that considerable variability exists between animals for the same exposures, e.g., Alexander and Githler (28) have presented data reflecting ranges on the order of 60 dB in ΔCM_{sens}. Qualitative differences are also often observed, i.e., in the shape of the input–output functions (not to mention the configuration of the electrical audiogram). In extreme cases, Lawrence (24,36) has observed nonmonotonic input–output functions following exposure. Price (12,13,17) has attempted to minimize variability by setting the level of exposures with reference to the SPL at which CM_{max} occurs, but a considerable spread of data is still observed. Furthermore, Wever and Smith (6) were not able to demonstrate a significant correlation between pre- and postexposure sensitivity. Whatever its exact basis, the variability in the CM data following acoustic trauma is not inconsistent with the variability often observed in the histological data, as discussed below.

RECOVERY OF COCHLEAR MICROPHONICS FROM TRAUMATIC SOUND EXPOSURES

Most of the cochlear electrophysiological data reported in the literature are from studies which were undertaken with the intent of causing demonstrable anatomical damage to the organ of Corti. Studies of the CM involving reversible impairments have been much less prevalent, but partial or complete recovery is observable in the microphonics. The time course of recovery appears to have an exponential characteristic, that is, rapid changes initially, and more gradual changes as recovery progresses (20). At least during the first few minutes following exposure, the recovery of CM sensitivity as a function of time approximates a straight line on a log–log plot in cases reminiscent of short-term temporary threshold shift (TTS) observed behaviorally. This can be seen in the data of Tonndorf et al. (34) and Price (17), as well as the data of Gisselsson and Sorenson (35) and Suga et al. (26) when recast in log–log coordinates. Tonndorf and Brogan (33) and Benitez et al. (32) have presented data reflecting similar recovery functions extending over fairly prolonged periods of recovery (i.e., over 2 hr). The possible involvement of multiple recovery stages is suggested by the findings of Aubry et al. (15), who reported nonmonotonic recovery functions suggestive of the "bounce" seen in the behavioral TTS data. There is little doubt that the time for complete recovery increases with intensity and duration of the exposure, but no definite relationships have emerged from the limited available data (14,15,35).

Even in cases of severe acoustic trauma, where substantial anatomical injury is expected, some structural repair may occur with time, and a degree of recovery might be observed (21,25,37). However, the detailed time course of recovery has not been pursued in such cases. It is interesting to note, nonetheless, that Lawrence and Yantis (21) found little correspondence between the initial or short-term recovery (i.e., partial recovery) and long-term recovery extending over a period of approximately 2 months.

OTHER INDICES OF ACOUSTIC TRAUMA: COMPARISON WITH EFFECTS ON CM

Electrophysiological Measures

Other electrophysiological measures have been studied in conjunction with the microphonic, so it is of interest to examine the relative effects of intense sound exposures on these different potentials. The emphasis here will be placed on data from studies in which the CM was examined in the same experiment. It is well known that altering the endocochlear potential (EP) will bring about a corresponding change in the CM. Consequently, a change in the EP following exposure could conceivably account for at least part of the observed change in the CM. Several investigators have questioned this possibility (23,25,33), but there has been surprisingly little research to determine the susceptibility of this potential to acoustic trauma. Benitez et al. (32) have examined the EP following exposures which caused a reduction in the cochlear potentials, but could not demonstrate any prevalence of abnormal EP. Dallos and Bredberg (38) have made similar observations. Furthermore, Johnstone and Sellick (39) found the EP to be potentiated following exposure to an intense pure tone. Still, the EP might well be depressed in cases in which Reissner's membrane is ruptured following exposure. Injuries of this sort have been reported (21,37), but there does not appear to have been any studies of the EP in such cases.

The whole-nerve action potential (AP) has received much more attention. With little exception (40) the AP has been found to be more susceptible to acoustic trauma than the CM (11,23,32,41–44). Eldredge et al. (8) found changes in the AP to be best correlated with changes in the CM monitored from the first turn, even though the exposure and test stimuli were low-frequency tones. This is consistent with the popular belief that the N_1 component (which is the component observed in these studies) is primarily a product of the activity of fibers innervating the base of the cochlea. The AP has perhaps not been as attractive a measure of the effects of acoustic trauma as it might be because of this belief and the further presumption that the AP contains little frequency-specific information.* However, recent efforts in clinical electrocochleography have stimulated the use of filtered

---

* Davis et al. (23) also felt that the AP is too "labile" for monitoring the effects of acoustic trauma leading to permanent impairment. The magnitude of the AP depends upon the synchrony of the nerve-fiber discharges, so it is the lack of adequate synchrony which may account (partly) for the apparently greater vulnerability of the AP, compared to the CM (32).

clicks, narrow-band masking, etc. to glean as much frequency information from the AP as possible. In a similar vein, Eldredge and his coworkers (45) have recently used partially masked AP responses to examine the effects of small lesions which were due to acoustic trauma, but without any concomitant decreases in behavioral thresholds. In contrast to the somewhat nonsystematic changes in the CM, the AP data very well ranked the degree of anatomical damage. The presently available data in the literature do not adequately describe the changes in AP as a function of the parameters of the exposure stimulus. Recovery of the AP has received some attention; the time course of recovery appears to resemble that which is typically seen in the behavioral TTS studies, that is an exponential-like function (44,46).

Some comparisons have also been made between postexposure changes in cortical or brainstem-evoked responses and the CM and/or AP. The results of these studies potentially suggest differential effects of traumatic sound exposures on the peripheral and central responses, but there does not appear to be a consistent picture as to which is more "vulnerable" (32,46–49).

Anatomical and Behavioral Indices

Numerous investigators have attempted to corroborate histological and electrophysiological indices of acoustic trauma (4,7,8,16,21,23,27–29,45,50). There is clearly a correspondence between the degree of anatomical injury and the reduction of CM sensitivity or output after exposure to traumatic sound stimuli. In a detailed correlative study of histological and electrophysiological measurements Eldredge et al. (8) found that the amount of loss in CM sensitivity precisely ranks the degree of anatomical destruction, although the greatest reliability in the CM as an indicator of the degree of injury was obtained within a given set of exposure conditions. Alexander and Githler (28) demonstrated fairly good correspondence between the loss in microphonic sensitivity and the percent of organ of Corti destroyed. The best-fitting line through the data points was found to be linear on a semilog plot (percent destroyed versus decibel loss) up to about a 40 dB loss where the function began to taper off. Thus, at this point, cases were observed which appeared to have quantitatively the same anatomical loss, but not the same loss of CM. The source of this variability seemed to be in the differences in the pattern of destruction between these cases. For the same percent destruction, damage involving the basal and middle turns produced greater CM depression than that confined mostly to the middle turns. Histological and electrophysiological indices also may not reflect the same degree of dependence on the parameters of the exposure. For instance, under conditions in which the changes in the CM tended to follow the equal energy relationship, Eldredge and his associates (7,8) have found the degree of anatomical injury to depend more on the SPL of the exposure per se. Finally, changes in the CM are not always accompanied by anatomical changes (37), that is, anatomical changes which are detectable via conventional microscopy.

Comparisons between cochlear electrophysiological and behavioral measurements obtained in the same experiment, or even in the same species, are largely lacking in this area of research. The findings of Simmons and Beatty (31) suggest considerable differences in the degree to which the CM and the behavioral thresholds may be correlated from one experiment to another. In some cases, the behavioral audiogram and the electrical audiogram were at least qualitatively similar, i.e., in configuration, while in others they were quite disparate. Quantitatively, the CM often underestimated the amount of hearing loss. On the other hand, Eldredge et al. (45) have recently observed decreases in the CM (and AP) in cases in which there were no significant hearing losses manifested behaviorally, as noted earlier. We anticipate that the rapidly expanding field of clinical electrocochleography will contribute to this area; a step has already been taken in that direction with regard to the AP. Sohmer and Pratt (46) have reported the effects of noise on the nerve response in humans. The recovery pattern of N_1 appeared to resemble that of the TTS. Pugh et al. (44) have examined the AP in monkeys and have found excellent correspondence between the N_1 magnitude and the animal's reaction time (in response to the test stimulus) during recovery. Interestingly, in these experiments the CM were not observed to be depressed, but rather enhanced in some cases following exposure.

ACOUSTIC TRAUMA AND THE SUMMATING POTENTIAL: PERSONAL OBSERVATIONS

Background

The summating potential (SP) has been shown to be quite sensitive to the effects of electrical, mechanical, and neural forms of biasing of the cochlear partition (51–53). This potential is, by definition, a form of nonlinearity, and it appears to arise from distortion in the microphonic transduction process. Whether the SP arises at the level of the hair cell due to electromechanical nonlinearities, or from hydromechanical nonlinearities occurring ahead of the transducer, has not been clearly resolved. The data from the biasing studies appear to reinforce the predominance of hair-cell distortion in the generation of the SP components recorded differentially, DIF^+ and DIF^- (53), which essentially correspond to the traditionally defined SP^+ and SP^-. Thus, any change in the hair-cell transduction process can potentially alter the production of SP. Other researchers have, in fact, demonstrated the effects of various adverse conditions on this potential, i.e., the influence of anoxia (54) or ototoxicity (55). On the other hand, the adverse effects of traumatic sound exposures on the SP have received very little attention. Eldredge et al. (16) presented data on the SP in one of their figures, but no description of their observations was given. Nevertheless, their data reflect substantial reduction in the SP following exposure, consistent with more recent observations of Dallos and Bredberg (39). We have undertaken experiments to determine the influence of intense sound exposures on the SP in the belief that this potential might serve as a valuable supplement to the electrophysiological study of noise-induced hearing loss. The main area of study thus far has been in the course of recovery from presumably reversible fatigue (although the possibility of at least partially permanent impairment could not be ruled out, since full recovery was not usually observed within the observation times of these acute experiments). The ultimate goal of this research is to contribute to the identification, on a cochlear electrophysiological basis, of the point at which irreversible damage is imminent.

The SP, CM, and, frequently, the AP were recorded utilizing differential electrodes in the guinea pig. Generally, only the negative SP component was monitored. The responses were recorded on magnetic tape before, and at various intervals following, exposures to intense tones. Tone-burst stimuli were used to elicit the responses and were presented at levels within the linear range of the CM input–output function. At least 1 hr was permitted to elapse between the surgical preparation and the first measurements, in the expectation of recovery from any acoustic trauma incurred during surgery.

Effects of Traumatic Pure-Tone Exposures on SP

During the early phases of this study, the cochlear responses were monitored in the first turn alone. The exposure stimuli were 5-kHz tones presented at intensities which were never in excess of 115 dB SPL for durations which were 45 min or less. The more intense stimuli were presented for shorter durations, e.g., 105 dB for 15 min or 110 dB for 5 min were typical. Such exposures were generally found to have minor, if any, effects on the CM. The SP, however, exhibited marked decreases following exposure, as shown in Fig. 2. The data are graphed in terms of the normalized magnitudes of the responses, that is the postexposure magnitude is divided by the preexposure magnitude of the respective potentials. (This parameter is utilized to fascilitate comparisons between the different responses which, in turn, are generally not equal in absolute magnitude.) The order in the degree of postexposure depression shown for the different responses is typical of this series of experiments; the SP was reduced proportionally more than the AP, and the AP more than the CM. This order was generally maintained throughout the course of recovery. Thus, the findings of these initial experiments suggested that substantial changes can be produced in the SP via acoustic trauma, even in cases in which the CM are hardly affected.

Since 5 kHz is tonotopically below the best frequency of the first-turn

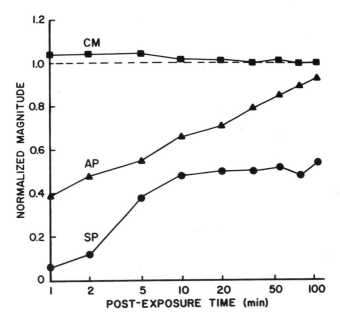

FIG. 2. Normalized magnitudes of CM, AP (N_1 component), and SP (negative component recorded differentially) elicited by a 5-kHz tone (65 dB SPL) at various times following exposure to a 5-kHz tone presented at 95 dB SPL (re 2×10^{-5} N/m²) for 30 min. The preexposure magnitudes of the responses were as follows: CM, 85 μV_{rms}; AP, 340 μV; and SP, 22 μV.

placement used in this investigation, it was questioned whether or not the apparent difference in the sensitivity of the CM and SP to acoustic trauma would be maintained if the frequency of the exposure tone were chosen more closely to the best frequency. (This situation places the hair cells which are presumably subjected to the greatest trauma within the primary pickup area of the differential electrodes.) It was questioned whether the same relative changes observed in the SP and CM would be observed in different cochlear turns. Consequently, it was necessary to effectively equalize the exposure frequency for each turn examined. This scheme is illustrated by Fig. 3. Median 1–μV–isopotential data are shown from 3 groups of animals ($N =$ 5/group) from which recordings were obtained in turns 1, 2, and 3 prior to any exposure. The frequencies of the tone later used to expose the animals in each group were 12,000, 2,828, and 750, respectively, as shown by the arrows in Fig. 3. In all cases the exposure stimuli were presented at 110 dB for 5 min (test stimuli at 60–75 dB).*

The data from 3 different animals, 1 from each turn-group, are shown in Fig. 4. (Data are shown for the animal that yielded the best overall approximation to the median recovery function for the SP and, when possible,

---

* Ideally, the exposure, and perhaps the test stimuli, should have been presented at levels which cause equal displacements of the basilar membrane at each frequency. However, this was not done in these experiments.

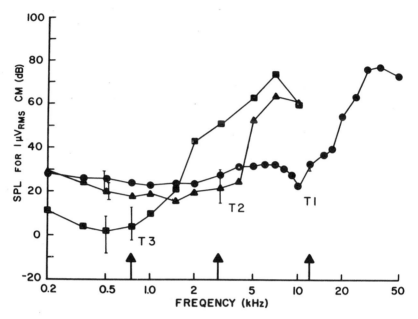

FIG. 3. Median 1–µV–isopotential data (CM) observed in turns 1, 2, and 3 in groups of 5 animals each per turn. Ranges are shown at a standard low test frequency and at a standard frequency at the frequency of the exposure stimulus (indicated by arrows) utilized later in the experiment.

the CM; this was not possible for the second turn-group.) Marked depression of the CM is seen following exposure in all 3 turns, and the overall effects seem to be comparable between turns. In contrast, the postexposure depression of the SP appears to be quite different in the 3 turns, at least during the first 10 or more minutes of recovery. There is a trend toward less depression in the SP from the lower to the upper turns. To better illustrate this, the data from 3 animals (not necessarily the same as shown in Fig. 4) are shown in Fig. 5 where the ratio of the normalized SP magnitude to the normalized CM magnitude (SP_N/CM_N) is plotted as a function of postexposure time. A value of SP_N/CM_N of less than 1.0 indicates that the SP was reduced proportionally more than the CM, whereas values greater than 1.0 indicate greater depression of CM. In first-turn animals in general the SP is usually depressed more than the CM, and in third-turn animals the opposite is nearly always observed, during the initial phase of recovery. The second-turn data tend to fall in the middle, that is a given animal may exhibit greater depression of either response.*

---

* Scrutiny of the actual preexposure magnitudes of the responses, indicated in the legends of Figs. 4 and 5, reveal that the ratio of SP to CM (SP/CM) diminishes in the upper turns, while SP_N/CM_N increases (at least during the initial recovery). Consequently, there is an apparent inverse relationship between SP_N/CM_N and SP/CM across turns. However, SP/CM per se is probably not the primary determinant of SP_N/CM_N. In the first turn SP/CM is much less at 5 kHz than at 12 kHz under comparable conditions, and yet SP_N/CM_N is less than 1.0 following a 5-kHz exposure, as it is following a 12-kHz exposure.

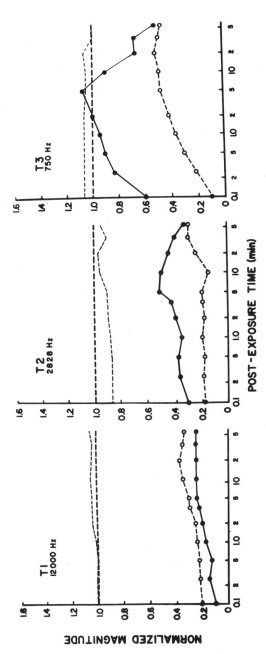

FIG. 4. Data from 3 representative animals from each turn-group showing normalized magnitudes of the SP (closed circles) and CM (open circles) as a function of postexposure time. The indicated exposure frequencies for each turn were presented at 110 dB SPL for 5 min. The responses were elicited at the same frequency as the exposure, and the fluctuation in the sound pressure of the test stimulus (monitored in front of the eardrum) is shown by the thin dashed line. The level of the test stimulus in each case and the preexposure magnitudes were as follows. T1: SP, 96 μV; CM, 21 μV$_{rms}$ at 60 dB. T2: SP, 65 μV; CM, 69 μV$_{rms}$ at 75 dB. T3: SP, 80 μV; CM, 245 μV$_{rms}$ at 70 dB.

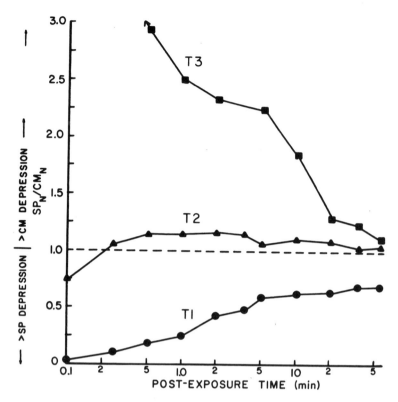

FIG. 5. Data from 3 animals showing representative plots of SP_N/CM_N (see text) as a function of post-exposure time. (Except for T3, not the same animals as shown in Fig. 4.) The turn from which the recordings were made is indicated. The level of the test stimulus in each case and the preexposure magnitudes of the SP and CM were as follows. T1: SP, 140 μV; CM, 27 μV_{rms} at 70 dB. T2: SP, 34 μV; CM, 30 μV_{rms} at 60 dB. T3: SP, 80 μV; CM, 245 μV_{rms} at 70 dB.

Supplementary Observations on the Cochlear Potentials

In the course of this research and some more recently initiated experiments, observations have been made on the CM, SP, and EP which are relevant to the findings of other researchers discussed earlier. We have observed the expected differential effects of traumatic sound exposure of CM_{sens} and CM_{max}. Furthermore, proportionally less reduction in the SP at 90 dB, compared to that recorded at 60 dB SPL, was seen in some first-turn animals. (90 dB is the level at or near that at which CM_{max} occurred; the input–output function of DIF⁻ SP is generally linear over the same range, but was not measured in these experiments.) The initial impression obtained, however, is that the level of the test stimulus is a less influential parameter in the observed effects of intense sound exposure on the SP than in the case of the CM. We have also observed the maximum CM depression to occur at a frequency below the frequency of exposure in first-turn preparations, but in second- and third-turn recordings the maximum reduction in the CM typically occurred in the vicinity of the exposure frequency, not below. Finally, the EP has been recorded under exposure conditions similar to those utilized for the first turn-group described above (i.e., 10–12 kHz at 110 dB for 15 min). The site of recording was in the same area as our typical differential electrode placement in the first turn. No significant postexposure changes in the EP were observed in cases in which the CM and SP were expected, if not directly verified, to be depressed.

ANALYSIS AND CONCLUSIONS

The results of the present investigation must be considered preliminary; much more experience is needed with the SPs under a wider range of exposure and test conditions. Perhaps more mysteries than insights have been revealed by these observations. The basis of the differential effects of intense sound exposures on the CM and SP and their relative courses of recovery observed in the different turns is not clear. It is clear, however, that more subtle effects of acoustic trauma are experienced by the organ of Corti, presumably the hair cells in particular, than is simply manifested in decreased microphonic sensitivity. It is tempting to suggest the involvement of a change in the operating characteristics of the hair-cell transduction system which, in turn, would be expected to alter the nonlinearities of the system. Still, there is no apparent reason for differences between turns.

On an empirical basis, some ground may have been gained. At least under some conditions, the SP may serve to extend the lower limits of sound exposure (intensity and duration) which can cause significant poststimulatory changes in the hearing organ, since the SP can be depressed under conditions in which little or no change is seen in the CM. The same could be said for the AP, but the problem then arises as to whether alterations in this potential are of cochlear or neural origin. Some basis is needed for clearly separating fatigue of cochlear origin and adaptation, or perhaps fatigue, of a neural origin. The SP suggests itself in this role. It should be noted for practical purposes that the usefulness of the SP in evaluating the effects of noise or other traumatic sound exposures is not limited to the use of intracochlear electrodes. The SP recorded via the round window and that recorded in the first turn via differential electrodes are comparably depressed by the same exposures and exhibit essentially the same time course of recovery.

Much has been made of the differential reduction in CM_{max} and CM_{sens} following exposure, to the point that the 2 parameters have come to be viewed as somewhat independent. Benitez et al. (32) have summarized the basis of this point of view. They suggest that a conductive lesion of middle ear and/or cochlear origin is responsible for the change in CM sensitivity. Presumably the efficiency of energy transfer to the hair cells is reduced, causing an overall shift of the input–output function toward higher sound intensities. This conductive lesion could conceivably involve anything up to and including the steady-state electrical resistance postulated by Davis (56). On the other hand, the change in maximum output is attributed to either a drop in the EP or a decreased range of resistance modulation, that is, something which could cause an overall shift in the output of the hair cell toward decreased magnitudes of response.

Interestingly, the CM sensitivity can be reduced in a totally and immediately reversible manner—by interference (57). In fact, when the post-exposure input–output function shown in Fig. 1 is shifted upward to correct for the loss of CM_{max}, the derived input–output function bears a striking resemblence to that observed under interference. At the other extreme, CM_{sens} can be reduced as the result of anatomical injury, such as the fracturing of the organ of Corti between the supporting cells and the sensory cells as described by Beagley (25). Injury of this sort readily suggests itself as a cochlear conductive lesion. Now the loci of the effects of interference, reversible fatigue, and permanent noise-induced impairment on the CM might well be different (58), and yet they are manifested in qualitatively the same manner, namely, decreased CM sensitivity. Certainly these different effects might be separable on a quantitative basis, but it takes little speculation to suggest that there may be too much overlap to provide distinct dividing lines between these phenomena. At least a change in CM_{max} seems to be limited to cases of fatigue or irreversible losses, but the separation of the two on a quantitative basis might not be too precise for the same reason. It would appear that CM_{max} can be reduced without any reduction in the EP following exposure, so it is tempting to attribute changes in the maximum output to hair cell dysfunction. However, the possible involvement of decreased EP in cases of severe acoustic trauma has yet to be ruled out, i.e., those involving injury to Reissner's membrane. In brief, the loss of CM sensitivity and maximum output appear to be rather limited indicators of the detailed mechanisms involved with acoustic trauma, based upon the currently available data.

In the final analysis, even the separation of CM_{sens} and CM_{max} is somewhat tenuous. There is a continued lack of understanding of the exact transduction process(es) involved in the generation of the CM. The theory outlined by Benitez et al. is predicated on the assumption that the gross CM recorded in the fluid spaces of the cochlea are reasonable facsimiles of the unit microphonics. This assumption has come under attack in recent years (59). Suffice it to say, there is ample indication that the gross CM only approximates the individual hair cell output under limited conditions (60). Any changes observed in the gross output, which reflects the combined output of many hair cells, will depend upon both the changes in the hair cells and the pattern of injury to the organ of Corti, as suggested by the observations of Alexander and Githler (28) discussed earlier. This is expected to affect the relative changes in sensitivity and the maximum output observed in the gross recording (24), as well as the configuration of the electrical audiogram.

In the normal cochlea the round window electrode provides a "view" of the hair cells which is weighted toward the population of hair cells in the base (60). As long as the damage to the base is no greater than that in the upper turns, the local generators in the base will dominate the recorded CM output, since the output from more distal hair cells are attenuated through the perilymph. This same situation contributes to the generally indiscriminate injury produced by tones of different frequencies and the typically flat electrical audiogram observed via the round window. The base is stimulated by nearly all frequencies within the range of hearing at high SPLs. While the differential electrodes are expected to give a selective or regional "view" of the hair cell output, this technique is limited by what Dallos (60) calls spatial resolving power. Thus, even when it is possible to place electrodes at different sites along the cochlear partition, it may not be possible to determine precisely the nature and extent of the lesion electrophysiologically utilizing the microphonic.

There are obvious problems and limitations in the use of the microphonic in the evaluation of noise-induced damage to the hearing organ, which may ultimately limit the potential for formulating a DRC on a purely objective (electrophysiological) basis. However, this does not necessarily limit the use of cochlear electrophysiology in general for such purposes. By cross-correlating the effects of noise on the CM, SP, AP, and EP it is not unreasonable to expect that it will ultimately be possible to differentiate underlying mechanisms as well. Much potential for an objective DRC has perhaps not been realized because sufficiently comprehensive analyses of the cochlear potentials have not been undertaken. Moreover, the full potential of the microphonic itself has probably not been realized. Various similarities have been demonstrated between behavioral TTS data and CM data. The dependence of the loss of CM sensitivity on the duration and intensity of the exposure appears to follow the same basic rules governing TTS. This is also true of the time course of recovery and growth of time for complete recovery. Even asymptotic TTS-like behavior is observable in the microphonic (32). However, the details of the underlying functions and the equally important differences between the TTS and CM data are generally difficult to evaluate because the cochlear electrophysiological data are just too limited. More direct comparisons are needed between the behavioral and electrophysiological data, including measurements in the same animal, since species differences may be significant (61). Cochlear electrophysiology can contribute much to an understanding of the effects of noise on cochlear function and can substantially contribute to the formulation and/or evaluation of DRCs simply by virtue of the fact that these potentials *are* intimately dependent upon the state of the hair-cell transduction system. That one may not always obtain a simple picture of pathological changes in the cochlea from recording the cochlear responses is a technical problem. While this is clearly troublesome for the researcher, it in no way mitigates the importance of studying the cochlear electrophysiological manifestations of the effects of noise on hearing.

ACKNOWLEDGMENTS

The author is indebted to Dr. James Saunders, University of Pennsylvania, for his helpful comments and criticisms. The preparation of this report and the research upon which it was in part based was supported by a grant from the Deafness Research Foundation.

REFERENCES

1. Wever, E. G., and Bray, C. W. (1930): Action currents in auditory nerve in response to acoustic stimulation. *Proc. Nat. Acad. Sci.,* 16:344–350.
2. Wever, E. G., Bray, C. W., and Horton, G. P. (1934): The problem of stimulation deafness studied by auditory nerve technique. *Science,* 80:18–19.
3. Hughson, W., and Witting, E. G. (1934): An objective study of auditory fatigue. *Acta Otolaryngol.,* 21:457–486.
4. Lurie, M. H., Davis, H. and Hawkins, J. E. (1944): Acoustic trauma of the organ of corti in the guinea pig. *Laryngoscope,* 54:375–386.
5. Davis, H., Derbyshire, A. J., Kemp, E. H., Lurie, M. H., and Upton, M. (1935): Functional and histological changes in the cochlea of the guinea pig resulting from prolonged stimulation, *J. Gen. Psychol.,* 12:251–277.
6. Wever, E. G., and Smith, K. R. (1944): The problem of stimulation deafness. I. Cochlear impairment as a function of tonal frequency. *J. Exp. Psychol.,* 34:239–245.
7. Eldredge, D. H., and Covell, W. P. (1958): A laboratory method for the study of acoustic trauma. *Laryngoscope,* 68:465–477.
8. Eldredge, D. H., Bilger, R. C., Davis, H., and Covell, W. P. (1961): Factor analysis of cochlear injuries and changes in electrophysiological potentials following acoustic trauma in the guinea pig. *J. Acoust. Soc. Am.,* 33:152–159.
9. Gerhardt, H.-J., and Wagner, H. (1962): Die Wirkung dosierter Geräuschbelastung auf die Mikrofonpotentiale der Meerschweinchenschnecke. *Arch. Otorhinolaryngol. (NY),* 179:459–472.
10. Wagner, H. and Gerhardt, H.-J. (1963): Die Wirkung dosierter Reintonbelastung auf die Mikrofonpotentiale der Meerschweinchenschnecke. *Arch. Otorhinolaryngol. (NY),* 181:82–106.
11. Jankowski, W., Ziemski, Z., Birecki, W., Cyrulewska-Orłowska, J., Praga, J., and Kowalewska, M. (1971): Wpływ ostrego urazu akustycznego i narkozy uretanowej na modelowanie biopotencjałów ucha wewnętrznego u świnek morskich. *J. Otolaryngol. Pol.,* 25:253–265.
12. Price, G. R. (1968): Functional changes in the ear produced by high-intensity sound. I. 5.0-kHz stimuation. *J. Acoust. Soc. Am.,* 44:1541–1545.
13. Price, G. R. (1972): Functional changes in the ear produced by high-intensity sound. II. 500-Hz stimulation. *J. Acoust. Soc. Am.,* 51:552–558.
14. Burgeat, M., and Burgeat-Menguy, C. (1964): Étude des modifications du potential microphonique cochléaire survenant á la suite des stimulation sonores intenses. *J. Physiol. (Paris),* 56:225–232.
15. Aubry, M., Pialoux, P., and Burgeat, M. (1965): Influence d'une stimulation acoustique intense sur la réponse de la cochlée. *Acta Otolaryngol.,* 60:191–196.
16. Eldredge, D. H., Covell, W. P., and Gannon, R. P. (1959): Acoustic trauma following intermittent exposure to tones. *Ann. Otol. Rhinol. Laryngol.,* 68:723–732.
17. Price, G. R. (1974): Loss and recovery processes operative at the level of the cochlear microphonic during intermittent stimulation. *J. Acoust. Soc. Am.,* 56:183–189.
18. Wagner, H., Berndt, H., and Gerhardt, H.-J. (1973): Zum Einsatz elektrophysio-

logischer Methoden in der Gehör-Lärmschadenforschung. *Z. Gesamte. Hyg.,* 19:18–21.

19. Wagner, H., and Gerhardt, H.-J. (1964): Weitere Untersuchungen zur kritischen Belastungschwelle des Meerschweinschens für kontinuierliche Töne und Geräusche. *Arch. Otorhinolaryngol. (NY),* 184:179–191.

20. Gerhardt, H.-J., and Wagner, H. (1965): Untersuchungen zur Ruckbildung von Minderungen des Mikrophonpotentials (MP) nach Schallbelastungen. *Arch. Otorhinolaryngol. (NY),* 184:461–472.

21. Lawrence, M., and Yantis, P. A. (1957): Individual differences in functional recovery and structural repair following overstimulation of the guinea pig ear. *Ann. Otol. Rhinol. Laryngol.,* 66:595–621.

22. Smith, K. R., and Wever, E. G. (1949): The problem of stimulation deafness. III. The functional and histological effects of a high-frequency stimulus. *J. Exp. Psychol.,* 39:238–241.

23. Davis, H., and Associates (1953): Acoustic trauma in the guinea pig. *J. Acoust. Soc. Am.,* 25:1180–1189.

24. Wever, E. G., and Lawrence, M. (1955): Patterns of injury produced by overstimulation of the ear. *J. Acoust. Soc. Am.,* 27:853–858.

25. Beagley, H. A. (1965): Acoustic trauma in the guinea pig. *Acta Otolaryngol.,* 60:437–451.

26. Suga, F., Snow, J. B., Preston, W. J., and Glomset, J. L. (1967): Tonal patterns of cochlear impairment following intense stimulation with pure tones. *Laryngoscope,* 77:784–805.

27. Alexander, I. E., and Githler, F. J. (1949): The effects of jet engine noise on the cochlear response of the guinea pig. *J. Comp. Physiol. Psychol.,* 42:517–525.

28. Alexander, I. E., and Githler, F. J. (1952): Chronic effects of jet engine noise on the structure and function of the cochlear apparatus. *J. Comp. Physiol. Psychol.,* 45:381–391.

29. Krejci, R., and Bornschein, H. (1951): Der Einfluss chronischer Lärmschädigung auf die Cochlearpotentiale von Meerschweinschen. *Acta Otolaryngol.,* 39:68–79.

30. Lawrence, M., Wolsk, D., and Burton, R. D. (1959): Stimulation deafness, cochlear patterns, and significance of electrical recording methods. *Ann. Otol. Rhinol. Laryngol.,* 68:5–33.

31. Simmons, F. B., and Beatty, D. L. (1962): The significance of round-window-recorded cochlear potentials in hearing: an autocorrelated study in the cat. *Ann. Otol. Rhinol. Laryngol.,* 71:767–801.

32. Benitez, L. D., Eldredge, D. H., and Templer, J. W. (1972): Temporary threshold shifts in chinchilla: electrophysiological correlates. *J. Acoust. Soc. Am.,* 52:1115–1123.

33. Tonndorf, J., and Brogan, F. A. (1952): Two forms of change in cochlear microphonics: parallel shift in stimulus intensity and truncation of gradient curves. *USAF Sch. Aviation Med.,* Proj. #21–27–001, Rep. #6.

34. Tonndorf, J., Hyde, R. W., and Brogan, F. A. (1955): Combined effect of sound and oxygen deprivation upon cochlear microphonics in guinea pigs. *Ann. Otol. Rhinol. Laryngol.,* 64:392–405.

35. Gisselsson, L., and Sørensen, H. (1959): Auditory adaptation and fatigue in cochlear potentials. *Acta Otolaryngol.,* 50:391–405.

36. Lawrence, M. (1958): Functional changes in inner ear deafness. *Ann. Otol. Rhinol. Laryngol.,* 67:802–823.

37. Eldredge, D. H., Covell, W. P., and Davis, H. (1957). Recovery from acoustic trauma in the guinea pig. *Laryngoscope,* 67:66–84.

38. Dallos, P., and Bredberg, G., personal communication.

39. Johnstone, B. M., and Sellick, P. M. (1972): Dynamic changes in cochlear potentials and endolymph concentrations. *J. Otolaryngol. Soc. Aust.,* 3:317–319.

40. Faltýnek, L., and Veselý, C. (1966): Vliv krátkodobého ohlušení na odpověd kochley morčete na click. *Česk. Otolaryngol.,* 15:65–67.

41. Rosenblith, W. A. (1950): Auditory masking and fatigue. *J. Acoust. Soc. Am.,* 22:792–800.

42. Rosenblith, W. A., Galambos, R., and Hirsh, I. J. (1950): The effect of exposure to

loud tones upon animal and human responses to acoustic clicks. *Science,* 111:569–571.

43. Mitchell, C., Brummett, R., and Vernon, J. (1973): Changes in the auditory nerve evoked potential after intense sound stimulation. *J. Acoust. Soc. Am.,* 53:326.

44. Pugh, J. E., Horwitz, M. R., and Anderson, D. J. (1974): Cochlear electrical activity in noise-induced hearing loss. *Arch. Otorhinolaryngol.,* 100:36–40.

45. Eldredge, D. H., Mills, J. H., and Bohne, B. A. (1973): Anatomical, behavioral, and electrophysiological observations on chinchillas after long exposures to noise. *Adv. Otorhinolaryngol.,* 20:64–81.

46. Sohmer, H., and Pratt, H. (1975): Electrocochleography during noise-induced temporary threshold shifts. *Audiology,* 14:130–134.

47. Benning, C., and Stange, G. (1971): Das Verhalten peripherer und zentraler akustischer Reizantworten des Meerschweinchens unter Sinustonbeschallung. *Arch. Otorhinolaryngol. (NY),* 199:529–533.

48. Benning, C. D. (1972): Periphere und zentrale akustische Reizantworten beim Meerschweinchen nach akuter Schallschädigung mit weißem Rauschen und Sinustonen. *Arch. Otorhinolaryngol. (NY),* 202:457–464.

49. Babighian, G., Moushegian, G., and Rupert, A. L. (1975): Central auditory fatigue. *Audiology,* 14:72–83.

50. Beck, C., and Michler, H. (1960): Feinstrukturell und histochemische Veränderungen an den Strukturen der Cochlea beim Meerschweinchen nach dosierter Reintonbeshallung. *Arch. Otorhinolaryngol. (NY),* 174:496–567.

51. Durrant, J. D., and Dallos, P. (1972): Influence of direct-current polarization of the cochlear partition on the summating potentials. *J. Acoust. Soc. Am.,* 52:542–552.

52. Durrant, J. D., and Dallos, P. (1974): Modification of DIF summating potential components by stimulus biasing. *J. Acoust. Soc. Am.,* 56:562–570.

53. Durrant, J. D., and Gans, D. (1975): Biasing of the summating potentials. *Acta Otolaryngol.,* 80:13–18.

54. Konishi, T., Butler, R. A., and Fernández, C. (1961): Effect of anoxia on cochlear potentials. *J. Acoust. Soc. Am.,* 33:349–356.

55. Davis, H., Deatherage, B. H., Rosenblut, B., Fernández, C., Kimura, R., and Smith, C. A. (1958): Modification of cochlear potentials produced by streptomycin poisoning and by extensive venous obstruction. *Laryngoscope,* 68:596–627.

56. Davis, H. (1965): A model for transducer action in the cochlea. *Cold Spring Harbor Symp. Quant. Biol.,* 30:181–190.

57. Wever, E. G., Bray, C. W., and Lawrence, M. (1940): The interference of tones in the cochlea. *J. Acoust. Soc. Am.,* 12:268–280.

58. Wever, E. G., and Lawrence, M. (1941): Tonal interference in relation to cochlear injury. *J. Exp. Psychol.,* 29:283–295.

59. Whitfield, I. C., and Ross, H. F. (1965): Cochlear-microphonic and summation potentials and the output of individual hair cell generators. *J. Acoust. Soc. Am.,* 38:126–131.

60. Dallos, P. (1973): *The Auditory Periphery: Biophysics and Physiology.* Academic Press, New York.

61. Drescher, D. G., and Eldredge, D. H. (1974): Species differences in cochlear fatigue related to acoustics of outer and middle ears of guinea pig and chinchilla. *J. Acoust. Soc. Am.,* 56:929–934.

DISCUSSION

J. Saunders: My question has two parts. First, after your considerable review of the literature, is the CM a receptor potential, and as such is it non-fatiguable; and second, if it is fatiguable, then are the changes in the CM only indicative of some kind of PTS type of phenomena—e.g., all of us have had the experience of tuning a wave analyzer, setting the sound to 85–95 dB(A) and letting it sit for hours and hours without a change. Then, at some point you can expose it to enough sound and suddenly you see changes in CM amplitude. Are these changes in CM indicative of a PTS, or can you get true TTS-type changes in CM?

J. Durrant: First, we still think that CM is a receptor potential, with a questionable relation to the initiation of the response of the 1st order neuron. Second, we can see the CM depressed by an exposure and then follow it back to where it was prior to an exposure. The factors which determine the amount of CM depression bear some resemblance to the basic parameters which we see determining TTS.

C. Trahiotis: When you're measuring SP you're measuring one sign of it, and I get confused by the SP with changing signs; could you be picking up changing signs as opposed to loss?

J. Durrant: You can pretty well select the polarity by picking the test frequency. SP is a positive at most levels, at least from 1 kHz down.

G. Price: We've noticed a systematic relationship between the intensity of the stimulus and the rate at which loss of CM accumulates. There are also recovery processes which are orderly. Recent data indicate that the early recovery processes in the CM are vital, because if you interrupt the early process, you get very large losses, perhaps twice as large as you would if you let the recovery process run its uninterrupted course.

Effects of Noise on Hearing, edited by Donald Henderson, Roger P. Hamernik, Darshan S. Dosanjh, and John H. Mills. Raven Press, New York © 1976

Temporary Sensorineural Hearing Losses and 8th Nerve Changes

E. F. Evans

Department of Communication, University of Keele, Keele, England

This chapter will be limited to changes observed in the behavior of single cochlear nerve fibers in animals under various conditions of cochlear pathology. Some of these are identical to, and others, it will be argued, may be related to, conditions giving rise to temporary (and ultimately) permanent sensorineural hearing loss in man.

The pioneering study of the behavior of single cochlear fibers in relation to permanent cochlear damage (arising from chronic exposure to ototoxic antibiotics) is that of Kiang et al. (1). The experiments reviewed here, however, form part of a series designed to investigate one important aspect of auditory function, namely, frequency selectivity. In normal hearing, this appears to be already determined, in large part at least, at the level of the cochlear nerve, as a result of a 2-stage frequency filtering process in the cochlea. The second stage of this filtering process appears to be particularly vulnerable to the deleterious effects of local damage, hypoxia, local and systemic administration of ototoxic agents, and complete drainage of the perilymph from the appropriate regions of the scala tympani. Under these conditions, the threshold and tuning of single cochlear fibers deteriorate, so that the normally sharp frequency selectivity is lost. These changes can be permanent, or, under certain conditions, reversible. They can account for such features of sensorineural hearing loss as recruitment.

The purpose of this chapter is to outline some of the evidence for the above statements in terms of their possible significance for sensorineural hearing losses in general, and temporary losses in particular.

METHODS OF ANALYSIS

These have been described in full elsewhere (2,34). Briefly, the responses of positively identified single fibers in the cochlear nerve of anesthetized cats, guinea pigs, and rats were recorded with micropipettes. For acoustic stimulation in a closed sound field, a compensated Bruel & Kjaer half-inch microphone was used as a source. The sound pressure was calibrated at the tympanic membrane.

In order to determine the response of these fibers as a function of frequency and intensity, a number of procedures were employed. Manual plotting (3) of the frequency threshold ("tuning") curve (FTC) is adequate under static conditions. Under the changing conditions of these experiments, however, this method is not sufficiently rapid and leads to bias. All of the data obtained here under changing conditions were therefore determined using a computer-controlled system which randomized the sequence of both frequency and intensity of a series of tone bursts (ca. 50 msec duration, 5/sec repetition rate). This system also counted the number of spike discharges corresponding to each frequency–intensity combination, and displayed the counts as the length of a vertical line positioned at the appropriate frequency–intensity locus (see Figs. 2,3,5,6). This frequency–response paradigm minimizes any systematic bias introduced by changing conditions, provides suprathreshold data, as well as allowing estimations of the FTC (interrupted lines around response area as in Figs. 2–7), and can give usable information in a short space of time. The full analysis of 1,024 points (64 frequency steps × 16 intensity levels) takes about 4 min; but quarter- or half-samples are sufficient to determine the FTC (e.g., Fig. 3B–F).

The state of the cochlea was monitored by recording the gross cochlear action potential (AP) with a wire electrode on the round window margin, and determining its thresholds and amplitude in response to click stimuli. The latter, and the cochlear microphonic (CM) were electronically gated out of the round window recorded response, and displayed continuously (insets of Figs. 3 and 6).

CONCEPT OF THE "SECOND FILTER"

There is now strong evidence for a frequency-sharpening mechanism in the cochlea, producing a considerably sharper neural frequency selectivity compared to that of the basilar membrane vibration. Comparisons of data within the same species have been carried out in guinea pig (2,4–6), squirrel monkey (7), and cat (8), with similar findings (see ref. 13). Figure 1 illustrates the differences between the FTCs of cochlear fibers in the guinea pig (2) with measurements of the amplitude of vibration on the cochlear partition by various workers (9–11). In contrast to the almost low-pass filter characteristic of the basilar membrane vibration, the neural FTCs are band-pass. Fibers with characteristic frequencies (CFs: the most sensitive frequency, i.e., at the tip of the FTC) above 1–2 kHz have asymmetrical curves having a steep high-frequency cutoff, becoming steeper with stimulus level, and a rather less steep low-frequency cutoff, becoming much less steep above about 80 dB SPL. The fibers with CFs above 2 kHz, therefore, have low-threshold sharply tuned segments extending 40–60 dB below a higher threshold segment with low-pass characteristic. The slopes of the cutoffs and the bandwidth of the low-threshold segments are substantially steeper and narrower, respectively, than those of the analogous basilar membrane measurements (for details see

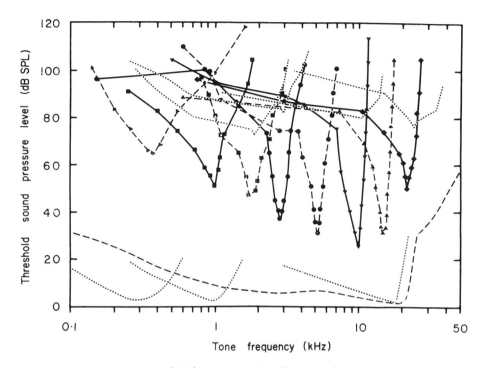

FIG. 1. Frequency threshold curves (FTCs) of single cochlear fibers recorded from normal and abnormal cochleae, compared with measurements of basilar membrane frequency response (guinea pig). Continuous and dashed lines through points: FTCs of 8 cochlear fibers from 6 normal cochleae. *Upper dotted curves:* FTCs of cochlear fibers from cochleae rendered abnormal by circulatory insufficiency (CFs at 1.9, 3, and 10 kHz). The curve of highest CF (24 kHz) was obtained in an otherwise normal cochlea in company with normally sharply tuned fibers. It may be related to sporadic hair cell loss found in normal guinea pigs (see ref. 2). *Lower dashed and dotted curves:* Frequency response curves derived from the measurements of the vibration amplitude of the guinea pig basilar membrane by von Békésy (9: dotted curves with tip at 0.3 and 0.95 kHz), by Johnstone et al. (10: dotted curve with tip at 18 kHz); and by Wilson and Johnstone (11: dashed curve with tip at 20 kHz). All curves are corrected to sound pressure level (in dB SPL) at the tympanic membrane under closed bulla conditions. The basilar membrane curves are positioned arbitrarily on the ordinate. (From refs. 2 and 34.)

refs. 2 and 13). For "intermediate" frequencies (7–14 kHz, corresponding to the most sensitive fibers in cat and guinea pig), the difference in bandwidth measured at 10 dB above the tip of the curves approaches an order of magnitude. Analogous comparisons in the squirrel monkey (7) and cat (12) yield quantitatively similar differences (13).

These differences are not simply a result of the different conditions under which the basilar membrane and neural measurements are usually taken. In particular, the need for high stimulus levels and surgical opening of the scala tympani for the basilar membrane measurements have been invoked to account for the differences observed. More recent basilar membrane measurements have been made in the guinea pig (11) at sound levels comparable to the thresholds of the cochlear fibers shown in Fig. 1. Others have been made

202 TEMPORARY 8TH NERVE CHANGES

in the squirrel monkey (7) at levels where comparison is possible with neural curves analogous to the FTCs, but constructed with higher than threshold discharge rate criteria (isorate contours). While *complete* drainage of the perilymph from the scala tympani can eliminate the low-threshold, sharply tuned segment from cochlear nerve FTCs (8,14), sharply tuned FTCs can be obtained under the same conditions of drainage for the basilar membrane measurements in the guinea pig (15), and have been recorded in simultaneous basilar membrane and cochlear nerve measurements in the cat (8). Furthermore, measurements of basilar membrane motion utilizing the Mössbauer technique have been made in the undrained condition (10,16).

Various lines of evidence have led to the proposal that the above discrepancy in sharpness of tuning is due to a "second filtering" process in the cochlea subsequent to that of the basilar membrane, the "first filter" (2,11,12). First, there is considerable variation in the sharpness of tuning from cochlear fiber to fiber even in the same cochlea and at the same CF (2,12,7). This would not be expected on the basis of sharp tuning properties of the basilar membrane, the tuning properties of which would be expected to be evenly distributed and therefore not to vary between neighboring points. A sharpening process "private" to individual fibers or groups of fibers, however, could account for this. Second, in guinea pig cochleae subjected to accidental hypoxia (through low systemic blood pressure or occlusion of the cochlear blood supply by the presence of the microelectrode in the internal auditory meatus), high-threshold, broadly tuned FTCs were obtained (2), which were similar in shape to the basilar membrane frequency response functions (upper dotted lines in Fig. 1; quantitatively compared in ref. 2). This suggested that the "second filter" was physiologically vulnerable, and that when its effects were eliminated, the cochlear fiber tuning merely reflected that of the "first filter," the basilar membrane. As will be indicated below, these effects can be obtained transiently and *reversibly* under a variety of ototoxic conditions, which would not be expected to affect basilar membrane motion. Further evidence for lack of alteration of basilar membrane response is given by the observation that, where the ototoxic effects are generalized over the cochlea (systemic hypoxia, intraarterial furosemide), the grossly recorded CM is not affected substantially (17,18,32; see Fig. 6). Third, certain distortion-type phenomena observed in cochlear fiber response patterns with stimulation by 2-tone combinations, e.g., 2-tone suppression (3,19,20), and excitation by the intermodulation distortion product $2f_1 - f_2$ (21), are consistent with a 2-stage model of cochlear filtering involving a nonlinearity "sandwiched" between a low-pass and band-pass filter (22,23). The absence of the intermodulation distortion product from the basilar membrane vibration patterns (24) and from the cochlear microphonic (25) point to its being generated prior to or in a subsequent more frequency-selective filter. Fourth, measurements on a patient with a notch hearing loss are consistent with this model (23; see discussion in ref. 13).

While in terms of its response to broadband and multicomponent noise stimuli the second filter behaves as if it were a linear filter (26–31,12), its mechanism of action and its situation remain obscure. What is clear is that it is a most delicate mechanism, easily disturbed by a variety of influences, many of which are known to be involved in pathological conditions of the human cochlea. The question is asked whether the second filter is a "final common path" (to borrow a term from another context!), for varieties of cochlear pathology including that induced by noise exposure?

VULNERABILITY OF THE SECOND FILTER

Long-term loss (that is, hours to days) of the normal sharpness of tuning of single cochlear fibers in several species has been encountered as a result of: chronic administration of ototoxic antibiotics (1); hypoxia (2,17,41); local administration of cyanide, furosemide (an ototoxic diuretic), α-adrenergic receptor blocking agents, and other toxic agents into the cochlea (18,32–34); systemic administration of furosemide (18); complete drainage of the appropriate part of the scala tympani (14,8); local damage to a small part of the cochlear partition (2). These changes are reflected in the elevation of threshold of the gross cochlear AP, but may or may not be accompanied by attenuation of the CM. Under these conditions, as has been mentioned above, the FTCs appear to have lost their low-threshold, sharply tuned segment, leaving behind the high-threshold more broadly tuned segment (as in Fig. 1). This is more clearly demonstrated in cases where the onset of the pathology is sudden, as illustrated in Fig. 2. Here are shown the effects of the introduction of inadvertently toxic artificial perilymph into the scala tympani, at the time of the bar in the center plot. Up to this point, normal minimum thresholds of single cochlear fibers were obtained (solid circles) in conjunction with a normal threshold for the gross cochlear AP response (solid square symbols). (The large scatter of single-fiber thresholds reflects the distribution of thresholds as a function of characteristic frequency, i.e., the threshold audiogram (see Fig. 3b of ref. 34 for a plot of these thresholds as a function of frequency). Within 30 min of instillation, the gross cochlear AP threshold rose rapidly, associated with consistently raised minimum thresholds of the 36 fibers obtained subsequently (open circles). The surrounding plots represent determinations of the response of 5 cochlear fibers as a function of frequency and intensity, randomized and displayed as described in the Methods of Analysis section. The dotted lines represent the FTCs for the fibers, 2 of which (A,B) were obtained before the cochlear contamination, the others after (C–E). Various degrees of loss of the low-threshold segment are seen, from partial (D,E) to complete (C).

A clearer demonstration still of the vulnerability of the second filter is afforded by experiments where reversible, *transient* loss of the low-threshold sharply tuned segment of the FTC was obtained, under the conditions out-

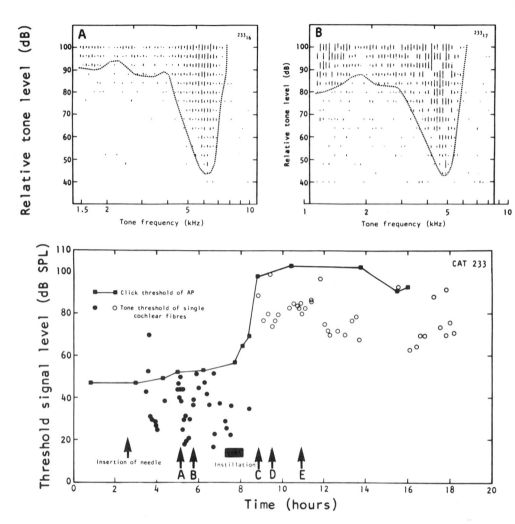

FIG. 2. Determinations of the frequency response of single cochlear fibers in the cat before and after toxic damage to the organ of Corti. *Center plot:* Minimum thresholds of 75 cochlear fibers some before (*solid circles*), and others after (*open circles*), toxic damage due to instillation of contaminated artificial perilymph into scala tympani. Instillation needle inserted at time indicated by first arrow. Instillation of artificial perilymph occurred during time indicated by bar. Fiber thresholds expressed in dB SPL at tympanic membrane. *Solid square points and continuous lines:* threshold of gross cochlear AP response recorded from round window to 50 μsec click stimuli (expressed in peak equivalent dB at 10 kHz). *Plots A–E:* Automatic determinations of frequency response of 5 cochlear fibers, A, B before, C, D, E after, onset of toxic effects. The frequency and intensity of ca. 50 msec tone bursts (presented at 5/sec) are randomized, and the number of spike discharges occurring during each tone are displayed as the length of the vertical bar at the appropriate frequency–intensity locus (see Methods of Analysis). Plots A, D, and E represent full determinations (1,024 points), whereas plots B and C represent half-point determinations (512 points). Dotted outlines represent FTC drawn by eye using an arbitrary "threshold" response. Note varying degrees of loss of low-threshold sharply tuned segment of FTC, in plots C-E. These frequency response data, and those of Figs 3, 5, and 6, have not been corrected for the characteristics of the sound system, but represent approximate ($+8\ -2$) dB SPL at the tympanic membrane. (From ref. 37.)

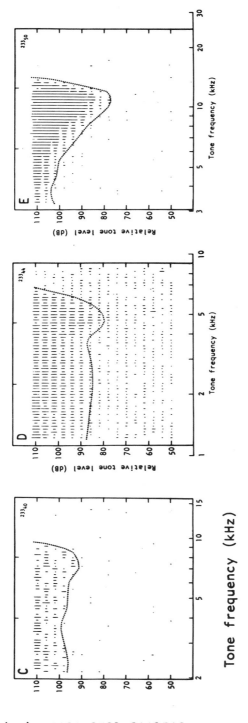

lined below. Although very different in nature, the conditions led to apparently identical effects on the threshold and suprathreshold properties of cochlear fibers.

Reducing the inspired oxygen concentration to 5% can produce marked attenuation in the gross cochlear AP without substantial changes in the CM, (35). This paradigm was used to examine the effects of brief (2–4 min) hypoxia on the discharge patterns of single cochlear fibers and particularly on their frequency selectivity (17,32,34).

Figure 3 shows these effects on a single cochlear fiber in the cat. The inset record displays the amplitude of the gross AP recorded by an electrode on the round window in response to repetitive click stimulation of constant intensity ($\sim$50 dB above AP threshold; repetition rate: 1/10 sec, interposed between the tone burst measurements illustrated in the surrounding plots). During the period indicated by the horizontal bar, the inspired oxygen concentration was reduced to 5%. After a delay of about 3 min, the amplitude of the gross AP decreased substantially. On restoring the oxygen supply, the AP returned to its former magnitude within about 5 min. Plot A represents a full determination of the frequency response of the cochlear fiber. The dashed outline therefore represents the FTC for the fiber in the control condition. Plots B, C, D, and E represent one-quarter-point determinations as the cochlear hypoxia progressively developed, and plot F shows a half-point determination during recovery before contact with the fiber was lost, as a result of extensive changes in blood pressure. (The sparseness of data points in B, C, D, and E result from the fact that only one-quarter of the points have been "addressed" in order to make rapid determinations; see Methods of Analysis section.)

The FTCs of Fig. 3 are shown superimposed in Fig. 4. During the period of hypoxia, the cochlear fiber progressively lost the low-threshold sharply tuned segment of the FTC (B,C,D), until after 2–3 min of cochlear hypoxia, only the high-threshold, broadly tuned segment remained (E). The low-threshold sharply tuned segment was partially restored (F) before the fiber was lost.

$\longrightarrow$

FIG. 3. Reversible effects of hypoxia on the tuning of a single cochlear fiber in the cat. Inset shows the time course of the gross cochlear AP amplitude in response to click stimuli of constant amplitude ($\sim$50 dB above threshold) presented every 10 sec. The thick bar indicates duration of reduction of inspired oxygen to 5%. (There is $\sim$2–3 min time delay before the effects become apparent on the cochlea.) The bars over the AP record indicate the times during which the frequency response plots illustrated in the main figure were determined. Each plot is determined in the manner described in Fig. 2. Plots B, C, D, and E represent determinations with only one-quarter of the available points, and plot F with half. Plot A: Control plot obtained before cochlear hypoxia developed. Plots B, C, D, and E obtained during cochlear hypoxia. *Plot F:* during partial recovery of response from hypoxia. (Cochlear fiber recovery lags slightly behind that of gross cochlear AP.) (From refs. 32 and 34.)

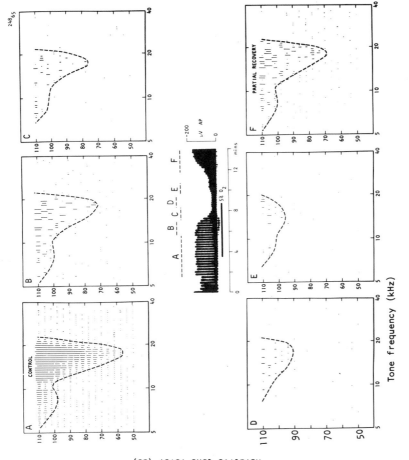

CONTROL

PARTIAL RECOVERY

Tone frequency (kHz)

Relative tone level (dB)

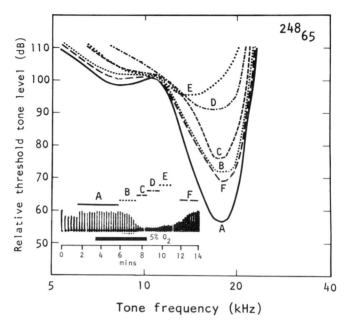

FIG. 4. Reversible effects of hypoxia on the tuning of single cochlear fiber in the cat. (Superimposition of FTCs obtained from data shown in Fig. 3.) For further explanation see legend of Fig. 3. Note loss and partial recovery of low-threshold, sharply tuned segment of FTC. (From ref. 32.)

Such changes could be observed without substantial changes in the CM (32).

With sufficient periods of recovery between trials of hypoxia, similar transient results were obtained in 13 consecutive fibers and 13 corresponding periods of hypoxia in 1 animal. With longer periods of hypoxia, however, the reversibility of the effects was reduced and fibers of progressively higher threshold would be encountered as the cochlea deteriorated (in a similar but more gradual manner to Fig. 2). Whether the cochlea would eventually recover, given more than the few hours possible in the present experiments, remains to be determined.

Intracochlear Instillation of Cyanide

These experiments were carried out in cats, in collaboration with R. Klinke, in order to examine ototoxic changes under the more controlled conditions of cochlear instillation (36). Through a needle inserted into the scala tympani of the first cochlear half-turn (via the round window membrane) KCN was introduced in approximately 0.5 mM concentration in artificial perilymph (cerebrospinal fluid). The effects are illustrated in Fig. 5.

Plots A–F (Fig. 5) represent full point determinations of the frequency re-

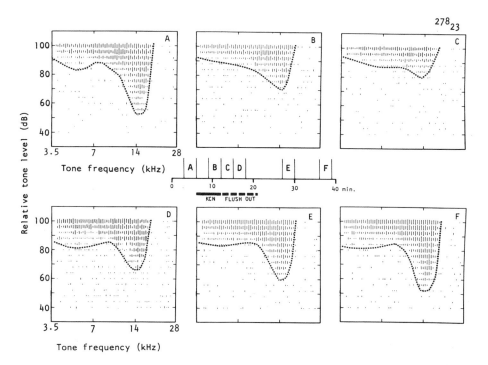

FIG. 5. Reversible effects on the response of cat cochlear fiber of instillation of potassium cyanide into cochlea. Inset indicates times of determinations of frequency response plots A–F in relation to instillation of 0.5 mM potassium cyanide in artificial perilymph into scala tympani, and subsequent "flushing out" with artificial perilymph. Time for agents to reach the cochlea at instillation rate of 7 μl per min: ~2 min. *Plot A:* Control determination of frequency response (for explanation of plot see legend to Fig. 2). *Plots B, C:* Progressive action of cyanide, eliminating lower threshold sharply tuned segment of FTC. *Curves D, E, F:* Progressive recovery of the lower threshold sharply tuned segment of the FTC, during and following flushing out of cyanide with artificial perilymph. Plot F shows almost complete recovery of FTC. (From refs. 18, 32, and 34.)

sponse of a single cochlear fiber. A is the control. Plots B and C were obtained during the action of the KCN (there is ~2 min delay before the instillation fluids reach the organ of Corti via the injection system). They show progressive loss of the low-threshold, sharply tuned segment of the FTC until in C, only the high-threshold, broadly tuned segment remains. Plots D, E, and F demonstrate progressive, but complete, recovery of the fiber from these effects, during and following "flushing" with artificial perilymph (see inset).

These effects were seen in all fibers originating in regions of the cochlea within range of the instillation (with CFs above 7 kHz).

It will be noted that, in Fig. 5, these changes occurred without substantial alteration in the spontaneous activity (the scattered points outside the FTC). On a few favorable occasions the following sequence of events has been observed (37): progressive loss of low-threshold, sharply tuned segment; reduction in evoked discharge activity; loss of spontaneous and evoked activity (presumably due to the action of the cyanide on the spike generation process itself); return of spontaneous activity, followed by progressive return of evoked activity (demonstrating the high-threshold broadly tuned FTC); finally, progressive restoration of the sharply tuned segment of the FTC, as in Fig. 5D,E,F. This strongly suggests that the effects on the frequency selectivity of the cochlear fibers can occur independently of effects on the cochlear fibers themselves.

Local and Systemic Injection of Furosemide (Fursemide)

Furosemide is a potent diuretic, which, like ethacrynic acid, has well-known ototoxic effects characterized by rapidity of onset (e.g., ref. 38). Given into the vertebral arterial supply, the agent produces transient attenuation of the gross cochlear AP (39).

Figure 6 shows the effects on a single cochlear fiber in the cat of 20 mg furosemide injected via the subclavian artery into the vertebral circulation (18,32,34). The inset shows the amplitude of the gross cochlear AP response and CM gated electronically out of the round window recorded response to constant click stimulation, approximately 40 dB above AP threshold. Two injections were made, the second of which being sufficiently vigorous to spill over into the cochlear circulation to produce the marked but transient depression in the recorded gross AP response (12–16 min). The CM was substantially unaltered. Frequency response plots A and F represent full point plots determined before and after the furosemide effects, respectively. Plots B, C, D, E represent one-quarter-point plots obtained as indicated in the inset during the development of and recovery from the effects of the furosemide. While the spontaneous discharge rate in this example does decrease somewhat during the action of the furosemide, the discharge rate in response to high-level stimulation does not (length of bars in top row of plots B–E). Again, it is the low-threshold, sharply tuned segment which is lost, leaving relatively unchanged the high-threshold broadly tuned segment.

It is interesting to note that, while instillation of ca. 0.5 mM furosemide in artificial perilymph into the cochlea produced identical changes to those obtained with intraarterial injection, the time course of recovery was very long,

---

→

FIG. 6. Reversible effects of furosemide, a potent ototoxic diuretic, on FTC of a cat cochlear fiber. *Inset:* Cochlear microphonic (CM) and gross cochlear AP response gated from round window recording of responses to constant amplitude clicks (as in Figs. 3 and 4). *Arrows:* Injection of 20 mg furosemide into the subclavian artery of the same side as the cochlea. Note transient but substantial reduction in AP following the second injection, compared with slight change in CM. *Plots A–F:* Frequency response determinations on single cochlear fiber at times indicated in the inset. (Explanation of analysis in legend of Fig. 2.) Plots B, C, D, and E represent determinations using only one-quarter of the total points (see Methods of Analysis section). *Plot A:* Control FTC. *Plots B, C:* During action of furosemide on cochlea. Note loss of low-threshold segment of FTC. *Plots D, E and F:* Recovery of normal frequency response. (From refs. 18, 32, and 34.)

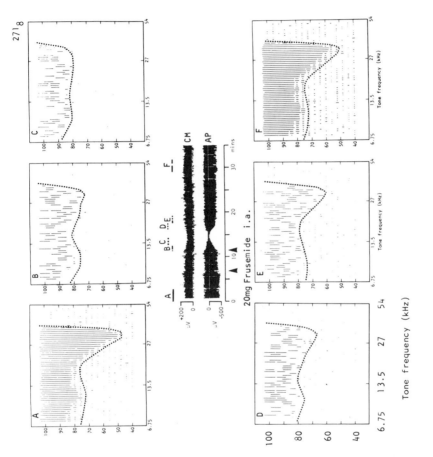

271

of the order of several hours. In one case, no obvious recovery of single fiber or gross cochlear AP responses occurred during the 7 hr of subsequent observation (37).

Other Factors

Transient occlusion of the internal auditory artery by the presence of the recording microelectrode in the cochlear nerve can cause deterioration in the threshold of tuning of cochlear fibers and of the gross cochlear AP response (guinea pig: ref. 2; rat: ref. 40). Similarly, *complete* drainage of the perilymph from the scala tympani of the first half-turn of the guinea pig (14) and cat cochlea (8), can reversibly eliminate the low-threshold, sharply tuned segment of FTCs in fibers from the affected regions of the cochlea. The high-threshold, broadly tuned FTCs thereby obtained closely resemble the basilar membrane amplitude frequency response curves obtained at the same time (8). [It should be emphasized that these data are not to be taken as evidence of damage to sharp basilar membrane tuning, as has been concluded (14). As indicated above, in the section detailing evidence for the existence of a second filter, these effects can be obtained without changes in the basilar membrane response recorded concurrently (8); sharp cochlear nerve FTCs can therefore be obtained under the same conditions in which the broadly tuned basilar membrane data are obtained.]

Significance

The question arises, what do these changes in frequency selectivity reflect? From changes in the FTCs of spiral ganglion cells in guinea pigs undergoing respiratory hypoxia similar to those described above, Robertson and Manley (41) concluded that the effects were dependent upon changes in the sensitivity of the cochlear neurons themselves, as indicated by the association with alterations in sensitivity and spontaneous activity in their data. That this is not the case, however, is indicated (i) by the analyses of suprathreshold responsiveness described above, where even under hypoxia, loss of the narrowly tuned FTC segment can occur without changes in the discharge rate in response to high-level tonal stimulation (32,34; see also Fig. 6 here); (ii) these changes in tuning can occur independently of effects on spontaneous activity (see "Intracochlear Instillation of Cyanide" above); (iii) the effects occur primarily on the low-threshold sharply tuned segment of the FTC, whereas the threshold and suprathreshold properties (e.g., discharge rate—intensity function) of the low-frequency "tail" of the FTC are relatively unmodified (32,34); (iv) local instillation of tetrodotoxin into the scala tympani can block cochlear fiber spike generation abruptly without any prior deterioration in tuning being evident, in contrast to the effects with cyanide, etc. (37). It is clear, however, that *excessive* administration of the agents or procedures producing loss of tuning can produce direct effects on the cochlear neurons themselves or on the transduction-spike initiation process in the hair cells. Under these conditions (observed in the present experiments under systemic hypoxia, and intracochlear administration of cyanide and furosemide) the fibers become inactive. This too, can be reversible (see "Intracochlear Instillation of Cyanide" above).

The simplest interpretation of these results therefore is that the observed deterioration in cochlear nerve frequency selectivity reflects a reduction in tuning of the second filter.

The fact that many of the deleterious influences on cochlear nerve tuning appear to have a preferential effect on the outer hair cells (e.g., refs. 42–47), whereas our recordings must be predominantly from fibers arising from the inner hair cells [which constitute about 95% of the fibers leaving the organ of Corti (ref 48)], raises the tempting speculation that the second filter process is determined by some form of interaction between the outer and inner hair cells of the organ of Corti, and/or their innervations (32,49). One possibility is that the FTC represents the sum of 2 separate excitatory processes, one related to the outer hair cells and responsible for the low-threshold sharply tuned segment (as a result of the action of the second filter following the first) and the other related to the inner hair cells, responsible for the broadly tuned high-threshold segment (reflecting basilar membrane properties alone. Several lines of data are consistent with this notion. First, in many cochlear fibers, the discharge rate–tone intensity functions for the low-threshold segment are different in slope from those of the low-frequency tails of the FTC (32,13). Second, whereas the latter rate–intensity functions are little affected by the procedures eliminating the low-threshold sharply tuned segment, the former are affected (32,34). Third, loss of the sharply tuned segment of the FTC is associated with a shift in the CF toward lower frequencies (32,34; see Figs. 4, 5, and 7). Outer spiral fibers innervate regions of the organ of Corti about 0.5 mm *basal* from those innervated by the inner radial fibers with which they come into contact in the habenular openings (50). Fourth, the presence of high-threshold, abnormally tuned fibers in the data of Kiang et al. (ref. 1, Figs. 10 and 14) coming from regions of the cochlea with abnormal outer hair cells but normal inner hair cells (to light microscopy at least) is consistent with the scheme. More clear-cut evidence of this has recently been obtained in the guinea pig (Harrison and Evans, *to be published*). This notion requires that the second filter process be located in the outer hair cells themselves or their innervation patterns, and the APs (presumably) propagated along the outer spiral fibres, to initiate or influence spike generation in the inner radial fibers. There appears to be ample opportunity for electrical cross-talk to occur between the 2 sets of fibers in the habenular opening (51,52), and it has been proposed for other purposes (e.g., refs. 53 and 20). The validity of this and the many other models which have been proposed for the second filter process (with and without inner

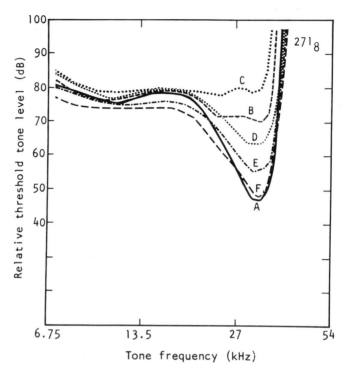

FIG. 7. Reversible effects of furosemide on FTC of a cat cochlear fiber. (Superimposition of FTCs from Fig. 6.) Each curve is identified by the same letters used in the plots and inset of Fig. 6. (From refs. 18, 32, and 34.)

and outer hair cell interaction) remains an open question and awaits further data; they are discussed elsewhere (12,13,34).

Conclusions for Sensorineural Hearing Loss

There is good evidence for the hypothesis that, to a first approximation at least, the normal frequency selectivity of the auditory system is already developed at the level of the cochlear nerve, and is determined by the tuning properties of individual fibers (12,32,54).

For signals with complex spectra, the cochlear fibers act as if they were linear filters with characteristics given by the shape of their pure-tone FTCs. This has been demonstrated for broadband noise (26–28,12), comb-filtered noise (29–31,12), for click stimuli (55); and by implication from measurements on cochlear nucleus cells by Møller (56; see discussion of this study in ref. 13). This means that in spite of the increase in width of the FTCs with signal level, the *effective* bandwidth remains constant, that is, in terms of the influence of certain frequencies in determining the pattern of activity in a given fiber, it is those frequencies within the effective bandwidth which are most significant. (The effective bandwidth is the width of the equivalent rectangular filter, and is derived by integrating the area under the FTC considered as an attenuation function in linear power and frequency coordinates; it is approximately the half-power—3 dB down—bandwidth.) This appears to be the case for signals at least up to 70–80 dB SPL; thereafter, there is some evidence that the cochlear filtering process becomes increasingly nonlinear or broadly tuned or both (see refs. 57 and 13 for reviews).

There is good quantitative agreement between the effective bandwidths of normal cochlear fibers in the cat and the analogous measure of human psychophysical frequency selectivity, the critical band (12,13). In addition, direct measurements of psychophysical frequency selectivity, using combfiltered noise signals, agree well with analogous measurements in normal cochlear fibres in the cat (30,13). Recent tone-on-tone masking paradigms have revealed the existence of human psychophysical "tuning curves," resembling the FTCs of cochlear fibers (54,58–60). Other properties of the critical band are consistent with the hypothesis (see ref. 13).

On the other hand, there are some recent behavioral data in cat which appear to suggest that the behavioral critical band may be larger than the effective bandwidths of cochlear nerve fibers by a factor as much as 2 (61). While there is no evidence of sufficient convergence at the level of the cochlear nucleus to account for this (62,63), lateral inhibitory mechanisms in the dorsal division of the cochlear nucleus do appear to preserve the frequency selectivity at the high stimulus levels at which it appears to deteriorate in the cochlear nerve (63). If this is the case, and whatever the exact relationship to the critical band, the cochlear second-filtering process and subsequent inhibitory mechanisms would appear to serve to establish and preserve, respectively, the normal peripheral frequency analysis, important for the processing of complex signals, particularly speech.

In view of its vulnerability to a wide variety of deleterious influences: metabolic, toxic, surgical, mechanical, etc., the second filter process may be one of the first functions to be affected in pathological conditions in man giving rise to sensorineural hearing loss, permanent and temporary (2,12, 32,34). This notion receives support from some psychophysical experiments indicating deterioration of the critical band in severe hearing loss of cochlear origin (64–66), and in deterioration in the perception of speech, resistant to amplification in cases of cochlear hearing loss above about 30 dB (67). Direct measurements of the effective bandwidths of cochlear fibers in the cat, under various types of experimentally induced cochlear pathology, e.g., under similar conditions to those illustrated in Fig. 2, indicate an increase in effective bandwidth to broadband signals by factors of 3 to 10 over the normal values (68). However, under conditions in which less complete loss of the sharply tuned segment was obtained, the effective bandwidths would appear to be little affected, thus accounting for reports of essentially normal speech perception in patients with mild cochlear hearing loss (67).

The hypothesis, however, affords a simple explanation for the phenomena, typically observed in cochlear hearing loss, of recruitment in loudness (69), and of recruitment in the gross cochlear AP recorded by the technique of electrocochleography in man (e.g., refs. 70 and 71), and in animals under ototoxic conditions (72), see Fig. 8 (2,34,82). There is no evidence (73,13) for 2 populations of cochlear fibers of low and high thresholds, respectively, the loss of 1 set of which could account in some way for recruitment, as in some theories (e.g., ref. 74). On the contrary, the data described above and the evidence of Fig. 2 indicates a single population of fibers whose normally sharp tuning and low-threshold properties deteriorate under conditions of cochlear pathology.

On the assumption that loudness, and the magnitude of the gross cochlear

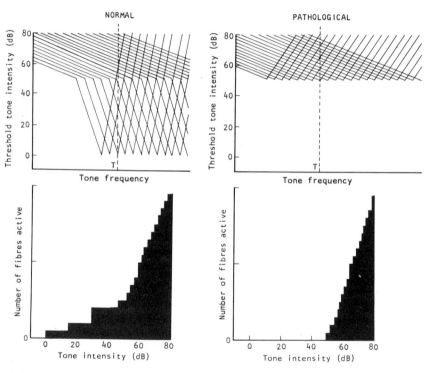

FIG. 8. Hypothetical scheme for recruitment. Schematic diagram illustrating rate of growth in number of active cochlear fibers with tone stimulus level, in normal and pathological cochleas. Tone frequency indicated by dashed line at T. *Upper half: left:* Sharply tuned FTCs of single cochlear fibers in normal cochlea; *right:* high-threshold, broadly tuned FTCs of pathological cochlea (as in Figs. 1–7). *Lower half:* Growth in number of active fibers with increasing tone level corresponding to the difference in sharpness and threshold of the cochlear fiber FTCs in normal (*left*) and pathological cochlea (*right*). Each new fiber is added to the active group as the tone level crosses its FTC. The scales in each plot are arbitrary. In the case of the tone intensity scales in particular, the dB values are given purely for convenience in relating the upper and lower plots, and are not intended to represent absolute threshold values. (From refs. 34 and 82.)

AP, is related to the number of fibers driven by a particular tone (T in Fig. 8), the rate of growth in these functions will be determined by the shapes, particularly the slopes of the cutoffs of the FTCs. In the case of the broadly tuned pathological fibers (right half of Fig. 8), once the elevated thresholds are reached, the size of the active group of fibers will grow more rapidly with intensity than in the normal situation (left half of Fig. 8). (It is, however, possibly unwise to seek simplistic or unitary explanations of gross AP phenomena; see refs. 13 and 72.) In addition to this effect, cochlear pathology serves to increase the steepness of the discharge rate–intensity functions at the CF of cochlear fibers (32,34). Lesions underlying sensorineural hearing loss of retrocochlear origin, even if they eliminated cochlear fibers, would not be expected to affect the cochlear filtering (unless the blood supply to the cochlea was impaired by the lesion), and recruitment would not occur, as appears to be the case (69). On the contrary, loss of cochlear fibers would be expected to reduce the loudness at all stimulus levels relative to the normal situation.

In summary, a distinction may need to be made between effects of cochlear pathology on the effective bandwidth and slopes of the cutoffs of cochlear fibers, respectively. Changes in the latter may be evident without substantial changes in the former, because the tips of the FTCs are more U than V shaped when detailed measurements are made (e.g., refs. 1,27, and 12). Thus, increase in the effective bandwidth of cochlear fibers and therefore deterioration of auditory frequency selectivity (reflected in critical band; peripheral analysis of speech signals) may not be appreciable until elevation of threshold above a certain level (e.g., 30–40 dB) occurs, whereas change in the cutoff slopes (particularly the low-frequency cutoff) would be expected to accompany any shift in threshold and be manifest in early signs of recruitment.

SIGNIFICANCE FOR NOISE EXPOSURE

"Pseudorecruitment" of loudness occurs in normal subjects during and following exposure to broadband noise. Studies of the effects of noise stimuli on the slopes of cochlear fiber FTCs (32) indicate that, while their effective bandwidth changes little, the cutoff slopes decrease with the higher levels of noise. Similar reduction in sharpness of tuning can follow exposure to intense tones at the CF (1).

These temporary effects, and those of higher levels of noise exposure producing permanent hearing losses, may themselves result from cochlear hypoxia. Several studies of noise-induced damage have implicated local reductions in cochlear blood flow and consequent oxygen availability to the organ of Corti (75–78). It is interesting in this respect also that the ototoxic antibiotics and diuretics inhibit the respiratory enzymes in the outer hair cells (47). The tuning and threshold properties of cochlear fibers appear to be extremely sensitive to any deficiencies in meeting the metabolic requirements of the organ of Corti; there appears to be little "reserve." These properties of cochlear fibers deteriorate within seconds of occlusion of the internal auditory artery (79,2,40), and of complete drainage of the perilymph from the appropriate part of the scala tympani (14,8), the latter presumably exerting its effects by restricting oxygen diffusion from the spiral artery into the organ of Corti.

It seems possible, then, in conclusion, that the metabolic requirements of the second filter form the "final common path" of cochlear pathology, ranging from noise-induced hearing loss, through the effects of ototoxic agents, to presbycusis. This notion could account for the synergistic effects of otherwise apparently unrelated agents, e.g., noise and ototoxic antibiotics (80). Alternatively, or in addition, the numerous adrenergic terminals in the spiral ganglion and habenular region of the cochlea (e.g., ref. 81) may be involved. It is interesting in this respect that the local instillation of α-adrenergic blocking agents produce similar, though long-term, changes in threshold and tuning, to the temporary changes described above (33).

ACKNOWLEDGMENTS

I am grateful to Drs. J. P. Wilson and R. Klinke for many helpful discussions, and to the former for criticisms of the manuscript. The work described has been supported in part by the Medical and Science Research Councils and the Deutsche Forschungsgemeinschaft (K1 219).

REFERENCES

1. Kiang, N. Y-s, Moxon, E. C., and Levine, R. A. (1970): Auditory-nerve activity in cats with normal and abnormal cochleas. In: *Sensorineural Hearing Loss,* edited by Wolstenholme and J. Knight, pp. 241–268. Churchill, London.
2. Evans, E. F. (1972): The frequency response and other properties of single fibres in the guinea-pig cochlear nerve. *J. Physiol. (London),* 226:263–287.
3. Kiang, N. Y-s, Watenabe, T., Thomas, E. C., and Clarke, L. F. (1965): Discharge Patterns of Single Fibres in the Cat's Auditory Nerve. MIT Press, Cambridge, Mass.
4. Evans, E. F. (1970): Narrow "tuning" of cochlear nerve fibre responses in the guinea pig. *J. Physiol. (London),* 206:14–15P.
5. Evans, E. F. (1972): Does frequency sharpening occur in the cochlea? In: *Hearing Theory 1972,* pp. 27–34. IPO: Eindhoven.
6. Wilson, J. P. (1974): Basilar membrane data and their relation to theories of frequency analysis. In: *Facts and Models in Hearing,* edited by E. Zwicker and E. Terhardt. Springer, Berlin.
7. Geisler, C. D., Rhode, W. S., and Kennedy, D. T. (1974): Responses to tonal stimuli of single auditory nerve fibres and their relationship to basilar membrane motion in the squirrel monkey. *J. Neurophysiol.,* 37:1156–1172.
8. Evans, E. F. and Wilson, J. P. (1975): Cochlear tuning properties: concurrent basilar membrane and single nerve fiber measurements. *Science,* 190: Dec. 19th.
9. Békésy, E. von (1944): Über die mechanische Frequenzanalyze in der Schnecke verschiedener Tiere. *Akust. Z.,* 9:3–11.
10. Johnstone, B. M., Taylor, K. J., and Boyle, A. J. (1970): Mechanics of the guinea pig cochlea. *J. Acoust. Soc. Am.,* 47:504–509.

11. Wilson, J. P., and Johnstone, J. R. (1975): Basilar membrane and middle-ear vibration in guinea pig measured by capacitive probe. *J. Acoust. Soc. Am.*, 57:705–723.
12. Evans, E. F., and Wilson, J. P. (1973): Frequency selectivity of the cochlea. In: *Basic Mechanisms in Hearing*, edited by A. R. Møller, pp. 519–557. Academic Press, New York.
13. Evans, E. F. (1975): Cochlear nerve and cochlear nucleus. In: *Handbook of Sensory Physiology*, edited by W. D. Keidel and W. D. Neff, Vol. 5, Part II, Chapt. 1. Springer, Berlin.
14. Robertson, D. (1974): Cochlear neurons: frequency selectivity altered by perilymph removal. *Science*, 186:153–155.
15. Evans, E. F. (1970): Narrow "tuning" of the responses of cochlear nerve fibres emanating from the exposed basilar membrane. *J. Physiol. (London)*, 208:75–76P.
16. Rhode, W. S. (1971): Observations of the vibration of the basilar membrane in squirrel monkeys using the Mössbauer technique. *J. Acoust. Soc. Am.*, 49:1218–1231.
17. Evans, E. F. (1974): Effects of hypoxia on the tuning of single cochlear nerve fibres. *J. Physiol. (London)*, 238:65–67P.
18. Evans, E. F., and Klinke, R. (1974): Reversible effects of cyanide and frusemide on the tuning of single cochlear fibres. *J. Physiol. (London)*, 242:129–131P.
19. Sachs, M. B., and Kiang, N. Y-s. (1968): Two-tone inhibition in auditory nerve fibres. *J. Acoust. Soc. Am.*, 43:1120–1128.
20. Arthur, R. M., Pfeiffer, R. R., and Suga, N. (1971): Properties of "two-tone inhibition" in primary auditory neurones. *J. Physiol. (London)*, 212:593–609.
21. Goldstein, J. L., and Kiang, N. Y-s. (1968): Neural correlates of the aural combination tone $2f_1$-f_2. *Proc. IEEE*, 56:981–992.
22. Pfeiffer, R. R. (1970): A model for two-tone inhibition of single cochlear nerve fibres. *J. Acoust. Soc. Am.*, 48:1373–1378.
23. Smoorenburg, G. F. (1972): Combination tones and their origin. *J. Acoust. Soc. Am.*, 52:615–632.
24. Wilson, J. P., and Johnstone, J. R. (1973): Basilar membrane correlates of the combination tone $2f_1$-f_2. *Nature*, 241:206–207.
25. Dallos, P. (1969): Combination tone $2f_1$-f_h in microphonic potentials. *J. Acoust. Soc. Am.*, 46:1437–1444.
26. De Boer, E. (1969): Reverse correlation II. Initiation of nerve impulses in the inner ear. *Koninkl. Ned. Akad. Wetenschap. Proc. Ser.*, 72:129–151.
27. Evans, E. F., Rosenberg, J., and Wilson, J. P. (1970): The effective bandwidth of cochlear nerve fibres. *J. Physiol. (London)*, 207:62–63P.
28. Evans, E. F., and Wilson, J. P. (1971): Frequency sharpening of the cochlea: the effective bandwidth of cochlear nerve fibres. *Proc. 7th Int. Cong. Acoust.*, 3:453–456.
29. Evans, E. F., Rosenberg, J., and Wilson, J. P. (1971): The frequency resolving power of the cochlea. *J. Physiol. (London)*, 216:58–59P.
30. Wilson, J. P., and Evans, E. F. (1971): Grating acuity of the ear: psychophysical and neurophysiological measures of frequency resolving power. *Proc. 7th Int. Cong. Acoust.*, Vol. 3:397–400.
31. Wilson, J. P., Evans, E. F., and Rosenberg, J. (1974): Linearity of the cochlear nerve fibre filter response: a test for the influence of two-tone suppression. *Proc. 8th Int. Cong. Acoust.*, 1:180.
32. Evans, E. F. (1974): Auditory frequency selectivity and the cochlear nerve. In: *Facts and Models in Hearing*, edited by E. Zwicker and E. Terhardt, pp. 118–129. Springer, Berlin, Heidelberg, New York.
33. Klinke, R., and Evans, E. F. (1975): Alpha-receptor blocking agents decrease cochlear potentials. *Pfluegers Arch.* 355:R115.
34. Evans, E. F. (1975): Normal and abnormal functioning of the cochlear nerve. In: *Sound Reception in Mammals:* Symp. Zoo. Soc., pp. 133–165, Vol. 197, No. 37. Academic Press, London.
35. Fernandez, C., and Alzate, R. (1959): Modifications of cochlear responses by oxygen deprivation. *Arch. Otolaryngol.*, 69:82–94.
36. Galley, N., Klinke, R., Oertel, W., Pause, M., and Storch, W-H. (1973): The effects of intracochlearly administered acetylcholine-blocking agents on the efferent synapses of the cochlea. *Brain Res.*, 64:55–63.

37. Evans, E. F., and Klinke, R. To be published.
38. Schwartz, G. H., David, D. S., Riggio, R. R., Stenzel, K. H., and Rubin, A. L. (1970): Ototoxity introduced by furosemide. *N. Engl. J. Med.* 282:1413.
39. Brown, R. D., and McElwee, T. W., Jr. (1972): Effects of intraarterially and intravenously administered ethacrynic acid and furosemide on cochlear N_1 in cats. *Toxicol. Appl. Pharmacol.,* 22:589–594.
40. Evans, E. F., and Vater, M. Unpublished data.
41. Robertson, D., and Manley, G. A. (1974): Manipulation of frequency analysis in the cochlear ganglion of the guinea pig. *J. Comp. Physiol.,* 91:363.
42. Davis, H., Deatherage, B. H., Rosenblut, B., Fernandez, C., Kimura, R., and Smith, C. A. (1958): Modifications of cochlear potentials produced by streptomycin poisoning and by venous obstruction. *Laryngoscope,* 68:596–627.
43. Kohonen, A. (1965): Effect of some ototoxic drugs upon the pattern and innervation of cochlear sensory cells in the guinea pig. *Acta Otolaryngol. [Suppl.] (Stockh.),* 208:1–70.
44. Hawkins, J. E. Jr., Beger, V., and Aran, J. M. (1967): Antibiotic insults to Corti's Organ. In: *Sensorineural Hearing Processes and Disorders,* edited by A. B. Graham, pp. 411–425. Little, Brown, Boston, Mass.
45. Mathog, R. H., Thomas, W. A., and Hudson, W. R. (1970): Ototoxicity of new and potent diuretics: a preliminary study. *Arch. Otolaryngol.,* 20:7–13.
46. Dallos, P., Billone, M. C., Durrant, J. D., Wang, C-y., and Raynor, S. (1972): Cochlear inner and outer hair cells: functional differences. *Science,* 177:356–358.
47. Kaku, Y., Farmer, J. C., and Hudson, W. R. (1973): Ototoxic drug effects on cochlear histochemistry. *Arch. Otolaryngol.,* 98:282–286.
48. Spoendlin, H. (1969): Innervation patterns in the organ of Corti of the cat. *Acta Otolaryngol. (Stockh.),* 67:239–254.
49. Zwislocki, J. J., and Sokolich, W. G. (1974): Neuro-mechanical frequency analysis in the cochlea. In: *Facts and Models in Hearing,* edited by E. Zwicker and E. Terhardt, pp. 107–117. Springer, Berlin, Heidelberg, New York.
50. Spoendlin, H. (1966): The organization of the cochlear receptor. *Adv. Otorhinolaryngol.,* 13:1–227.
51. Smith, C. A., and Dempsey, E. W. (1957): Electron microscopy of the organ of Corti. *Am. J. Anat.,* 100:337.
52. Spoendlin, H. (1974): Neuroanatomy of the cochlea. In: *Facts and Models in Hearing,* edited by E. Zwicker and E. Terhardt, pp. 18–32. Springer, Berlin, Heidelberg, New York.
53. Lynn, P. A., and Sayers, B. McA. (1970): Cochlear innervation, signal processing, and their relation to auditory time-intensity effects. *J. Acoust. Soc. Am.,* 47:525–533.
54. Zwicker, E. (1974): On a psychoacoustical equivalent of tuning curves. In: *Facts and Models in Hearing,* edited by E. Zwicker and E. Terhardt, pp. 132–140. Springer, Berlin, Heidelberg, New York.
55. Goldstein, J. L., Baer, T., and Kiang, N. Y-s. (1971): A theoretical treatment of latency, group-delay and tuning characteristics for auditory-nerve responses to clicks and tones. In: *Physiology of the Auditory System,* edited by M. B. Sachs, pp. 133–141. National Educational Consultants, Baltimore, Md.
56. Møller, A. (1970): Studies of the damped oscillatory response of the auditory frequency analyzer. *Acta Physiol. Scand.,* 78:299–314.
57. Pfeiffer, R. R., and Kim, D. O. (1973): Considerations of nonlinear response properties of single cochlear nerve fibers. In: *Basic Mechanisms in Hearing,* edited by A. R. Møller, pp. 555–587. Academic Press, New York.
58. Small, A. M., Jr. (1959): Pure tone masking. *J. Acoust. Soc. Am.,* 31:1619–1625.
59. Rodenburg, M., Vershuure, J., and Brocaar, M. P. (1974): Comparison of two masking methods. *Acustica,* 31:99–106.
60. Vogten, L. L. M. (1974): Pure tone masking; a new result from a new method. In: *Facts and Models in Hearing,* edited by E. Zwicker and E. Terhardt, pp. 142–155. Springer, Berlin, Heidelberg, New York.
61. Pickles, J. O. (1974): The origin of critical bands in the cat. *J. Physiol. (London),* 242:131–132P.

62. Kiang, N. Y-s. (1965): Stimulus coding in the auditory nerve and cochlear nucleus. *Acta Otolaryngol. (Stockh.)*, 59:186–200.
63. Evans, E. F., and Palmer, A. R. (1975): Responses of units in the cochlear nerve and nucleus of the cat to signals in the presence of bandstopnoise. *J. Physiol.*, 252: 60–62.
64. de Boer, E. (1959): Measurement of critical band-width in cases of perception deafness. *Proc. 3rd Int. Cong. Acoust.*, 1:100–102.
65. Scharf, B., and Hellman, R. P. (1966): Model of loudness summation applied to impaired ears. *J. Acoust. Soc. Am.*, 40:71–78.
66. Martin, M. C. (1974): Critical bands in sensori-neural hearing loss. *Scand. Audiol.*, 3:133–140.
67. Hood, J. D., and Poole, J. P. (1971): Speech audiometry in conductive and sensorineural hearing loss. *Sound*, 5:30–38.
68. Evans, E. F. (1976): The effective bandwidths of individual cochlear nerve fibres from pathological cochleas in the cat. *Proceedings of the Second British Conference on Audiology*, Academic Press, London, New York.
69. Dix, M. R., Hallpike, C. S., and Hood, J. D. (1948): Observations upon the loudness recruitment phenomenon with especial reference to the differential diagnosis of disorders of the internal ear and VIII nerve. *Proc. Roy. Soc. Med.*, 41:516–526.
70. Aran, J-M. (1971): The electrocochleogram: recent results in children and in some pathological cases. *Arch. Otorhinolaryngol. (NY)*, 198:128–141.
71. Eggermont, J. J., and Odenthal, D. N. (1974): Electrophysiological investigation of the human cochlea. Recruitment, masking and adaptation. *Audiology*, 13:1–22.
72. Aran, J-M., and Darrouzet, J. (1975): Observation of click evoked compound VIII nerve responses before during and over seven months after kanamycin treatment in the guinea pig. *Acta Otolaryngol. (Stockh.)*, 79:24–32.
73. Kiang, N. Y-s. (1968): A survey of recent developments in the study of auditory physiology. *Ann. Otol. Rhinol. Laryngol.*, 77:656–676.
74. Portmann, M., Aran, J-M., and Lagourgue, P. (1973): Testing for "recruitment" by electrocochleography: preliminary results. *Ann. Otol. Rhinol. Laryngol.*, 82:36–43.
75. Koide, Y., Yoshida, M., and Kouno, M. (1960): Some aspects of the biochemistry of acoustic trauma. *Ann. Otol. Rhinol. Laryngol.*, 69:661–697.
76. Lawrence, M., Gonzalez, G., and Hawkins, J. E., Jr. (1967): Some physiological factors in noise-induced hearing loss. *Am. Ind. Hyg. Assoc. J.*, 28:425–430.
77. Hawkins, J. E., Jr. (1971): The role of vasoconstriction in noise-induced hearing loss. *Ann. Otol. Rhinol. Laryngol.*, 80:903–013.
78. Schnieder, E-A. (1974): A contribution to the physiology of the perilymph: Pt. III on the origin of noise-induced hearing loss. *Ann. Otol. Rhinol. Laryngol.*, 83:406–412.
79. Konishi, T., Butler, R. A., and Fernandez, C. (1961): The effect of anoxia on cochlear potentials. *J. Acoust. Soc. Am.*, 33:349–356.
80. Dayal, V. S., Kokshanian, A., and Mitchell, D. P. (1971): Combined effects of noise and kanamycin. *Ann. Otol. Rhinol. Laryngol.*, 80:897–902.
81. Densert, O., and Flock, Å., (1974): An electron-microscopic study of adrenergic innervation in the cochlea. *Acta Otolaryngol. (Stockh.)*, 77:185–197.
82. Evans, E. F. (1975): The sharpening of cochlear frequency selectivity in the normal and abnormal cochlea. *Audiology*, 14:419–442.

DISCUSSION

J. Tonndorf: Considering the innervation of both inner hair cells (IHC) and outer hair cells (OHC), is it possible that the sharply tuned low-threshold segment is due in the main to the activity of the OHC and whether the high-threshold, low-pass segment is due mainly to the activity of the IHC?

E. Evans: This is a tremendously interesting speculation, because many of the phenomena we have been describing, e.g., furosemide has a specific inhibiting effect on the respiratory enzymes of the OHC. You begin to see that the most sensitive elements in the cochlea are the OHC. And if the fibers from which we are recording are almost entirely coming from the IHC, and not the OHC, then how is it the properties of all these fibers appear to be determined by the properties and the susceptibilities of the OHC? This leads to the speculation that some kind of interaction is occurring. My favorite place for the interaction is at the habenular opening, where you could get some form of electrical cross talk. One of the outcomes of this speculation would be, if you eliminate the activity of the OHC, leaving behind the frequency selectivity of the IHC, then the CF of the tuning curves should shift about one-fifth of an octave toward lower frequencies.

A. Møller: May I add that Zwislocki and Sokolich (*Facts and Models in Hearing* (1974), edited by E. Zwicker and E. Terhardt, Springer, Berlin) proposed an interaction between the OHC and IHC in their model.

H. Spoendlin: On the interaction between OHC and IHC, there is no anatomical evidence for such interaction. Also, there is no, let's say practical possibility of an electrical interaction, because these fibers are practically always separated by a supporting structure.

E. Evans: But you showed that they are very close together at the habenula.

H. Spoendlin: If you look quite carefully, the distance where the fibers for the OHC and the fibers from the IHC are actually in close approximation is very minimal. They have a tendency to separate immediately after the habenular opening. This interaction is on weak grounds.

I wonder whether this loss of sharpening following hypoxia could also be due to a change of the dendrites to the IHC. Because, as both we and B. Bohne have found, these dendrites are extremely sensitive to hypoxia. In fact, after hypoxia the swollen dendrites are the only obvious change.

D. Dunn: Do you completely discount the efferent system in this tuning?

E. Evans: Yes, completely, and on very strong grounds. (1) All these experiments are carried out under deep pentabarbital anesthesia, and (2) you can show, as Aage Møller [*Acta Physiol. Scand.* (1970), 78:299–314] has shown, that the cochlear filtering properties are already established to click stimuli, and there is no time for information to go up the routes and back. However, it is interesting, whether the local presence of the efferent fibers in the cochlea might, by local interactive mechanisms, produce something.

D. Dunn: I asked, because there had been some work recently where severing of the fibers had resulted in changes in the bandwidth.

E. Evans: Not in cochlear nerve fibers. Cochlear nerve fibers show very clearly that if you cut the nerve and record peripherally, to the site of the incision, you can record quite normally tuned cochlear fibers.

C. Trahiotis: On the point of frequency resolution being pretty much determined at least in the cochlea: One of the facts about frequency discrimination is that it gets decidedly better at higher sensation levels. This should be well up on the tuning curves. And on animals, Elliot (*Ann. Otol. Rhin. Laryngol.* (1960), 70:582–598) has shown that the intensity and frequency discrimination in an animal with a sensory neural loss is essentially normal.

E. Evans: You're confusing two separate functions. You're confusing frequency discrimination, which is our ability to distinguish the differences in frequencies, i.e., C sharp and C, and frequency selectivity, which is what I'm talking about, which is the ability to separate out, or resolve the individual frequency component of a complex signal. For example, the individual notes of a chord on the piano. Now, narrow frequency selectivity doesn't get better, it hardly changes, slightly deteriorates at higher levels, and that we could predict on the basis of other data which I don't have time to go into. But frequency discrimination does include the level, and I don't know what your theory of frequency discrimination is, but mine is that it's based on the slope of the high frequency cutoffs of the tuning curves, which will demarcate an area of active and inactive fibers somewhere in the auditory system. Now, those slopes, as we saw from the first slide, get steeper as you increase level, so that that would fit with frequency discrimination, but if you're specifically referring to frequency selectivity that's a different thing.

W. Ward: Well, let's talk about pitch. Your model, if its going to apply to both TTS and PTS conditions, would predict pitch changes and at high intensities we should return to normal pitch.

E. Evans: I haven't been making any predictions about pitch changes at all, yet. What one might infer from the shift in the CF of fibers downward, is that, in cases of localized areas of sensorineural damage in the cochlea, you might get pitch shifts in the upward direction. I gather that this is in fact found, is it not?

G. Manley: We have similar recordings from the spiral ganglion in the guinea pig, which show the loss of the very sharply tuned segment of the basal turn fibers. We found that under the various conditions that we used, e.g., perilymph drainage or minor damage to the cochlea accidental, but sometimes fortuitous in producing poorly tuned fibers. The 2-tone inhibitory phenomena always disappears concomitant with the drop in sensitivity and the loss of the sharply tuned segment. When the tuning is relatively good, the 2-tone inhibition is weak; when tuning is bad, 2-tone inhibition is totally absent.

Effects of Noise on Hearing, edited by Donald Henderson,
Roger P. Hamernik, Darshan S. Dosanjh, and John H. Mills.
Raven Press, New York © 1976

Eighth Nerve Responses and Permanent Sensorineural Hearing Loss

Robert L. Smith

Institute for Sensory Research, Syracuse University, Syracuse, New York 13210

The 8th nerve is the most peripheral portion of the mammalian auditory system from which single-unit recordings can presently be obtained. Its responses form the inputs to the central nervous system and provide important boundary conditions for the perception of sound. However, there are several considerations that limit the application of 8th-nerve studies to the formulation of noise damage risk criteria. From the practical point of view, there exist at present no recordings from animals having permanent noise-induced hearing losses. In addition, 2 sets of basic questions must be more fully answered in order to interrelate noise-induced changes in cochlear anatomy, 8th-nerve responses, and hearing. The first set concerns the roles of the various cochlear structures in producing 8th-nerve responses. For example, what changes can be expected in responses from fibers innervating regions devoid of outer hair cells? The second set concerns the functional significance of the various measureable parameters of 8th-nerve responses, i.e., what kinds of changes in hearing are produced by changes in these parameters? For example, how strict a correspondence can we expect between the characteristic frequencies of units suffering a loss in sensitivity and the sound frequencies for which abnormal hearing occurs? This chapter reviews some of the 8th-nerve results that may be relevant to these issues and that may suggest fruitful avenues for future research. The considerations are not necessarily new [e.g., Stevens and Davis (1)], but have received new support from recent experimental findings.

A REVIEW OF SOME SIMPLE RESPONSE PROPERTIES

The systematic studies of Kiang and associates (2–6) established the existence of a homogeneous population of auditory-nerve fibers with similar response properties. Since that time, a large body of experimental results has been devoted to obtaining additional details of the stimulus–response relationships in an effort to understand both cochlear mechanisms and encoding properties in normal animals. This section aims at reviewing some of the experimental findings and resulting questions which, in the opinion of the author, will ultimately be important for understanding the basic mechanisms and effects of noise damage. The section is organized in terms of the 3 physical parameters that describe a simple tonal stimulus—its intensity, frequency, and duration.

Intensity Characteristics

When a unit is stimulated at its characteristic frequency (CF), i.e., the frequency of maximum sensitivity, firing rate is typically an S-shaped function of sound pressure level (SPL). The rate first increases and then becomes negatively accelerated, asymptotically approaching a saturation value within 20–40 dB. Although the degree of the saturation varies somewhat from unit to unit (7), it would appear that saturation severely limits the useful operating range of a unit. Since the distribution of sensitivities among units with similar CFs is limited to a small range of about 25 dB (4,8,9), the question arises as to how the auditory system is able to operate over a large dynamic range of over 120 dB. An answer to this question appears to be required in order to understand the physiological basis for psychophysical loudness and differential sensitivity in both normal and abnormal ears.

One possibility that should be considered is that a unit operating in its saturated region, as determined with constant intensity stimuli, may still be able to transmit useful auditory information about dynamic or time-varying stimuli. For example, some of the results of Rose et al. (10) led them to suggest that a sensitivity control mechanism might be operating in the auditory periphery. A typical set of their results are shown by the period histograms in the upper portion of Fig. 1. These histograms were each obtained with a different stimulus intensity and describe the average temporal distribution of spikes relative to a period of the 1.1 kHz stimulus. They have a 92 μsec binwidth and illustrate the phase-locking generally encountered in responses to low-frequency stimulation—spikes occur only during a preferred half-cycle of the stimulus. Rose et al. (10) interpret the shape of the histograms as reflecting the "effective stimulating waveform." They point out that the shape of the period histograms remains relatively unaltered, even at intensities that produce a saturation of the average firing rate. For example, the SPL used for histogram d produced little change in average firing rate relative to histogram c, as can be observed in the intensity function in the lower portion of Fig. 1. Nevertheless, the corresponding period histogram shows none of the flattening that might be expected from a simple saturation. It is as if a renormalization of the unit's range of sensitivity occurred, allowing the unit to continue to transmit the same information about the shape of the stimulating waveform while producing a saturation of the average response. Similar conclusions can be drawn from observations of some of the responses to amplitude-modulated tones in cochlear-nucleus units (11).

In contrast to the above results, the envelope properties of neural responses measured with poststimulus-time (PST) histograms do not appear

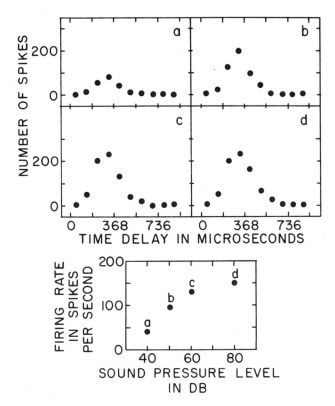

FIG. 1. Above: Period histograms of the responses of an auditory-nerve fiber to a CF tone. SPL increases in going from *a* to *d*. Stimulus frequency, 1.096 kHz; stimulus duration, 5 sec; histogram binwidth, 92 μsec; species, squirrel monkey. [Redrawn from Rose et al. (10), unit 67–253–3.] Below: Firing rates and SPLs corresponding to histograms *a* to *d*.

to reflect any renormalization at high intensities. This can be seen, for example, in the PST histograms in the upper portion of Fig. 2. These histograms are based on 5-msec binwidths which are more than an order of magnitude larger than those of Fig. 1. The histograms describe the average firing rate during the course of a 220-msec stimulus which consisted of a CF tone burst beginning at time 0 and a 6-dB increment in intensity occurring at a time delay of 150 msec. At the lower intensities, a and b, the intensity increment produced a large response increment. However, at the higher intensities, c and d, the incremental response was substantially reduced, even though the incremental intensity was constant in decibels relative to the pedestal, so that the relative shape of the stimulus envelope was unaltered. As in Fig. 1, histogram d corresponds to a SPL that produced a saturation of average firing rate. However, in this situation it appears that the same saturation limits both the steady-state and incremental responses (12,13). Hence, if changes in SPL are encoded by changes in neural firing rate, a sensitivity

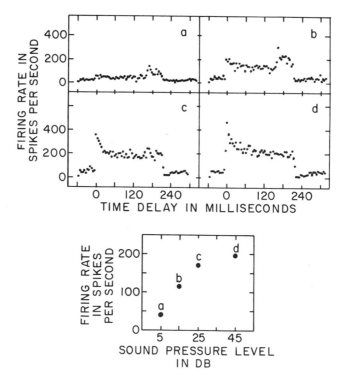

FIG. 2. Above: Poststimulus-time histograms of responses of an auditory-nerve fiber to a CF tone with a superimposed intensity increment. The increment occurs at a delay of 150 msec from the pedestal onset and produces a 6-dB increase in intensity. SPL increases in going from a to d. Stimulus frequency, 0.66 kHz; histogram binwidth, 5 msec; species, Mongolian gerbil. [From Smith (*unpublished results*), unit Ge-17–8.] Below: Steady-state firing rates and pedestal SPLs corresponding to histograms a to d.

control mechanism does not appear to aid in the transmission of this information. Another explanation for the large dynamic range of the auditory system will be considered after reviewing some effects of sound frequency.

Frequency Characteristics

Frequency selectivity is a well-established property of both mechanical and neural responses of the auditory periphery. There are several aspects of the selectivity, as can be seen by comparing the 3 families of curves in Fig. 3. The data come from squirrel monkeys and are redrawn from Geisler et al. (14). The upper curve is an isoamplitude contour—it shows the SPL at the eardrum necessary to maintain a constant displacement amplitude at 1 point of the basilar membrane as a function of sound frequency. The middle curves are isorate contours for an auditory-nerve fiber presumably innervating the same region of the cochlea. They show the SPLs necessary to maintain a constant firing rate as a function of sound frequency. The lowest of

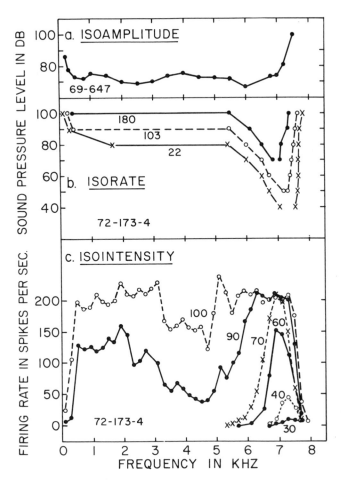

FIG. 3. Three aspects of peripheral frequency selectivity. a: An isoamplitude contour of basilar-membrane displacement. b: Isorate contours for a single auditory-nerve fiber. The parameter is firing rate in spikes per second. c: Isointensity contours for the fiber in b. The parameter is sound pressure level in dB. Species, squirrel monkey. [Redrawn from Geisler et al. (14).]

these isorate curves, shown by crosses, is basically a threshold tuning curve and indicates that the unit has a CF of approximately 7.3 kHz. As can be seen, the isorate curves exhibit considerably more frequency selectivity than do the mechanical curves, an observation that has been made many times before, but never quite so explicitly. The difference is most apparent in the low-frequency portions of the curves where an approximately constant SPL maintains a constant amplitude of displacement, whereas the SPL must be greatly increased to maintain a constant firing rate. Three questions immediately arise concerning the sharpening of frequency selectivity: How does it come about, what is its functional significance, and how is it affected by cochlear damage? These questions have been addressed by Evans (*this volume*) and will be returned to below.

Another aspect of the neural frequency response is illustrated in the lowermost family of curves. The data come from the same unit as in the middle curves, but the responses are plotted in terms of isointensity contours. The contours show firing rate versus sound frequency for various constant SPLs. They illustrate that the neural tuning seen in the isorate curves is not invariant. As SPL increases, the neuron responds over wider and wider frequency ranges, i.e., the effective bandwidth increases. For example, if the SPL is raised to 90 dB, which is 60 dB above the threshold SPL, the unit can provide substantial responses over the entire frequency range below its CF. The shapes of the various curves differ because firing rate is a nonlinear function of sound intensity and, perhaps to a lesser extent, of sound frequency.

Interaction Between Intensity and Frequency

A second possibility for explaining the overall dynamic range of hearing is implicit in the lower curves of Fig. 3. The results imply that the operating range of a unit depends on stimulus frequency. At frequencies below the CF the operating range in decibels is roughly the same as at CF, but has shifted to higher SPLs. A shift also occurs for a small range of frequencies above the CF, but this is generally accompanied by a substantial decrease in the slope of the intensity function (7,14). Accordingly, as the intensity of a tone is increased and units stimulated at their CF become saturated, additional units begin responding at frequencies below and, to a lesser extent, above their CFs. Subjective loudness could depend on a summation of firing rates of all the responding nerve fibers and continue to increase even though the most sensitive units have saturated. In response to increments in sound intensity, different units could provide incremental responses or differential sensitivity for different background SPLs—a sort of sensitivity control mechanism distributed over the population of nerve fibers. A unique mapping would therefore not exist between the frequency of an increment and the subpopulation of units responding to the increment. According to this interpretation, the low-frequency sharpening may serve to extend the overall dynamic range of the system by preventing units from firing at low intensities below their CFs. (For additional data and references, see refs. 12 and 15; and for theoretical treatments, see refs. 16 and 17.)

Based on these considerations, one can attempt to evaluate the functional hearing changes that occur when the population of neurons like the one illustrated undergoes a loss in sensitivity. Loudness recruitment and improved differential sensitivity would presumably occur for frequencies near 7 kHz, as is discussed further below. In addition, the physiological loss would appear to influence the encoding of some suprathreshold signals at significantly lower frequencies.

However, a major difficulty remains in accounting for the large dynamic range of the auditory system in the presence of wideband noise. Such noise presumably excites most units even at low intensity levels. Indeed, in recent psychophysical experiments with maskers specifically designed to prevent any spread of excitation (18,19), the overall dynamic range was not significantly reduced. It is likely that additional response properties, such as 2-tone suppression and response fine-time structure, play a significant role in the encoding of such masked signals and other complex signals, but the full extent of these phenomena is just beginning to be explored (15,20,21).

It may also be of interest to mention at this point a possible relationship between neural isointensity contours and psychophysical frequency discrimination. Let us assume that the sound frequency is sufficiently high so that periodicities in firing play a minor role in pitch determination. Let us also ignore the systematic decreases in the frequency of maximum response with SPL that apparently occur in 36% of the fibers with CFs above 4 kHz (14). Imagine a fiber, such as the one in Fig. 3, responding at its CF and a given SPL. When the SPL is low, the firing rate decreases as sound frequency is either increased or decreased. As SPL is increased, the response areas eventually become steeper on the high-frequency side and shallower on the low-frequency side. In other words, the unit becomes more sensitive to increases in frequency but less sensitive to decreases in frequency. On the other hand, the psychophysically determined difference limen (DL) for frequency decreases with sensation level (22). This seems to imply that units stimulated slightly above their CFs play a major role in frequency discrimination. As frequency is changed, the mechanical pattern of stimulation moves along the cochlea, and the firing rates of these units are the most significantly altered. The central nervous system may utilize this change to detect a change in sound frequency. If this view is correct, the low-frequency sharpening exhibited by the isorate curves appears to play a minor role in determining this particular aspect of overall auditory-frequency sensitivity. It should also be noted that the units involved in frequency discrimination are not necessarily those which determine the sensation of pitch. For example, as intensity increases, the pitch of a high-frequency tone increases (23). This may be related to the decrease in the frequency of maximum response that occurs in some units, i.e., more basal units become maximally excited (24). Accordingly, the locus of maximum excitation can determine the subjective pitch, as in the classical place theory, while changes in the apical gradient of excitation determine the frequency DL. In addition, the existence of a gradient may be a necessary condition for the generation of pitch sensation, as is discussed further below.

It appears ultimately necessary that, for any stimulus configuration, the responses of the population of auditory-nerve fibers must be evaluated in terms of their potential significance to the central nervous system. This should lead to a determination of the relative importance of the nonlinear effects outlined above and elsewhere (25), and the linear filtering properties also known to be present (e.g., ref. 26, and Evans, *this volume*). In situations involving moderate to high SPLs and/or background tones and noise, units stimulated at their CFs would be saturated. Consequently, in the presence of cochlear damage, changes in hearing might occur over significantly different frequency ranges than those exhibiting losses in threshold sensitivity. Additional aspects of cochlear damage are discussed after considering some effects of stimulus duration.

Stimulus Duration

Perstimulatory Effects

In response to a stimulus of constant sound intensity, auditory-nerve fibers exhibit a maximum firing rate at the onset, followed by a monotonic decrease toward a steady level. This adaptation in firing rate can be considered as the simplest indication that changes occur during ongoing acoustic stimulation. The adaptation is composed of several phases—a rapid decay occupying the first 15 msec, a short-term adaptation lasting about 150 msec, a "moderate" term decay lasting several seconds, and long-term effects occurring over many minutes (2,12,27). During the course of adaptation, the response of a unit can decline from an onset rate exceeding 600 spikes/sec to a quasi-steady-state value of less than 150 spikes/sec, and most of this decay occupies the first few seconds. The extent to which the various decay rates reflect different underlying processes and the possible sites of the processes have not been determined. However, the limitation of the maximum steady-state firing rate appears to occur peripherally to neural spike generation, since sustained firing rates exceeding 600 spikes/sec can be obtained with electrical stimulation (28). In addition, during the period of short-term adaptation both onset and steady-state intensity functions have the same shape and appear to be controlled by the same peripheral saturating process (12,13). Note that the decrease in rate during adaptation does not necessarily imply a change in the information transmitting capabilities or differential sensitivity of a neuron. For example, when intensity increments are superimposed on tonal pedestals, the resulting changes in firing are the same before and after short-term adaptation (12,13). Some other effects of adaptation can be observed by applying a test tone after an adapting tone, as is discussed next.

Poststimulatory Effects

At the termination of a sufficiently strong adapting stimulus, spontaneous firing is suppressed and gradually returns to its unadapted value (2). Responses to a test stimulus are also reduced, as can be seen in the PST histograms of Fig. 4 (29). The middle and upper histograms show responses to a brief test stimulus and to a short-adapting stimulus of moderate intensity.

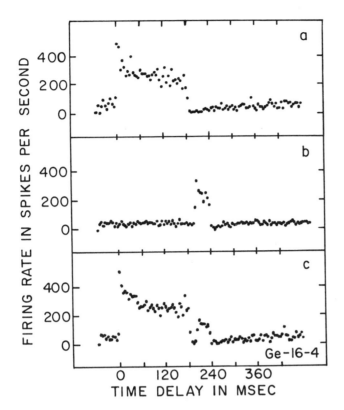

FIG. 4. Poststimulus-time histograms of response to a: a 200-msec adapting tone; b: a 40-msec test tone; and c: both stimuli applied in succession. All stimuli are at 4.35 kHz, the CF of the unit. Adapting SPL, 37 dB; test SPL, 18 dB; histogram binwidth, 5 msec; species, Mongolian gerbil. [From Smith (29).]

To obtain the lowermost histogram both stimuli were applied in succession. The response to the test stimulus was substantially reduced. As adapting intensity and/or duration are increased, the decrement might be expected to grow in amount and temporal extent and approach the condition of a permanent sound-induced loss. However, the available information suggests that increases in the exposure parameters invoke a hierarchy of different processes, making extrapolation difficult.

Short-term adapting stimuli appear to produce relatively simple after-effects. When the stimuli have durations of up to 300 msec and SPLs within 60 dB of a unit's threshold, the aftereffects last for several hundred milliseconds [(2) and Smith, *unpublished data*]. Some typical aftereffects are illustrated by the CF intensity functions of Fig. 5 (29). The unfilled and filled circles indicate the onset and steady-state responses to a 230-msec adapting tone. The crosses show the onset responses to a constant-intensity test tone occurring 19 msec after the adapting tone. The triangles show the decrement in test response as a function of adapting intensity level. As the

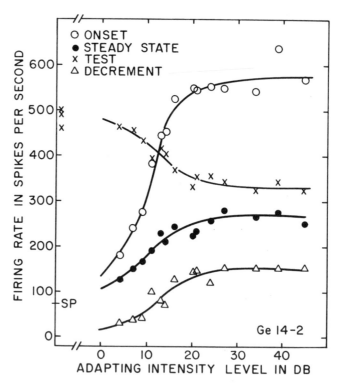

FIG. 5. Some effects of adapting intensity level. The unfilled and filled circles indicate the onset and steady-state responses to a 230-msec adapting tone. The crosses indicate the onset responses to a 15-dB test tone occurring 19 msec after the adapting tone. The 3 leftmost crosses correspond to test responses in the absence of the adapting tone and obtained at the beginning, middle, and end of the data run. The triangles indicate the decrements in test response and were obtained by subtracting the test responses from the appropriate control response. SP indicates the spontaneous firing rate. Onset responses were computed using 10 msec bins. All stimuli were at the unit's CF of 6.6 kHz. The 0-dB intensity level corresponds to approximately 3 dB SPL re 0.0002 dynes/cm² in the ear canal. Species, Mongolian gerbil. [From Smith (29).]

level increases, the response to the adapting tone increases to an asymptote. The decrement in test response shows a similar variation, i.e., the test response first decreases, then remains fixed at a reduced value. The decrement in test response is a saturating function of adapting intensity, which is approximately proportional to the intensity function for the adapting tone (Smith, *unpublished results*). In the saturation region, although adapting intensity is increased by a factor of 316, i.e., 25 dB, the responses to the test and adapting stimuli show no further signs of adaptation. Accordingly, it appears that a peripheral saturation precedes the adaptation process and effectively shields the neural elements from the effects of high intensity. This is consistent with the perstimulatory effects on incremental responses described briefly above (12,13,29).

For longer durations and/or more intense stimuli, the above description no longer applies. Young and Sachs (27) applied adapting tones about 1-min long at intensities up to 80 dB above a unit's threshold. Recovery from adaptation occurred over 10s of seconds. When they increased the adapting intensity, the test response continued to decrease well beyond the saturation region of the adapting stimulus. This led them to conclude that the energy of the adapting stimulus determined the severity of the poststimulatory effect and that the poststimulatory adaptation mechanism is located peripherally to the rate-saturating mechanism, i.e., the reverse of the sequence fitting short-term adaptation. Their findings illustrate the danger of a priori judging poststimulatory effects from perstimulatory effects, and of extrapolating from one situation to another.

Accordingly, short-term and moderate-duration exposures appear to reflect qualitatively different and perhaps anatomically distinct processes. It is not clear what additional processes become involved as exposure duration and intensity are increased. For example, will longer-term, more intense sound exposures result in poststimulatory effects that can resemble temporary threshold shifts (TTS) extending over hours? There are few data available to answer this question but the preliminary results of Parkins and Henderson (30) suggest that the answer is negative. They concluded that a 7½-min exposure to 115 dB SPL white noise produced little change in test response beyond the first few minutes. This short-duration aftereffect seems consistent with the results of Kiang (2) showing that spontaneous activity recovers within a few minutes after exposure to 13-min-long tones. However, it has been shown behaviorally (31) that the same noise exposure produces substantial TTS, lasting for many hours, in cats. Accordingly, it appears that at least some forms of TTS may have central origin (e.g., see Salvi, *this volume*). Ultimately, of course, sufficient exposure can produce irreversible cochlear changes and permanent threshold shifts that would undoubtedly be reflected in 8th-nerve changes. Unfortunately, as mentioned above, relevant 8th-nerve data do not yet exist. However, some data do exist with respect to the permanent changes produced by ototoxic drugs, as is discussed next.

PERMANENT EFFECTS OF OTOTOXIC DRUGS

An Experimental Alternative to Noise Exposure?

Several studies have dealt with the irreversible changes in 8th-nerve response produced by kanamycin sulfate, an ototoxic antibiotic (32,33). Their results may be of relevance in predicting some kinds of permanent noise-induced changes, but a word of caution seems in order. Although drug- and noise-induced damages potentially share common mechanisms, it may be misleading to directly extrapolate from one condition to the other, even if similar cochleograms are produced. A comparison of the findings of Henderson et al. (34,35) and Ryan and Dallos (36) based on noise damage and kanamycin, respectively, can serve to underscore this warning. Both studies used chinchillas and both treatments produced cochleograms with substantial loss of outer hair cells and unaltered inner hair cell counts. The drug treatment produced behavioral threshold losses on the order of 45 dB in the region of outer hair-cell loss—in qualitative agreement with single-unit sensitivity shifts observed in other species (32,33). In contrast, the noise-damaged animals often sustained little permanent threshold shift, as measured with evoked responses and recently confirmed behaviorally (37).

A possible interpretation of these results is that normal inner hair cells are sufficient for a normal threshold—a conclusion that runs counter to currently prevailing opinion and is discussed further below. Kanamycin may have produced functional damage in inner hair cells or elsewhere, that was unobservable under the light microscope (e.g., 38,39). The noise exposure, on the other hand, may have produced a "pure" outer hair-cell lesion, leaving the rest of the cochlea functionally unaltered. In this regard, the 8th-nerve results of Sokolich et al. (33) also suggest that ototoxic agents can have subtle effects that are not revealed in surface preparations. They showed, in kanamycin-treated gerbils, an alteration and/or loss of sensitivity in the responses of some of the fibers innervating apparently normal regions of the cochlea. Furthermore, even noise-exposed chinchillas sometimes exhibit frequency regions with apparently equal losses of hair cells, but substantially different behavioral threshold shifts (e.g., 37). Hence, the presence of hair cells, as revealed in a surface preparation, does not necessarily imply normal hair-cell functioning.

Single-Unit Results and Hearing Changes

With the above caveats in mind, it is of importance to review the experimental results obtained on kanamycin-poisoned animals. Kiang et al. (32) described some of the 8th-nerve changes and discussed their implications for the encoding of auditory information. A fundamental finding was that, in regions of outer hair-cell loss, fibers responsive to sound exhibited raised thresholds and abnormal, broadened tuning curves with relatively unaltered low-frequency "tails." Some of their results are summarized in Fig. 6. The unfilled circles specify the coordinates of the threshold intensities and CFs for a number of fibers in a normal animal. The filled circles do the same for a kanamycin-damaged animal. This animal exhibited negligible loss of inner hair cells over the illustrated frequency range. The approximate loss of outer hair cells is specified along the upper abscissa. The solid and dashed curves indicate portions of tuning curves from the normal and damaged animals, respectively. It should be noted that most of the shift in the low-frequency thresholds of the damaged animal was attributed to a conductive hearing loss. Otherwise, these thresholds approached those in a normal animal. On the

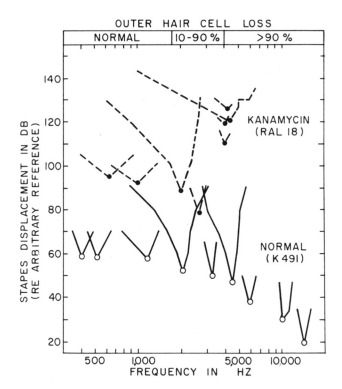

FIG. 6. Tuning curves from normal (*solid lines*) and kanamycin-treated (*dashed lines*) cats. The reference stapes displacement is 10^{-8} μm peak to peak for the normal cat. The kanamycin-treated cat suffered a conductive loss of ~40 dB, causing a corresponding shift in the reference stapes displacement. [Redrawn from Kiang et al. (32).]

other hand, an abnormal rise in thresholds and broadened tuning curves near the apical border of the lesion was a reproducible effect of the drug treatment. Those abnormal fibers with measurable CFs generally exhibited a normal distribution of spontaneous activity, and showed a normal growth of firing rate with SPL, once their thresholds were exceeded. More severe abnormalities were also encountered in many fibers presumably innervating the damaged region. The fibers had no spontaneous activity, did not respond to sound, and could only be driven by electrical stimulation. Based on these results, Kiang et al. (32) discussed possible physiological bases for loudness recruitment and tinnitus.

The results of Kiang et al. (32) are consistent with the hypothesis that loudness recruitment and increased differential sensitivity can be caused by an elevation of thresholds of primary fibers. The explanation for recruitment depends on 3 assumptions. First, as already mentioned, the subjective loudness of a tone must depend on summated activity of all the responding nerve fibers. Second, fibers having CFs near the frequency of stimulation must undergo changes similar to those illustrated in Fig. 6, i.e., raised thresholds, shifted intensity functions, and approximately normal CFs. Third, although not true in these results, fibers innervating more apical regions of the cochlea must have nearly normal low-frequency response areas. As SPL increases, the thresholds of the "damaged" fibers are exceeded. They begin to respond, as do fibers with higher CFs. This abnormal increase in the number of responding fibers causes an abnormally rapid growth of loudness with intensity. Similarly, when increments in intensity are applied, an increase in overall sensitivity can occur, reflecting the increase in the number of fibers producing an incremental response.

Kiang et al. (32) also speculate that some forms of tinnitus may be caused by "the existence of distinctly different distributions of activity in tonotopically adjacent elements of the auditory nerve." In their results, units from the most basal cochlear regions are characterized by the absence of spontaneous activity, whereas those in adjacent regions may have normal spontaneous activity. This produces a substantial gradient of neural firing rate in the absence of stimulation, which may cause an apparent pitch sensation. Davis et al. (40) proposed a similar explanation for diplacusis in which, in the presence of a tonal stimulus, the border of an unresponsive zone creates a spatial gradient of response that generates an anomalous pitch sensation. Note that the results of Kiang et al. (32) correspond to a gradient in which firing rate is absent in units innervating the base of the cochlea, the reverse of the dominant gradient produced by a pure tone. Hence, the explanation would seem to more readily apply to a lesion that also has a basalward border. In any case, it seems reasonable to expect that the abnormal patterns of activity produced by cochlear damage would be subject to misinterpretation by the central nervous system. The changes in response also have important implications for cochlear mechanisms discussed next.

Implications for Cochlear Mechanisms

Since 95% of the afferent cochlear neurons innervate inner hair cells (41), the results of Kiang et al. (32) raise a key question. Why does the destruction of outer hair cells produce changes in the tuning and sensitivity of fibers presumably ending only on inner hair cells? Two of the possible explanations are: (i) kanamycin may produce damage to inner hair cells, radial nerve fibers, or other cochlear structures that a cochleogram does not reveal, and (ii) outer hair cells may normally interact with inner hair cells in producing nerve-fiber responses. The latter hypothesis has been the subject of much speculation (e.g., 42–48). In this regard, some recent studies of 8th-nerve responses in normal and kanamycin-treated gerbils (46,47,33) appear to provide the most direct evidence to date that both of the above explanations apply.

Figure 7 illustrates some results obtained by Sokolich et al. (33) in a

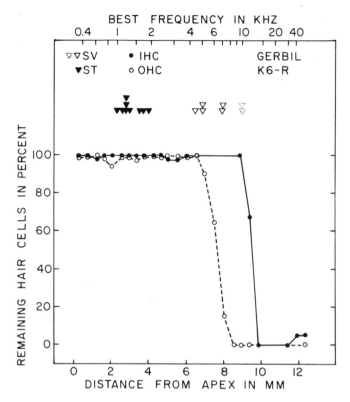

FIG. 7. Cochleogram showing the hair-cell population in a kanamycin-treated Mongolian gerbil. The un-filled and filled triangles give the CFs of units that responded with increased firing during motion and/or displacement of the basilar membrane toward scala vestibuli and scala tympani, respectively. The dotted triangles correspond to 2 SV units whose CFs were indirectly estimated, based on the latencies of their responses to acoustic clicks. [From Sokolich et al. (33).]

kanamycin-treated gerbil. It includes a cochleogram of the hair-cell loss pro-duced by the treatment. The abscissa is labeled in terms of distance along the cochlea (below) and frequency of maximum sensitivity (above) as revealed by cochlear microphonic measurements. The region of outer hair-cell loss extends more apically than the region of inner hair-cell loss so that a signifi-cant region exists where only inner hair cells are present. Sokolich et al. (33) applied an especially designed 40-Hz stimulus in order to produce trapezoidal displacements of the basilar membrane. Based on their responses to the trape-zoids, the abnormal 8th-nerve units in the kanamycin-treated animals fell into 2 classes. The units of 1 class responded with increased firing rate during motion and/or displacement of the basilar membrane toward scala vestibuli, and decreased rate during the alternate half-cycle. These units invariably innervated regions of the cochlea that contained only inner hair cells. Their CFs are indicated by the locations of the unfilled triangles, labeled SV. Units of the second class produced a reversed firing pattern, i.e., an increased firing rate during the motion and/or displacement toward scala tympani (ST). The CFs of these units are indicated by the filled triangles. They innervated regions showing normal counts of both inner and outer hair cells. Many of the abnormal units exhibited decreased sensitivity and broad tuning. In addition, relatively normal response properties occurred in some of the fibers innervating the regions of the cochlea with a full complement of hair cells.

Viewing the responses in kanamycin-treated gerbils, Zwislocki (46) and Zwislocki and Sokolich (47) concluded that inner hair cells produced excitation of auditory-nerve fibers during the motion and/or displacement of the basilar membrane toward scala vestibuli. The cochleograms of Sokolich et al. (33) supported this conclusion. The reversed polarity, i.e., ST response, was interpreted as being caused by the inputs from outer hair cells, which apparently often predominated over inner hair cells in the regions containing both cell types. Hence, the assumption was made that outer hair cells influenced the firing of radial nerve fibers and were in polarity opposition to the inner hair-cell contributions. These results confirmed the earlier studies in normal gerbils. There it was shown that responses to trapezoidal motion of the basilar membrane could be explained in terms of 2 components in polarity opposition (46). The kanamycin studies supported the earlier hypothesis that the opposing components were produced by inner and outer hair cells, respectively. Nevertheless both Zwislocki and Sokolich (47) and Sokolich et al. (33) point out that quantitative differences occur between the responses to trapezoids in normal and kanamycin-treated animals. In the normal animals the 2 components must be of nearly equal magnitude, whereas in the kanamycin-treated animals 1 component often appears to predominate, even where both types of hair cells are present. In addition, the responses are generally more phasic in nature in the kanamycin-treated gerbils. Hence, kanamycin appears to alter the specific response waveforms and the hypothesized balance between inner and outer hair cells throughout the cochlea, even where the cochleogram is reasonably normal. Zwislocki and Sokolich (47) speculate that the predominance of outer hair cells in apical regions may be an early sign of the apical damage of inner hair cells produced by kanamycin (49).

If we accept the hypothesis that inner and outer hair cells interact and are in polarity opposition, an interesting possibility arises for explaining the sharpening seen in neural isorate curves. Zwislocki (46) assumes that the interaction occurs between radial and spiral fibers sharing the same habenular opening and that the hair-cell responses at low stimulus levels are proportional to basilar-membrane displacement at the appropriate cochlear locations. Because of the basalward course of the outer spiral fibers, the frequency characteristic of the outer hair cells is shifted toward higher frequencies relative to that of the inner hair cells. If the frequency response of radial fibers represents the sum of the 2 opposing responses, it can exhibit considerable sharpening compared to a mechanical curve (46,47,50,51). Under these conditions the neural stimulus–response relationship can still exhibit "linear" frequency selectivity (e.g., 26) to the extent that the difference between hair-cell responses does. The broad tuning and threshold shifts produced by various ototoxic agents (32,33,48, and Evans, *this volume*) would then be accounted for by two effects—an alteration of hair-cell interaction and an overall loss of sensitivity. In addition, this model may be able to account for normal neural response properties such as 2-tone suppression and the widening of response areas at high SPLs.

Among the criticisms that may be leveled at this scheme of interaction between the inner and outer hair cells are the following. First, no firm anatomical basis for interaction has yet been described (52,53). Second, inner and outer hair cells are required to have approximately equal sensitivities. As mentioned above, there is some behavioral evidence that inner hair cells alone are sufficient for normal threshold sensitivity, but relevant single-unit data are not yet available. Third, in response to high-frequency stimuli, outer hair cells are required to produce a net inhibition in radial fibers, since high-frequency phase information is presumably not transmitted by the relevant neural structures. Direct evidence for this proposition does not seem immediately forthcoming since the appropriate cochlear lesions are not readily attainable. It remains for future experimental evidence to either validate or invalidate the described model. At present, it is still possible that mechanical rather than physiological factors play a major role in phenomena such as sharpening and 2-tone suppression [e.g., various papers and discussions in Zwicker and Terhardt (54)], but purely mechanical models do not seem able to explain polarity reversals in kanamycin-treated animals. Accordingly, a resolution of the questions relating to hair-cell interaction seems particularly important for an understanding of the mechanisms of noise damage as well as 8th-nerve response properties in normal animals.

CONCLUSIONS

The title of this chapter could just as well have been "Eighth-Nerve Responses and Normal Hearing" or "Eighth-Nerve Changes and Permanent Sensori-Neural Hearing Loss." As I have attempted to illustrate, the two topics are inextricably intertwined. Until we obtain a better understanding of the significance of the spatiotemporal patterns of 8th-nerve responses in normal hearing, we cannot hope to understand the effects of changes in these patterns. Similarly, an understanding of the changes in 8th-nerve responses produced by ototoxic agents awaits a clearer knowledge of the normal cochlear mechanisms producing the responses. Fortunately, there are reasons to believe that, in the near future, integrated studies involving cochlear lesions, 8th-nerve responses, and behavioral changes will provide conclusive insights into the normal and abnormal functioning of the auditory periphery.

ACKNOWLEDGMENTS

I thank Dr. J. J. Zwislocki for his comments and discussions concerning various aspects of this manuscript. Supported by NIH grant NS 03950.

REFERENCES

1. Stevens, S. S., and Davis, H. (1938): *Hearing, Its Psychology and Physiology.* Wiley, New York.
2. Kiang, N. Y. S., Watanabe, T., Thomas, E. C., and Clark, L. F. (1965): *Discharge Patterns of Single Fibers in the Cat's Auditory Nerve.* M.I.T. Press, Cambridge, Mass.
3. Kiang, N. Y. S., Sachs, M. B., and Peake, W. T. (1967): Shapes of tuning curves in single auditory-nerve fibers. *J. Acoust. Soc. Am.,* 42:1341–1342.
4. Kiang, N. Y. S. (1968): A survey of recent developments in the study of auditory physiology. *Ann. Otol. Rhinol. Laryngol.,* 77:656–675.
5. Sachs, M. B., and Kiang, N. Y. S. (1968): Two-tone inhibition in auditory-nerve fibers. *J. Acoust. Soc. Am.,* 43:1120–1128.
6. Wiederhold, M. L., and Kiang, N. Y. S. (1970): Effects of electric stimulation of the crossed olivocochlear bundle on single auditory-nerve fibers in the cat. *J. Acoust. Soc. Am.,* 48:960–965.
7. Sachs, M. B., and Abbas, P. J. (1974): Rate versus level functions for auditory-nerve fibers in cats: tone-burst stimuli. *J. Acoust. Soc. Am.,* 56:1835–1847.
8. Wiederhold, M. L. (1970): Variations in the effects of electric stimulation of the crossed olivocochlear bundle on cat single auditory-nerve-fiber responses to tone bursts. *J. Acoust. Soc. Am.,* 48:966–977.
9. Evans, E. F. (1972): The frequency response and other properties of single fibers in the guinea-pig cochlear nerve. *J. Physiol. (London),* 226:263–287.
10. Rose, J. E., Hind, J. E., Anderson, D. J., and Brugge, J. F. (1971): Some effects of stimulus intensity on response of auditory nerve fibers in the squirrel monkey. *J. Neurophysiol.,* 34:685–699.
11. Møller, A. R. (1972): Coding of amplitude and frequency modulated sounds in the cochlear nucleus of the rat. *Acta Physiol. Scand.,* 86:223–238.
12. Smith, R. L. (1973): *Short-Term Adaptation and Incremental Responses of Single Auditory-Nerve Fibers.* Special Rpt. LSC-S-11, Laboratory of Sensory Communication, Syracuse University, Syracuse, New York.
13. Smith, R. L., and Zwislocki, J. J. (1975): Short-term adaptation and incremental responses of single auditory-nerve fibers. *Biol. Cyb.,* 17:169–182.
14. Geisler, C. D., Rhode, W. S., and Kennedy, D. T. (1974): Responses to tonal stimuli of single auditory nerve fibers and their relationship to basilar membrane motion in the squirrel monkey. *J. Neurophysiol.,* 37:1156–1172.
15. Kiang, N. Y. S., and Moxon, E. C. (1974): Tails of tuning curves of auditory-nerve fibers. *J. Acoust. Soc. Am.,* 55:620–630.
16. Siebert, W. M. (1968): Stimulus transformations in the peripheral auditory system. In: *Recognizing Patterns,* edited by P. A. Kolers and M. Eden, pp. 104–133. M.I.T. Press, Cambridge, Mass.
17. Goldstein, J. L. (1974): Is the power law simply related to the driven spike response rate from the whole auditory nerve? In: *Sensation and Measurement,* edited by H. R. Moskowitz, B. Scharf, and J. C. Stevens, pp. 223–229. D. Reidel, Dordrecht, Holland.
18. Viemeister, N. F. (1974): Intensity discrimination of noise in the presence of band-reject noise. *J. Acoust. Soc. Am.,* 56:1594–1600.
19. Hellman, R. P. (1974): Effect of spread of excitation on the loudness function at 250 Hz. In: *Sensation and Measurement,* edited by H. R. Moskowitz, B. Scharf, and J. C. Stevens, pp. 241–249. D. Reidel, Dordrecht, Holland.
20. Abbas, P. J., and Sachs, M. B. (1974): Two-tone suppression in cat auditory-nerve

fibers: comparison of frequencies above and below fiber CF. *J. Acoust. Soc. Am.,* 55:466 (A).

21. Rose, J. E., Kitzes, L. M., Gibson, M. M., and Hind, J. E. (1974): Observations of phase-sensitive neurons of anteroventral cochlear nucleus of the cat: nonlinearity of cochlear output. *J. Neurophysiol.,* 37:218–253.

22. Shower, E. G., and Biddulph, R. (1931): Differential pitch sensitivity of the ear. *J. Acoust. Soc. Am.,* 3:275–287.

23. Stevens, S. S. (1935): The relation of pitch to intensity. *J. Acoust. Soc. Am.,* 6:150–154.

24. Terhardt, E. (1974): Pitch of pure tones: its relation to intensity. In: *Facts and Models in Hearing,* edited by E. Zwicker and E. Terhardt, pp. 353–360. Springer, Berlin.

25. Pfeiffer, R. R., and Kim, D. O. (1973): Considerations of nonlinear response properties of single cochlear nerve fibers. In: *Basic Mechanisms in Hearing,* edited by A. R. Møller, pp. 555–591. Academic Press, New York.

26. Evans, E. F., and Wilson, J. P. (1973): The frequency selectivity of the cochlea. In: *Basic Mechanisms in Hearing,* edited by A. R. Møller, pp. 519–554. Academic Press, New York.

27. Young, E., and Sachs, M. B. (1973): Recovery from sound exposure in auditory-nerve fibers. *J. Acoust. Soc. Am.,* 54:1535–1543.

28. Moxon, E. C. (1968): Auditory nerve responses to electric stimuli. *M.I.T. Quart. Prog. Rept.,* 90:270–275.

29. Smith, R. L. (1975): Recovery from short-term adaptation in single auditory-nerve fibers. *Ann. Res. Rpt. ISR-20,* pp. 13–17. Institute for Sensory Research, Syracuse University, Syracuse, New York.

30. Parkins, C. W., and Henderson, D. (1971): Noise induced temporary threshold shift recorded in single neurons of the cat's eighth nerve. Paper read to the American Academy of Ophthalmology and Otolaryngology, Las Vegas, Nevada.

31. Miller, J. D., Watson, C. S., and Covell, W. P. (1963): Deafening effects of noise on the cat. *Acta Otolaryngol. [Suppl.] (Stockh.),* 176.

32. Kiang, N. Y. S., Moxon, E. C., and Levine, R. A. (1970): Auditory-nerve activity in cats with normal and abnormal cochleas. In: *Sensorineural Hearing Loss,* edited by G. E. W. Wolstenholme and J. Knight, pp. 241–273. Churchill, London.

33. Sokolich, W. G., Hamernik, R. P., Zwislocki, J. J., and Schmiedt, R. (1976): Inferred response polarities of cochlear hair cells. *J. Acoust. Soc. Am.*

34. Henderson, D., Hamernik, R. P., and Sitler, R. (1974): Audiometric and anatomical correlates of impulse noise exposure. *Arch. Otolaryngol.,* 99:62–66.

35. Henderson, D., Hamernik, R. P., and Sitler, R. W. (1974): Audiometric and histological correlates of exposure to 1-msec noise impulses in the chinchilla. *J. Acoust. Soc. Am.,* 56:1210–1221.

36. Ryan, A., and Dallos, P. (1975): Effect of absence of cochlear outer hair cells on behavioral auditory threshold. *Nature,* 253:44–46.

37. Hans, J., Henderson, D., and Hamernik, R. P. (1975): Effects of impulse noise on the temporal integration function of the chinchilla. *J. Acoust. Soc. Am.,* 57:S41 (A).

38. Hawkins, J. E., Jr. (1970): Biochemical aspects of ototoxicity. In: *Biochemical Mechanisms in Hearing and Deafness,* edited by M. M. Paparella, pp. 323–339. Charles C Thomas, Springfield, Ill.

39. Wersäll, J. (1973): Problems and pitfalls in studies of cochlea hair cell pathology. In: *Basic Mechanisms in Hearing,* edited by A. R. Møller, pp. 235–256. Academic Press, New York.

40. Davis, H., Morgan, C. T., Hawkins, J. E., Jr., Galambos, R., and Smith, F. W. (1950): Temporary deafness following exposure to loud tones and noise. *Acta Otolaryngol. [Suppl.] (Stockh.),* 88.

41. Spoendlin, H. (1966): *The Organization of the Cochlear Receptor.* Karger, Basel, New York.

42. Lynn, P. A., and Sayers, B. McA. (1970): Cochlear innervation, signal processing, and their relation to auditory time-intensity effects. *J. Acoust. Soc. Am.,* 47:525–533.

43. Nieder, P. (1971): Addressed exponential delay line theory of cochlear organization. *Nature*, 230:255–257.
44. Davis, H. (1973): The cocktail hour before the serious banquet. In: *Basic Mechanisms in Hearing*, edited by A. R. Møller, pp. 259–271. Academic Press, New York.
45. Zwislocki, J. J., and Sokolich, W. G. (1973): Velocity and displacement responses in auditory nerve fibers. *Science*, 182:64–66.
46. Zwislocki, J. J. (1974): A possible neuro-mechanical sound analysis in the cochlea. *Acustica*, 31:354–359.
47. Zwislocki, J. J., and Sokolich, W. G. (1974): Neuro-mechanical frequency analysis in the cochlea. In: *Facts and Models in Hearing*, edited by E. Zwicker and E. Terhardt, pp. 107–117. Springer, Berlin.
48. Evans, E. (1974): Auditory frequency selectivity and the cochlear nerve. In: *Facts and Models in Hearing*, edited by E. Zwicker and E. Terhardt, pp. 118–131. Springer, Berlin.
49. Engström, H., and Kohonen, A. (1965): Cochlear damage from ototoxic antibiotics. *Acta Otolaryngol. (Stockh.)*, 59:171–178.
50. Zwislocki, J. J., and Sokolich, W. G. (1974): Model of neuromechanical filtering in the cochlea. *J. Acoust. Soc. Am.*, 56:S21 (A).
51. Zwislocki, J. J., and Sokolich, W. G. (1975): Neuromechanical frequency analysis in the cochlea. *Ann. Res. Rpt. ISR-20*, pp. 17–25. Institute for Sensory Research, Syracuse University, Syracuse, New York.
52. Perkins, R. E. (1973): Innervation patterns in cochleas of cat and rat: study with rapid Golgi techniques. *Anat. Rec.*, 174:410(A).
53. Spoendlin, H. (1974): Neuroanatomy of the cochlea. In: *Facts and Models in Hearing*, edited by E. Zwicker and E. Terhardt, pp. 18–32. Springer, Berlin.
54. Zwicker, E. and Terhardt, E., editors (1974): *Facts and Models in Hearing*. Springer, Berlin.

DISCUSSION

J. Hawkins, Jr.: I think it is important, if we're going to use kanamycin for hair cell elimination, to say at what time the animal was tested after the kanamycin treatment. Even though it disappears from the blood in hours, it probably takes days to leave the cochlea. Therefore, to be sure you're dealing with hair cell elimination and not with an ototoxic agent slopping around in the endocochlear fluids.

R. Smith: That time was exceeded.

J. Miller: One of the keys to understanding how the auditory system works in temporary and permanent threshold shift is this fact of the ½ octave shift. Now, if you select an exposure carefully, you can produce a large threshold shift at frequencies above the exposure stimulus, and almost no threshold shift at the exposure frequency. It is easy to find a general upward shift; and you go to the bird as Dooling and Saunders (*Proc. Nat. Acad. Sci.* (1974), 71:1962–1965) did, you do not find this. It seems to me that those 2 facts have to be incorporated into your models and, further, may lead to data that will help decide among models.

J. Mills: Bob, do you know if anyone looked carefully at the inner hair cells (IHC) that were remaining in the area of the outer hair cells (OHC) loss? The gerbil is an animal which has a progressive loss of both OHC and IHC.

R. Hamernik: Cochleas were evaluated at 400× magnification and a decision was made only as to the presence or absence of hair cells. Since a long time had elapsed between kanamycin treatment and sacrifice, i.e., on the order of a month or more, the remaining IHC as well as OHC did not appear unusual in the surface view. A more critical anatomical study was not undertaken.

C. Trahiotis: It seems that there might be a 90° difference between the data of Dallos (*Science* (1972), 177:356–358) and yours.

R. Smith: The difference may not be in the data as much as in their interpretation. In the kanamycin-treated animals, single-fiber responses are classified as scala tympani or scala vestibuli according to the polarity or deflection of the basilar membrane which produces excitation. Each classification encompasses excitation during velocity and/or displacement in the relevant direction. Since there is a permanent velocity component in the responses of nearly all fibers associated with inner hair cells, the data does not conflict with Dallos' microphonic recordings.

Discussion

A. Møller: I think this session has taught us many things and was fruitful for 2 reasons: To give us a better understanding of what actually happens when the auditory system is damaged in one way or the other by sound or drugs, but I think that we have also seen that there are very good prospects for being able to study many important features in the normal auditory system using well-controlled lesions. As I said in the beginning, this type of study has not been very common in the past, and I hope that this session will show that this is a very useful way of studying many things.

We have heard about the CM. I think for many people, CM potentials are a mystery, and of course that, in itself, is appealing. Is it artifact? Then we should at least want to know where this artifact comes from and what the rules are.

We are seeing, as we saw yesterday, that almost any change we can think of in the cochlea will increase the threshold; that is not remarkable; what is interesting is that it will also increase the width of the tuning. It might very well be that 2 people with the same audiogram will not have the same speech intelligibility score. It's important to assess this sort of thing from a practical point of view. But it's important from a theoretical point of view also. What is it that is common for all those lesions in the cochlea that deteriorate the tuning? Is it possible that, for example, the mechanical characteristics of the basilar membrane are changed in some way? After all, we know very little about which of the mechanical properties of a biological membrane are important for the very small vibrations that we are concerned with. Perhaps the forces keeping together the basilar membrane will be affected by the lack of O_2, by chemicals, etc. The only way to assess such things is to experiment.

I'm very happy to hear, as Dr. Smith pointed out, that it's very important to consider what happens when sound changes either in the amplitude or frequency domain. We have had a fixation with tones having constant frequency and intensity. Honestly, I don't know where that comes from, because we don't find such sounds in nature anywhere. We use stationary signals to measure the hearing of ordinary people. It's strange enough that it works, but it's really not a very natural stimulus, and I think it's extremely important to study how the auditory system processes small changes in intensity, frequency of sound tone, etc. It's also very important to find out what it is that we call temporary threshold shift (TTS). That this may very well be partially a different phenomenon from what is called permanent threshold shift (PTS), that the TTS may very well be a fatiguing of the nervous system. And if we then try to extrapolate values of TTS into PTS, we will not be successful. We also have the practical implications of this type of research. We badly need a method by which we can evaluate the effects of a noise on human hearing, and since we don't need or like to make deaf people experimentally, it is extremely important to know if such phenomena as TTS can really be used in assessing the effect of noise on hearing. Because, as many people unfortunately seem to forget, we all know noise is very detrimental, we can't just assign a single figure to describe the traumatic potential of a given noise.

Effects of Noise on Hearing, edited by Donald Henderson,
Roger P. Hamernik, Darshan S. Dosanjh, and John H. Mills.
Raven Press, New York © 1976

Central Components of the Temporary Threshold Shift

Richard J. Salvi

*State University of New York, Department of Otolaryngology and Communication Sciences, Upstate
Medical Center, Syracuse, New York 13210*

Excessive sound stimulation can temporarily modify several auditory processes, such as pitch discrimination, loudness growth, and localization. However, the primary symptom of auditory fatigue is the change in absolute sensitivity or the temporary threshold shift (TTS) in hearing. Although the operational definition of TTS is straightforward, it appears to be a rather complex phenomenon as illustrated by the TTS recovery curves shown in Fig. 1. The 3 recovery curves were produced by: an impulse noise; a long duration noise exposure that produced an asymptotic level of TTS; and a short duration noise exposure. Each of these traumatic exposures produces nearly the same amount of TTS ($\sim$22 dB) 2 min after the exposure. However, the time course for TTS recovery is significantly different for each noise exposure. This point is very important because it suggests that the physiological processes involved in TTS may vary with the type of acoustic exposure.

Physiological processes which have been implicated in TTS include: a diminished cochlear blood supply (4); detachment of the tectorial membrane from the hair cells (5); an edema-like reaction in the supporting and sensory cells in the cochlea (6); altered permeability of structures within the cochlear partition (7); and cochlear hypoxia (8). These events are believed to be involved with the depressed cochlear potentials that often accompany TTS (9).

There is also circumstantial evidence which links TTS to the cochlea. For example, the audiological disorders associated with TTS include the abnormally rapid growth of loudness (loudness recruitment), a ringing or rushing sensation in the absence of sound (subjective tinnitus) and a compression of the function which relates the threshold of a tone to its duration (a reduction of auditory temporal summation) (10–12). These audiological signs and symptoms are consistent with a hearing loss of cochlear origin.

Although the concensus has been that TTS is strictly a cochlear phenomenon, this chapter will present evidence which suggests that the central auditory system is involved in TTS. However, the conditions for central auditory involvement appear to depend on the nature of the acoustic exposure. Hence, the following discussion will focus on changes in the central auditory system following long-duration exposures that produce an asymptotic level of TTS and those following low-level, short-duration exposures. Several questions

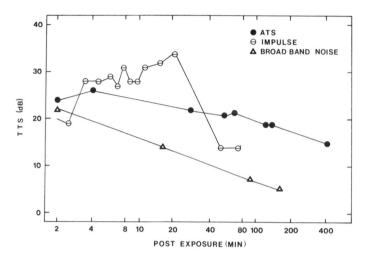

FIG. 1. The TTS recovery curves are shown for humans exposed to: impulse noise (⊖, gunfire, 155 dB SPL, 5 impulses); a long-duration, octave band of noise that produces an asymptotic level of TTS (●, 29.5 hr, 375–750 kHz, 92.5 dB SPL); and a short-duration, broadband noise (△, 12 min, 106 dB SPL). The hearing loss was measured at 4.0 kHz for the impulse noise and the short-duration broadband noise exposure. Threshold was measured at 750 Hz for the long-duration exposure. (From refs. 1, 2, and 3.)

will be explored. For example, how are the discharge properties of central auditory neurons affected by TTS exposures? Is the auditory system's overall loss in sensitivity determined only by changes in the cochlea or does the central auditory system contribute to TTS? Is there any evidence that different sound exposures generate different physiological changes? The first section of this paper will examine the central auditory changes during asymptotic TTS.

ASYMPTOTIC TTS

One advantage of long-duration sound exposures is that they lead to an asymptotic level of TTS that is quite predictable. The hearing loss from asymptotic TTS is also relatively stable for several hours postexposure which makes it possible to record and compare several different physiological measures. Benitez et al. (8) have measured a subset of auditory potentials during the slow recovery from asymptotic TTS. They used a 95-dB sound pressure level (SPL) octave band of noise (375–750 Hz) that produced a 48-dB asymptotic level of TTS at 715 Hz. Figure 2 summarizes the behavioral data along with salient electrophysiological results. The sound exposure did not appear to affect the DC endocochlear potential which has its source in the stria vascularis. However, the cochlear microphonic (CM), which depends on the integrity of the hair cells, showed a loss in sensitivity and a reduction in maximum voltage. The reduction in CM sensitivity was 24 dB in the second turn of the cochlea and 48 dB in the third turn at 5 hr postexposure. The average loss in CM sensitivity computed from the second and third turn CM

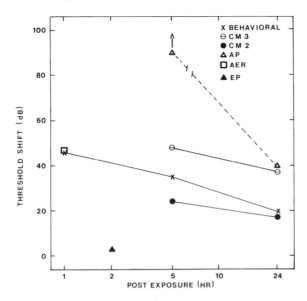

FIG. 2. Behavioral and electrophysiological data obtained from Benitez et al. (8). Behavioral threshold shifts (✗) were measured at 715 Hz. Threshold shifts for the AER (☐) and the 8th nerve AP (△) were derived from the visual detection levels for each potential. The AP could not be elicited with clicks 90 dB above the normal VDL. The threshold shift for the CM recorded from the second (●) and third (⊖) turn of the cochlea was defined as the lateral shift of the CM input–output function to a 200 Hz tone. The DC endocochlear potential (▲) from the noise-exposed animals was nearly the same as in normal animals. Small differences in the endocochlear potential could not account for more than a few decibels loss in sensitivity.

was nearly the same as the behavioral threshold shift at 715 Hz. Attempts at measuring the 8th nerve action potential (AP) 5 hr postexposure were unsuccessful. The AP could not be elicited even with wide-band clicks 90 dB above the normal threshold. At 24 hr postexposure, the AP threshold shift was approximately 40 dB and the maximum AP voltage was reduced. The chinchilla's auditory evoked response (AER), which originates in the inferior colliculus (14), was the only index of central auditory function. Within 1 hr after exposure, the AER threshold shift averaged across 3 animals was approximately 46 dB. The AER threshold shift was in close agreement with behavioral data.

A comparison across all the preceding measures suggests that the primary dysfunction for TTS is in the hair cells, because the CM shows a large loss in sensitivity, while the DC endolymphatic potential remains normal. The CM, which is a cochlear measure, and the AER, which is a central measure, both show a loss in sensitivity that is approximately the same as the behavioral TTS data. The similarity across measures suggests that asymptotic TTS is basically a cochlear phenomenon.

The 8th nerve measurements are rather paradoxical considering that the AP threshold shifts are at least 40 dB greater than those obtained with the

CM, AER, or behaviorally. The lack of an AP could occur because individual 8th nerve fibers do not respond or, alternatively, because the neurons in the 8th nerve do not respond with the proper degree of synchrony. Benitez et al. (8) favored the latter explanation because behavioral and AER thresholds were manifested at lower sound levels than the AP.

Recent experiments by Henderson and Møller (15) suggest that the AP grossly overestimates the changes in sensitivity that occur at the single-neuron level. They exposed rats to a broadband noise from 4–6 days. The octave band levels between 2.0 and 16.0 kHz were approximately 80 dB, while the levels outside this frequency range were less than 50 dB. After the exposure, they recorded from neurons in the cochlear nucleus. Figure 3 compares the single-unit thresholds from normal and noise-exposed animals. When units with characteristic frequencies (CF) above 20.0 kHz or below 3.5 kHz are compared, the thresholds from the noise-exposed animals are found to be similar to those from normal animals. However, in the noise-exposed animals, the neurons with CFs between 3.5 and 20.0 kHz had thresholds which were 20–40 dB higher than similar units from normal animals. Behavioral data on asymptotic TTS is lacking for the rat, but in the chinchilla, an 80-dB octave band of noise between 3.0 and 6.0 kHz will produce 30–50 dB of TTS 1–4 hr postexposure (16). The TTS values from chinchilla are approximately the same magnitude as the single-unit threshold shifts in the rat's cochlear nucleus.

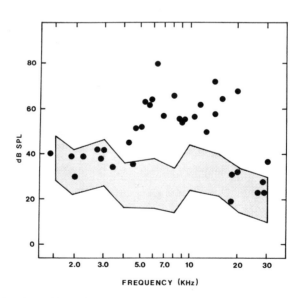

FIG. 3. Filled circles, thresholds at CF for neurons in the rat's cochlear nucleus during asymptotic TTS. Shaded area, normal thresholds for units in the rat's cochlear nucleus. Note that the neurons from the noise-exposed ear have higher thresholds than those from the normal ear between 3.5 and 20.0 kHz. (From ref. 15.)

The asymptotic TTS exposure not only elevates threshold, but it also influences the frequency–threshold response area or tuning curve of a neuron. Figure 4 is a schematic which compares the tuning curves from a normal and a noise-exposed animal. In the normal animal, the excitatory region of the tuning curve is quite narrow for tones within 30 dB of the threshold at CF. In the noise-exposed animal, the tuning curve shows a 20–40 dB threshold shift for frequencies near CF. The high threshold units have tuning curves that are much wider than those from normal animals. The tuning curve bandwidth has increased in the noise-exposed animal because the slope of the tuning curve below CF is shallower than normal. The high-frequency slope of the tuning curve is normal. The tuning curves from the noise-exposed animals appear to be quite similar to those from the 8th nerve when there is evidence of some type of cochlear dysfunction (17–19).

In the cochlear nucleus, a unit's response to a tone at CF can be inhibited by a second tone of the proper frequency and intensity. These inhibitory effects were studied during asymptotic TTS by exciting a neuron with a tone at CF, while a second probe tone was swept through the response area of the neuron. Normally, the sweep tone will produce a pronounced inhibitory effect when the sweep-tone frequency is slightly above or below CF and when the sweep-tone intensity is 5–15 dB above the unit's threshold at CF. However, in the high-threshold neurons, the 2-tone inhibitory effects were often com-

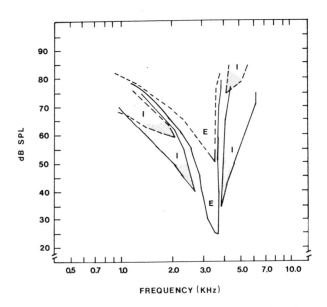

FIG. 4. Typical single unit tuning curves from the rat's cochlear nucleus are shown for normal (*solid lines*) and noise-exposed (*dashed lines*) rats. The inhibitory (I) regions of the tuning curves show a larger loss in sensitivity than the excitatory (E) regions. The bandwidth of the excitatory region is wider in the noise-exposed animals than in normals. (From ref. 15.)

pletely lacking or they could be elicited only at very high sound levels. The 2-tone inhibitory effect appears to show a greater loss in sensitivity than does the threshold at CF.

When the animals were in a state of TTS, the intensity characteristics of a number of cochlear nucleus units were studied. The dynamic properties of the high-threshold units were tested by modulating the amplitude of a tone at CF with pseudorandom noise. The modulated response from these neurons was found to be within normal limits.

We have also obtained preliminary data from single units in the inferior colliculus of the chinchilla during asymptotic TTS. The exposure was a 3–6 kHz octave band of noise at 86 dB sound pressure level (SPL). Figure 5 shows the expected free-field behavioral thresholds for the chinchilla at the termination of the exposure (16). Figure 5 also compares the thresholds (SPL measured at the tympanic membrane) of inferior colliculus units that were obtained from normal and noise-exposed chinchillas. The thresholds from the noise-exposed animals are consistently higher than those from nor-

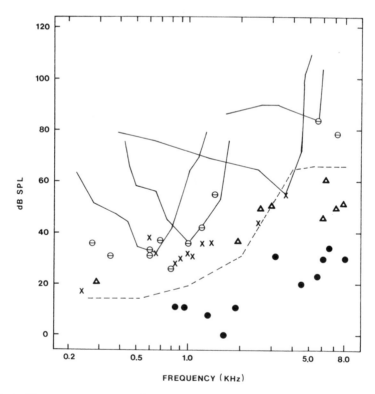

FIG. 5. Dashed line, expected thresholds (measured free field) for chinchilla after exposure to a 3.0–6.0 kHz band of noise at 86 dB SPL for 3 days (From ref. 16). The thresholds for single units in the inferior colliculus are shown for normal (●) and noise-exposed chinchilla (⊖, 1–5 hr; ✕, 5–10 hr; and △, 10–15 hr postexposure).

mal animals, particularly at higher frequencies. Between 1 and 5 hr postexposure, the thresholds from the noise-exposed animals are 30–60 dB higher at the midfrequencies than those from normal animals. Note that single-unit thresholds improve with time after exposure.

Figure 5 also contains the tuning curves from several colliculus units during the asymptotic TTS. The high-threshold units above 1.0 kHz have very wide tuning curves because the slope of the tuning curve below CF is quite shallow. The tuning curves from the high-threshold units are similar to those obtained in the cochlear nucleus during asymptotic TTS (15). The units with low CFs have relatively normal thresholds and their tuning curves are similar to those from normal animals.

From the foregoing, it is possible to summarize some of the central auditory changes during asymptotic TTS. First, the excitatory region of the tuning curve shows a greater loss in sensitivity near CF than below CF, consequently the low-frequency slope of the tuning curve becomes shallower than normal and the tuning curve bandwidth is increased. Second, 2-tone inhibitory effects are abolished, or show a loss in sensitivity that are greater than in the excitatory region of the tuning curve. Finally, the CM, AER, and single units from the cochlear nucleus and inferior colliculus show a loss in sensitivity which is similar to behavioral TTS data. The changes in sensitivity at central auditory sites are similar to those that occur at the cochlea which implies that asymptotic TTS is primarily a cochlear phenomenon. In the next section, a review of the literature suggests that there is a central component to TTS when the sound exposure is of low level and short duration.

LOW-LEVEL, SHORT-DURATION EXPOSURE

A few early experiments using low-level, short-duration exposures suggest that central auditory structures are particularly susceptible to auditory fatigue. Rose et al. (20), for example, showed that units in the cochlear nucleus became less sensitive after being stimulated for less than 20 min by tones that were within 40 dB of a unit's threshold. These exposures were capable of reducing the sensitivity of units in the cochlear nucleus for more than 3 min. This is rather surprising considering the benign nature of the exposure. They hypothesized that very loud sound exposures would reduce the sensitivity of units in the cochlear nucleus for several hours.

Recent evidence by Saunders and Rhyne (21) indicates that there may be rather large threshold shifts in the cochlear nucleus following a mild TTS exposure. They subjected cats to a 95 dB SPL broadband noise for 15 min and measured the threshold shifts at the cochlear nucleus using the frequency following response (FFR). The FFR reflects the volleying action of many neurons that are responding synchronously to low-frequency tones (below 3.0 kHz). The exposure generally produced threshold shifts in the FFR that were between 5 and 20 dB. However, the threshold shifts were sometimes as large as 32 dB. The largest threshold shifts often required more than 3 hr to recover. The authors considered the threshold shifts at the cochlear nucleus to be relatively large compared to behavioral TTS values obtained from cats.

Starr and Livingston (22) have also reported long-lasting changes in central auditory structures following a low-level noise exposure. They subjected cats to a broadband noise at 85 dB for 2 hr and measured changes in a potential which reflects the spontaneous activity summed over many neurons. The potential was recorded at several auditory sites. Figure 6 summarizes the major findings of their experiments. The spontaneous potential measured at the round window of the cochlea or at the 8th nerve remained at the control

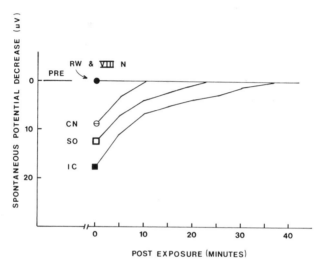

FIG. 6. Schematic diagram of the recovery of the summed "spontaneous potential" after a 2-hr broadband noise at 85 dB SPL. The recording sites were at the round window or 8th nerve (●), the cochlear nucleus (⊖), superior olive (□), and inferior colliculus (■). (From ref. 22.)

level following the exposure. However, the noise exposure depressed the spontaneous potential from the cochlear nucleus for as long as 10 min. There was a further reduction of the potential and a lengthening of the recovery period at the superior olive and the inferior colliculus. The exposure had negligible effects on the spontaneous potential recorded from more central auditory sites such as the medial geniculate and auditory cortex. These findings suggest that mild noise exposures can produce long-lasting changes at retrocochlear nuclei without affecting the cochlea.

Later, Starr (23) was able to provide support for a central component to TTS with the help of binaurally excitable neurons in the trapezoid body. He first established the ipsilateral and contralateral preexposure thresholds for binaurally excitable units and then exposed only the ipsilateral ear to a long-adapting tone. At the end of the exposure, both the ipsilateral and contralateral thresholds were elevated. This implied that the loss in sensitivity was occurring proximal to the 8th nerve where there is binaural interaction. If the exposure had elevated only the ipsilateral threshold, then the neuron's loss in sensitivity could be attributed to a loss in sensitivity at the cochlea.

We have recently obtained data which suggest that there is a central component to TTS with low-level, short-duration exposures. Chinchilla were used in 3 series of experiments. Each animal was given a standard TTS exposure at a frequency between 0.4 and 8.0 kHz. The standard exposure was always

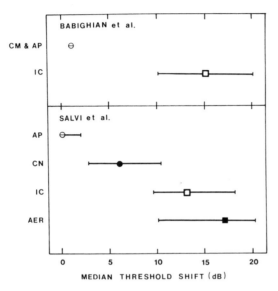

FIG. 7. Lower: Median threshold shift and interquartile range after an 8-min pure-tone exposure at 95 dB SPL. Threshold shifts for the 8th nerve action potential (AP, $\ominus$, N = 41) and auditory evoked response (AER, ■, N = 30) were based on the visual detection level. Threshold shifts for single units in the cochlear nucleus (CN, ●, N = 51) and inferior colliculus (IC, □, N = 12) were based on the lateral shift of the discharge rate intensity function. Upper: Approximate threshold shifts obtained by Babighian et al. (13) for the CM and 8th nerve action potential ($\ominus$) input–output function and the inferior colliculus (□) input–output function.

on for 8 min at 95 dB SPL (near the tympanic membrane). The AER was measured in 1 group using tone bursts. The AER threshold shift was always recorded at the TTS exposure frequency. In a second group, the 8th nerve AP was measured with clicks and single units from the cochlear nucleus were studied with tone bursts at CF. Only units with CFs between 0.4 and 8.0 kHz were selected for study. Spontaneous activity and the discharge rate—intensity function were measured for each unit pre- and postexposure. The frequency of the TTS exposure was at the CF of the neuron. In a third group, single units from the inferior colliculus were studied with the procedures outlined for the cochlear nucleus.

Figure 7 contains the median threshold shift and interquartile range for each set of measurements during the first 10 min postexposure. The TTS exposure has no effect on the visual detection level for the 8th nerve AP when it was measured ~7 min postexposure. The median threshold shift for the AP was 0 dB and the interquartile range was 0–2 dB. The threshold shifts for the cochlear nucleus units were measured in terms of the lateral shift of the discharge rate–intensity function. The threshold shifts have been collapsed across units with different best frequencies since the threshold shift did not systematically vary with CF. The median threshold shift for all cochlear nucleus units was 6.8 dB ($N = 51$) with an interquartile range of 2.9–10.4 dB. The threshold shift for the units from the colliculus was measured in the same manner as for units in the cochlear nucleus. The median threshold shift for the colliculus neurons was 13 dB ($N = 12$) with an interquartile range of 9–18 dB. It is important to note that all units in the colliculus exhibited a threshold shift of 6 dB or greater, whereas some units in the cochlear nucleus failed to show any loss in sensitivity. The lack of a threshold shift in some of the cochlear nucleus units implies that the 8th nerve fibers innervating these cells were unaffected by the exposure.

The threshold shifts for the AER were nearly constant across 6 different exposure frequencies between 0.5 and 8.0 kHz. Thus, TTS values have been collapsed across frequency in Fig. 7. The overall median threshold shift for the AER was 17 dB with an interquartile range of 10–20 dB. Figure 7 also contains recent TTS data from Babighian et al. (13). They used a TTS exposure that was almost identical to ours and found a 10–20 dB threshold shift in a frequency-tuned evoked potential from the inferior colliculus. They reported virtually no change in the CM or AP input–output function from the cochlea. It is clear that our results are nearly identical to those of Babighian et al. (13). Both sets of data indicate that low-level exposures produce a progressively larger loss in sensitivity from the cochlea to more central auditory sites.

The TTS exposure produced several systematic effects in single-unit activity. During the exposure, the Chopper, Pauser, Flat Primarylike and Primarylike units from the cochlear nucleus displayed high rates of driven activity. After the exposure, their spontaneous discharge rates were depressed below the preexposure level. Similar effects have been observed by Starr (23) at the cochlear nucleus and by Goldberg et al. (24) at the superior olive. The on units responded somewhat differently than other functional categories in the cochlear nucleus. The on units gave an "off" response during the exposure, i.e., their discharge rates fell below the spontaneous level. After the exposure, their spontaneous rates were equal to or temporarily greater than the preexposure level. Similar, but less pronounced, effects have been observed for units in the inferior colliculus.

Figure 8 (upper) shows the effects of the TTS exposure on the discharge rate–intensity function of units from the cochlear nucleus. The exposure generally displaced the function to the right without significantly altering its

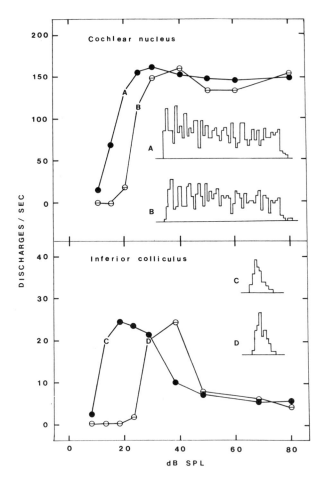

FIG. 8. Pre- (●) and postexposure (⊖) discharge rate intensity functions for a typical neuron from the cochlear nucleus (upper) and inferior colliculus (lower). Pre- and postexposure poststimulus-time histograms are shown for 50-msec tone bursts. The pre- and postexposure histograms from the cochlear nucleus (A vs B) and inferior colliculus (C vs D) are nearly identical when the loss in sensitivity is compensated for.

slope or maximum discharge rate. Figure 8 (lower) gives the typical effect of the exposure on a colliculus neuron's discharge rate–intensity function. Most of the time, the TTS exposure simply displaced the function to the right as in Fig. 8 (lower), but occasionally, the maximum discharge rate was reduced by more than 50%.

The tone-burst discharge patterns were also examined to determine if the exposure had altered the firing patterns of the units. Figure 8 contains the pre- and postexposure histograms for a typical unit from the cochlear nucleus and inferior colliculus. The pre- and postexposure histograms for the same sound pressure level are different due to the loss in sensitivity. However, when the loss in sensitivity is compensated for, the histograms are virtually identical in terms of latency and shape. The TTS exposure does not appear to significantly alter the firing patterns of units in the cochlear nucleus or the inferior colliculus.

ANALYSIS

In summary, the TTS exposures reduce the sensitivity of central auditory neurons. The slope of the excitatory region of the tuning curve becomes shallower below the neuron's CF and the bandwidth of the tuning curve becomes wider. Two-tone inhibitory effects are also reduced or abolished during TTS. Although a neuron's sensitivity is reduced, its input–output properties remain the same after the exposure. A few units in the inferior colliculus, however, show a large reduction in the maximum discharge rate during TTS. The input-output properties of the high-threshold units are paradoxical because loudness grows at an abnormally rapid rate during TTS. Furthermore, the input–output function for the 8th nerve AP can show an abnormally rapid growth during TTS (Pugh et al., 25). The dynamic properties of single neurons in the cochlear nucleus and inferior colliculus do not appear to be correlated with either of these phenomena.

Although TTS exposures affect the sensitivity of a neuron, they do not seem to alter its firing pattern over time when the loss in sensitivity is compensated for. This finding is somewhat surprising because the psychophysical function which relates the threshold of a tone to its duration is known to be reduced during TTS. The reduced threshold–duration functions have been thought to result from an abnormally rapid decay in the neural output of the cochlea near threshold (26). This abnormal decay should be reflected in the discharge patterns of units from the cochlear nucleus; however, effects of this nature have not been observed.

TTS exposures also tend to reduce spontaneous activity in most neurons from the cochlear nucleus and inferior colliculus. This finding is also somewhat of an enigma because descriptive explanations for subjective tinnitus or "head noise" are based on elevated rates of spontaneous neural activity in the 8th nerve. One should therefore expect to find elevated rates of spontaneous activity in the cochlear nucleus during TTS. However, only the on units from the cochlear nucleus show a temporary elevation of spontaneous activity after the exposure. Other neurons from the cochlear nucleus and the inferior colliculus show a reduction in spontaneous activity.

Finally, the physiological results from long duration exposures suggest that the primary disorder for TTS is in the cochlea. With low-level, short-duration exposures, the major loss in sensitivity appears to occur at central auditory sites. These seemingly opposite findings can be reconciled by a simple descriptive model which we propose for the auditory system. Our explanation assumes that the auditory system is organized as a series of cascaded stages. The output of each stage is assumed to be a function of the input to that stage and also the gain and sensitivity of that stage. The first stage (i.e., the sensory cell) in this system is unique because the input signal (basilar membrane motion) can be held constant by external stimuli. The output of the first stage, therefore, depends *only* on its gain and sensitivity (or, conversely, on the amount of fatigue). The output of the succeeding stages depends on both the incoming signal level (or, the output of the preceding stage) and the gain and sensitivity of that stage. The important point is that the output of the second (or succeeding) stage can be reduced by fatigue at a more peripheral site.

Consider the hypothetical response of this system following a long-duration exposure. The exposure will produce considerable fatigue at the first stage which lowers its sensitivity. This lowers the output of the first stage which, in turn, reduces the possibility for adaptation at succeeding stages in the system. Thus, the loss in sensitivity at the first stage will tend to determine the overall loss in sensitivity of the entire system. Under these conditions, the threshold shift at the first stage (i.e., the cochlea) will match the threshold shift at later stages in the auditory system.

The response of our hypothetical system will be different with low-level, short-duration exposures. Such exposures will produce a high output at each stage of the system because none of the stages can be completely fatigued by the exposure. This leads to a small amount of fatigue at each stage. Thus, the overall output (or overall loss in sensitivity) of the system will depend on the net output (loss) at each stage. Consequently, the measured loss in sensitivity will increase from the cochlea to more central sites within the auditory system.

In summary, different TTS exposures are likely to produce different patterns of physiological fatigue even though the final behavioral measures of TTS may be identical. Evidence from previous studies indicates that long-duration exposures may primarily affect the cochlea. Our results indicate that low-level, short-duration exposures may primarily fatigue retrocochlear structures.

ACKNOWLEDGMENTS

Part of the work described here was supported by grants: 2-R01-04-00364, NIOSH, PHS, Dept. HEW; 1-R01-ES00969, NIEHS, Dept. HEW; and the Deafness Research Foundation, New York.

I am grateful to Phyllis DiRaddo and Helen Hayes who assisted with the manuscript and figures.

REFERENCES

1. Ward, W. D., Glorig, A., and Sklar, D. L. (1959): Relation between recovery from temporary threshold shift and duration of exposure. *J. Acoust. Soc. Am.,* 31:600–602.

2. Mills, J. H., Gengel, R. W., Watson, C. S., and Miller, J. D. (1970): Temporary changes of the auditory system due to exposure to noise for one or two days. *J. Acoust. Soc. Am.*, 48:524–530.
3. Luz, G. A., and Hodge, D. C. (1971): Recovery from impulse noise-induced TTS in monkeys and men: a descriptive model. *J. Acoust. Soc. Am.*, 49:1770–1777.
4. Lawrence, M., Gonzales, G., and Hawkins, J. E. (1967): Some physiological factors in noise induced hearing loss. *Am. Ind. Hyg. J.*, 28:425–430.
5. Crane, H. D. (1966): Mechanical impact: a model of auditory excitation and fatigue. *J. Acoust. Soc. Am.*, 40:1147–1159.
6. Wüstenfeld, E. (1957): Experimentelle untersuchungen zum problem der schallanalyse im innenohr. *Z. Mikrosk. Anat. Forsch.*, 63:327–387.
7. Misrahy, G. A., Spradley, J. F., Dzinovic, S., and Brooks, C. J. (1961): Effects of intense sound; hypoxia and Kanamycin on the permeability of cochlear partitions. *Ann. Otol. Rhinol. Laryngol.*, 70:572–581.
8. Misrahy, G. A., Shinabarger, E. W., and Arnold, J. E. (1958): Changes in cochlear endolymphatic oxygen availability, action potential and microphonics during and following asphyxia, hypoxia, and exposure to loud sounds. *J. Acoust. Soc. Am.*, 30:701–704.
9. Benitez, L. D., Eldredge, D. G., and Templer, J. W. (1972): Temporary threshold shifts in chinchilla: electrophysiological correlates. *J. Acoust. Soc. Am.*, 52:1115–1123.
10. Jerger, J. F. (1955): Difference of stimulus duration on the pure tone threshold during recovery from auditory fatigue. *J. Acoust. Soc. Am.*, 27:121–124.
11. Hickling, S. (1967): Hearing test patterns in noise induced temporary hearing loss. *J. Audit. Res.*, 7:63–76.
12. Loeb, M., and Smith, R. (1967): Relation of induced tinnitus to physical characteristics of the inducing stimuli. *J. Acoust. Soc. Am.*, 42:453–455.
13. Babighian, G., Moushegian, G., and Rupert, A. L. (1975): Central auditory fatigue. *Audiology*, 14:72–83.
14. Rothenberg, S., and Davis, H. (1967): Auditory evoked response in chinchilla. *Percept. Psychophys.*, 2:443–447.
15. Henderson, D., and Møller, A. (1975): Effects of asymptotic threshold shift in the neural firing patterns of the rat cochlear nucleus. *J. Acoust. Soc. Am.*, 57:S53.
16. Mills, J. (1973): Temporary and permanent threshold shifts produced by nine-day exposures to noise. *J. Speech Hear. Res.*, 16:426–438.
17. Kiang, N. Y. S., Moxon, E. C., and Levine, R. A. (1970): Auditory-Nerve activity in cats with normal and abnormal cochleas. In: *Sensorineural Hearing Loss*, edited by G. E. W. Wolstenholme and J. Knight, pp. 241–268. Churchill, London.
18. Evans, E. F. (1972): The frequency response and other properties of single fibers in the guinea-pig cochlear nerve. *J. Physiol. (London)*, 226:263–287.
19. Robertson, D. (1974): Cochlear neurons: frequency selectivity altered by perilymph removal. *Science*, 186:153–155.
20. Rose, J. E., Galambos, R., and Hughes, J. R. (1959): Microelectrode studies of the cochlear nuclei of the cat. *Johns Hopkins Med. J.*, 104:211–251.
21. Saunders, J. C., and Rhyne, R. L. (1970): Cochlear nucleus activity and threshold shift in cat. *Brain Res.*, 24:336–339.
22. Starr, A., and Livingston, R. B. (1963): Long-lasting nervous system responses to prolonged sound stimulation in waking cats. *J. Neurophysiol.*, 26:416–431.
23. Starr, A. (1965): Suppression of single neuron activity in the cochlear nucleus of the cat following sound stimulation. *J. Neurophysiol.*, 26:416–431.
24. Goldberg, J., Adrian, H. D., and Smith, F. D. (1964): Response of neurons of the superior olivary complex of the cat to acoustic stimuli of long duration. *J. Neurophysiol.*, 27:706–749.
25. Pugh, J. E., Horowitz, M. R., and Anderson, D. J. (1974): Cochlear electrical activity in noise-induced hearing loss. *Arch. Otolaryngol.*, 100:36–40.
26. Wright, H. N. (1968): Clinical measurements of temporal auditory summation. *J. Speech Hear. Res.*, 11:109–127.
27. Atherly, G. R. C., Hempstock, T. I., and Noble, W. G. (1968): Study of tinnitus induced temporarily by noise. *J. Acoust. Soc. Am.*, 44:1503–1506.

DISCUSSION

C. Trahiotis: What I'm worried about is the relationship between TTS measured by the AER and the AP. What was the duration of the tone that was used to measure the AER. Is it possible that the magnitudes are even greater than they appear to be in terms of differences in threshold shift?

R. Salvi: The AP was elicited with clicks, because that is one of the most appropriate stimuli for eliciting it. The AER was obtained with 20-msec tone bursts and the single units were studied with 50- or 100-msec tone bursts. These auditory responses have different properties and they are influenced by different stimulus parameters, consequently it is difficult to make a quantitative comparison regarding the loss in sensitivity at different auditory sites. Yes, I would predict a larger TTS if we measured the behavioral threshold using long-duration signals. However, we feel that the qualitative trends in the data are important. That is, with low-level, short-duration exposure, we get a progressively larger loss in sensitivity from the cochlea to more central auditory sites.

W. Melnick: An old design for trying to differentiate whether an event has peripheral or has a central component involved is to use a contralateral exposure and then measuring the effect on the ipsilateral side. Did you try that?

R. Salvi: No, we didn't, but there is an old experiment by Starr (*J. Neurol. Physiol.* (1965), 33:137–147), where he records from binaurally sensitive neurons in the trapezoid body. He measured the contralateral and ipsilateral thresholds for these units before and after a mildly fatiguing sound. The fatiguing sound was presented only to the ipsilateral ear. If TTS is just simply a cochlear phenomenon then threshold should rise only in the exposed ear. These units showed a threshold shift to stimuli delivered to both ears. I should add that these were relatively moderate exposures, where I don't think you expect to see any cross talk.

J. Saunders: You might ask what sort of mechanisms might be involved in this sort of central auditory system fatigue. An interesting guide line to answering that question comes from laboratories far removed from our own work dealing with the spinal cord of the crayfish and the somata sensory system of the cat. Basically, these experiments take a presynaptic neuron and electrically excite it and record from a postsynaptic neuron. The remarkable findings are that, in some cases, 5 min of electrical stimulation can produce as much as 8 hr of abnormal responses, postsynaptically postexposure. The contextural framework in which these experiments are carried out is the concept of synaptic depletion and it may be that under sustained auditory stimulation, central nervous system synapses also undergo the types of depletion that are discussed in these particular systems.

R. Smith: With low-level, short-duration exposure you showed the loss of threshold progressively increasing as you recorded more centrally. Have you determined the transition between long- and short-duration exposures; that is, do you expect to see that progression change as you increase the exposure duration? Would you see the greatest shift in threshold move back into the periphery?

R. Salvi: We have not conducted the experiments to determine the transition point, but I would expect to see the changes you mentioned.

E. Evans: I'm interested to see the effects on tuning of the CN cells. I think that you should be very cautious in drawing the analogy between effects on CN cells compared with the reduction in 2-tone suppression, because these 2 phenomena are totally different. You obtained your inhibitory areas from single-tone stimulation.

R. Salvi: No, the experiments by Henderson and Møller (*J. Acoust. Soc. Am.* (1975), 57:S53A) were done with 2 tones; a tone fixed at the CF and a second tone that was swept across CF.

E. Evans: That's a different question then, because normally in the CN you can demonstrate these low-pass inhibitory side bands with single tones, but of course you can't in primary fibers.

R. Butler: Have you considered using lower level exposures, e.g., 10–20 dB SL, to determine if you can get threshold shifts at these low levels?

R. Salvi: That's a good suggestion, but I wouldn't expect the effects to last very long. I usually try to use exposures that produce effects lasting more than a few minutes, so that I can measure several different response properties from a neuron.

E. Evans: Qualitatively you see these changes, certainly in the cortical areas. They habituate exceedingly rapidly.

W. Ward: I like Butler's comment. Because Selters' (*J. Acoust. Soc. Am.* (1964), 36:2202–2209) have shown, inferentially at least, that lower level adaptation and that ordinary fatigue probably exists at different places, because they're additive, and it would be interesting to see if you can isolate one of those.

J. Tonndorf: I'm bothered by your model of a spillover into higher levels, because it seems to me that if the peripheral auditory system shuts down, then that should protect the central auditory system. With kanamycin it's different. You can knock the hair cells without affecting the higher levels, because the drug is brought to the hair cells by the bloodstream. When the stimulus is reduced peripherally, how can things spill over into the higher levels?

R. Salvi: In the beginning of a low-level, TTS-producing exposure, the peripheral auditory system cannot protect the more central auditory sites because the periphery does not immediately shut down. During the beginning of an exposure it is possible to activate the central auditory system. The longer the exposure remains on, the greater the fatigue at the peripheral. Eventually we get this protective action that you mentioned. We could also get this protective action near the onset of a TTS-producing exposure if we use very high level sounds, e.g., 125 dB. This could have a dramatic and immediate effect on the exposure. The TTS-producing exposures that we have used are 95 dB or less.

Part IV
Experimental Studies of Noise-Induced Hearing Loss
Introduction

Noise, as a pollutant, has not received as systematic an evaluation as other environmental pollutants. Typically, most pollutants are evaluated both in animal experiments and through systematic demographic surveys. Hearing function is difficult to measure in animals; consequently, few animal studies have been published. Moreover, because of the ambiguity involved when generalizing from animals to man, the few studies that do exist have had little impact on the development of noise criteria. Animal noise research, however, is bound to take a more prominent place in future noise research for a number of reasons. Human demographic data is becoming more difficult to obtain. The enactment of noise control legislation should insure that individuals will now be exposed to significantly less traumatic noise. Furthermore, human temporary threshold shift (TTS) experiments are becoming more difficult to justify to committees that monitor human experimentation.

There are numerous examples that can be chosen to demonstrate the value of animal noise research. Perhaps the greatest value is that animal experiments can include histological confirmation of the noise trauma. Specifically, recent animal experiments have shown that (a) noise exposures can cause relatively large lesions in the cochlea without appreciably altering the animal's quiet threshold; (b) for a given noise exposure level, there appears to be an asymptotic value of TTS that an animal will develop, regardless of the duration of the exposure; and (c) the effects of a continuous noise can be potentiated by the addition of either "safe" doses of ototoxic drugs or impulse noise at "safe" levels.

An exact quantitative extrapolation of the above findings to humans is probably impossible at present. However, the phenomena are so clear that they are almost certainly operative in all human noise data and should be reckoned with.

Effects of Noise on Hearing, edited by Donald Henderson,
Roger P. Hamernik, Darshan S. Dosanjh, and John H. Mills.
Raven Press, New York © 1976

Threshold Shifts Produced by a 90-Day Exposure to Noise

John H. Mills

*Department of Otolaryngology, Medical University of South Carolina,
Charleston, South Carolina 29401*

Most studies of temporary threshold shifts (TTS) produced by exposure to sound have evolved from an interest in the occupational problems of noise-induced permanent threshold shifts (PTS), and from a desire to predict the facts of PTS from the facts of TTS. Although the efforts have been large in number, dividends in the form of quantitative and qualitative relations between TTS and PTS have been minimal. Indeed, it is believed in some quarters that TTS and PTS may be unrelated phenomena.

In the present chapter, an attempt is made to relate TTS to PTS. This attempt is based upon experiments conducted over the past several years at the Central Institute for the Deaf (1–9). In most of these experiments monaural chinchillas, trained in behavioral audiometry, were exposed to octave bands of noise for durations as short as a few hours and as long as 21 days. Auditory sensitivity for pure tones was measured before the exposure, during quiet periods interspersed within an exposure, and at periodic intervals after an exposure. A comparison of final postexposure audiograms with preexposure audiograms revealed PTSs produced by the exposure. After completion of the behavioral audiometry, cochlear microphonics and action potentials of the 8th nerve were measured. Animals were then sacrificed and the cochleae were subjected to anatomical study. While the total product of these researches speaks to the effects of noise on hearing as well as to behavioral, anatomical, and physiological relations and correlations, this chapter is restricted to the effects of noise as indicated by behavioral data.

A major finding of the behavioral studies is that threshold shifts, measured at postexposure times of about 4 min (TS_4) or about 11 min (TS_{11}), increase for the first 24 hr of exposure and then remain constant. Threshold shifts measured after about 24 hr of exposure, therefore, have been considered to be asymptotic. The levels and durations of exposure for which the asymptote can be maintained have not been determined; however, it is clear that the asymptote can be maintained for as long as 21 days when the magnitude of TS_4 is 30 dB (3,4) and for as long as 9 days when the magnitude of TS_4 is 80 dB (6).

The notion that threshold shifts reach an asymptote is critical to hypotheses about the relations between temporary and permanent threshold shifts (6,11). One hypothesis states, for example, that if TTSs produced by a sound of fixed level and spectrum truly reach an asymptote, then the threshold shifts at asymptote are an upper bound on the PTS that can be produced by that sound regardless of the duration or scheduling of exposures. This hypothesis must be true if threshold shifts reach a true asymptote rather than a plateau and do not increase after termination of the exposure. While the latter is unlikely, the former seems to be a realistic possibility. It is important, therefore, to determine if threshold shifts reach a true asymptote and not just a plateau. Thus, the duration of exposure was extended to 90 days in the present study.

METHOD

The subjects were 4 chinchillas who had been rendered monaural by surgical destruction of their left cochlea (10). Each animal was required to have normal hearing, to be easy to train and test, and to be in good general health. At a postexposure time of 6 months the age of the animals ranged from 30 months to 34 months with a mean age of 33 months.

The animals were trained by the method of instrumental avoidance conditioning and testing was done using a modified method of limits. The stimulus paradigm for a single trial consisted of a series of 3 tonal pulses with each pulse 750 msec in duration and with rise–fall times of 50 msec. Interpulse interval was 500 msec, and intertrial interval was varied randomly between 5 and 10 sec. Additional details of the training methods, testing procedures, and audiometric apparatus are given elsewhere[4,10].

After training, and after each animal had been shown to have normal hearing, extensive preexposure audiometry was conducted. For each animal 15 measurements of auditory thresholds were made at each frequency from 2.0 to 16.0 kHz in one-half octave steps, and 10 measurements were made at each frequency from 0.25 to 1.0 kHz in one-octave steps.

The animals were exposed as a group in a diffuse sound field on 2 occasions to an octave-band noise centered at 4.0 kHz. The level of the noise was 80 dB sound pressure level (SPL). The first exposure was only 2 days in duration and was conducted to insure that these particular animals were typical with respect to the growth and decay of threshold shifts. The second exposure was initiated about 2 weeks after the first and lasted 90 days.

To follow the growth of threshold shifts each animal was removed from the noise at specified times, placed in a test room where auditory thresholds were measured, and then returned to the noise chamber. The exact test schedule was as follows: Animals were tested daily during the first 9 days of the exposure; then daily over 5-day periods centered at 15, 27, 55, and 87 days. On days when animals were not tested, they were removed from the noise exposure and given 20-min dust baths. Body weights were also recorded at this time. Thus, during the 90-day exposure to noise animals were actually in the noise for about 23.5 hr/day. After termination of the exposure thresholds were measured at regular intervals. At a postexposure time of about 150 days audiograms were obtained and compared with preexposure audiograms to determine the presence and magnitude of any PTSs. Of course, the procedure used for the postexposure audiograms, including the number of measurements, were identical to those used for the pre-exposure audiograms.

RESULTS

Growth of Threshold Shifts

The growth of threshold shifts at 5.7 kHz is shown in Fig. 1 as a function of the duration of exposure. These measurements were made at a post-exposure time of about 4 min (TS_4). The solid symbols are the present data; the open symbols are the means of data reported in other studies (5–7). The dotted line is a best fit, by eye, to the 2 sets of data. For durations greater than 9 days the dotted line has been extended with no change in slope, and the data points are the means of measurements made over 5-day periods centered at durations of 15, 27, 55, and 87 days.

Threshold shifts increase for the first 24 hr of exposure, remain constant, or nearly so, from about 24 hr to 15 or 30 days, and then increase 5 dB during the remainder of the exposure. While the difference in threshold shifts of about 5 dB between 1 and 5 days of exposure and 85 to 90 days of exposure is significant ($p < 0.05$) by appropriate statistical tests, effects

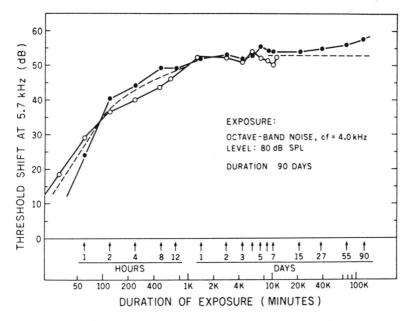

FIG. 1. Growth of threshold shifts at 5.7 kHz during exposure to an octave-band noise with a center frequency of 4.0 kHz. These measurements were made at a postexposure time of 4 min. The filled datum points are an average from those reported in refs. 5–8.

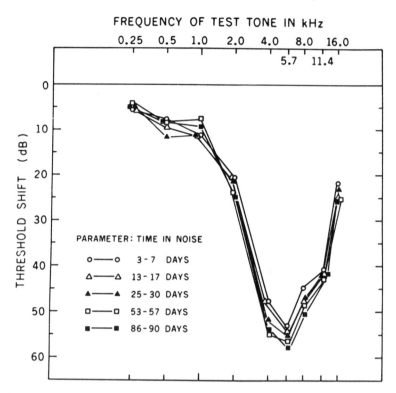

FIG. 2. Threshold shifts as shown by the audiogram. The parameter is the time in noise. These measurements were made at postexposure times of about 11 min. Each datum point is the group mean of measurements made daily over 5-day periods.

on the order of 5 dB are about equal to the precision of measurement and to response criteria of the animals.

The data in Fig. 2, which were obtained at a postexposure time of about 11 min (TS_{11}), indicate that threshold shifts are maximal in and slightly above the frequency region of the noise, that is, from 4.0 to 8.0 kHz, and decrease as the frequency of the test tone is increased or decreased. As the exposure duration is increased from about 5 days to 90 days, TS_{11} increases by about 5 to 7 dB. While this increase is not large, it is very systematic, especially for test tones from 4.0 to 8.0 kHz. Thus, the data of Fig. 2 in combination with the data of Fig. 1 suggest that TS_{4-11} increases from about 53 dB to about 58 dB between exposure durations of 5 days and 90 days.

Decay of Threshold Shifts and Permanent Threshold Shifts

Decay of threshold shifts at 5.7 kHz is shown in Fig. 3 for an exposure of 2 days and for an exposure of 90 days. Whereas the threshold shifts

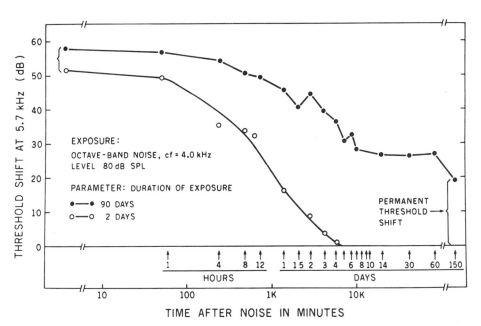

FIG. 3. Decay of threshold shifts for a tone of 5.7 kHz after exposure to an octave-band noise with a center frequency of 4.0 kHz. The parameter is the duration of exposure.

produced by the 2-day exposure decay to zero in about 3 to 5 days, the threshold shifts produced by the 90-day exposure do not decay to zero. A PTS of about 20 dB was measured. The shapes of the decay curves of Fig. 3 are consistent with earlier results (4,6) with 1 exception. The exception is the improvement in thresholds between postexposure times of 60 and 150 days which occurred for all animals.

Threshold shifts at several test frequencies are shown on Fig. 4 where the parameter is postexposure time. Several factors should be noted in Fig. 4. PTSs are maximal at 5.7 kHz and decrease to zero as the frequency of the test tone is increased to 16.0 kHz or decreased to 1.0 kHz. PTSs are largest in the frequency region where TS_4 was largest. Thus, both TS_4 and PTSs were largest in and slightly above the frequency region encompassed by the noise. Closer inspection of Fig. 4, especially at test frequencies not encompassed by the exposure noise, reveals some irregularities in the correspondance between the TS_4 results and the PTS results. For example, TS_4 is equal at 2.0 kHz and 16.0 kHz, but PTS is about 8 dB at 2.0 kHz and 0 dB at 16.0 kHz. Also, while PTS at 2.0 kHz and at 8.0 kHz is nearly equal (within 1 dB), TS_4 was 52 dB at 8.0 kHz but only 25 dB at 2.0 kHz. Apparently at test frequencies remote from the frequency region encompassed by the exposure noise, predictions of TS_4 from PTS or predictions of PTS from TS_4 could err significantly. Between 60 and 150 days postexposure thresholds improved for test tones from 1.0 to 16.0 kHz, but remained es-

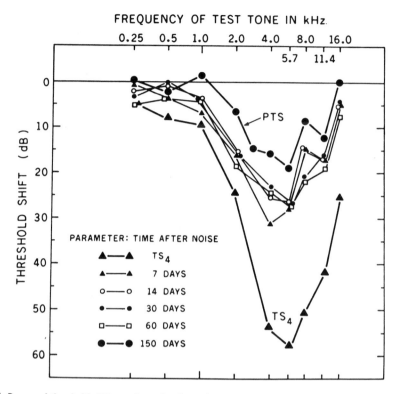

FIG. 4. Decay of threshold shifts as shown by the audiogram after exposure for 90 days to an octave-band noise with a center frequency of 4.0 kHz. The parameter is the time after cessation of the exposure.

sentially unchanged at 0.25 and 0.5 kHz. Since the unexpected improvement in thresholds between 60 and 150 days did not occur at all test frequencies, it may reflect additional repair of the inner ear rather than just measurement error.

As can be ascertained from Fig. 3, Fig. 4, and previous results (6), a 90-day exposure at 80 dB produced a PTS of about 20 dB at 5.7 kHz, whereas a 2-day or 9-day exposure at 80 dB did not produce PTSs. In different words, while TS_4 may have increased from about 53 dB to about 58 dB at durations greater than 9 days, PTSs increased from 0 dB to 20 dB. Thus, the preliminary indication may be that a tenfold increase in duration produces a 20-dB increase in PTS. Additional data are needed, of course, to specify this relation.

ANALYSIS

Growth and Decay of Threshold Shifts

For durations up to 9 days the present results are consistent with earlier results in several respects. From 1 to 9 days TS_4 remains constant or nearly so; the magnitude of TS_4 at 5.7 kHz is very close to that predicted by the equation.

$$TS_4 = 1.7 \ (SPL - A)$$

where $A = 47.0$ (6); and TS_{4-11} is maximal in and slightly above the frequency region encompassed by the noise.

The results observed when the duration is extended from 9 to 90 days are difficult to interpret. On the one hand, the results were obtained from only 4 animals, and an increase in threshold shifts as small as 5 dB approaches the precision of measurement. On the other hand, the fact that the increase in threshold shifts between 15 and 90 days of exposure occurred very systematically at some test frequencies, but not at others, suggests that the increase may be more than just measurement error. In light of this equivocal result several hypotheses about the growth of TS_{4-11} will be considered in the following section.

With 1 exception the decay of threshold shifts after the 90-day exposure at 80 dB is consistent with the decay of threshold shifts after 9-day exposures where the levels were 86, 92, or 98 dB and where PTSs of 10–40 dB were produced (6). The exception, as stated earlier, is the improvement in thresholds between 60 and 150 days of recovery. This result is difficult to interpret, given results for chinchilla which show no improvement in thresholds between 15 and 90 days of recovery (6), and results for cat which show no improvement in thresholds between 56 and 84 days (12). In these other studies, however, the duration of the exposure was never more than 9 days in the case of chinchilla and usually was only a few hours or a few minutes in the case of cat. The present results, therefore, can be interpreted in at least 3 ways. One is that the repair of the inner ear can occur for as long as 150 days after the exposure. A second way is that repair of the inner ear after a 90-day exposure occurs over longer periods of time than the repair of the inner ear after exposures of a few hours or a few days. A third way is that the improvements in auditory sensitivity between 15 and 150 days of recovery represent nothing more than measurement error. Of course, one may wish to temper this third interpretation in light of the fact that the improvements did not occur at all test frequencies.

Relations Between TS_4 and Permanent Threshold Shifts

An old issue in the study of noise-induced hearing loss is the relation or correlation between TTS and PTS. In the context of the present paper the concern is with the relation between TS_4, that is threshold shifts measured at a postexposure time of 4 min, and PTS, that is, threshold shifts measured at a postexposure time of 15–150 days. To look at possible relations between TS_4 and PTS it is necessary to specify the growth curve for TS_4 and the growth curve for PTS. This is not a simple task. The present data show that there are uncertainties regarding the growth of TS_4, and there are so few data from which to estimate the growth of PTS. Accordingly, we proceed to develop hypothetical growth curves for both TS_4 and PTS. These hypothetical growth curves must not be regarded as scientific fact. They should be regarded as limiting cases in some instances and as realistic possibilities in others. Indeed, the forte of these hypothetical growth curves may not prove to be their quantitative accuracy, but rather their value in the design of future experiments and in conceptualizing certain aspects of the problem of noise-induced hearing loss.

Three possible hypothetical growth curves for TS_4 are shown in Fig. 5 (solid lines) where the noise is an octave band centered at 4.0 kHz, its level is 80 dB SPL, and the frequency of the test tone is 5.7 kHz. The first hypothetical possibility is labeled $ATS_{(1)}$ and represents the situation described earlier. That is, TS_4 reaches an asymptote after 24 hr of exposure and the asymptote is sustained indefinitely. The second possibility, labeled $ATS_{(2)}$, is that TS_4 reaches a plateau after 24 hr of exposure, the plateau is sustained for about 5–30 days, and then TS_4 increases at a rate of about 0.05 dB/day. After about 1,000 days of exposure, TS_4 reaches an asymptote, $ATS_{(2)}$. This asymptote is equal to and determined by the masked threshold of a 5.7 kHz tone, where the spectrum and level of the masker is identical to the spectrum and level of the exposure noise. Thus, the threshold of a tone *in the presence* of a noise of fixed level and spectrum (masked threshold of TS_0) is an upper bound on the threshold shift (TS_4) that can be produced by that noise. Moreover, it is assumed that if the masked threshold or TS_0 can be indefinitely, then $ATS_{(2)}$ can be sustained indefinitely also. The third possibility is that TS_4 does not reach an asymptote, but increases without bound as the exposure is continued. This hypothetical possibility, labeled TS_4 nonasymptotic on Fig. 5, has ominous implications. It suggests that after 300 to 1,000 days of continuous exposure to noise, both the masked threshold (TS_0) and TS_4 increase without bound. An increase in the masked threshold without an increase in the level of the noise suggests that the integrity of the organ of Corti and sensory cells is not maintained, and the inner ear is in a state of "disintegration" either at selected regions of the cochlea or perhaps along its entire growth. In summary, the solid lines of Fig. 5 indicate that there are at least 3 limiting conditions for the growth of TS_4—a true asymptote which is reached after 24 hr of exposure, a true asymptote which is reached after years of exposure and which is equal to the masked threshold, and unlimited growth of TS_4. Which of the possibilities, if any, is correct can only be determined by conducting a lengthy animal investigation.

Developing hypothetical possibilities for the growth of PTS may be somewhat presumptuous, given the few PTS data available and given the uncertainties regarding the growth of TS_4. Nevertheless, several logical possibilities emerge from the 3 limiting cases developed for TS_4.

The hypothetical possibilities for the growth of PTSs (dotted lines) are

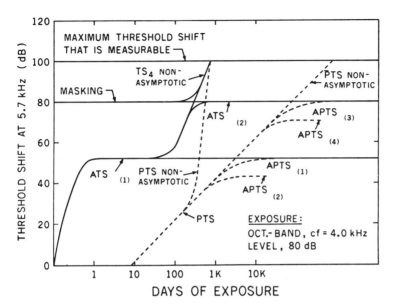

FIG. 5. Hypothetical possibilities for the growth of threshold shifts measured at a postexposure time of 4 min (*solid lines*), and hypothetical possibilities for the growth of threshold shifts measured at a post-exposure time of 150 days (PTS, *dotted lines*).

given in Fig. 5. The first possibility is that PTSs increase without bound as the duration of exposure is increased. The increase in PTS is plotted in accordance with the suggested finding that PTS increases 20 dB for every decade increase in duration of exposure. This first hypothetical possibility is used here as a stepping stone to other hypothetical possibilities where the growth of PTS is dependent upon the growth of TS_4.

The second and third possibilities for the growth of PTSs are dependent upon the existence of $ATS_{(1)}$. That is, ATS must reach a true asymptote, $ATS_{(1)}$, which becomes an upper bound on the PTS. Thus, as an exposure is increased beyond 9 days, PTSs increase and then reach an asymptote. The magnitude of the PTS asymptote may be equal to or is determined by the magnitude of $ATS_{(1)}$. This possibility is called $APTS_{(1)}$. If, after termination of the exposure, a constant amount of recovery occurs at postexposure times greater than 4 min, then an APTS will be produced that is always less than $ATS_{(1)}$. This possibility is labeled $APTS_{(2)}$ in Fig. 5. The existence of $APTS_{(1)}$ or $APTS_{(2)}$ depends upon the existence of $ATS_{(1)}$ as well as upon mechanisms common to both TS_4 and PTS.

The next 2 possibilities for PTS, labeled $APTS_{(3)}$ and $APTS_{(4)}$ in Fig. 5, are dependent upon the existence of $ATS_{(2)}$. As stated earlier $ATS_{(2)}$ is determined by the threshold of the tone in the presence of the noise (TS_0). Thus, TS_0 forms an upper bound on PTS as well as on TS_4. Note from Fig. 5 that PTS increases and then reaches an asymptote, $APTS_{(3)}$. The magnitude of $APTS_{(3)}$ is equal to the magnitude of TS_0 (masking) and $ATS_{(2)}$. If, after termination of the exposure, a constant amount of recovery occurs at post-exposure times greater than 4 min, then a PTS asymptote will be formed, $APTS_{(4)}$, that is always smaller than $APTS_{(3)}$, $ATS_{(2)}$, or TS_0. The existence of $APTS_{(3)}$ or $APTS_{(4)}$ depends upon $ATS_{(2)}$, the assumption that the masked threshold remains constant as a function of time, and that there are mechanisms common to TS, PTS, and masking. Of course, as Fig. 5 has been constructed, the duration required to produce $APTS_{(3)}$ or $APTS_{(4)}$ eliminates any application to practical situations.

The last possibility to be discussed for the growth of PTS is related directly to the notion that TS_4 is nonasymptotic, and that, after 300 to 1,000 days of exposure, both TS_4 and TS_0 (masking) increase rapidly. As stated earlier, an increase in masking without an increase in the level of the noise is an indication that the organ of Corti and sensory cells are in a stage of "disintegration." Thus, in Fig. 5 PTS increases gradually, and then between 300 and 1,000 days of exposure PTS increases more rapidly to converge on nonasymptotic values for TS_0 and TS_4. The extent of the increase in PTS depends upon the extent to which the structures involved in TS_0 and TS_4 repair themselves after termination of the exposure. In Fig. 5, it has been assumed that very little, if any, repair occurs.

Again it may be desirable to state that Fig. 5 and its discussion are speculation—nothing more, nothing less. They should be used principally to assist in the design and evaluation of future animal studies wherein the exposures last for months and years. Indeed, it is difficult to imagine the development of the quantitative facts of noise-induced hearing loss and the specification of the relations between TTS and PTS in the absence of definitive data from long-exposure studies with animals.

ACKNOWLEDGMENTS

This research was supported by Program Project Grant NS03856 from the National Institute of Neurological Diseases and Stroke, U.S. Public Health Service, Department of Health, Education and Welfare to the Central Institute for the Deaf.

This study was part of a series of studies in a research program on the effects of noise under the supervision of Drs. James D. Miller and D. H. Eldredge. Ms. Seija A. Talo assisted in the data collection and training of animals. Surgery was supervised by Dr. Eldredge.

REFERENCES

1. Peters, E. (1965): Temporary shifts in auditory thresholds of chinchilla after exposure to noise, *J. Acoust. Soc. Am.* 37:831–833.
2. Miller, J. D., Rothenberg, S. J., and Eldredge, D. H. (1971): Preliminary observations on the effects of exposure to noise for seven days on the hearing and inner ear of the chinchilla. *J. Acoust. Soc. Am.*, 50:1199–1203.

3. Carder, H. M., and Miller, J. D. (1971): Temporary threshold shifts produced by noise exposure of long duration. *Trans. Am. Acad. Opthalmol. Otolaryngol.*, Nov.–Dec.:1346–1354.
4. Carder, H. M., and Miller, J. D. (1972): Temporary threshold shifts (TTS) produced by noise exposures of long durations. *J. Speech Hear. Res.*, 15:603–623.
5. Mills, J. H., and Talo, S. A. (1972): Temporary threshold shifts produced by exposure to high-frequency noise. *J. Speech Hear. Res.*, 15:624–630.
6. Mills, J. H. (1973): Temporary threshold shifts produced by nine-day exposures to noise. *J. Speech Hear. Res.*, 16:426–438.
7. Mills, J. H., Talo, S. A., and Gordon, G. S. (1973): Decay of temporary threshold shifts in noise. *J. Speech Hear. Res.*, 16:267–270.
8. Mills, J. H. (1973): Threshold shifts produced by exposure to noise in chinchillas with noise-induced hearing losses. *J. Speech Hear. Res.*, 16:700–708.
9. Eldredge, D. H., Miller, J. D., Mills, J. H., and Bohne, B. A. (1973): Behavioral physiological and anatomical studies of hearing loss in animals: Relations to human data. *Proc. Int. Cong. Noise Public Health Problem.* EPA Doc. 550/9-73-008, 237–256.
10. Miller, J. D. (1970): Audibility curve of the chinchilla. *J. Acoust. Soc. Am.*, 48:513–523.
11. Mills, J. H., Gengel, R. W., Watson, C. S., and Miller, J. D. (1970): Temporary changes of the auditory system due to exposure to noise for one or two days. *J. Acoust. Soc. Am.*, 48:524–530.
12. Miller, J. D., Watson, C., and Covell, W. (1963): Deafening effects of noise on the cat. *Acta Otolaryngol. [Suppl.] (Stockh.),* 176:91.

DISCUSSION

D. Moody: I'd like to comment on a 90-day exposure that we did in monkeys, to 90 dB noise. We, also, saw the animals reach an asymptote in about 12 hr for the 90 dB noise; about a 20 dB asymptote; after 15 days we started to see some variability in the threshold, and at 20 days the animals increased their plateau or asymptote (this is what we decided to call it) by about 10 more dB.

J. Mills: As I recall that data, there's a slight increase after a few days that puttered around, but my recollection was that there was roughly a 10-dB increment, and that you were using a 10-dB step attenuation to measure it.

D. Moody: After about 70 days we switched to a 5-dB step attenuation. It made perhaps 1–2 dB difference in mean threshold, and increased the variability somewhat.

Effects of Noise on Hearing, edited by Donald Henderson,
Roger P. Hamernik, Darshan S. Dosanjh, and John H. Mills.
Raven Press, New York © 1976

Human Asymptotic Threshold Shift

William Melnick

Department of Otolaryngology, Ohio State University, Columbus, Ohio 43210

Ethical consideration and the need for procedures which are unpleasant
have limited the experimental conditions available for investigating the effects of prolonged noise exposure on human subjects. Noise levels have been
restricted to those which would produce threshold shifts not exceeding 30–40
dB. Conditions producing threshold shifts greater than 40 dB have been
assumed to be hazardous and capable of causing permanent hearing loss.
Up until the 1970s, investigations of threshold shifts with human subjects
had been limited to durations of 8 hr or less. The experiments of Carder and
Miller (1) and of Mills et al. (2) prompted a renewed interest in the effects
of exposure durations longer than 8 hr on threshold shifts. The military were
particularly interested in these experiments because of the unusual environments encountered in prolonged missions involving submarines, aircraft, and
spacecraft.

The number of investigations using human subjects has increased over the
past 5 years. Duration of noise exposure for the most part has been limited
to 24–48 hr. Few, if any, experiments have used noises which lasted for the
extended periods endured by chinchillas, periods of up to 21 days (1). Ac-
quisition of human subjects for experiments using noise exposures lasting
more than a day or two would be difficult, and extremely expensive. The
experiments described in this review, therefore, have limited exposure durations from 16 to 48 hours (2–10). These experiments of prolonged noise
exposure with human subjects have indicated, without exception, that threshold shift will plateau if the noise exposure is of sufficient duration. The
experiment of Mills et al. (2), in which Mills was exposed to an octave band
of noise centered at 500 Hz for 48 hr at 81.5 dB SPL, and for 29.5 hr at
92.5 dB SPL, indicated that an asymptotic level of threshold shift (ATS)
was achieved sometime between 8 and 16 hr of exposure. Melnick (4), in a
study which exposed adult male subjects continuously for 16 hr to an octave
band of noise 300–600 Hz at octave-band levels 80–95 dB, concluded that
the 16-hr duration was not long enough to establish firmly that an asymptote
in threshold shift had been reached. A subsequent experiment, which extended
the exposure period to the same octave band of noise at 90 dB for 24 hr (6),
indicated that the asymptotic levels were reached by 12 hr of exposure.

Johnson et al. (3), in an experiment which used 2 exposure periods (24 and 48 hr) to a pink noise measured at 85 dB(A), provided evidence that the asymptote occurred after noise durations of 8–16 hr. Ward (9), in an experiment which exposed 10 normal-hearing college students to an octave band of noise centered at 4 kHz for as long as 24 hr, summarized that the asymptote was always reached in the period between 8 and 12 hr. In graphs showing threshold shifts for his group of subjects, Ward showed that, with a noise level of 75 dB SPL, his subjects apparently achieved asymptote after only 2 hr of exposure. When the octave band level was shifted to 80 dB, the asymptote was reached by 4 hr of exposure, and, in an abbreviated experiment using an 85-dB exposure level, Ward's data indicated that the asymptote may or may not have been reached by 8 hr. Data available thus far vary from experiment to experiment, but asymptotic threshold levels were

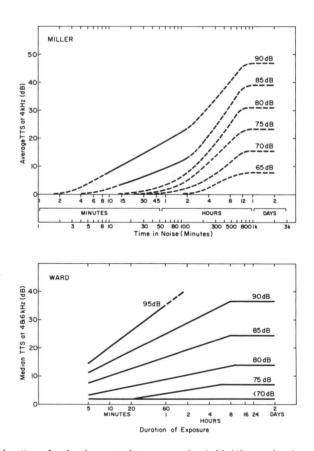

FIG. 1. Proposed patterns for development of temporary threshold shift as a function of exposure level and duration. The top graph is an adaptation of curves proposed by Miller (10) for TTS$_2$ at 4 kHz when the noise is an octave band centered at 4 kHz. The bottom graph is an adaptation of similar growth curves for TTS averaged 4 and 6 kHz proposed by Ward (9).

definitely observed in human subjects if noise exposures were of sufficient duration. Although there are individual variations, it is probable that threshold shift for the average human subject will plateau between 8 and 12 hr of exposure.

GROWTH PATTERN

Data from human experiments thus far have led to at least 2 postulated growth patterns for temporary threshold shift (TTS). These 2 patterns of development are indicated in Fig. 1. The top graph is an adaptation of Miller's (10) hypothetical growth curves for TTS_2 at 4 kHz as a function of the level of an octave band of noise centered at 4 kHz. This adaptation of Miller's curves shows only those conditions which have been used with humans. The bottom graph shows an idealized set of curves that have been proposed by Ward (9). These curves differ in several aspects; however, for the time being, we shall concentrate merely on the pattern of TTS development up to the point of the asymptote. Miller's curves indicate a triphasic growth pattern with a very slow rate during the early portions of the prolonged exposure, a time period of rapid development, and finally, a plateau. Miller's contours suggest that this triphasic growth pattern is particularly noticeable at very low levels of exposure, and that as the level

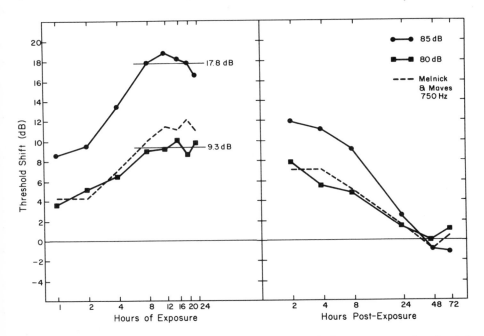

FIG. 2. Growth and recovery curves for 9 subjects for 4 kHz as a result of exposure to an octave band of noise centered at 4 kHz for 24 hr at 80 and 85 dB. These data are indicated by the solid lines and filled squares (80 dB) and filled circles (85 dB). Similar data for 10 men are shown for 750 Hz resulting from a 24-hr exposure to a 300–600 Hz octave band of noise at 90 dB [Melnick and Maves (6)].

of the noise increases, the duration of the early slow phase decreases until, at noise levels of 85 dB, it is difficult to detect any slow component. Ward's set of curves suggests a simple exponential growth of TTS. He proposes that during the rapid growth phase, TTS increases linearly with log time. This is a familiar proposal which was developed earlier from investigations which used shorter noise durations and higher exposure levels. Ward rightly points out that the triphasic nature of the low-level curves proposed by Miller were chiefly the result of an experiment on 1 human subject, that of Mills (2). However, data from subsequent experiments also indicate a slow component in TTS growth curves. Figure 2 shows the growth and recovery data from 24-hr exposures to 300–600 Hz, reported by Melnick and Maves (6), and 24-hr exposures to an octave band of noise centered at 4 kHz at 80 and 85 dB, reported by Melnick (5). Threshold shift here was measured at 750 Hz for the low-frequency exposure and at 4 kHz for the high-frequency noise. As can be seen from the growth curves in the left-hand figure, in these experiments there was a slow growth phase of TTS over the first 2 hr of exposure, then a rapid growth period for 4–8 hr, and a subsequent leveling off at the asymptote. Ward (9) himself, in displaying data from earlier 8-hr noise exposures to a 4 kHz noise, indicated a slow growth phase between 1 and 2 hr of exposure, and then a rise in growth rate. If data concerning longer exposures can be applied to these 8-hr exposures, we would then expect to see an asymptotic level a short while after 8 hr. Results from other experiments, including those of Mosko et al. (7) and Johnson et al. (3), do not show an early slow component and would support a simple exponential growth pattern for TTS.

RELATIONSHIP OF MAGNITUDES OF ATS TO EXPOSURE LEVEL

One of the results of the experiments with chinchillas, Carder and Miller (1), Mills and Tallo (11), and Mills (12), indicates that the magnitudes of ATS in the frequency region of maximum effect can be described by the equation: $ATS = 1.6 \times (OBL - C)$. The substracted constant C depends on the spectrum of the noise exposure and on the species of the subject. It is a lower level for high-frequency noise and seems to be less for chinchillas than for man (13). The growth rate of 1.6 dB for every decibel increase in level of noise seems also to hold for man. Figure 3 shows an adaption of Miller's (10) hypothetical curves and data from experiments by Ward (9) and by Melnick (5), which used similar experimental conditions. The data actually observed in the experiments by Ward and by Melnick fit a linear function with a slope of 1.6 rather well. The hypothetical functions of Ward (9) indicated in Fig. 1 would lead to the belief that the growth rate with the level of noise is not constant, but would increase as the level of the exposure noise increases. It certainly would be fortuitous for prediction if there were a single growth rate, but there are not sufficient data available to provide a definitive description. As a matter of fact, in Melnick's (4) earlier experiments using 16 hr of exposure to a 300–600 Hz octave band of noise, the slope of the growth function observed with increase in exposure level varied from approximately 1.0 at 750 Hz to 1.3 at 1,500 Hz.

Nixon et al. (8) report data that would show a growth factor of 0.6, rather than 1.6, per decibel of increase in the noise-exposure level. Their data were gathered using a ⅓ octave band of noise centered at 1,000 Hz and noise levels of 80, 85, and 90 dBA. Their growth factor was determined for an average of the TTS developed at 3 test frequencies, 1,000, 1,500, and 2,000 Hz, rather than simply at the frequency which showed peak ATS. This may account for the relatively small growth rate reported by these investigators. The predictive equation was developed to account for the magnitude of ATS at the maximally affected frequencies, and not for all frequencies which show any threshold shift. There is no reason to believe that the growth of TTS at the fringe frequencies would show the same growth rate as that observed for those frequencies which were maximally affected. In any case, there is ample indication of variability in the relationship of peak ATS to the exposure level. The present state of knowledge does not

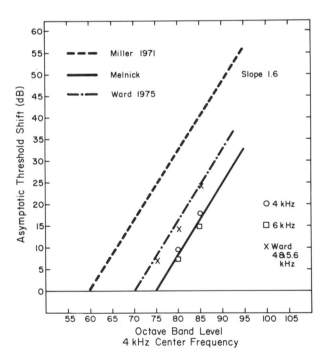

FIG. 3. Growth of ATS as a function of exposure level of maximally affected frequencies. The dotted line represents an adaptation from the hypothetical curves of Miller (10) for 4 kHz. The slope of all 3 lines is 1.6. The data of Ward (9) are represented by the symbol X. The data of Melnick are plotted as open circles for 4 kHz and open squares for 6 kHz.

warrant using any particular growth rate in prediction of the minimum exposure level which will produce any TTS.

Examination of Fig. 3 shows that the magnitude of ATS at 4 kHz, predicted by Miller's hypothetical functions (10), is much greater than that which was actually measured in experiments by Melnick (5) and Ward (9). The discrepancies amount to ~20 dB. Miller would predict that threshold shift begins to occur when an octave band of noise centered at 4 kHz is ~60 dB. Our data would indicate that threshold shifts would begin at 75 dB, while Ward's data are closer to 70 dB than 75 dB. At first, the reason postulated for the discrepancy between Miller's predictions and our own data was the sample of subjects which we used in our experiments. These were adult males in their third, fourth, and fifth decades, and we speculated that perhaps these subjects came from the resistant, less susceptible portion of the overall human population. However, data gathered independently by Ward using a different group of subjects, namely, that of young college students, indicate closer agreement to the results which we obtained than those predicted by Miller. It may be that the discrepancy between Ward's data and our own could be attributed to susceptibility differences of the subjects, but it is now doubtful that this factor could be solely responsible for the difference between the hypothetical amplitudes of ATS of Miller and those which we have observed.

FREQUENCY EFFECT

The dependence of threshold shift at various frequencies on the spectrum of the exposure noise, or the fatiguing noise, is similar to that observed with shorter exposure durations. Figure 4 contrasts the effects of a low-frequency octave band 300–600 Hz exposure (4) and an exposure to an octave band centered at 4 kHz (5). When frequency is plotted in the usual log fashion, the low-frequency exposure seems to have a broader frequency effect than the 4-kHz noise. For the 300–600 Hz octave band, significant threshold shift was observed at 500, 750, and 1,000 Hz, with insignificant threshold shifts at other frequencies. Threshold shifts observed with the 4-kHz noise seemed to be sharply restricted to the frequencies 4 and 6 kHz, with some noticeable threshold shift at 3 and 8 kHz, and no significant change for the other test frequencies. Mills (2) showed a greater spread to higher frequencies when he was exposed to an octave band of noise centered at 500 Hz. Significant threshold shifts were observed at 1,500, 2,000, and 3,000 Hz in that experiment. Nixon et al. (8), using a ⅓ octave band centered at 1,000 Hz, showed maximum threshold shift at 1,500 Hz, with noticeable significant threshold shifts at 1,000 nd 2,000 Hz, and little or no change in threshold at 500, 4,000, and 8,000 Hz. Ward (9) reported from his experiments using an octave band centered at 4 kHz that the maximum effect occurred at 4

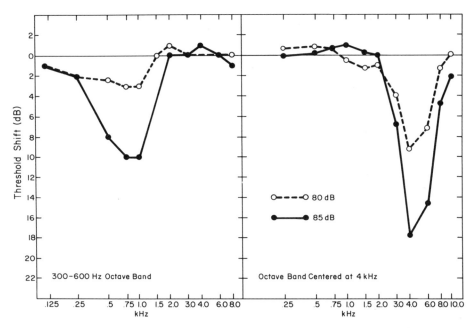

FIG. 4. Frequency dependence of threshold shift on spectrum of noise. The left graph displays ATS for 16-hr exposures to a 300–600 Hz band of noise at 80 and 85 dB (Melnick (4)). The right graph shows ATS from 24-hr exposures to an octave band centered at 4 kHz at similar octave-band levels.

and 5.6 kHz, with equal amounts of threshold shift at each of those test frequencies.

Mosko et al. (7) and Johnson et al. (3) used broadband exposure noises. Johnson and his colleagues used a pink noise at 85 dB(A). The pink noise had equal sound pressure levels in the octave bands from 125 to 4,000 Hz. Threshold shifts measured at 24 hr of exposure in that experiment are shown in Fig. 5. Peak threshold shifts were observed at 3, 4, and 6 kHz, while at the test frequencies 0.5, 1, and 2 kHz, the magnitude of threshold shift was 5 dB or less.

The noise used by Mosko et al. (7) was constructed to approximate that produced by armored vehicles in the military. Essentially, that noise was flat at frequencies 250 Hz and below, and decreased by 10 dB per octave for the higher frequencies. As a result of their 48-hr exposure to that noise, the 17 male subjects showed a maximum threshold shift of 15 dB at 2,000 Hz and 13 dB at 500 Hz. At the test frequencies of 4, 8, 12, and 16 kHz, there was threshold shift of 5–8 dB. The usually reported maximum effect at the frequencies 4,000 and 6,000 Hz in industrial and military noises probably results from the fact that the spectra of these environmental noises are broadband and relatively flat, much like that used by Johnson et al. (3), and not

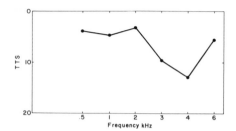

FIG. 5. TTS measured following 24-hr exposure to pink noise at 85 dB(A) [Johnson et al. (3)].

because of some peculiar susceptibility of cochlear elements responsible for detection of these frequencies.

RECOVERY FROM ATS

Almost unanimously, the human studies that have used exposure times of sufficient duration to develop ATS have shown delayed recovery patterns. Mills et al. (2) reported a recovery period of 3–6 days for the relatively small levels of threshold shift produced in their experiments. In the experiments conducted in our laboratory, both with the 300–600 Hz noise exposure (6) and the exposure noise centered at 4 kHz (5), prolonged recovery times requiring 1–2 days for complete recovery to preexposure threshold levels were revealed. The graph showing recovery in Fig. 4 illustrates the prolonged recovery time. This was the case even though the magnitude of threshold shifts at some frequencies was less than 5 dB.

Nixon et al. (8) and Mosko et al. (7) indicate a rapid recovery phase somewhere between 2 and 30 min postexposure, then a leveling off up to 8 hr postexposure, and finally a fairly rapid recovery phase from 8 to 24 hr postexposure. Miller's hypothetical recovery curves would indicate a relatively flat recovery function (10) from 2 min postexposure until approximately 4–8 hr of exposure, then a rapid decline thereafter to either preexposure levels or to levels of permanent hearing loss. Mills (2) did not show a rapid recovery in threshold shift at 750 Hz within the first hour of his recovery period. His data would more nearly approximate those represented by Miller. Ward (9) also showed a delay in his recovery function following 24-hr exposure to noise centered at 4 kHz. His subjects, exposed to 75 and 80 dB, completely recovered by 16 hr postexposure. It was only in his abbreviated experiment using an 85-dB exposure level that the subjects required as much as 24 hr to complete the recovery. The prolonged exposure experiments with humans, as well as laboratory animal experiments, support the observation that recovery not only depends on magnitude of threshold shift, but also depends upon how that threshold shift was developed. Duration of exposure is undoubtedly an important variable in the production of TTS, and probably is equally important in the development of permanent hearing loss.

INFLUENCE OF DURATION AT ASYMPTOTE ON RECOVERY

Mills (11), in his study with chinchillas, reported that the recovery pattern was clearly dependent on duration of the exposure when the ATS was 55 dB or greater. However, Carder and Miller (1) reported earlier that when the ATS was 30 dB or less, there was no difference in recovery pattern when the exposure periods varied from 2 to 21 days. Johnson et al. (3) were particularly concerned with this observation. These investigators were curious about whether Carder and Miller's observation would hold with human subjects. Therefore, 12 subjects were exposed for 24 and 48 hr to a pink noise at 85 dBA. The results of this study are shown in Fig. 6. Their subjects

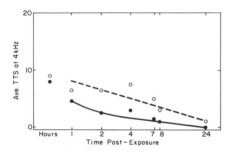

FIG. 6. Recovery of sensitivity at 4 kHz measured as threshold shifts at selected times following 24-hr (filled circles) and 48-hr (open circles) exposure to pink noise at 85 dB(A). [adapted from Johnson et al. (3).]

showed a significantly longer recovery time following the 48-hr exposure than was observed following the 24-hr period. This difference persisted over 24 hr of recovery time. These data would not support the hypothesis of Carder and Miller that the ATS probably represents an equilibrium between fatiguing and restorative processes.

PROCEDURE ARTIFACT

Nixon et al. (8) were concerned that the procedures of previous experiments, which had interruptions of the continuous noise exposure for various times during the 24-hr exposure period, would lead to a reduction in the magnitude measured for ATS. Nixon and his coworkers investigated the effects of measuring threshold shifts in 1 group of subjects following 8, 16, and 24 hr of exposure to a ⅓ octave band of noise centered at 1 kHz, while a smaller group of subjects was measured solely following the completion of the 24-hr exposure period. Those subjects involved in the uninterrupted exposure period showed greater threshold shift by 8 dB. Unfortunately, this group of subjects had better preexposure hearing levels than the group that was involved in the interrupted condition. When the experimenters compared a group of subjects in the interrupted condition with similar hearing levels to those in the uninterrupted condition, the differences in threshold shift became insignificant. The answer to the question of whether the interruption for measuring threshold is a significant procedural artifact, especially following the prolonged exposure periods, remains for a future experiment which eliminates the confounding variables of preexposure hearing levels.

INTERSUBJECT VARIABILITY

A hallmark of all threshold shift experiments with human subjects has been the considerable variance among subjects in the susceptibility to the effects of noise exposure. The data reported from the animal experiments would lead one to believe that there is considerable stability in the measures of ATS. The data from the human experiments would indicate the contrary. Without exception, in the experiments which used prolonged noise exposures in human subjects, there was considerable intersubject variability. Figure 7 shows standard deviations measured at various times during and following the exposure, exemplifying this variability. These data came from a 24-hr exposure of 9 men to an octave band centered at 4 kHz at the octave-band levels 80 and 85 dB. With the 85 dB noise, there was an increase in intersubject variability as the duration of exposure increased up to 24 hr. The standard deviation at 1 hr was ~7 dB, while at the 24-hr measurement the standard deviation was increased to 10 dB. As the recovery progressed, the magnitude of intersubject variance decreased with the standard deviation, finally approximating intrasubject variation of about 2 dB at 72 hr postexposure.

Another example of subject variability is indicated in Fig. 8. Individual data points for each of 9 subjects which were exposed to an octave band centered at 4 kHz at 85 dB are displayed. There were some subjects who

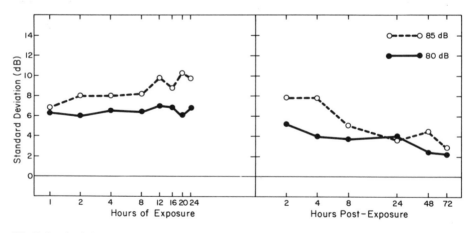

FIG. 7. Standard deviation of threshold shifts for 9 men at 4 kHz following 24-hr exposure to an octave band centered at 4 kHz at 80 (filled circles) and 85 (open circles) dB.

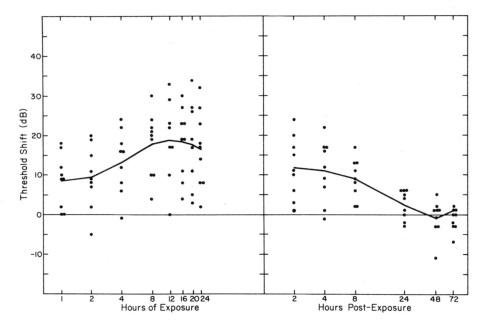

FIG. 8. Individual data points for 9 men showing threshold shifts at 4 kHz resulting from exposure to an octave band of noise centered at 4 kHz. The line represents the mean.

showed less than 5 dB of threshold change at 4 kHz during the entire 24-hr exposure period. One of these subjects showed absolutely no change at all. On the other hand, another subject showed as much as 35 dB from exposure to this same noise. The recovery period showed reduction in variance as the postexposure time increases, but still there was considerable variability. These observations cannot be considered atypical, and are probably representative of the findings of other investigators who have been involved in similar studies.

SUMMARY

The following points summarize the findings of investigations of prolonged continuous noise exposures using human subjects:

1. These experiments indicate that ATS is observed for moderate levels of exposure to continuous noise.

2. Although there is considerable individual variability, on an average the ATS is reached between 8 and 12 hr.

3. The recovery from levels of ATS 30 dB or less is prolonged when compared with recovery from similar magnitudes of threshold shift produced by short-term, high-level exposure. Often, recovery is not complete to pre-exposure levels prior to 24 hr of recovery.

4. Most of the experiments indicate that after some threshold noise level has been exceeded, TTS will grow at a rate greater than dB per dB, as the noise level is increased. Many of the available data indicate an approximate growth rate of 1.6 dB per dB exposure level.

5. The minimum noise level effective in producing threshold shift varies with frequency.

6. The magnitude of threshold shift and the frequencies affected by a given noise depends upon the noise spectrum. Generally, when the energy of the exposure noise is concentrated in the low frequencies, it has a broader effect on the test frequencies than when the energy is concentrated in a high-frequency band.

7. Exponential growth and recovery patterns from prolonged continuous noise exposure represent good first approximations to the observed data.

8. The inter- and intrasubject variability previously reported for short-term TTS experiments continues to be a common finding with prolonged noise exposure.

REFERENCES

1. Carder, H. M., and Miller, J. D. (1972): Temporary threshold shifts from prolonged exposure to noise. *J. Speech Hear. Res.*, 15:603–623.
2. Mills, J. H., Gengel, R. W., Watson, C. S., and Miller, J. D. (1970): Temporary changes of the auditory system due to exposure to noise for one or two days. *J. Acoust. Soc. Am.*, 48:524–530.
3. Johnson, D. L., Nixon, C. W., and Stephenson, M. R. (1975): Asymptotic behavior of temporary threshold shift during exposure to long duration noises. Aerospace Medical Specialists Meeting, Advisory Group for Aerospace Research and Development (AGARD), North Atlantic Treaty Organization (NATO), Toronto, Canada.
4. Melnick, W. (1974): Human temporary threshold shift from 16-hour noise exposures. *Arch. Otolaryngol.*, 100:180–190.
5. Melnick, W. (1975): TTS in man from a 24-hour exposure to an octave band of noise centered at 4 kHz. Aerospace Medical Specialists Meeting, Advisory Group for Aerospace Research and Development (AGARD), North Atlantic Treaty Organization (NATO), Toronto, Canada.
6. Melnick, W., and Maves, M. (1974): Asymptotic threshold shift (ATS) in man from 24-hour exposure to continuous noise. *Ann. Otol. Rhinol. Laryngol.*, 83:820–829.
7. Mosko, J. D., Fletcher, J. L., and Luz, G. A. (1970): Growth and recovery of temporary threshold shifts following extended exposure to high level, continuous noise. U.S. Army Medical Research Laboratory, Ft. Knox, Kentucky, Report 911.
8. Nixon, C. W., Krantz, D. W., and Johnson, D. L. (1975): Human temporary threshold shift and recovery from 24-hour acoustic exposures. Aerospace Medical Research Laboratory, Wright-Patterson AFB, Ohio, Report AMRL-TR-74.101.
9. Ward, W. D. (1975): Studies of asymptotic TTS. Aerospace Medical Specialists Meeting, Advisory Group for Aerospace Research and Development (AGARD), North Atlantic Treaty Organization (NATO), Toronto, Canada.
10. Miller, J. D. (1971): Effects of noise on people. U.S. Environmental Protection Agency, NTID, 300.7, 16–24.
11. Mills, J. H., and Talo, S. A. (1972): Temporary threshold shifts produced by exposure to high frequency noise. *J. Speech Hear. Res.*, 15:624–631.
12. Mills, J. H. (1973): Temporary and permanent threshold shifts produced by nine-day exposures to noise. *J. Speech Hear. Res.*, 16:426–438.

13. Mills, J. H. (1973): Further data on the pattern of threshold shift produced by prolonged noise in animals and man. In: *A Basis for Limiting Noise Exposure for Hearing Conservation,* Appendix 12, technical report for Environmental Protection Agency, EPA 550/9–73–001–A, compiled by J. C. Guignard.

DISCUSSION

W. Ward: Bill, on the one slide on which you show both 300–600 and 4,000 Hz, you have the legend 80–85; that wasn't the case for the 300–600, was it?

W. Melnick: No, that is true, the 300–600 was strictly 90 dB. As a matter of fact, when you adjust for preexposure difference, the magnitude of ATS you get from the low-frequency exposure is predictable from the 4 kHz data.

Effects of Noise on Hearing, edited by Donald Henderson,
Roger P. Hamernik, Darshan S. Dosanjh, and John H. Mills.
Raven Press, New York © 1976

The Potentiation of Noise by Other Ototraumatic Agents

Roger P. Hamernik and Donald Henderson

SUNY Upstate Medical Center and Syracuse University, Syracuse, New York 13210

A diversity of ototraumatic agents are known, and their deleterious effects
on hearing are well documented. These agents include not only a variety of
classes of noise, and drugs such as the aminoglycoside antibiotics, the diuretics,
and the analgesics, but also nature's own ototraumatic agent, aging. Hawkins
(1) has made the case that noise, drugs, and aging may produce indistinguishable cochlear pathology and audiological symptoms. However, the pathway to this common set of conditions is undoubtedly different for many of the
ototraumatic agents. The issue to be explored in this paper is: do combinations of drugs and noise, as well as combinations of the different classes of
noise, interact to produce cochlear pathologies and hearing losses? To understand the interaction of the 2 classes of ototraumatic agents, as well as to
gain insight into the basis for an interaction, one should first delineate the
effects of noise and ototoxic drugs.

In the generic sense, excessive noise can injure the cochlea mechanically
and biochemically. The details of various hypothesized mechanisms have been
discussed in some of the previous chapters. Mechanically, the first signs of
acoustic trauma may be a rupture of tight cell junctions of the reticular lamina,
which leads to an alteration in the biochemistry of the spaces of Neul (2), or
a dislocation of various supporting cellular masses, which could change the
mechanical response of the basilar membrane (3). As exposures become
more intense, there can be swelling of the afferent dendrites (4) and buckling
of both sensory and supporting cells. At high levels of exposure, inertial forces
can virtually wrench the organ of Corti from the basilar membrane (5). In
addition to the changes in the organ of Corti, noise is responsible for a general
"sludging" and capillary malfunction throughout the cochlea (6). In fact,
lower level, long-term exposures primarily affect the lateral wall of the cochlea and thus indirectly influence the organ of Corti via biochemical changes.

Mechanical changes are not a primary factor when ototoxic drugs are considered. Drug toxicity, typified by the action of the aminoglycosidic antibiotics, affects nearly all cellular subsets in the cochlea (7). Perhaps the
earliest changes can be seen in the cells and capillaries of the lateral wall and
the stria vascularis, and only after increased dosages are sensory cells lost.
The long-term aftereffects of the aminoglycosidic antibiotics, however, are
virtually indistinguishable from the effects of noise exposure. The effects of

certain drugs differ completely from those of noise, in that they are almost exclusively TTS-producing (ethacrynic acid, salicylates, etc.). Their action is thought to be localized to the secretory cells of the stria vascularis and the capillaries of the lateral wall (8).

In summarizing the ototraumatic effects of drugs and noise, both classes of agents can induce parallel changes in the vascular network of the cochlea. However, noise differs in an important dimension, in that it can mechanically damage the organ of Corti directly. Thus, in combination studies, the individual ototraumatic agents can compete among themselves for a particular site of action and not precipitate a synergistic interaction, or they might focus their effect on 2 separate cochlear processes and possibly set up the potential for a strong interaction.

A number of combination studies can be imagined: noise/noise; noise/drug; and drug/drug. By further including the possible potentiating factor of aging, the diversity of experiments is great. Of particular interest in the area of public health standards are interactions between normally temporary threshold shift (TTS)-producing agents which have the potential to generate a permanent threshold shift (PTS). Considering the variety of interactions, comparatively few studies are available in the literature. The following is a review of most of the available studies which have been directed at the potentiating effects of ototraumatic agents administered in combination. This review does not include in any detail the drug on drug interactions, since these are, for the most part, beyond the scope of this volume.

NOISE AND DRUGS

Ototoxic drugs can be broadly divided into 2 classes: (i) generally TTS-producing; even with excessive dosages, patients, as well as experimental animals, suffer only temporary losses in hearing sensitivity. Whereas individual cases of permanent damage have been reported, the tendency is definitely toward temporary effects only. Drugs in this class include quinine, salicylates, ethacrynic acid, furosemide, etc. Their histological changes are primarily localized to the vascular elements of the lateral wall and to the cells of the stria vascularis. (ii) PTS-producing (e.g., the family of aminoglycoside antibiotics). Dosages necessary for use in clinical treatments can cause permanent changes in hearing thresholds and cochlear sensory cell populations. In the last few years, there have been clinical reports (9–11) and laboratory studies (12,13) showing a synergistic effect within the large family of ototoxic drugs, e.g., patients have developed permanent hearing losses from ethacrynic acid therapy when they were also receiving kanamycin therapy. The issue to be discussed now is: to what extent do the ototoxic drugs interact synergistically with various types of noise exposure, and do such interactions constitute a sufficient hazard to warrant consideration in public health standards?

PTS-PRODUCING DRUGS AND NOISE

A subset of the aminoglycoside antibiotics have been shown to act as a potentiating agent for noise exposure. Gannon and Tso (14) studied the interaction of kanamycin and impulse noise. Guinea pigs were given subcutaneous doses of kanamycin of 15, 50, and 250 mg/kg/day for 21 days. Further, each day a group of animals received 2 impulses in "rapid succession" [intensities were not specified, but can be assumed to be in the range of 140–160-dB peak sound pressure level (SPL)]. The group of animals that received as little as 15 mg/kg/day with the impulses, developed a much larger lesion than either control group. Increasing the dosage still further increased the interaction effect. These results have a general significance since the 15 mg/kg dose is consistent with the recommended clinical dosage of kanamycin. Dayal et al. (15) found a similar interaction in guinea pigs exposed to low-frequency incubator noise (68–72 dB) and a modest ototoxic regimen (either 15, 50, or 100 mg/kg/day for 3–5 weeks). In the animals in all the interaction groups, small, but identifiable, apical hair cell lesions developed, in spite of the relatively benign nature of the treatments. This is a surprising result, because the normal site for the initial signs of the destructive action of kanamycin is in the base of the cochlea, whereas the low-frequency noise should have affected the apical region of the cochlea. It seems reasonable to assume that kanamycin establishes a condition of vulnerability throughout the cochlea, and that permanent changes in hair cell populations can be generated virtually anywhere in the cochlea, depending upon the frequency of the noise exposure. The data of Dayal, however, are somewhat confounded by the "normal" inner and outer hair cell losses usually seen in the apical end of the cochlea of guinea pigs. Jauhiainen et al. (16), using neomycin and octave-band noise, found a potentiating interaction similar to the results of the kanamycin exposure. Neomycin was administered in dosages of 200 mg/kg/day intramuscularly for 7 days, followed by a 70-hr exposure to 115-dB, 8-kHz octave-band noise. Using cochlear microphonics (CM) as an index of the physiological integrity of the cochlea and the surface preparation to quantify hair cell populations, they found that: "The combined effect shows far greater damage than might be expected on the basis of simple addition of the two effects." In the most recent study, Marques et al. (17) studied the temporal aspects of the noise/kanamycin interaction and found that its maximum interaction occurred when the noise exposure was concurrent with the kanamycin treatment. The interaction also occurred, but was less severe, when the cochlea was recovering (from either noise or drugs) and the second agent was introduced. Their measure of cochlear performance was the CM, while irreversible changes in cochlear anatomy were measured using cochleograms. Figure 1 summarizes their results. The median loss in the maximum CM_{RW} voltage for 1 kHz is plotted as a function of the level of the interacting noise.

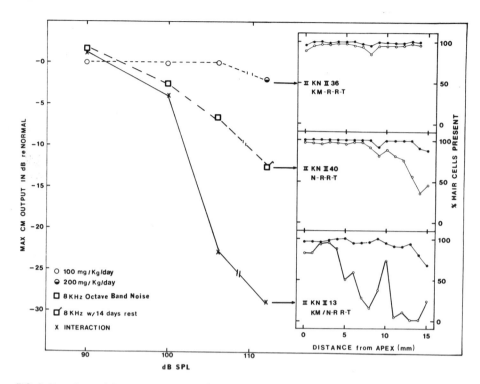

FIG. 1. The effects of the interaction of kanamycin and noise on the round window cochlear microphonics (median data) and cochlear anatomy of the guinea pig. The cochleogram inserts at the right are for 3 individual animals exposed to the most severe paradigm of drug (⬤), noise (☐), and the combination (✕). [Redrawn from Marques et al. (17)].

For the 100 mg/kg dosage, increasing the noise also increases the interaction effect as compared to the noise alone group. The points at the extreme right are based on 250 mg/kg of kanamycin. The inserted cochleograms correspond to the drug, noise, and interaction group, respectively, for the most traumatic paradigm. Together, the CM depression and losses in the hair cell population show that the interaction of the 2 agents produces more damage than the simple addition of effects from each agent alone.

When surveying the results on aminoglycosides and noise interaction, all the studies are limited because there are no clear behavioral changes that one can use to put the CM and cochlear lesion into perspective. Nevertheless, the aminoglycosides do potentiate the effects of noise; the nature of the potentiation appears to be a general cochlear process that predisposes the cochlea to damage from low-frequency, high-frequency, and impulse noise. The implications of this interaction are that persons working or living in high-level noise environments may run an increased risk of auditory damage when they are on a schedule of aminoglycoside antibiotic therapy.

SALICYLATES AND NOISE

The ototoxicity of salicylates is well known and the consensus is that the effects of the drug are temporary and not additive with repeated doses. However, because of the known interaction between aminoglycosides and noise, it is worthwhile to investigate the possibility that salicylates and noise interact, especially when one considers the large quantity of salicylates (in the form of aspirin) that are ingested yearly by the general population and, in particular, by the subset of arthritic patients.

Woodford et al. (18) systematically studied the interaction between sodium salicylates and short-duration high-level noise, sodium salicylate, and an asymptotic threshold shift (ATS)-producing noise, and finally, sodium salicylate and impulse noise. The levels of the noise were chosen so as to produce a level of TTS in the chinchilla that would recover in 24–48 hr. The median (N = 5) audiograms at the point of maximum TTS (irrespective

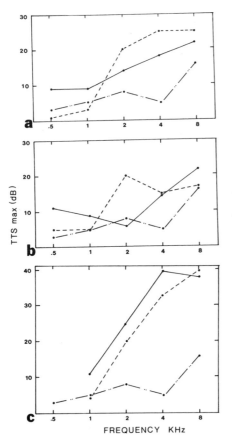

FIG. 2. The median evoked response audiometric data for the interaction of sodium salicylate and 3 classes of noise. The experimental animal was the chinchilla. a: ---, Noise 2–4 kHz 95 dB SPL 1 hr; —··—, Na salicylate (400 mg/kg); ——, interaction. b: ---, 40 μsec A—duration, 50 impulses —158 dB; —··—, Na salicylate (400 mg/kg); ——, interaction. c: ---, 4 kHz octave noise, 80 dB SPL 96 hr; —··—, Na salicylate (400 mg/kg); ——, interaction.

TTS max (dB)

FREQUENCY KHz

of the time at which TTS_{max} occurred) for the controls and the interaction groups are shown in Fig. 2. The negative results are striking across all 3 types of noise. The agent that is producing the largest hearing loss at a particular frequency appears to dominate in the interaction group. On the basis of this data, as well as similar findings by Mitchell (19), it would seem that salicylates pose no additional hazard to an individual working in a noise environment.

The lack of an interaction between noise and the TTS-producing drug, sodium salicylate, raises the question of the mechanism of the interaction between noise and any ototoxic drug. It is known that sodium salicylate induces changes in the lateral wall vasculature which are similar to the vascular changes observed after exposure to noise; Marques et al. (17) have suggested that noise potentiates the effects of kanamycin by altering the permeability of the stria vascularis or external sulcus, or both, either by facilitating the entry or retarding the uptake of the drug by the cochlear vascular system. One possible test of this hypothesis would be to see if salicylates interacted with kanamycin in the same manner in which noise interacts with kanamycin.

NOISE/NOISE INTERACTION

Combinations of impulse and continuous noise are commonly found in industrial and military environments. Damage risk criteria (DRC) have been developed for both classes of noise, but no proviso exists for evaluating the traumatic power of both classes of noise in combination. This omission is probably the result of not recognizing the potential differences between impulse and continuous noise. In fact, Kryter (20) states that when impulse frequency spectra are considered, the audiometric effects of impulse noise are essentially the same as continuous noise. He proposed a scheme for converting impulse noise into its approximate A-weighted value. Atherly and Martin (21), using a different strategy, proposed to evaluate impulse noise in terms of its equivalent energy value. Since the original proposals by Kryter, Atherly, and Martin, 2 sets of data have been published that bring into question the view that impulse and continuous noise have basically similar effects: (i) McRobert and Ward (22) demonstrated the concept of "critical level" for impulse noise. Subjects were exposed to trains of impulses that were adjusted in intensity so as to produce a criteria level of $TTS_{30\ sec}$. When the criteria level was established, the exposure was repeated, but at successively lower intensities and with concomitantly longer pulse trains, thereby maintaining equal energy. In all cases, a drop of 3 dB from the criterial level (with, of course, a doubling in number of impulses) resulted in significantly less TTS. The data also hint that a drop of 6 or 9 dB would create an impulse level that an individual could be exposed to safely, an infinite number of times. Clearly, at the low level of the intensity scale, the

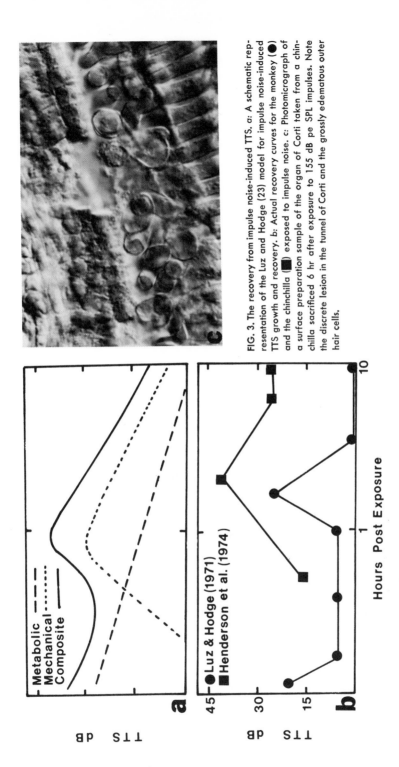

FIG. 3. The recovery from impulse noise-induced TTS. a: A schematic representation of the Luz and Hodge (23) model for impulse noise-induced TTS growth and recovery. b: Actual recovery curves for the monkey (●) and the chinchilla (■) exposed to impulse noise. c: Photomicrograph of a surface preparation sample of the organ of Corti taken from a chinchilla sacrificed 6 hr after exposure to 155 dB pe SPL impulses. Note the discrete lesion in the tunnel of Corti and the grossly edematous outer hair cells.

equal energy principle is not working for impulse noise. (ii) Several years ago, Luz and Hodge (23), after analyzing recovery from impulse noise, published a descriptive model of TTS from impulse noise (Fig. 3). They postulated that there were 2 mechanisms involved in the production of TTS; the first was presumed to be a process of metabolic depletion and was assumed to be similar to the processes underlying TTS from continuous noise. The second mechanism was assumed to be an edematous reaction such as one sees in soft tissue trauma. At the cessation of a brief exposure to impulse noise, the metabolic processes in the cochlea are assumed to begin to recover. By contrast, the edematous reaction has a slower time constant and may actually be growing after the cessation of the trauma. The actual value of TTS is hypothesized to be the product of both classes of effect. Consequently, recovery from impulse noise may proceed in a triphasic course; an initial recovery (due to recovery of metabolic equilibrium), a rebound to higher levels of TTS (due to a delayed or prolonged edematous reaction), and then a final monotonic course of recovery. There are several lines of data that support the Luz and Hodge model. Chinchilla (24) exposed to impulse noise routinely have nonmonotonic recovery curves, but more importantly, their cochleas during the state of impulse-generated TTS show mechanical lesions and grossly edematous hair cells (Fig. 3).

Given that there are basic differences in the course of the physiological processes underlying TTS from impulse and continuous noise, an obvious question to be asked is whether the 2 classes of noise interact. The experimental literature is divided into 2 camps.

Cohen et al. (25) measured the TTS after exposure to continuous noise (75–1,200-Hz band of 90–110 dB for 15 min), impulse noise (133-msec duration at 124–127 dB, 1.3/sec), and a combination of the 2 classes of noise. The impulse alone produced the greatest TTS, while the addition of the 90 or 100 dB background noise to the impulse actually reduced the level of TTS. Cohen et al. reasoned that the acoustic reflex provided the reduction in TTS with the combination exposure. Walker (26) and Lutman (27) both verified the results of Cohen et al., and found that the level of TTS produced by impulses (up to 132-dB SPL) was reduced when background noise [78–96 dB(A)] was added.

Hamernik, Henderson, and Crossley (28) demonstrated a dramatic synergistic interaction between individually safe levels of impulse and continuous noise. The experiments were conducted on monaural chinchilla. The animal's hearing was estimated using the auditory evoked response technique, and their cochleae were analyzed using the surface preparation. The various exposure groups are outlined in Fig. 4. The 3 control groups are: 50 exposures to 40 μsec "A" duration impulses, 1/min at 158 dB and 175 dB pe SPL, and the 1-hr exposure to 2–4 kHz octave-band noise at 95-dB SPL. The initial experiments involved simply a combination of the 158-dB impulse and the continuous noise. The reaction of the chinchilla to the combination exposure

Impulse

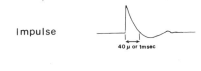

40 μ or 1msec

Continuous

FIG. 4. Schematic of the impulse–continuous noise interaction experiments. The peak of the impulse noise was varied between 175 and 137 dB and the continuous noise was presented at either 95- or 89-dB SPL, 2–4 kHz for 1 hr.

1 Min

Combination
Exposure
Impulse+Continuous

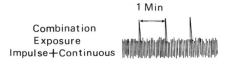

was consistent and devastating. In 8 out of 9 animals, there were large lesions in both the outer hair cell and inner hair cell populations, along with median PTSs of ~40 dB across a broad range of test frequencies. An example of a typical lesion and the corresponding audiograms for an individual chinchilla are shown in Fig. 5. The median PTS for the interaction and control groups are shown in Fig. 6. The PTS values across the 8 animals in the combination groups were greater than the PTS that developed in the chinchilla when exposed to 50 of the same impulses alone, but at 175 dB pe SPL.

The results suggest a number of practical and theoretical questions: what are the limits of the interaction, i.e., how much background noise is necessary to potentiate the 158-dB impulse or vice versa; what is the mechanism responsible for the interaction, i.e., is it simply a local cochlear process requiring overlapping spectra of the impulse and continuous noise, or is it the product of a more general potentiating effect?

Obviously, these 2 questions open up an almost infinite number of experi-

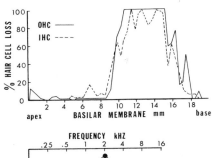

FIG. 5. Typical evoked response audiogram and cochleogram for a chinchilla exposed to the 158-dB impulse in combination with the 95-dB background noise.

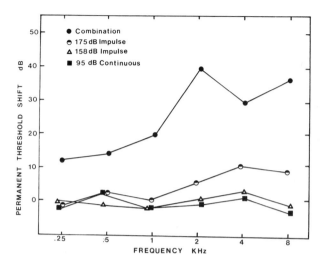

FIG. 6. Median PTS (30 days after exposure) for the 158-dB impulse plus 95-dB background noise and the 3 control groups. Note that the interaction group is not only significantly higher than either control group, but is also higher than the group exposed to 175-dB impulses.

mental permutations. A start has been made on determining the limits of the interaction of the 40-μsec impulse and the 2–4 kHz noise. Hunt et al. (29) exposed groups of chinchilla to combinations of the 1-hr 2–4 kHz, 95-dB SPL continuous noise and 50 impulses having 40 μsec "A" durations at 147, 142, and 137 dB pe SPL. The median TTS recovery curves at 4 kHz for all groups in this exposure paradigm are shown in Fig. 7. The 158-dB impulse alone, or the 95-dB continuous exposure alone, produce a TTS of approximately 25 and 45 dB, respectively, at 1-hr postexposure, but neither exposure

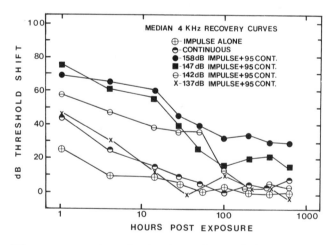

FIG. 7. Median TTS recovery curves for various impulse–continuous noise interaction groups for which the impulse intensity was gradually lowered.

produces a PTS. The animals recovered to normal hearing thresholds within 100 hr after exposure. When the 158-dB impulse is combined with the 95-dB continuous exposure, there is a 70-dB TTS 1 hr after exposure which eventually leads to a 30 dB PTS 30 days postexposure. The 158-dB impulse plus the 95 dB continuous exposure gave the largest PTS across all frequencies tested. The interaction effect was found to be a reliable and systematic effect; as we decrease the level of the impulse in the combination exposure, there is an orderly reduction in the magnitude of both TTS and PTS. The combination exposure with the 147-dB impulse produced a 75-dB TTS 1 hr postexposure, which resolved to a 15-dB PTS by the end of 30 days. The final audiogram for this group showed a gradually sloping loss which peaked at 4 kHz. The

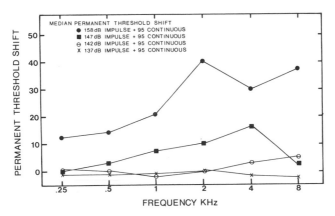

FIG. 8. Median PTS for various impulse–continuous noise interaction groups for which the impulse intensity was gradually lowered.

combination exposure with the 142-dB impulse gave a somewhat smaller TTS (58 dB at 1 hr postexposure) but essentially no PTS. The interaction effect with the 142-dB impulse exposure was marginal. When the impulse in the combination exposure was lowered to 137 dB, the median values show no interaction effect, i.e., the combination exposure gives nearly the same threshold shifts as the 95-dB exposure alone. The median values are somewhat misleading, however, as some animals in the lowest impulse exposure showed 60-dB TTS at some frequencies 1 hr postexposure. Thus, even for the 137-dB impulse and continuous exposure, there may be an interaction in the animals with greater susceptibility.

Figures 8 and 9 summarize the audiometric and histological data for all 4 combination groups. The audiometric data are the median PTS for each group and cochleograms are actual cochleograms for a representative animal from that exposure group. It appears for the 95-dB 2–4-kHz 1-hr exposure, the impulse has to be between 137 and 142 dB pe SPL to trigger a significant interaction effect. However, it should be noted that, although the chinchilla in

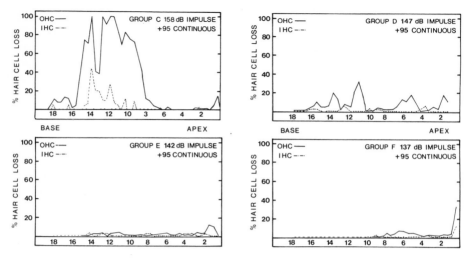

FIG. 9. Cochleograms for individual animals that were typical of their respective interaction groups. These cochleograms correspond to the interaction groups whose TTS recovery is shown in Fig. 7.

the 137-dB group showed no outstanding loss of sensitivity and all had recovered to preexposure thresholds, their cochleae all showed losses of sensory cells in excess of that seen in normal non-noise-exposed animals.

The converse of this experiment is in progress. The objective is to determine the level of background noise that is necessary to potentiate the effects of the 158-dB impulse. Preliminary results at 4 kHz test frequency are shown in Fig. 10 and are compared with the results of the constant background noise paradigm. When the continuous 2–4 kHz background noise is dropped 6

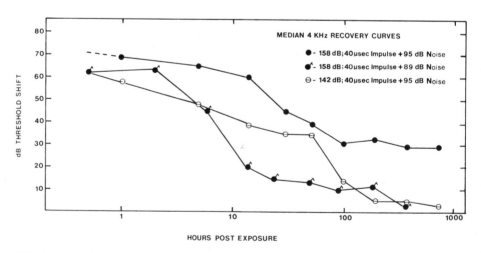

FIG. 10. Median 4-kHz recovery curves showing the relative effect on the interaction of impulse and continuous noise of decreasing the intensity of the 2–4 kHz background noise by 6 dB.

dB from 95 to 89-dB SPL, the interaction effect persisted and was most noticeable when evaluated in terms of TTS. One hour after exposure, thresholds for the 158-dB impulse and 89-dB continuous background noise group were elevated 62 dB, while for the 158-dB impulse and 95-dB continuous noise group, the corresponding threshold was up by 69 dB. Thus, the initial TTS is similar for both groups. After 2 hr postexposure, the 89-dB group begins to recover rapidly and, by 400 hr, has returned to near-normal thresholds, while the 95-dB group ends up with a 30-dB PTS after 30 days. The picture is relatively similar for the other test frequencies. Since the animals have not completed their recovery period, no comment can be made as to PTS or hair cell integrity. The 4-kHz recovery curve for the 158-dB impulse plus 89-dB continuous group is qualitatively similar to that of the 142-dB impulse plus 95-dB continuous group both in terms of TTS and PTS; thus, at the 4-kHz test frequency, a reduction of 16 dB in the peak of the impulse is nearly equivalent to a 6-dB reduction of the background noise. In conclusion, combinations of 158-dB 40 μsec impulses with 89-dB 2–4-kHz background noise do demonstrate an interaction, but the effect is considerably lessened when PTS values are compared.

The experiments that have just been described have impulse and continuous noises that are both primarily biased toward high frequencies. It is important to know if this spectral match is necessary for the interaction effect. In a preliminary study, chinchilla were exposed to 140-dB reverberant impulses (the impulses had a 1-msec "A" duration) that had a predominant low-frequency (200–400 Hz) component in combination with 2–4 kHz, 95-dB SPL continuous noise in the same noise paradigm as previously described.

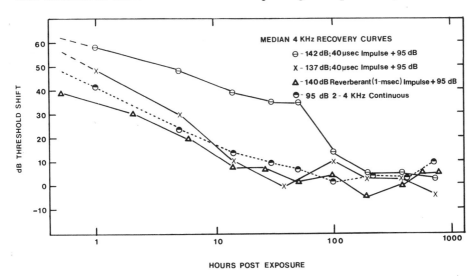

FIG. 11. Median 4-kHz recovery curves showing the relative effect of greatly mismatched spectra of the impulse and continuous noise on the interaction phenomena.

This was the first attempt at studying the interaction phenomena for noises whose spectra were not matched. Figure 11 shows the median TTS recovery curves at 4 kHz for the 2 control groups and the combination groups. The presence of the background noise does not increase the level of TTS that would have been produced by the impulse alone. These data are preliminary, and no attempt has been made to equalize the traumatic power of the noise components of this experiment with the noise used in the original interaction studies; nevertheless, there is no obvious interaction. However, there are not enough data to decide on the spectral requirements for the interaction effect.

All the data that support the notion of an interaction between continuous and impulse noise came from laboratory experiments with chinchilla. Admittedly, the chinchilla is more sensitive to acoustic trauma than is man; nevertheless, the laboratory situation is ideal to localize the interaction effect and, clearly, both the size and consistency of the interaction is impressive. The next question is, does the interaction effect play a role in the process of industrial noise-induced PTS? This is a difficult question to answer because the available data from audiometric and noise surveys do not lend themselves to a systematic *ex post facto* analysis of noise interactions. However, 2 observations appear to support the interaction hypothesis: (i) Walden et al. (30) reported that in 215 army personnel with 10 years' active duty in the armor branch, 63% had sustained hearing losses. In fact, 41% had losses in excess of 50 dB at 4–6 kHz (a handicap that warrants duty limitation). Comparable hearing losses in other branches of the army were 23% in the infantry, 29.8% in the artillery, and 16.3% in aviation. Personnel in the armor branch are subjected to noise levels that are similar to other branches of the service. What may be significant about these statistics is that the armor personnel are more likely to be exposed to a combination of continuous noise and impulse noise to a much greater extent than personnel in other branches of the military. (ii) The most commonly cited functions for relating the dB(A) level to HL are Passchier-Vermeer's (31) synthesizations of several industrial hearing level surveys (Fig. 12). If one compares the growth of PTS at 4 kHz with the similar function published by Burns and Robinson (32), the Passchier-Vermeer curve has a slightly lower intercept, but, more importantly, a considerably steeper slope. One possible explanation for this difference is given by Burns and Robinson who stated, "For the most part, the environments selected were steady noises, unvarying for long periods of time and, except in a few cases, devoid of markedly impulsive characteristics." Consequently, the Burns and Robinson curves are perhaps representative of the growth of PTS from prolonged continuous noise exposure, while the Passchier-Vermeer data may be influenced by the impulse–continuous noise interactions that are in a number of studies she uses. This point is supported when the data from Taylor's (33) survey of Weavers, and the Kuzniarz et al. (34) survey of metal workers are plotted with the 2 functions. The noise environment in the studies of both Taylor and Kuzniarz is a combination of continuous and impulse

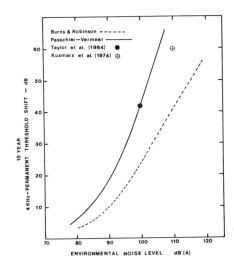

FIG. 12. The relationship between the dB(A) level of a noise environment, and the 4-kHz hearing level of a population exposed for 10 years based upon 2 different noise surveys. (See text for further discussion.)

noise, consequently, the Passchier-Vermeer curve is a much better predicter of the hearing loss than the Burns and Robinson curves.

The military hearing survey and the difference between Burns and Robinson vs. Passchier-Vermeer are cited as possible real-life examples of the continuous–impulse noise interaction. The experimental data provide a much stronger support for the case of the interaction between impulse and continuous noise. In fact, the interaction is potentially dangerous enough to warrant special consideration when evaluating a given noise environment.

ACKNOWLEDGMENTS

This research was supported in part by the National Institute of Environmental Health Sciences Grant ES-OH-00969 and the National Institute of Occupational Safety and Health, Grant 1RO1-OH-00364, Department of Health, Education and Welfare.

REFERENCES

1. Hawkins, J. E. (1973): Comparative otopathology: Aging, noise, and ototoxic drugs. *Adv. Otorhinolaryngol.* 20:125–141.
2. Bohne, B. A. (1974): Mechanism for continuing degeneration in the organ of corti. *J. Acoust. Soc. Am.,* 55:S77 (A).
3. Beagley, H. A. (1965): Acoustic trauma in the guinea pig I. Electrophysiology and histology. *Acta Otolaryngol.,* 60:(A) 437–451.
4. Spoendlin, H. (1962): Primary structural changes in the organ of corti after acoustic overstimulation. *Acta Otolaryngol.,* 71:166–176.
5. Hamernik, R. P., and Henderson, D. (1974): The morphological changes underlying temporary threshold shift produced by impulse noise. *Proc. 8th Int. Cong. Acoustics,* London, England.
6. Hawkins, J. E. (1971): The role of vasoconstriction in noise-induced hearing loss. *Ann. Otol. Rhinol. Laryngol.,* 80:903–914.

7. Hawkins, J. E., Johnsson, L. G., and Preston, R. E. (1972): Cochlear microvasculature in normal and damaged ears. *Laryngoscope,* 82:1091–1104.
8. Falk, S. A. (1972): Combined effects of noise and drugs. *Environ. Health Perspect.,* 1:1–22.
9. Matz, G. J., and Beal, D. D. (1969): Ototoxicity of ethacrynic acid demonstrated in a human temporal bone. *Arch. Otolaryngol.,* 90:152.
10. Mathog, R. H., and Klein, W. J. (1969): Ototoxicity of ethacrynic acid and aminoglycosid antibiotics in uremia. *N. Engl. J. Med.,* 280:1223.
11. Johnson, A. H., and Hamilton, C. H. (1970): Kanamycin ototoxicity—possible potentiation by other drugs. *South. Med. J.,* 63:511.
12. West, B. A., Brummitt, R. E., and Himes, D. L. (1973): Interaction of kanamycin and ethacrynic acid. *Arch. Otolaryngol.,* 98:32.
13. Hawkins, J. E., Marques, D. M., Clark, C. S., and Preston, R. E. (1975): Ototoxic potentiation between ethacrynic acid and aminoglycoside antibiotics in guinea pigs. *J. Acoust. Soc. Am.,* 57:S60 (A).
14. Gannon, R. P., and Tso, S. S. (1969): The occult effect of kanamycin on the cochlea. *Excerpta Medica,* 189:98.
15. Dayal, V. S., Kokshanian, A., and Mitchell, D. P. (1971): Combined effects of noise and kanamycin. *Ann. Otol. Rhinol. Laryngol.,* 80:1–6.
16. Jauhiainen, T., Kohoren, A., and Jauhiainen, M. (1972): Combined effects of noise and neomycin on the cochlea. *Acta Otolaryngol.,* 73:387–390.
17. Marques, D. M., Clark, C. S., and Hawkins, J. E. (1975): Potentiation of cochlear injury by noise and ototoxic antibiotics in guinea pigs. *J. Acoust. Soc. Am.,* 57:S1 (A).
18. Woodford, C. M., Henderson, D., and Hamernik, R. P. (1974): Effect of combinations of sodium salicylate and noise on the auditory thresholds of the chinchilla. *J. Acoust. Soc. Am.,* 56:S2 (A).
19. Mitchell, C., Brummitt, R., and Vernon, J. (1973): Interaction between agents which produce temporary hearing threshold shifts: Intense sound and sodium salicylate. *J. Acoust. Soc. Am.,* 54:S2 (A).
20. Kryter, K. D. (1970): *The Effects of Noise on Man,* pp. 207–239. Academic Press, New York.
21. Atherly, G. R. C., and Martin, A. M. (1971): Equivalent-continuous noise level as a measure of injury from impact and impulse noise. *Ann. Occup. Hyg.,* 14:11–28.
22. McRobert, H., and Ward, W. D. (1973): Damage risk criteria: The tracking relation between intensity and the number of reverberant impulses. *J. Acoust. Soc. Am.,* 53:1297–1301.
23. Luz, G. A., and Hodge, D. C. (1970): Recovery from impulse noise-induced TTS in monkeys and men: A descriptive model. *J. Acoust. Soc. Am.,* 49:1770–1777.
24. Henderson, D., Hamernik, R. P., and Sitler, R. W. (1974): The audiometric and histological correlates of exposure to 1 msec noise impulses in the chinchilla. *J. Acoust. Soc. Am.,* 56:1210–1221.
25. Cohen, A., Kylin, B., and LaBenz, P. J. (1966): Temporary threshold shifts in hearing from exposure to combined impact/steady state noise conditions. *J. Acoust. Soc. Am.,* 40:1371–1380.
26. Walker, J. G. (1972): Temporary threshold shift caused by combined steady-state and impulse noise. *J. Sound Vib.,* 24:493–504.
27. Lutman, M. E. (1972): The effect of steady state and impulse noise combinations on temporary threshold shift. Thesis, Univ. of Southampton, 1SVR, Southampton, England.
28. Hamernik, R. P., Henderson, D., Crossley, J. J., and Salvi, R. (1974): Interaction of continuous and impulse noise: audiometric and histological effects. *J. Acoust. Soc. Am.*
29. Hunt, W., Hamernik, R. P., and Henderson, D. (1975): Effect of impulse level on the interaction between impulse and continuous noise. *J. Acoust. Soc. Am.,* 57:SP 1 (A).
30. Walden, B. E., Worthington, D. W., and McCurdy, H. W. (1971): The extent of hearing loss in the army—A survey report. Walter Reed Army Medical Center Rep. No. 21.

31. Passchier-Vermeer, W. (1974): Hearing loss due to continuous exposure to steady-state broad band noise. *J. Acoust. Soc. Am.,* 56:1585–1593.
32. Burns, W., and Robinson, D. W. (1970): An investigation of the effects of occupational noise on hearing. In: *Sensorineural Hearing Loss,* edited by G. E. W. Wolstenholme and J. Knight. Williams and Wilkins, Baltimore, Md.
33. Taylor, W., Pearson, J., and Mair, A. (1964): Study of noise and hearing in jute weaving. *J. Acoust. Soc. Am.,* 38:113–120.
34. Kuzniarz, J. J., Swierczynski, Z., and Lipowczaw, A. (1974): Impulse noise-induced hearing loss in industry. Paper presented at symposium on the Effects of Impulse Noise, sponsored by Institute for Sound and Vibration Research, Southampton, England.

DISCUSSION

J. Tonndorf: I would like to mention a third possibility, for interactions, that is, general stress combined with noise. During World War II, I saw submarine personnel who had 14 to 15 missions over 4 or 5 years, who had sustained very mild losses, who would then show a steep decline in high frequencies. These men had what is usually called "battle fatigue." So signs of stress superimposed on the noise exposure produced the same traumatic interaction effect. This is another combination you can look into.

H. von Gierke: Did you measure middle ear muscle activity during these exposures?

R. Hamernik: The impulses we presented had total durations of approximately 140 μsec and would have gotten through before the reflex had a chance to act. Also, we presented the impulses at a rate of 1/min, so impulse activity should have adapted out before the second and subsequent impulses were presented. More importantly, however, muscle activity would serve to give a less traumatic exposure.

Effects of Noise on Hearing, edited by Donald Henderson, Roger P. Hamernik, Darshan S. Dosanjh, and John H. Mills. Raven Press, New York © 1976.

Noise-Induced Hearing Loss in the Monkey

David B. Moody, William C. Stebbins, Lars-Göran Johnsson, and Joseph E. Hawkins, Jr.

Kresge Hearing Research Institute, University of Michigan Medical School, Ann Arbor, Michigan 48109

Permanent impairment of hearing as a result of exposure to intense noise has generally been examined by one of two approaches—audiometric surveys of large industrial populations and experimental studies with animals in the laboratory. Recent legislation restricting industrial noise levels to which workers may be exposed has reduced the sampling population for audiometric surveys which, by their nature, have suffered from lack of control over off-the-job exposures as well as other potentially relevant variables. As human experimentation is inadvisable, there has been increased emphasis on the need for carefully done animal experiments. Central to such experiments, however, is the question of the degree to which the results can be extrapolated to man. For example, chinchillas exposed to a band of noise at 123 dB for 15 min have shown temporary hearing loss in excess of 70 dB and permanent losses in excess of 50 dB (1). Similar exposures in humans have resulted in temporary losses of only 20 to 30 dB (2) and minimal, if any, permanent impairment. Similarly, less sound pressure is required to produce a given asymptotic threshold shift in the chinchilla (3,4) than in man (5). The sensitivity of these animals to noise does not necessarily make them less suitable models for hearing loss studies, particularly where the interest is in the relation of cochlear damage to hearing loss. The results of such studies, however, must always be viewed as coming from a model with at least some characteristics which are different from man.

In our laboratory (6,7) and several others, noise-induced hearing loss is being studied in nonhuman primates. Because these animals are phylogenetically as close to man as laboratory models can be, we believe they are ideal for generalization of the results to humans. Although comparative laboratory studies in which man and monkey are given identical exposures have not been carried out, the results that are available do support the appropriateness of the nonhuman primate model for experiments on noise-induced hearing loss.

We have adopted positive reinforcement behavioral testing procedures because we believe the results they produce are more nearly comparable to audiometric data from man than are the results of indirect indices of sensory function such as cochlear microphonics or average evoked responses. Although these procedures are time-consuming, their precision and reliability enables the use of a smaller number of subjects on which to base conclusions.

The present chapter details some of our findings on the relationships between noise exposure, hearing loss, and cochlear pathology in the monkey. Particular emphasis is placed on a series of exposures carried out with bands of noise at 117–120 dB SPL for 20 days. Results from a 90-day continuous exposure to noise at 90 dB are also mentioned.

METHOD

Subjects

The data presented were obtained from members of the genus *Macaca,* species *nemestrina, mulatta,* and *fascicularis,* or from the baboon (*Papio papio*). We have found no consistent differences in susceptibility to noise among these species. The estimated ages of the subjects were from 2 to 9 years and their weights ranged from 3 to 9 kg. They were individually housed and received a restricted food ration at the conclusion of each daily testing session.

Apparatus

Threshold testing was carried out with the monkey seated in a primate restraining chair inside a double-walled IAC room. Earphones (Permoflux PDR-600 with MX 41AR cushions) were carefully fitted over the opening to the ear canals. Since this arrangement enabled the 2 ears to be tested separately, many of the acoustical problems associated with free-field stimulation were avoided. The monkey's head was restrained, and a food delivery chute was placed so that 190-mg banana-flavored food pellets (Noyes) could be delivered directly to the animal's mouth (8).

Also mounted in front of the monkey at eye level was a hollow metal cylinder, 44 mm in diameter and 70 mm long, in the center of which was a red light. The monkey's response consisted in making contact with the metal cylinder and was detected by a circuit which responded to a very small current flow from the restraining chair through the monkey to the cylinder.

Experimental contingencies were controlled and data recorded by a small digital computer (PDP 8/L). The computer produced a punched paper tape for later off-line analysis. Pure-tone stimuli produced by 1 of 9 oscillators (H-P 204C) were attenuated by a programmable attenuator and were gated by a tone switch having a rise–fall time of 50 msec.

The earphones were calibrated 2 ways: on a standard 6-cc coupler and on the monkey's ear with a probe-tube microphone inserted through the cushions so that the opening of the tube was adjacent to the external meatus. Because the coupler method yielded the more reproducible results, it was used to determine the final calibration values.

Sound exposures were carried out in a specially treated IAC sound room which was lined with 1/8-in. masonite held in place with 1-in.² struts placed randomly across the smooth surface. The room was equipped with 2 Altec-Lansing "Voice-of-the-Theater" speaker systems (511B horn, 808-8A driver, 416-8A low-frequency speaker, N501-8A crossover). These were driven by a McIntosh MC 2105 power amplifier which was fed noise produced by a GR 1382 noise generator and filtered by an Allison 2 BR variable band-pass filter.

The 90-day continuous exposure was carried out in a different room in which 4 wire-mesh primate cages could be placed. The room was lined with ceramic tile and sound was provided by a system similar to that described above except that University horns and drivers were the transducers and they were driven by a Heathkit amplifier.

These systems produced octave bands which were flat (± 5 dB) within the band, and a wide-band spectrum which was flat (± 10 dB) from 100 Hz to 10 kHz.

Procedure

Training and Normal Threshold Testing

The basic behavioral training procedures have been outlined in detail elsewhere (9) and only the final conditions will be reviewed here. In the presence of a flashing red light, the animals would make and maintain contact with the response device, and cause the light to go from flashing to steady. From 1 to 9 sec later a 2.5-sec trial was presented, which was either a tone trial or a catch trial; 33% of the trials were catch trials. Releases during tone presentation resulted in the delivery of a food pellet. All releases, including those which were reinforced, resulted in the light being terminated for 5 sec. Any response while the light was off postponed light onset for 5 sec.

Releases during tone presentations were counted as correct detections and resulted in the attenuation of the tone by 10 dB; failures to release during a 2.5-sec tone trial were counted as misses and resulted in a 10-dB increase in the tone. This "staircase" or tracking procedure was continued until threshold was crossed ("yes" to "no" or vice-versa) 10 times. Then a new frequency was presented. The sound pressure levels (SPLs) of the last 8 crossings were averaged to determine the threshold, and 9 frequencies were tested each day for each ear.

Sound Exposure

When the thresholds were stabilized to a criterion of less than 5 dB difference at any frequency for 2 of the last 3 days, sound exposure was begun. The 10 animals used in the high-level exposure study were exposed to one of 4 octave bands of noise (center frequencies = 0.5, 2, 4, or 8 kHz; 2 animals

each) or to a wide band of noise (2 animals). The animals were placed in
their restraint chairs in the exposure room for 8 hr/day, 5 days/week for 4
weeks: a total of 160 hr of exposure. The exposure level was 120 dB SPL
except for the 8 kHz group, for which the maximum level available was 117
dB SPL. The animals were tested at the conclusion of each daily exposure.

The low-level (90 dB) exposure animals lived in cages in the exposure room
at all times except during threshold testing. This exposure was continued for
90 days, with the animals being tested at least daily during that period.

Recovery

All animals were allowed to recover for 30 days following the last exposure.
Testing was continued on a daily basis.

Histological Examination

After the final audiogram was taken at the end of the 30-day recovery
period, the animals were sacrificed. The membranous labyrinth was fixed and
stained *in situ* by perilymphatic perfusion of 1% OsO_4 solution (Zetterqvist).
Cochlear tissues were prepared by microdissection (10), and whole-mounts
of the basilar membrane and organ of Corti were examined by phase-contrast
illumination. Noise-induced injury was assessed by making a complete count
of the hair cells throughout the length of the cochlea and plotting, in the form
of a cytocochleogram, the percentage of hair cells missing from each row per
millimeter of the length of the basilar membrane. In counting, a decision was
made as to whether each hair cell was present or absent, and there was no
attempt to assess lesser degrees of change which might be thought to signify
a reduced ability of a given cell to respond to sound.

RESULTS AND DISCUSSION

The results of the octave-band exposures are summarized in Fig. 1. Each
point represents the median threshold for both ears of both animals (4 values).
The compound threshold shift (CTS) function represents the data obtained
after the first 8-hr exposure. These losses are referred to as compound rather
than temporary because of the likelihood that they contain permanent as well
as temporary components. We have found that, almost without exception,
threshold shift is never greater, and often less, than that measured on the first
day, and we have data which indicate that a significant amount of permanent
damage was done in the first 8 hr, both in terms of behaviorally determined
hearing loss and cochlear histopathology. The permanent threshold shift (PTS)
functions shown in Fig. 1 represent the data obtained 1 month after the last

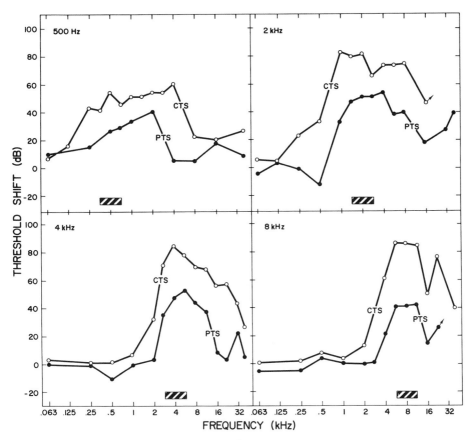

FIG. 1. Compound and permanent threshold shift functions from the 120 dB SPL octave-band exposures. The compound functions represent threshold shifts after the first 8 hr of exposure and the permanent functions represent threshold shifts after 30 days of recovery. Each point is a median over both ears of the 2 subjects in each group. The blocks along the lower edge of each function represent the frequency limits of the exposure band.

exposure. In all examples of octave-band exposure, the data accurately summarize the individual cases they represent; losses were similar between ears and between animals.

Several features of the data are apparent from this figure. First, the CTS functions are similar to but more extreme than the PTS functions and do a moderately good job of predicting the eventual shape of the permanent loss function. This prediction is especially good for the 2-, 4-, and 8-kHz noise bands. The second striking feature of the data is that higher frequency exposure results in narrower hearing loss functions than the lower frequency exposures, with the exception of the PTS function for the 500-Hz exposure band which is narrower than the 2-kHz PTS function. The 500-Hz band also differed in that it produced the least CTS of any of the octave bands. The reduced effectiveness of the 500-Hz band is consistent with previous data obtained from humans (2) and from the chinchilla (3,11).

The 2-, 4-, and 8-kHz noise bands all produced a maximum CTS of about 80 dB, but the frequency at which this maximum occurred was not necessarily at the center of the exposure band. For the 500-Hz band, the maximum compound loss was at 4 kHz, 3 octaves above the center of the band, while for the 2-kHz band, the maximum compound loss occurred at the 1-kHz test frequency. For both of these bands, and also for the 8-kHz band, the CTS functions show near-maximum losses at several frequencies, and specification of an exact frequency for the maximum is difficult. In the PTS data, however, the frequency of maximum loss is always at, or slightly above the center of the

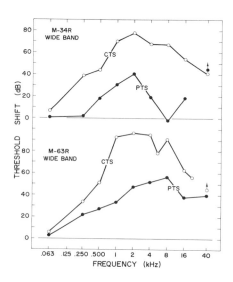

FIG. 2. Compound and permanent threshold shifts from the right ears of the two 120 dB SPL wideband exposure animals. The compound functions represent shifts measured after the first 8 hr of exposure and the permanent functions represent shifts after 30 days of recovery.

exposure band. As the center frequency of the exposure band is increased, starting from 500 Hz, the maximum loss occurs closer to the center of the band until with the band centered at 8 kHz, nearly identical losses occur at 5.6, 8, and 11.2 kHz. Thus, there is no uniform evidence of an upward shift in the frequency at which maximum loss occurs relative to the exposure band; rather, the tendency seems to be for a shift toward the midrange frequencies which suggests the familiar 4-kHz notch typical of noise-induced loss in human audiograms.

We had hoped to clarify this tendency somewhat with the wide-band exposures. The results of these are shown in Fig. 2 which presents the right ear audiograms for each of the subjects. The individual data are presented since the 2 subjects showed quite different PTS functions. These differences might not be predicted from the CTS functions, which have similar shapes. For animal M-63 (lower panel), however, the maximum CTS was 96 dB; 18 dB more than for animal M-34, and losses in excess of 90 dB occurred at 4 of the 5 frequencies between 1 and 8 kHz. This CTS was greater than that observed in any of the other 120-dB exposures and may reflect a hypersensitivity to noise in this subject.

Although the wide-band PTS functions are different from each other, neither is especially different from those observed with octave-band exposures. The function for animal M-34 resembles the sharply peaked functions observed with several of the other exposures and clearly demonstrates the mid-frequency "notch" typical of noise-induced hearing loss in man. For animal M-63, a rather broad PTS function is observed which resembles the PTS functions obtained from the 2-kHz exposure band monkeys. This pattern is less like those usually observed with noise-induced loss than is the pattern of animal M-34.

Comparison of these data with those obtained by other experimenters is difficult because of differences in species or exposure conditions, or both. Although the work of Davis et al. (2) differs in both of these features, it might be compared with our findings. These authors exposed human subjects to both pure-tone and wide-band noise at levels comparable to those reported here, but for shorter durations. Subjects showed losses after pure-tone exposures which were broader for low-frequency exposure than for high, and which showed maximum losses at or above the exposure frequency. The spectral function for the wide-band noise in their experiment was sharply peaked in the 0.5-kHz region with a second peak slightly above 4 kHz. The average loss produced was quite broad, but individual subjects showed considerable variability.

The above data demonstrate several features of noise-induced hearing loss, but the levels of exposure may be more severe than those in many industrial situations. In an attempt to reproduce the intensity characteristics of such exposures more closely, Scheib et al. (12) carried out a study on the effects of a long-term exposure to a 90-dB, 2-kHz octave band. One of the purposes of this study was an attempt to assess "asymptotic temporary threshold shift (TTS)" (3–5) as a predictor of eventual PTS. A primary advantage of this lower level of exposure is that the threshold shift develops over a more extended period of time and its development can be more easily studied.

The results of the first 100 hr of the 90-dB SPL exposure are shown in Fig. 3. TTS increases very slowly for the first 4 hr and then quite rapidly for the 4th through 8th hour. After the 8th hour there is no evidence of further growth in the hearing loss. In this experiment 3 of 4 animals showed similar growth functions typically reaching an "asymptote" of 19 to 21 dB of loss after 8 to 12 hr of exposure. The 4th subject was quite atypical in that he reached an "asymptote" of 56 dB only after 200 hr of exposure.

The continuation of this function is shown in Fig. 4, on a linear time scale. Point (a) represents the beginning of data not shown in Fig. 3. It is readily apparent that the asymptote observed after 8 hr of exposure is not a true

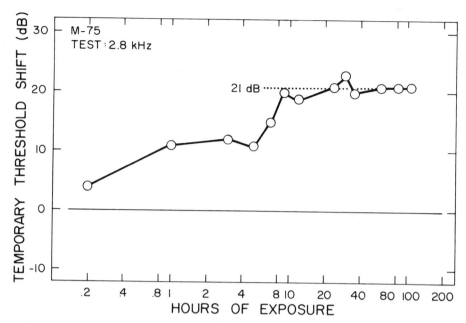

FIG. 3. Threshold shift of a 2.8-kHz tone as a function of time in a 90 dB SPL 2 kHz octave band.

asymptote at all, but rather a plateau in the function. Beginning at about 15 days of exposure, the threshold shift begins to become variable, and eventually stabilizes at a new level about 10 dB above the original plateau. At point (b) in the function, the step size used in the tracking procedure was switched from 10 dB to 5 dB because of our own concern that the shift was almost exactly equal to the step size. This switch caused about a 2–3 dB decrease in the threshold shift and a concurrent increase in variability. This increase in variability is frequently observed with the tracking method in animals when trials are concentrated around threshold, and probably reflects a slight disturbance of behavioral stimulus control.

After 90 days of continuous exposure, the animal was allowed to recover; the data from this recovery are shown in Fig. 5. There is almost no recovery in the first hour after exposure, followed by a gradual recovery to about 4 dB of threshold shift at 60 hr, and perhaps 1 or 2 dB additional recovery during the remainder of the 30-day period. This essentially complete threshold recovery was the pattern observed in 2 of the 4 subjects. A third subject showed about a 15-dB PTS, and the fourth subject (the sensitive one) about a 25-dB PTS.

For all exposure groups, the animals were sacrificed 1 month after the exposures were completed and their ears were examined histologically. It is impossible to present all of the details of this examination given the constraints on length of this chapter, so we will categorize our major findings and attempt

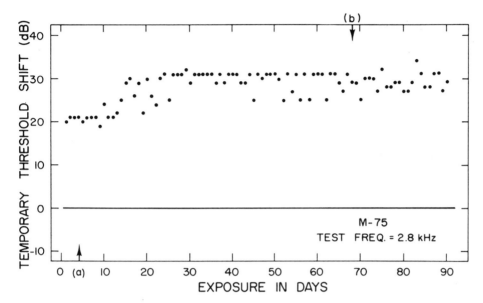

FIG. 4. Threshold shift of a 2.8-kHz tone as a function of number of days in a 90 dB SPL 2 kHz octave band. Point (a) indicates the continuation of the data presented in Fig. 3, and point (b) indicates a change from 10 dB to 5 dB steps in the tracking procedure.

to present an example of each category. The most typical pattern of hair cell loss observed with the octave-band monkeys was a reasonably discrete lesion of the third row of outer hair cells. The location of this lesion on the basilar membrane corresponded to the behavioral audiogram and to the previous findings on frequency localization in the cochlea. In most subjects, the first and second rows of outer hair cells showed scattered loss, if any, and the inner

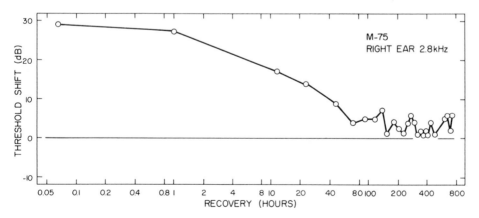

FIG. 5. Threshold shift of a 2.8-kHz test tone as a function of time after termination of a 90 dB SPL 2 kHz octave band to which the subject had been exposed for 90 days continuously.

hair cells were almost completely normal. In addition, there were severe losses of both outer and inner hair cells in the extreme basal end, usually in the first millimeter, and sometimes extending into the second. Figure 6 presents the hair cell counts together with the final audiograms from one of the 2-kHz exposure band animals and is typical of the loss pattern described above. This animal showed a severe basal turn loss, yet still had measurable hearing at 32 and 40 kHz.

The locus of hair cell loss agrees fairly well with our previous findings in monkeys with abrupt high-frequency losses from ototoxic aminoglycosides (13), but the positioning of the audiogram with respect to the cytocochleogram in this and subsequent figures is arbitrary, since the audiogram is plotted on

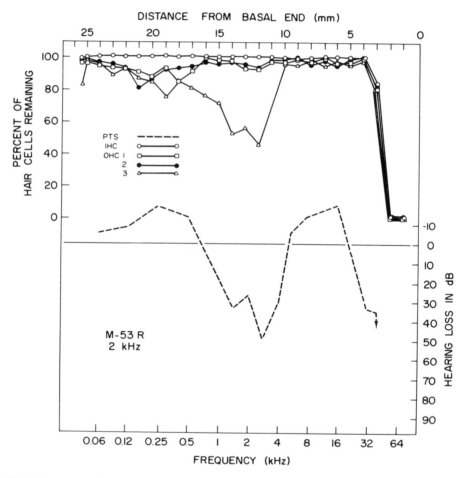

FIG. 6. Percentage of remaining hair cells as a function of location on the basilar membrane (upper) and permanent threshold shift measured after 30 days of recovery (lower) for one of the 120 dB SPL 2 kHz octave-band exposure subjects. For this subject, damage was largely restricted to the third row of outer hair cells.

conventional 4-cycle semilogarithmic coordinates. The correspondences shown are approximate at best, and no attempt has been made to indicate a more precise localization of frequencies along the basilar membrane. If this were done in accordance with the earlier findings, 2 kHz would correspond to a point 15 mm from the basal end of the cochlea, and 8 kHz would be localized at about 8 mm. Later studies showed 4 kHz to be localized at about 11 mm. Thus the frequencies from 2 kHz to 45 kHz should be shown as more widely spaced, occupying the lower 15 mm of the cochlea, with frequencies below 2 kHz crowded into the upper 10–12 mm.

In this animal, a hair cell loss between 11 and 18 mm corresponds to a hearing loss between 1.4 and 4 kHz. A normal hair cell pattern below 10 mm cor-

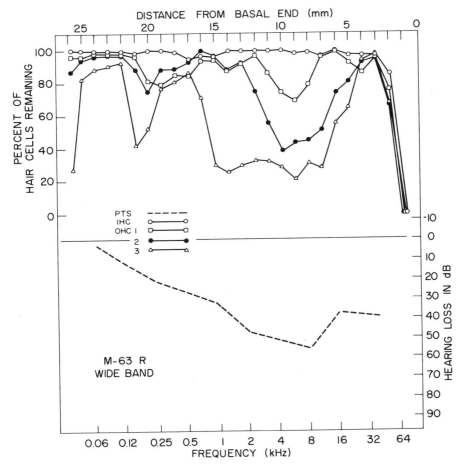

FIG. 7. Percentage of remaining hair cells as a function of location on the basilar membrane (upper), and permanent threshold shift measured after 30 days of recovery (lower) for one of the 120 dB SPL wide-band exposure subjects. Note the graded loss of outer hair cells from the third to the first row.

responds to supranormal hearing between 5.6 and 16 kHz. Since this animal was the only subject showing substantial improvement in hearing outside the region of loss, it is difficult to know what significance to attach to this finding. Hair cell loss as great as 20% appears not to affect low-frequency sensitivity. Loss patterns involving mostly the third row of outer hair cells were observed in all monkeys from the 0.5- and 2-kHz exposure groups.

A second loss pattern is shown in Fig. 7 which presents data from one of the wide-band exposure animals. The hair cell counts show a severe loss which is greatest for the third row of outer hair cells, and progressively less severe for the second and first rows, and an almost normal inner hair cell pattern. Again, as in the previous figure, there is a complete loss of hair cells at the extreme basal end.

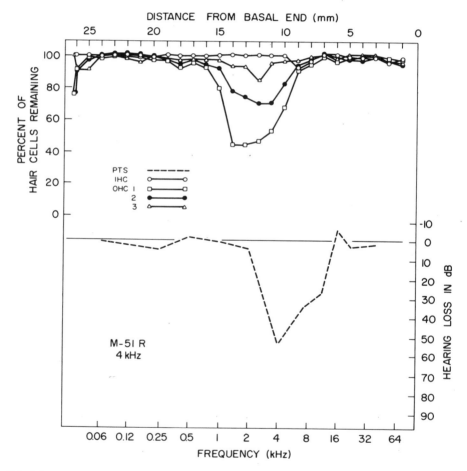

FIG. 8. Percentage of remaining hair cells as a function of location on the basilar membrane (upper), and permanent threshold shift measured after 30 days of recovery (lower) for one of the 120 dB SPL 4 kHz octave-band exposure subjects. For this subject the hair cell loss was graded from the first to the third row of the outer hair cells.

There is good agreement between the behaviorally determined hearing loss and the hair cell counts, but with such a broad loss, comparisons of exact cochlear loci with the audiograms are difficult. The most severe behavioral loss at 8 kHz corresponds fairly well with the locus of the maximum loss of hair cells in the 8–9 mm region of the cochlea and the graded decrease in hair cell loss corresponds to an increase in hearing sensitivity.

A pattern of graded involvement of all 3 rows of outer hair cells was observed in both of the wide-band animals and in one of the 8-kHz exposure band animals. The second 8-kHz animal and one of the 4-kHz animals showed involvement of all 3 rows of outer hair cells as well, but in those 2 animals, all 3 rows were about equally affected. There is no feature of the behavioral audiogram which would permit a prediction of degree of outer hair cell involvement, but it is tempting to speculate that such differential effects might yield some instructive recruitment functions. Unfortunately, we did not obtain such functions on these animals.

The last 4-kHz exposure subject yielded a pattern of hair cell loss not typical of either of the above 2 examples. The pattern, shown in Fig. 8, was a graded loss of outer hair cells with the first row, rather than the third, most severely damaged, followed by the second and the third. This animal showed neither high-frequency hearing loss nor hair cell loss in the extreme basal turn. The locus of the outer hair cell loss at 10–15 mm along the membrane agrees fairly well with the behaviorally determined loss with a maximum at 4 kHz and with our previous findings. Because this animal is the only example of a baboon (*Papio papio*) among our subjects, we cannot at this point rule out a species difference. However, another baboon also exposed to octave-band noise showed losses in the third row of outer hair cells only.

Preliminary examination of the cochleas of the 90-dB long-term exposure monkeys has shown a scattered loss of hair cells in the region we would expect to be affected by a 2-kHz exposure. Although the magnitude of this loss is greater than that observed in the unexposed controls, it is consistent with the recovery to near baseline observed in this animal.

CONCLUSIONS

We would like to draw several tentative conclusions from the present studies:

1. CTS functions can serve to some extent as a predictor of the shape of PTS functions and can set an upper limit for the amount of the permanent loss.

2. An upward shift of the frequencies involved in hearing loss relative to the center frequency of the octave band occurred only after exposure to the lower frequency bands; there was no evidence of such a shift after exposure to an 8-kHz band.

3. A single 8-hr exposure at 120-dB SPL is sufficient to produce maximum CTS. Although we do not have sufficient data for a firm conclusion, it is likely that such exposures also result in some permanent loss.

4. For 90-dB continuous exposure, a plateau in the CTS functions is reached at about 8–12 hr, but this loss increases again after about 20 days of exposure. After 90 days in the 90-dB SPL sound field, 2 of 4 subjects showed a permanent hearing loss.

5. There is a reasonably good correlation between the location of outer hair cell loss on the basilar membrane and the frequencies at which hearing is most impaired. The third row of outer hair cells was often most affected, but this was not invariably true.

ACKNOWLEDGMENTS

This research was supported by research grants NS-05077 and NS-05065 and by program project grant NS-05785 from the National Institutes of Health.

REFERENCES

1. Clark, W. W., Clark, C. S., Moody, D. B., and Stebbins, W. C. (1974): Noise-induced hearing loss in the chinchilla, as determined by a positive reinforcement technique. *J. Acoust. Soc. Am.,* 56:1202–1209.
2. Davis, H., Morgan, C. T., Hawkins, J. E., Galambos, R., and Smith, F. W. (1950): Temporary deafness following exposure to loud tones and noise. *Acta Otolaryngol. Suppl.,* 88:1–57.
3. Carder, H. M., and Miller, J. D. (1972): Temporary threshold shifts from prolonged exposure to noise. *J. Speech Hear. Res.,* 15:603–623.
4. Mills, J. H. (1973): Temporary and permanent threshold shifts produced by nine day exposures to noise. *J. Speech Hear. Res.,* 16:426–438.
5. Melnick, W., and Maves, M. (1974): Asymptotic threshold shift (ATS) in man from 24-hour exposure to continuous noise. *Ann. Otol.,* 83:820–828.
6. Stebbins, W. C., Moody, D. B., Coombs, S., Johnsson, L.-G., Clark, C. S., and Hawkins, J. E. (1974): Acoustic trauma in monkeys related to frequency spectrum of the noise. (abs) *J. Acoust. Soc. Am.,* 55:416.
7. Stebbins, W. C., and Coombs, S. (1975): Behavioral assessment of ototoxicity in non-human primates. In: *Behavioral Toxicology,* edited by B. Weiss and W. G. Laites. Plenum Press, New York.
8. Moody, D. B., Stebbins, W. C., and Miller, J. M. (1970): A primate restraint and handling system for auditory research. *Behav. Res. Meth. Inst.,* 2:180–182.
9. Moody, D. B., Beecher, M. D., and Stebbins, W. C. (1975): Behavioral methods in auditory research. In: *Handbook of Auditory and Vestibular Research Methods,* edited by J. A. Vernon and C. A. Smith. Charles Thomas, Springfield, Ill., pp. 439–495.
10. Hawkins, J. E., and Johnsson, L.-G. (1975): Microdissection and surface preparations of the inner ear. In: *Handbook of Auditory and Vestibular Research Methods,* edited by J. A. Vernon and C. A. Smith. Charles Thomas, Springfield, Ill.
11. Mills, J. H., and Talo, S. A. (1972): Temporary threshold shift produced by exposure to high frequency noise. *J. Speech Hear. Res.,* 15:624–631.
12. Scheib, B. T., Stebbins, W. C., and Moody, D. B. (1975): Temporary threshold shifts in non-human primates resulting from chronic exposure to a 2-kHz octave band of noise. (abs) *J. Acoust. Soc. Am. Suppl.,* 57:S41.
13. Stebbins, W. C., Miller, J. M., Johnsson, L.-G., and Hawkins, J. E. (1969): Ototoxic hearing loss and cochlear pathology in the monkey. *Ann. Otol.,* 78:1007–1025.

DISCUSSION

K. Henson: Could you speak for a moment about the efficacy of your paradigm for obtaining thresholds? Specifically, do the advantages of the positive reinforcement paradigm outweigh the disadvantages of requiring too much time to get a stable threshold?

D. Moody: We believe they do, and we stick with positive reinforcement after having tried avoidance conditioning for various paradigms. I think there is a good deal of stability involved in a positive reinforcement paradigm.

J. Miller: Two comments. First, I seem to recall some earlier data of Stebbins' group effort where the correspondence between hair cell counts and audiometric data was not so nice as it appeared today, and I surmise from your conclusion that, in the primates, you find a good correspondence. Second, you show missing hair cells in the third row only, for which you also show sizeable hearing losses. Have you focused down below the reticular lamina of the other 2 rows to note any changes in the remaining outer hair cells (OHC)?

D. Moody: To answer question 1: I think the earlier data you refer to was obtained with a lower level of exposure, where we found that the PTS does not correspond as well with the hair cell counts. That was one of the reasons we went to the higher level exposures.

J. Hawkins, Jr: To answer question 2: those hair cell counts were made solely on the basis of the presence of phalangeal scars. We have not attempted to make judgments in this case about distortion in the hair cells, or nuclear swelling, etc., which, by the way, we do not see as often in primates as in guinea pigs. I suspect that the presentation to which you are referring, where there was not such good correspondence between sensory cells and thresholds, is one in which the losses in terms of decibel change was small, i.e., there was some TTS and a minor amount of PTS. In fact, our findings correspond quite well with those of Ivan Hunter-Duvar, [*J. Acoust. Soc. Am.* (1972), 52:1181–1192] which he obtained in the squirrel monkey. However, if you go to the extent of exposing monkeys for the periods of time and levels that Moody just discussed, and produce a PTS, then you will see a distribution of scars that will correspond quite closely to the audiometric changes. But, if you are dealing with losses of 20–30 dB, which may, in fact, be reversible, you'll see very little change. In one of our earliest papers involving the aminoglycosides rather than noise, we saw an admirable correspondence. There were lesions with extremely sharp cutoffs and a corresponding abrupt high-tone loss. It was on that basis that we first set up the tentative frequency scale for the monkey cochlea.

J. Miller: It is my general impression, and I think it agrees with yours, that for a given amount of threshold shift, the monkey seems to have less gross loss of hair cells than you see in the cat or the chinchilla. For example, with a 30-dB shift in the cat, you're going to find considerable loss of hair cells, while in the monkey, not nearly as much. While you have a nice agreement in the animals shown here today, it doesn't really make a whole lot of sense that the loss of the third row of outer hair cells should do so much to thresholds.

H. Spoendlin: I wonder if it would be possible in your material to go back and look at the inner hair cells (IHS) under the electron microscope. I wonder if you would not find that there just might be changes in the stereocilla of the IHC. Quite frequently I find that after exposures to 120 dB for several hours, the only observable change is a bending, or disturbance of the inner hair cell stereocilia. It would be very interesting if, in this case, where you have an audiometric loss which is hard to explain on the basis of third row losses, you found a similar type of change at the IHC.

J. Hawkins, Jr: That's entirely possible. We have seen that same type of collapse of IHC hairs in G.P. treated not with noise, but with a single dose of kanamycin and ethacrynic acid. So this seems to be an almost characteristic reaction of the IHC to some ototraumatic agents. Do not let me leave the impression that we are trying to promote the idea that the third row of OHC are particularly sensitive. We just want to point out that often the third row of OHC does show a greater loss and that this loss is sometimes just confined to the third row. There are exceptions, as Moody has pointed out, where the reverse is obtained.

W. Melnick: Was this collapse always in the same direction?

J. Hawkins, Jr.: Yes, in the radial direction toward the stria.

C. Trahiotis: I compared, as best I could, considering small differences across experiments, data on the cat by Miller, Watson, and Covell, [*Acta Otolaryngol* [*Suppl.*] (*Stockh.*) (1963), 176.] human data, some data on chinchillas and some data reported from your (Hawkins') laboratory on the effects of drugs and noise. It turns out there are about 10-dB differences, say roughly between amounts of TTS produced by about 1½ to 2-hr exposures. The human is the least affected, followed by the cat, followed by the chinchilla, then followed by the monkey, which has, by far, the most TTS. I'd like to know what you think of the problem of deciding what a good correlation is between the cochleogram and the audiogram, in terms of the problems of the traveling wave. Once you get losses of 60 and 70 dB (obviously we're going to be stimulating quite a bit of cochlea, especially basalward), how do you handle this problem of evaluating whether you have a good correlation or not?

D. Moody: By correlation, I was referring to our findings on the ototoxic drugs where a sharply defined lesion on the basal membrane can be identified with a sharp cutoff on the audiogram, i.e., we can label the frequency of that audiometric cutoff with the locus of the lesion on the membrane. I'm talking about a distance correlation rather than an amplitude or an amount of hair cell loss correlation when I say that.

C. Trahiotis: With the very abrupt lesion that you produce using drugs, it seems reasonable that you are sampling the apical slopes of the traveling wave, or some portion of it. What I don't understand is how you separate distance from magnitude when you are attempting to relate the hearing loss to the anatomy.

D. Moody: I think that's a valid point. We don't know which part of the traveling wave is producing the sensation and the resultant response from the animal.

R. Smith: Is it fair to say that people are in agreement that the hair cell count, as revealed in the cochleogram, may not reveal the full extent of the functional damage?

J. Hawkins, Jr.: Yes, that's quite true.

Effects of Noise on Hearing, edited by Donald Henderson, Roger P. Hamernik, Darshan S. Dosanjh, and John H. Mills. Raven Press, New York © 1976.

A Comparison of the Permanent Deleterious Effects of Intense Noise on the Chinchilla Resulting from Either Continuous or Intermittent Exposure

Terrence R. Dolan, Robert J. Murphy, and Harlow W. Ades*

*Parmly Hearing Institute, Loyola University of Chicago, Chicago, Illinois 60626; and *BioAcoustics Laboratory, University of Illinois, Urbana, Illinois 61801*

This chapter is a brief description of some early results obtained in an ongoing investigation concerned with the permanent behavioral and anatomical effects of continuous and intermittent noise exposures on the auditory system of the chinchilla. The study is designed to address a simple question: if the chinchilla is exposed to an intense noise for a single 8-hr period, does the temporal pattern of the exposure influence the magnitude or quality of the deleterious effects produced? Stated differently, is the equal-energy hypothesis applicable in the consideration of the effects of a single exposure to an intense, 8-hr noise?

The general strategy of the investigation is a common one. Following surgery to render the animal monaural, the chinchilla is trained to avoid shock at the onset of a tone in a double-grill box. After training, the minimum sound pressure level (SPL) to which the animal will reliably respond is determined at several frequencies. The animal (unanesthetized, but restrained in a yoke-like device) is then subjected to a noise exposure and then behaviorally reexamined for a period of several weeks. After the postexposure audiogram has stabilized, the animal is sacrificed and the cochlea anatomically examined to ascertain the extent of damage that resulted from the exposure.

The hearing losses that will be reported are permanent threshold shifts, in decibels, that remained after several weeks of postexposure testing. The cochleograms to be shown are the results of hair cell counts using a phase-contrast technique.

For all of the data, the exposure was a 2-octave band-pass noise, 600–2,400 Hz. The patterns being examined are illustrated in Fig. 1. There are 3 patterns that contain equal energy: (i) a single, 8-hr continuous exposure; (ii) a temporal pattern of 1-hr on, 1-hr off for a total elapsed time of 15 hr (8-hr actual exposure time, and referred to as the 8-hr intermittent exposure); and (iii) a 1-hr a day for 8-days exposure (referred to as the 8-day intermittent exposure). A fourth exposure is simply a 1-hr exposure, and is being examined to estimate the extent of the deleterious effects caused in the first hour of each of the other exposures. At each temporal pattern, there are 5 different band

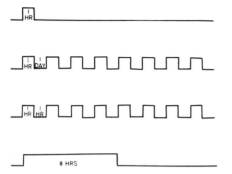

FIG. 1. Illustration of the temporal patterns being examined in the present study.

levels of noise: 126, 123, 120, 117, and 114 dB SPL. This combination of intensities and temporal patterns determines 20 separate exposures, and they are depicted in Fig. 2. Also in Fig. 2, the number of animals thus far exposed at each intensity is shown, currently 26.

Figure 3 depicts the behavioral data obtained thus far at 126 dB SPL for 3 exposure patterns: the intermittent 8-day exposure, the intermittent 8-hr exposure, and the continuous 8-hr exposure (again, all have equal energy). The coordinates are the permanent threshold shifts, in decibels, caused by the exposure as a function of frequency. The 3 exposure patterns caused generally similar changes in audiometric performance. That is, the animals were either incapable of response to a tone at any frequency, or indicated partial hearing only at the very low frequencies. We have exposed another animal that is not indicated in the figure. This exposure was at 126 dB for 1 hr, and similar results were obtained. That is, the animal was not able to respond to any frequency. These results indicate, then, that the hearing loss caused by both the intermittent and continuous exposures at 126 dB probably occurs as the result of damage sustained in the first hour of the exposure.

Figures 4–6 show cochleograms of animals subjected to each of these exposures. The coordinates on the graphs are percent of hair cells present (on the ordinate) and percent of length in cochlea proceeding from base to apex (on the abscissa). The 2 functions of the graph indicate the percentages of remaining inner (IHC) and outer (OHC) hair cells.

	114 dB	117 dB	120 dB	123 dB	126 dB
1 HR		1	1	1	
1 HR –8 DAY		1			1
INTERMITTENT	1	2	2	2	3
CONTINUOUS	1	2	2	3	3

FIG. 2. Number of animals examined at each combination of intensity and temporal pattern. Total number of animals exposed = 26.

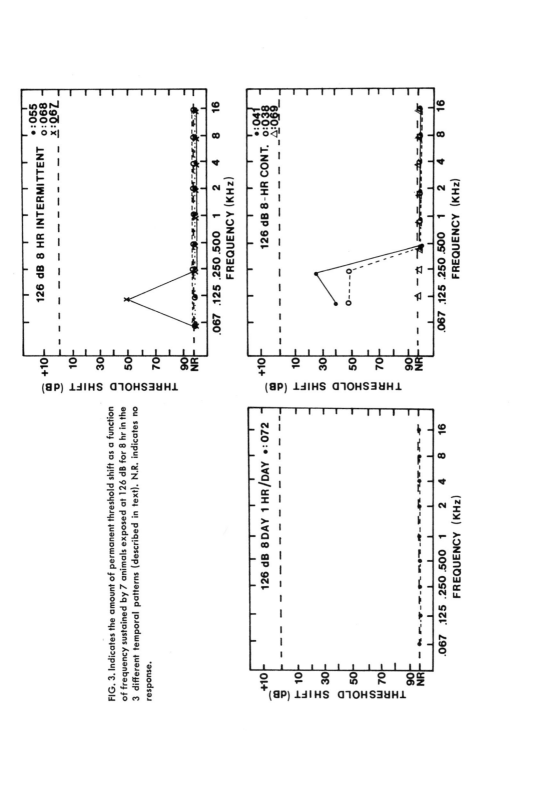

FIG. 3. Indicates the amount of permanent threshold shift as a function of frequency sustained by 7 animals exposed at 126 dB for 8 hr in the 3 different temporal patterns (described in text). N.R. indicates no response.

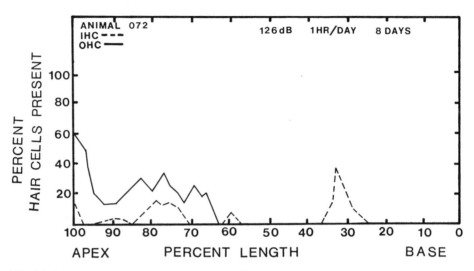

FIG. 4. Indicates percent of remaining inner hair cells (IHC, —) and outer hair cells (OHC, ●) as a function of percent of length of cochlea from base to apex. Results are for animal 072, exposed at 126 dB in the 8-day intermittent exposure.

The results obtained on animal 072, exposed to the intermittent 8-day exposure at 126 dB, are shown in Fig. 4. The exposure caused a severe lesion which eliminated all OHC and all but a small island of IHC in the basal 70% of the cochlea. Even in the apical portion of the cochlea, only a reduced number of hair cells remained. It is mildly surprising that the animal showed no behavioral response at low frequencies, since some IHCs and OHCs remained in the apical portion of the cochlea. It has been our experience, however, that the postexposure behavioral audiogram rarely reflects the condition of either the OHCs or the IHCs in the apical tip of the cochlea.

Figure 5 illustrates the anatomical results obtained on animal 055, also exposed at 126 dB, but in the intermittent 8-hr pattern. The same general results were obtained. The basal portion of the cochlea was clear of any hair cells and the apex sustained severe damage.

Figure 6 shows that similar results were obtained as a result of the 8-hr continuous exposure at 126 dB (animal 038). With the exception of a small island of IHCs in the basal portion of the cochlea, only a fractional number of hair cells in the apex remained.

The behavioral results obtained at 123 dB SPL for 3 different exposure patterns are shown in Fig. 7. The 3 patterns are: 1-hr only, 8-hr intermittent exposure, and the 8-hr continuous exposure. As can be seen, the 3 exposures again lead to generally similar results—no response at the high frequencies, and either no response or severe hearing loss at low frequencies (the variability in the responses indicated by the 3 animals exposed to the 8-hr continuous exposure is not uncommon at these intensities, and points out the

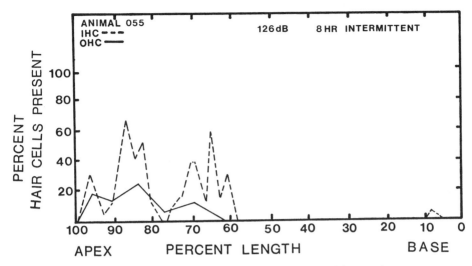

FIG. 5. Anatomical results for animal 055, exposed at 126 dB in the 8-hr intermittent exposure.

hazards of evaluating the effects of an exposure before it is replicated on other animals). A comparison of the results obtained in the single-hour exposure and those obtained in the 8-hr continuous exposure again suggest that much of the damage caused by the 8-hr exposure is occurring in the first hour. A comparison of the effects of the single-hour exposure to the 8-hr exposure, however, indicates perhaps a more interesting finding. That is, there appears to be no additive effects when the damaging single-hour exposure at 123 dB

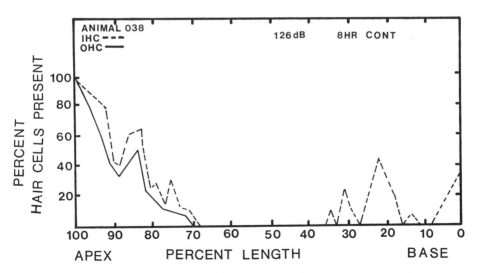

FIG. 6. Anatomical results for animal 038, exposed at 126 dB continuously for 8 hr.

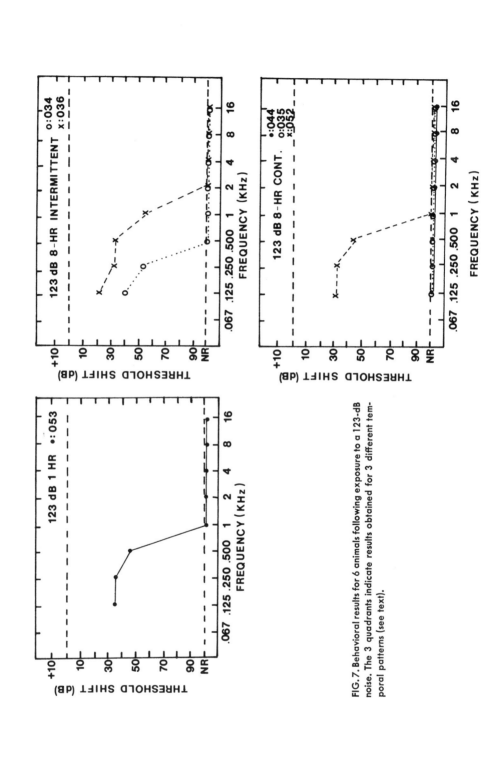

FIG. 7. Behavioral results for 6 animals following exposure to a 123-dB noise. The 3 quadrants indicate results obtained for 3 different temporal patterns (see text).

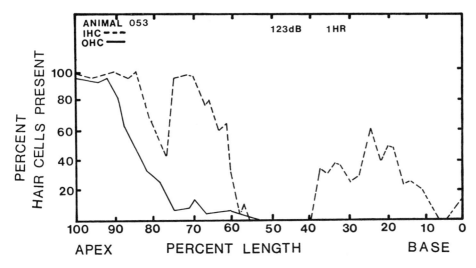

FIG. 8. Anatomical results for animal 053, exposed at 123 dB for 1 hr.

is repeated 7 more times. The partial hearing that is retained at the low frequencies after the first hour of exposure is unaffected by further exposures.

In summarizing the behavioral effects produced by exposures at 123 dB, then, it again appears there are not significant differences in the behavioral effects caused by intermittent and continuous exposures if each subexposure is 1 hr or longer. The primary reason for the similarity in the effects produced by the 2 types of exposures at this intensity seems to be the combination of lack of additivity of effects and the severity of damage caused in the initial hour of the exposure.

Figures 8–10 show anatomical data for animals at each of these 3 exposures. Animal 053 was exposed for a single hour; 036 was exposed intermittently for 15 hr; and 052 was exposed continuously for 8 hr. In general, the 3 exposures caused similar cochlear lesions with severe damage in the basal end, but nearly all of the OHCs and IHCs were present in the apical end of the cochlea.

At an exposure intensity of 117 dB, however, a slightly different result may be emerging, although variance in the magnitude of the exposure effects and a limitation in the number of animals thus far exposed make it difficult to ascertain. Figure 11 illustrates the behavioral data at 117 dB for 3 exposure patterns: the 8-day intermittent exposure, the 8-hr intermittent exposure, and the 8-hr continuous exposure. Both animals exposed continuously for 8 hr (066 and 064) showed complete lack of response at frequencies beyond 1 or 2 kHz, whereas the animal exposed over an 8-day period (071) showed only moderate hearing loss at frequencies less than 16 kHz. The 2 animals exposed to the 8-hr intermittent pattern, 057 and 059, were less homogeneous in their responses. One animal (057) indicated postexposure

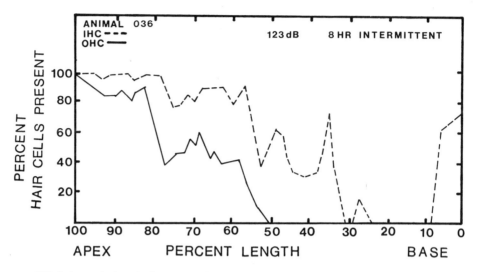

FIG. 9. Anatomical results for animal 036, exposed at 123 dB in the 8-hr intermittent pattern.

behavior similar to the results obtained on the animal in the 8-day exposure, while 059 indicated audiometric performance similar to animals exposed continuously for 8 hr.

The anatomical data, as shown in Figs. 12–15, suggest conclusions similar to those suggested by the behavioral data. Figure 12 shows the cochlea for the animal (071) exposed over the 8-day period. As you can see, OHCs and IHCs remained throughout the cochlea. Figure 13 shows the cochleogram for one of the animals (064) exposed continuously for 8 hr. Only a small num-

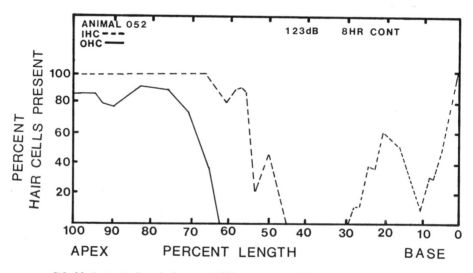

FIG. 10. Anatomical results for animal 052, exposed at 123 dB continuously for 8 hr.

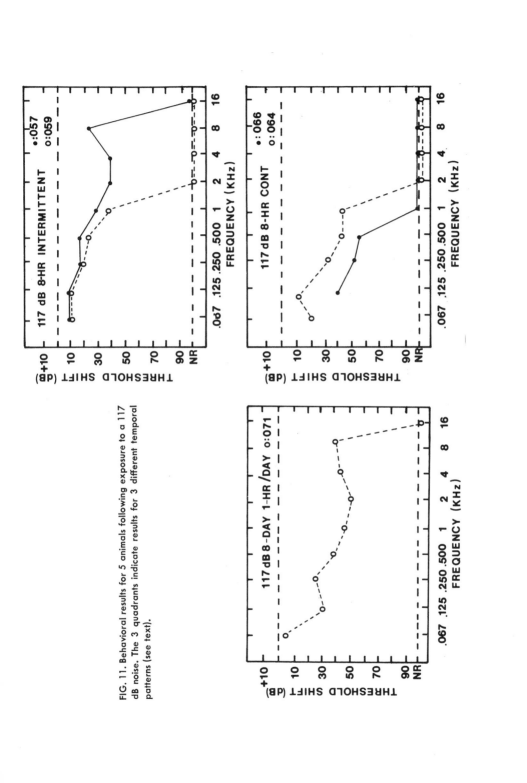

FIG. 11. Behavioral results for 5 animals following exposure to a 117 dB noise. The 3 quadrants indicate results for 3 different temporal patterns (see text).

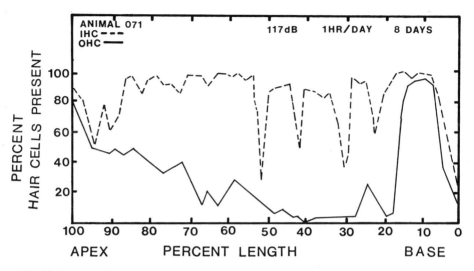

FIG. 12. Anatomical results for animal 071, exposed at 117 dB in the 8-day intermittent exposure.

ber of IHCs remained in the basal portion of the cochlea, and most hair cells were present in the apical portion. The cochleograms for the 2 animals exposed in the 8-hr intermittent condition are shown in Figs. 14 and 15. The animal that showed only moderate hearing loss at high frequencies (057) is shown in Fig. 14. Again, hair cells remain throughout the cochlea. The animal (059) that showed no behavioral response at the high frequencies is shown in Fig. 15. Again, the cochlea is almost bare in the basal half.

The behavioral results for 2 temporal patterns at 114 dB are shown in Fig.

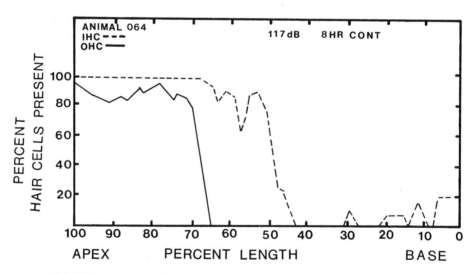

FIG. 13. Anatomical results for animal 064, exposed at 117 dB continuously for 8 hr.

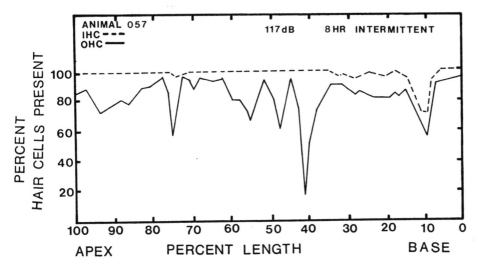

FIG. 14. Anatomical results for animal 057, exposed at 117 dB in the 8-hr intermittent exposure.

16. Both the intermittent exposure and the continuous exposure caused much less hearing loss relative to the results obtained at the higher intensities. Further, although only 1 animal has been exposed in each condition, it appears that the continuous exposure caused a slightly greater amount of hearing loss at most frequencies than did the intermittent exposure. Figures 17 and 18 show the anatomical data for these 2 animals. Figure 17 shows the cochleogram of the animal (074) exposed in the intermittent condition. Since the animal sustained only a moderate amount of hearing loss, it is not surprising that OHCs

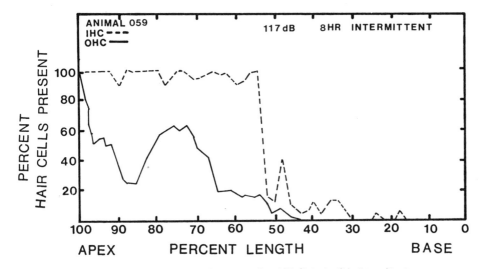

FIG. 15. Anatomical results for animal 059, exposed at 117 dB in the 8-hr intermittent exposure.

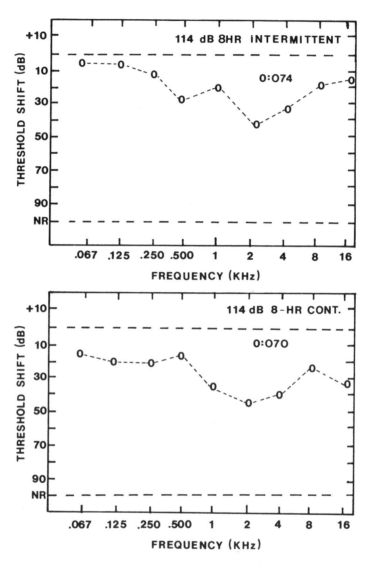

FIG. 16. Behavioral results for 2 animals exposed to a 114 dB noise for 8 hr. (*upper half*): indicates results for animal 074, exposed in the 8-hr intermittent condition; (*lower half*): indicates results for animal 070, exposed continuously for 8 hr.

remained throughout much of the cochlea. Figure 18 shows the anatomical results for the animal (070) exposed in the continuous condition. The damage to the OHCs appears to be more severe than that sustained by the intermittently exposed animal.

In conclusion, this chapter was limited to a brief description of early results of an investigation concerned with the effects of continuous and inter-

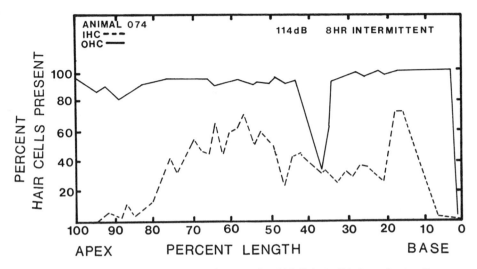

FIG. 17. Anatomical results for animal 074, exposed at 114 dB in the 8-hr intermittent pattern.

mittent noise exposures. The data obtained thus far do not support the constant-energy hypothesis when considering effects caused by a single 8-hr exposure. The data gathered at 117 dB, for example, indicate that continuous exposures cause a greater amount of hearing loss in hearing at higher frequencies and more severe damage in the basal half of the cochlea than intermittent exposures. The finding that the intermittent and continuous exposures of equal energy at 126 and 123 dB caused similar behavioral and anatomical results was due, at least partially, to the severity of damage in the first hour of

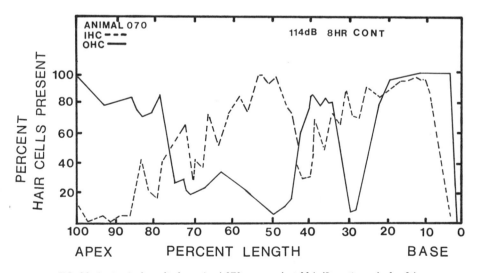

FIG. 18. Anatomical results for animal 070, exposed at 114 dB continuously for 8 hr.

the exposure and the lack of additivity of effects. Since the damage caused by the 114-dB exposure apparently is not limited to the first hour, however, the results obtained at that intensity may provide a more appropriate evaluation of the equal-energy hypothesis. Unfortunately, results have not yet been obtained on a sufficient number of animals at 114 dB to warrant any conclusions. Further, an examination of exposure effects at even lower intensities at longer durations is necessary before the present results can be utilized in practical applications.

DISCUSSION

D. Lipscomb: I am curious about your last few animals. Both of them showed rather large amounts of inner hair cell loss, especially at the apex. Were there any other special changes that accompany these odd lesions?

T. Dolan: No. Certainly the relation between the amount of damage as a function of intensity is not a very straight line. It is our experience that the audiogram maps the first 80% of the cochlea very well; the last 20% of the cochlea often isn't represented in the audiogram, at least not down to 67 Hz.

Effects of Noise on Hearing, edited by Donald Henderson,
Roger P. Hamernik, Darshan S. Dosanjh, and John H. Mills.
Raven Press, New York © 1976.

Application of Animal Data to the Development of Noise Standards

Constantine Trahiotis

Department of Psychology, University of Illinois, Champaign, Illinois 61820

Experiments performed on animal subjects have provided a substantial portion of our knowledge concerning hearing impairments produced by intense auditory stimulation. These studies have been relatively well-controlled attempts toward assessment of permanent and temporary effects as revealed by behavioral, electrophysiological, and anatomical methods.

The purpose of this chapter is to present and to assess a representative amount of this literature in terms of its potential use in development of noise standards. It is probably worth mentioning at the outset that current "damage-risk criteria" and "equinoxious contours" are heavily influenced and determined by studies of temporary threshold shifts (TTS) in human subjects. Undoubtedly, the belief that TTS and noise-induced permanent threshold shifts (NIPTS) are linearly related is incorrect, but constitutes a foundation for our best working hypotheses. [The reader is referred to excellent discussion of these issues by Ward (1) and Eldredge and Miller (2).]

INDICES OF AUDITORY IMPAIRMENT

Behavioral Measures

The most used behavioral index of auditory functioning is the threshold of detection. Typically, a variant of the method of limits or method of constant stimuli is used to determine the sound pressure level (SPL) that is related to a detection rate of 50%. Most modern investigators have employed an instrumental conditioning paradigm accompanied by negative or positive reinforcement. In many studies, an animal must make a response, such as moving from one side of a cage to another upon presentation of auditory stimulation. If the animal moves within some criterion time limit, shock is avoided, the signal is terminated and the next trial starts within some short, randomly determined time interval. Those who utilize positive reinforcement usually have an animal make a response by pressing or releasing a "response key" following the presentation of a tone, and reward the animal for correct detections by presenting banana-flavored food pellets (or some equivalent). Some studies have used bar pressing in combination with avoidance conditioning. Perhaps the major advantage of the reward technique comes from its ease of adaptation to other equipment that allows the stimulus presentation to be produced by earphones as compared to "free-field" stimulus presentation used almost exclusively by those who use negative reinforcement. Typically, "false-alarm responses" or responses during an intertrial interval are punished by "time-out" periods accompanied by total darkness of the test chamber. Occasionally, some experiments have utilized "countershock" to persuade an animal to sit still between trials in avoidance-conditioning paradigms.

The overwhelming majority of experimenters seem to agree that false-alarm responses are to be minimized. As recently discussed by Shusterman (3), there is reason to believe that the most popular techniques have essentially produced "Neyman–Pearson" animal subjects who are attempting to maximize the percentage of correct detections while maintaining a very low and constant false-alarm rate. One might well wonder about the degree to which the data reflect the high criteria "programmed" into the subject, and whether behavioral sensitivity as measured by conventional methods could be significantly improved by the use of more modern methods such as those embodied in signal detection theory. Suffice to say that experiments on humans (4,5) and chinchillas (6) agree that a criterion-free measure of behavior (e.g., d' of 1.00) only leads to about a 3–4 dB lowering of threshold. The literature that we will be reviewing primarily will concern TTS and PTS of 10 dB or greater and typically on the order of 20–80 dB. (The use of criterion-free measures may not be of minimal import for other purposes, however.)

Experimenters concerned with the ability to resolve intensive and frequency differences have employed shock-avoidance and have cautioned others about the difficulty in securing stable response measures in tasks which demand that the subject make discriminations between closely spaced physical stimuli (7).

Recently, a number of studies have employed the subject's reaction time as their principle dependent variable. The subject (typically, a monkey) must press a bar during the presentation of a neutral stimulus and, following presentation of a tone, release the bar to obtain reinforcement. The time elapsing between the start of the tone and the release of the response bar has been used as an indicant of performance for suprathreshold and threshold stimulation levels. Data will be discussed below which indicate that measures of reaction time to suprathreshold stimuli appear to reflect the loudness of the auditory input and may enable an experimenter to produce and to study "loudness recruitment" in an experimental animal. The use of reaction times to measure detection threshold has been reported in one recent study. This reviewer fails to understand how the percentage of reaction times longer than a criterial amount can be related uniquely to the sensitivity of the animal. The interested reader may wish to consult an excellent article by Emmerich et al. (8) which deals with reaction-time measures on human subjects who are performing a detection task.

ELECTROPHYSIOLOGICAL MEASURES

The most frequently used electrophysiological indices of auditory functioning monitor activity generated by sensory hair cells and the first-order auditory nerve fibers. The cochlear microphonic (CM) potential has been recorded from an electrode placed on or around the round-window membrane or between 2 electrodes placed in opposition in scala tympani and scala vestibuli. There is little doubt that the round window-measured CM reflects activity in the most basal portion of the cochlea and cannot be used to assess, in a precise manner, lesions which extend apically. Pairs of differential electrodes have contributed valuable data concerning hair cell functioning, and some of these data will be discussed below.

The most used measure of nerve fiber activity has been the action potential (AP) which is conceded to be a voltage generated by the synchronous discharge of neurons innervating the basal half or so of the cochlea. This potential has been measured from electrodes placed in, on, or around the round window, on the promontory, or from differential electrodes placed in one or another cochlea turn. In a very recent article, Pugh et al. (9) discussed the APs measured from the horizontal semicircular canal.

Few data have been collected from single units in animals exposed to fatiguing sounds. One major study of 8th nerve activity in a region where hair cells have been damaged by ototoxic drugs will be discussed because of its possible importance.

The final electrophysiological measure to be discussed is the so-called auditory evoked potential. This review will focus primarily upon the potential measured from the tentorium which presumably reflects activity occurring in the inferior colliculus. As discussed by Henderson and his colleagues, these potentials reflect the very early portions of the auditory stimulus (1–6 msec) and should be differentiated from the potentials which are typically recorded from scalp or dura (10). Cortical evoked potentials will not be considered further in the review.

ALTERATIONS OF ANATOMICAL STRUCTURES

Investigators have assessed deleterious effects of intense sounds by noting abnormalities in sensory epithelium, stria vascularis, Reissner's membrane, and the tectorial membrane. Some have reported loss of spiral ganglion cells of the organ of Corti (11).

Perhaps the majority of the inner ears of animal subjects have been evaluated with the aid of the phase-contrast microscope. Most of the detailed reports of damage in these studies are confined to statements about the integrity of the inner and outer sensory hair cells. Discussion of the various techniques and their limitations are to be found in Engstrom et al. (12) and in discussions in this volume by Bohne and Spoendlin.

TEMPORARY AND PERMANENT EFFECTS OF INTENSE ACOUSTIC STIMULATION

A monograph published in 1963 by Miller et al. (13) contained a host of data concerning temporary and permanent impairments produced by broadband and octave-band noises. Cats exposed to broad-band noise of 105 dB SPL for 15 min were found to have maximal TTS_{30} at 4 kHz. No TTS was observed at 2 kHz and below and about 20 dB TTS was measured at 8 kHz. When the level of the noise was increased to 115 dB and duration reduced to 7.5 min, TTS increased to about 45 dB at 4 kHz, 20 dB at 2 kHz, and about 27 dB at 8 kHz. Repeated exposures of 115 dB noise for 7.5 min demonstrated at least 2 important relations: (i) If time between exposures were maintained at 24 hr, maximal TTS decreased at 4 kHz (but not at 2 kHz) by about 15–20 dB over the first 4 exposures, and (ii) when the time between exposures was reduced to 1 or 6 hr, TTS began to increase. After the fourth to sixth exposure, TTS at 2 kHz had grown to equal that at 4 kHz. These conditions lead to a sizeable amount of PTS.

These investigators compared the TTS obtained in cats to those calculated to occur for humans presented with the same stimulus conditions (broad-band noise, 105 dB SPL, 15 min). They concluded that TTS for the cat exceeded that projected for man by about 22–28 dB.

Further experiments in cats exposed to an octave band of noise centered at 500 Hz at an overall level of 105 dB for either 8 or 48 hr revealed TTS of 20–30 dB from 2 to 8 kHz and *no PTS*. However, these animals did have injuries in the upper basal and lower middle portions of their cochlea. The observation that normal audiograms could be measured in animals that are shown to have anatomical and/or electrophysiological impairments has great practical import for damage-risk criteria and will be discussed later.

Interestingly, when chinchillas were exposed to the 500-Hz centered octave band of noise stimulus conditions for 48 hr, TTSs of 40–45 dB were measured at frequencies of 2, 4, and 8 kHz (14). The greater TTS found in the chinchilla does not appear to be explained in terms of time of testing after exposure.

Prolonged exposure to noise have been systematically investigated in a series of experiments conducted by Miller and Mills and their associates. Utilizing chinchillas as subjects, they have investigated impairments produced by octave bands of noise centered at either 500 Hz or 4 kHz. Only a portion of their voluminous results will be discussed. Miller et al. (15) found that TTS produced by an octave band or noise centered at 500 Hz, and presented at an average level of 100 dB SPL, and delivered for 7 days, produced TTS that reached an asymptotic value of about 60 dB or so after about 24 hr of exposure when measured at 715 Hz. TTS did not increase when the exposure continued to 7 days. Threshold shifts of 35 dB or more were obtained at frequencies from 125 Hz to 8 kHz. Total recovery of TTS for the midrange frequencies required about 5 days. Anatomical and electrophysiological abnormalities were noted. Small CM reductions were observed with differential electrodes placed in the first and second turns of the cochlea. APs elicited by a broad-band click were at the lower limits of normality at their higher level. The authors report a diffuse loss of outer hair cells in the second and third cochlear turns. One animal had many missing hair cells for 0.2 mm at a distance of 8.2 mm from the base of the cochlea.

Carder and Miller (14) investigated the relationship between octave-band level and the amount of asymptotic threshold shift for noises which were presented for 2, 7, or 21 days. Asymptotic TTS at 715 Hz produced by 500-Hz octave bands of 75, 85, 95, and 105 dB were about 17, 31, 49, and 63 dB, respectively. Asymptotes were reached in about 24 hr with greatest increases in TTS occurring from 4 to 24 hr. TTS produced by an 85-dB level noise remained asymptotic for a 21-day exposure. TTS at frequencies between 250 Hz and 8 kHz increased with band level and reached 50 dB or greater when the band level of the noise was 105 dB SPL. TTS at high frequencies reached asymptote in 2 days. These subjects showed only about 10 dB of recovery in the first 3 hr following termination of the noise and were within 5 dB of preexposure audiograms 2–5 days later. Animals held at asymptote for 2–21 days displayed virtually identical recovery functions. Growth and recovery of TS produced by an octave band of noise centered at 4 kHz was very similar to that produced by an octave band around 500 Hz at a level of 85 dB SPL. Recovery to TTS produced by the 4-kHz band of noise was complete in about 2 days. These subjects were also found to have some hair cell losses in spite of their normal audiograms.

Further experiments (16) indicate that subjects exposed to 4-kHz octave-band noises will reach an appropriate asymptotic level of TTS when the noise level increases from 57 to 80 dB over a 24-day period. These subjects were not permitted the luxury of recovery until 24 days had elapsed. In essence, asymptotic shift to any level is independent of the prior exposure. These subjects proceeded from one asymptotic TTS to another in 24 hr, which is the time required to go from zero TTS to an asymptotic level of 40 dB. However, recovery to near zero TTS required 12–28 days and these subjects were found to have missing outer hair cells. One subject had about 250 missing hair cells, less than normal AP voltages, and CM slightly decreased when measured from electrodes in the base of the cochlea (17). As a matter of interest, Mills and Talo attempted to explain the greater amount of TTS at high frequencies by the acoustic properties of the external ear and head and the notion that "more noise is effective" at high frequencies as shown by the relation of critical ratio and frequency. Threshold shifts greater than 40 dB were measured at frequencies from 2 to about 12 kHz.

Subsequent experiments (18) revealed that recovery to a lower asymptote from a higher one may take from 3 to 7 days, while recovery to zero TTS in the quiet [30 dB(A)] requires 2–4 days.

Chinchillas exposed for 9 days to 4-kHz entered octave-band levels of 86 dB or more recovered to a PTS value that was reached in about 15 days. PTS greater or equal to 30 dB from 2 to 16 kHz were produced by the 98 dB SPL noise. The rapid rise in PTS (about 22 dB) when the noise level was increased from 92 to 98 dB is reminiscent of experiments discussed earlier by Hayden (19).

Finally, Mills (20) showed that TTS produced in animals that had noise-induced hearing loss reached essentially the same levels as seen in normals (referred to normal audiograms). The threshold shifts of those with hearing impairment were smaller than normal, but the shifted thresholds were like those obtained in normal animals. Viewed in this way, the ear with the sensorineural hearing loss is not more susceptible to noise than is the normal ear.

Electrophysiological changes in chinchilla cochlear potentials following exposure to a 500-Hz centered octave band of noise presented at an overall level of 95 dB for 2 or 3 days were reported by Benitez et al. (21). CM changes measured in the 3 cochlea turns corresponded quite closely to the behavioral TTSs 5, 24, and 48 hr postexposure. However, APs could not be measured about 5 hr postexposure when a 90 dB SPL wide-band click was presented. APs measured 24–48 hr postexposure were of very low voltage and had a threshold of about 50 dB SPL. The average evoked responses paralleled the CM measures and behavioral thresholds in revealing about a 50 dB TTS at 30 min postexposure. These authors conclude that the losses revealed in the AP must reflect a lack of synchrony of discharge of nerve fibers in the basal portion of the cochlea.

Stebbins et al. (22) measured TTS in monkeys following exposure to octave bands of noise of 100 dB SPL. One monkey exposed to an octave band around 500 Hz for 2 hr suffered between 30 and 40 dB TTS over the frequency range 500 Hz and 2 kHz when tested immediately following noise termination. Recovery appeared to be complete in 48 hr. Another monkey stimulated by an octave band centered at 2 K obtained 40–50 dB TTS at frequencies from 2 to about 6 kHz. Two days following exposure, "TTS" was reported to be 15 dB at 3 kHz. TTSs measured in 3 monkeys stimulated by octave bands of noise centered in octave steps from 500 Hz to 4 kHz revealed that TTS produced by the lower frequency bands effected a broad range of test frequencies. When the data obtained from the monkeys exposed to an octave band centered around 500 Hz are related to those obtained by Miller et al. for the chinchilla, it becomes apparent that the monkey shows a *greater* TTS by about 12–15 dB and that the frequency spread of TTS is not decidedly different for the 2 species. I find this state of affairs rather perplexing. The critical ratios for the 2 species appear to be very similar (within 3 or 4 dB) at these low frequencies (23,6).

Apparently, TTS measured for quite similar conditions in man, cat, chinchilla, and monkey indicates that the amount of TTS *increases* in the order indicated. Perhaps those who prefer to use monkeys because they apparently are "closer" to man than the other species would like to challenge this assessment. Perhaps Stebbins et al. (22) would not agree to these comparisons. They do not state their reasons for completely omitting all reference to the work of Miller and his associates in their article.

Hunter-Duvar and Elliott (24) repeatedly exposed squirrel monkeys to pure tones of 120 dB SPL for 9–15 min. These animals were shown to have a TTS_{30} of about 16–23 dB at frequencies at, or one-half octave above, the stimulation frequencies. Diffuse outer hair cell losses were found in experimental and control ears. One animal who had relatively severe hair cell loss in the first row of outer hair cells (of both ears) required 2–3 days to return to normal threshold. The most spectacular finding in this study was PTS of 10–20 dB with no clear anatomical correlates.

In their discussion, Hunter-Duvar and Elliott refer to a number of instances in which behavioral and anatomical indices of impairment are at variance. Since these issues are discussed at length by Bredburg and Hunter-Duvar in a book soon to be published (25), they will not be pursued in toto here.

INTERPRETATION OF ANIMAL STUDIES AND THEIR POSSIBLE RELATION TO HUMAN DAMAGE-RISK CRITERIA

Behavioral thresholds measured in animals before or after exposure to noise typically appear to approach the precision of those measured in humans by similar procedures. Unpublished observations made in our laboratory indicate that NIPTS measured at 3–4 month intervals are extremely stable and bear strong resemblance to data on humans published by Ward and Glorig (26).

The question of predictive validity of these indices is quite complicated. One indication of validity would be similarity of effects when data from animals are compared to those obtained from humans. Mills et al. (27) subjected Mills to an octave band of noise centered at 500 Hz for 48 hr. The overall noise level was 81.5 dB SPL. Mills reached an asymptotic TTS value of 10.5 dB in about 12 hr when tested at 715 Hz. He recovered from this exposure to 0 dB TTS in about 3 days. Five weeks later, Mills was exposed to a 92.5 dB SPL octave-band noise centered at 500 Hz for 29.5 hr. An asymptotic TTS of 27.5 dB was reached in 8–12 hr. Recovery to 0 dB TTS took about 4–7 days. As Mills et al. point out, these data suggest that recovery from TTS is dependent on the manner it was produced. Apparently Mills and chinchillas appear to have the same relation between magnitude of TTS at asymptote and level of exposure, except for a difference in the level which would produce zero TTS if presented for long durations (which Miller et al. refer to as their subtractive constant in the formula $TTS_\infty = 1.55(SPL - k)$. Several other observations were made during TTS including (i) frequency discriminations were unaffected; (ii) recruitment of loudness for signals above 50 dB SPL; and (iii) the time constant of temporal integration was reduced at 750 Hz. These findings appear to be very important. They corroborate previously reported data concerning frequency discriminations in deafened cats reported by Elliott (28) and are similar to evidence for loudness recruitment in monkeys reported by Moody (29). The temporal integration findings will be discussed somewhat later.

Asymptotic threshold shifts in humans have also been reported by Melnick and Maves (30). They investigated a 24-hr exposure to a 500-Hz centered octave band of noise at 90 dB SPL. An asymptotic threshold shift of about 11 dB was reported to have occurred after about 12 hr in the noise. Recovery was not complete until about 24 hr following termination of the noise. The relatively small amount of TTS may have been due to prior NIPTS. The shifted threshold of their subjects appear to line up quite well with Mills' data and are fit quite nicely by the summary formula developed by Carder and Miller.

Another facet of validity concerns the relations between postexposure audiograms and anatomical and physiological data. For many years, it had been felt that behavioral deficits produced by intense sound were to be accounted for peripherally (within the cochlea) and that the *outer* hair cells were the receptors providing information at behavioral threshold levels. Matters appeared to get complicated when Spoendlin reported that 90–95% of the innervation of the cochlea is to the *inner* hair cells (31). This observation makes matters difficult for many of us who attempt to make transitions from psychophysical to physiological data and vice versa. More importantly for our topic, Ward and Duvall (32) reported that chinchillas deprived of all outer hair cells in the first and for most of the second cochlear turns had normal audiograms. All inner hair cells appeared to be normal except for some fused cilia. Subsequent investigations by three laboratories replicated the anatomical findings and showed that chinchillas with these large lesions suffered PTSs of 60 dB or more above 1 kHz (33,34). Some of Ward's animals were tested in our laboratory and, with our testing procedure, displayed PTS indistinguishable from those obtained by other investigators. Contrary to the belief of Clark et al. (34) the conflicting results are *not* produced by type of reinforcement or test procedure. We still do not know what accounts for Ward's aberrant findings.

The vast majority of the data on humans presented by Bredberg (11) appear to indicate that outer hair cell density is more closely related to hearing loss than is the density of inner hair cells.

Prior belief that *inner* hair cells have thresholds some 40–50 dB above thresholds of outer hair cells was supported by Ryan and Dallos (35). Animals treated with kanamycin were shown to have total outer hair cell destruction in the basal portions of the cochlea, while the inner hair cells were microscopically normal. Behavioral threshold shifts of 40–50 dB were measured for test frequencies above 3 kHz. A low-pass filtered noise with a rolloff of 84 dB per octave at 3 kHz was set at a level which produced about 40 dB of masking for low frequencies. The behavioral thresholds at *high* frequencies were unaffected by the masking noise. These data appear to be as internally consistent as any we can marshal to bear on the issue. The field still has to come to grips with Spoendlin's findings and this may entail a good deal of effort. In retrospect, however, the finding that cats could have normal audiograms, in spite of severe spiral ganglion losses, seems acceptable (36).

Perhaps *outer* hair cells are intimately involved in normal temporal integration of energy. A number of experiments have indicated a reduction in ability to integrate energy at threshold levels as a consequence of TTS and PTS (37–46). These findings are quite important independent of theory. The amount of TTS would appear to be *reduced* when *SPL* measures of threshold are used to determine the preexposure audiogram. That is, the auditory system requires greater SPLs at shorter durations for threshold response. When this latter value is subtracted from the SPL value of threshold under TTS or PTS the amount of impairment appears to be reduced. Fortunately, all behavioral studies have used fairly long test signals. One could speculate that animals deprived of their outer hair cells and having normal inner hair cells would show little or no temporal integration. Of course, it is possible that the particular neural circuitry following the respective hair cells (and not the hair cells *per se*) is critical. The very close correspondence regarding the lack of temporal integration in subjects with TTS found by Henderson (37) in chinchillas, and Jerger (46) and Mills et al. (27) in humans, is another example of the similarity in effects across species.

A host of studies published by Henderson and Hamernik and their associates (47–50) appear to indicate that the auditory evoked response (AER) measure should not be considered a substitute for behavioral testing. Losses in the AER appear to be related to inner hair cell damage much more readily than to outer hair cell damage. Data from one animal, CBE2, appear to contradict this generalization (48, p. 1214). However, in the text of the article, Henderson et al. point out that the inner hair cells, although present, were not normal and were disarranged. It appears that the AER is produced by the early portions of a short acoustic event and represents the integrated activity of a great number of neurons. Since most of the neurons appear to innervate inner hair cells, the obtained relationships appear to be consistent. However, we must cope with the idea that inner hair cells have a lower threshold by some 40 dB or so than outer hair cells and explain how AER thresholds in the normal animal can be only 20 dB or so poorer than the behavioral thresholds. It seems plausible that the physical spread of energy during the first 6 or 8 msec of the acoustic event could account for the data. From this point of view, the changing of the fundamental frequency should not change normal thresholds very much and, apparently, it does not. These comments are certainly not intended to be an indictment of the AER procedure. On the contrary, this procedure appears to be a relatively efficient indicator of peripheral trauma.

Another area in which data obtained from animals compare favorably with those obtained in people concerns the effects of masking on impaired ears. Experiments in our laboratory revealed that masked audiograms obtained at several levels of masking noise could differentiate between animals who had normal or damaged outer hair cells on the apical side of severe basal lesions (51). Simply put, damaged hair cells did not respond to low levels of noise sufficiently to produce masking typically obtained in normals at low levels of the masking noise. The data also indicated that the 20 dB SPL spectrum level of broadband noise produced masked thresholds indistinguishable from normal. Similar findings in humans with TTS were reported by Parker and Tubbs (52). They interpreted their data to mean that TTS decreased in the noise. We interpreted our data in terms of shifted thresholds. The issue is similar to that discussed above with regard to temporal integration.

The fact that noise-shifted thresholds in the subject with hearing exposures are essentially identical to those in the normal subject may be difficult to explain. One approach to the problem would be to consider the masking function as an example of Weber's law. Many experiments have indicated that the normal human masking data essentially obey Weber's law over an intensity range of about 80 dB. Physiological evidence concerning the short dynamic range of single 8th nerve units leads to the conclusion that nerve fibers distributed over a large area must be involved in the discrimination. However, the results of an experiment by Viemeister (53) are difficult to reconcile with this point of view. Apparently, Viemeister forced his subjects to utilize information in a narrow band of frequencies to perform intensity discrimination in noise. Weber's law held over a great intensity range in this experiment. Perhaps all that is needed is that the neurons be driven to their saturation rates and the "sensation level" of the masker is irrelevant.

The literature concerning masking in humans with NIPTS points to some disparities which will eventually have to be faced. Masked thresholds may be abnormally great in some patients with NIPTS (54–56). Some patients appear to have abnormal spread of masking when attempting to detect tones placed between 2 bands of noise. Clues concerning the differences between patients who display normal masking functions and those that do not are lacking.

A perplexing problem that may deserve discussion concerns the magnitudes of PTS observed in some animal experiments. It seems clear that 1–2 mm localized lesions of the organ of Corti may be accompanied by only 20 dB or so PTS (2). Apparently the traveling wave leads to stimulation of healthy cells to either side of the lesion and they provide the information used by the animals.

It is well known that chinchillas with severe basal lesions do not suffer nearly as much PTS as cats, monkeys, or people. Examination of CM data differentially recorded from 3 turns in the guinea pig raised the hope that the apical end of the traveling wave in the chinchilla was shallower than that of other animals. To elicit a 1-mV CM response in the third turn by a 5 kHz signal the SPL was found to be about 70 dB. This SPL value if very close to the shifted threshold for high frequency in chinchillas that have large basal lesions and essentially normal apical regions of the cochlea. It seemed that the high-frequency information was getting down to the upper middle and apical reaches of the cochlea. Unfortunately, the CM data may simply reflect the remote CM responses picked up by the differential electrode. The notion that the apical portion of the traveling wave *does reach* apically situated hair cells is supported by the masking data in chinchillas reported above. Some sort of unequivocal physiological evidence would be quite welcome.

The assumption that hearing impairments produced by intense noise reflect abnormalities in the peripheral portion of the auditory system seems to be almost universally accepted. Recent data indicate that neural responses measured in the cochlear nucleus (57) and the inferior colliculus (58) may be abnormal following intense sound exposure. The interpretation of these data in terms of alteration in *central* processing depends upon demonstration that the peripheral portions of the auditory system (i.e., hair cells) are not the site of the impairment. CM measured in the round window and whole-nerve AP represent *regions* of activity and may not provide adequate controls.

A thorough investigation of auditory nerve activity in cats by Kiang et al. (59) treated with kanamycin revealed abnormal tuning curves recorded from neurons innervating the lesioned area of the cochlea. The neurons displayed marked reductions of sensitivity to tonal frequencies near the "characteristic frequency" of the fibers. Perhaps a major finding of the study was that single units with abnormally high thresholds did not show any evidence of correlates of loudness recruitment. Input–output functions were reported to show no abnormally abrupt acceleration. Kiang et al. conclude that spatial distributions of activity and activity in populations of neurons must be addressed theoretically.

RECENT OBSERVATIONS WHICH MAY BEAR DIRECTLY ON DAMAGE-RISK CRITERIA

A thorough examination of the effects produced by the *interaction* of continuous and impulsive noise was provided by Hamernik et al. (47). They found that 2 noise exposures, which were "safe" when presented alone, produced severe traumatic effects when presented cotemporally. These data should be quite significant for standards concerning certain industrial and military environments.

Future noise standards may also be influenced by the observations of Jauhianinen et al. (60) regarding the traumatic effects produced by combinations of noise and neomycin treatment. CM measures and histological examination revealed that the effects of the 2 treatments were very much more than their linear combination.

Kellerhals (61) has recently published an article that may have great practical value. Guinea pigs and humans exposed to short-duration high-intensity stimuli were shown to benefit greatly from intravenous infusions of *low* molecular weight dextran. The guinea pigs treated with dextran were found to have a much smaller number of destroyed inner and outer hair cells. Humans treated with dextran following an explosion in a chemical plant were found to have less NIPTS 1 month following exposure than did control subjects. The data clearly indicate that dextran treatment may enable the sensory cells to maintain a metabolic level necessary for survival. These findings should certainly stimulate others to conduct research that will verify these findings and shed light on the details of the mechanisms involved. Generalizations from animal data to humans are most satisfying when the effects have such extreme social value.

In closing, it may be worth mentioning that the variance in magnitudes of hearing impairment across species will undoubtedly be difficult to reconcile. A recent article published by Drescher and Eldredge (62) is addressed to the factors that combine to make the chinchilla more sensitive than the guinea pig to sounds below 5 kHz. This excellent article should be read by those who believe that simple answers about species differences only await our discovery.

ACKNOWLEDGMENTS

The preparation of this manuscript was supported by NINCDS Grant NS 12501 to the Eye and Ear Hospital of Pittsburgh, Pa. The manuscript was completed while the author was Visiting Associate Professor of Otolaryngology at the University of Pittsburgh Medical School. The secretarial assistance of Nancy Stenson and Maria Feigel is greatly appreciated. Slides for the oral presentation at the symposium were prepared by Joseph Wisniewski. Special thanks are due Dr. Robert C. Bilger and Mark Stiegel for helpful discussions.

REFERENCES

1. Ward, W. D. (1969): Effects of noise on hearing thresholds. Proceedings of the Conference. *Noise as a Public Health Hazard.* ASHA Report #4:40–48.
2. Eldredge, D. H., and Miller, J. D. (1969): Acceptable noise exposures-damage risk criteria. Proceedings of the Conference. *Noise as a Public Health Hazard.* ASHA Report 4:110–120.
3. Schusterman, R. J. (1974): Low false-alarm rates in signal detection by marine mammals. *J. Acoust. Soc. Am.,* 55:845–848.
4. Watson, C. S., Franks, J. R., and Hood, D. C. (1972): Detection of tones in the absence of external masking noise. I. Effects of signal intensity and signal frequency. *J. Acoust. Soc. Am.,* 52:633–643.
5. Reed. C. M., and Bilger, R. C. (1973): A comparative study of S/No and E/No. *J. Acoust. Soc. Am.,* 53:1039–1044.
6. Seaton, W. H., and Trahiotis, C. (1975): Comparison of critical ratios and critical bands in the monaural chinchilla. *J. Acoust. Soc. Am.,* 57:193–199.
7. Elliott, D. N., and McGee, T. M. (1965): Effect of cochlear lesions upon audiograms and intensity discrimination in cats. *Ann. Otol. Rhinol. Laryngol.,* 74:386–408.

8. Emmerich, D. S., Gray, J. L., Watson, C. S., and Tanis, D. C. (1972): Response latency, confidence, and ROCs in auditory signal detection. *Percept. Psychophysiol.*, 11:65–72.
9. Pugh, J. E., Horwitz, M. R., and Anderson, D. J. (1974): Cochlear electrical activity. *Arch. Otolaryngol.*, 100:36–40.
10. Henderson, D., Onishi, S., Eldredge, D. H., and Davis, H. (1969): A comparison of chinchilla auditory evoked response and behavioral response thresholds. *Percept. Psychophysiol.*, 5:41–45.
11. Bredberg, G. (1968): Cellular pattern and nerve supply of the human Organ of Corti. *Acta Otolaryngol. [Suppl.] (Stockh.)* 236:1–135.
12. Engstrom, H., Ades, H. W., and Andersson, A. (1966): *Structural Pattern of the Organ of Corti.* Almqvist and Wiksell, Stockholm.
13. Miller, J. D., Watson, C. S., and Covell, W. P. (1963): Deafening effects of noise on the cat. *Acta Otolaryngol. [Suppl.] (Stockh.)* 176.
14. Carder, H. M., and Miller, J. D. (1972): Temporary threshold shifts (TTS) produced by noise exposures of long duration. *J. Speech Hear. Res.*, 15:603–623.
15. Miller, J. D., Rothenberg, S. J., and Eldredge, D. H. (1971): Preliminary observations on the effects of exposure to noise for seven days on the hearing and inner ear of the chinchilla. *J. Acoust. Soc. Am.*, 50:1199–1203.
16. Mills, J. H., and Talo, S. A. (1972) Temporary threshold shifts produced by exposure to high-frequency noise. *J. Speech Hear. Res.*, 15:426–630.
17. Eldredge, D. H., Mills, J. H., and Bohne, B. A. (1973): Anatomical behavioral and electrophysiological observations on chinchillas after long exposures to noise. *Adv. Otorhinolaryngol.*, 20:64–81.
18. Mills, J. H., Talo, S. A., and Gordon, G. S. (1973): Decay of temporary threshold shift in noise. *J. Speech Hear. Res.*, 16:267–270.
19. Hayden, Jr., R. C. (1967): Effects of intense auditory stimulation in animals. In: *Sensorineural Hearing Processes and Disorders,* edited by A. B. Graham, pp. 191–200. Little, Brown, Boston, Mass.
20. Mills, J. H. (1973): Threshold shifts produced by exposure to noise in chinchillas with noise-induced hearing losses. *J. Speech Hear. Res.*, 16:700–708.
21. Benitez, L. D., Eldredge, D. H., and Templer, J. W. (1972): Temporary threshold shifts in chinchilla: Electrophysiological correlates. *J. Acoust. Soc., Am.*, 52:1115–1123.
22. Stebbins, W. C., Clark, W. W., Pearson, R. D., and Weiland, M. G. (1973): Noise and drug induced hearing loss in monkeys. *Adv. Otorhinolaryngol.*, 20:42–63.
23. Gourevitch, G. (1970): Detectability of tones in quiet and in noise by rats and monkeys. In: *Animal Psychophysics,* edited by W. C. Stebbins. Appleton-Century-Crofts, New York.
24. Hunter-Duvar, I. M., and Elliott, D. N. (1972): Effects of intense auditory stimulation: Hearing losses and inner ear changes in the squirrel monkey. *J. Acoust. Soc. Am.*, 52:1181–1192.
25. Hunter-Duvar, I. M., Personal communication.
26. Ward, W. D. and Glorig, A. (1961): A case of firecracker-induced hearing loss. *Laryngoscope,* 71:1590–1596.
27. Mills, J. H., Gengel, R. W., Watson, C. S., and Miller, J. D. (1970): Temporary changes of the auditory system due to exposure to noise for one or two days. *J. Acoust. Soc. Am.*, 48:524–530.
28. Elliott, D. N. (1961): The effect of sensorineural lesions on pitch discrimination in cats. *Ann. Otol. Rhinol. Laryngol.*, 70:582–598.
29. Moody, D. B. (1973): Behavioral studies of noise-induced hearing loss in primates: loudness recruitment. *Adv. Otorhinolaryngol.*, 20:82–101.
30. Melnick, W., and Maves, M. (1974): Asymptotic threshold shift (ATS) in man from 24 hours exposure to continuous noise. *Ann. Otol.,* 83:820–828.
31. Spoendlin, H. (1966): The organization of the cochlear receptor. *Adv. Otorhinolaryngol.*, 13.
32. Ward, W. D., and Duvall, A. J. (1971): Behavioral and ultrastructural correlates of acoustic trauma. *Ann. Otol. Rhinol. Laryngol.*, 80:881–896.
33. Hunter-Duvar, I. M., and Bredberg, G. (1974): Effects of intense auditory stimu-

lation: hearing losses and inner ear changes in the chinchilla. *J. Acoust. Soc. Am.,* 55:795–801.

34. Clark, W. W., Clark, C. S., Moody, D. B., and Stebbins, W. C. (1974): Noise-induced hearing loss in the chinchilla, as determined by a positive-reinforcement technique. *J. Acoust. Soc. Am.,* 56:1201–1209.

35. Ryan, A., and Dallos, P. (1975): Effect of absence of cochlear outer hair cells on behavioral auditory threshold. *Nature,* 253:44–46.

36. Schuknecht, H. F., and Woellner, R. C. (1955): An experimental and clinical study of deafness from lesions of the cochlear nerve. *J. Laryngol.,* 69:75–97.

37. Henderson, D. (1969): Temporal summation of acoustic signals by the chinchilla. *J. Acoust. Soc. Am.,* 46:474–475.

38. Miskolczy-Fodor, F. (1953): Monaural loudness-balance-test and determination of recruitment-degree with short sound-impulses. *Acta Otolaryngol. (Stockh.),* 43:573–595.

39. Harris, J. D., Haines, H. L., and Myers, C. K. (1958): Brief-tone audiometry. *Arch. Otolaryngol.,* 67:699–713.

40. Watson, C. S., and Gengel, R. W. (1969): Signal duration and signal frequency in relation to auditory sensitivity. *J. Acoust. Soc. Am.,* 46:989–997.

41. Broadbent, D. E., and Stephens, S. D. G. (1970): Alternations to threshold measurement in the assessment of hearing. In: *Ciba Foundation Symposium in Sensorineural Hearing Loss,* edited by G. E. W. Wolstenholme and J. Knight, pp. 157–176. Churchill, London.

42. Gengel, R. W. (1973): Temporal effects in frequency discrimination by hearing-impaired listeners. *J. Acoust. Soc. Am.,* 54:11–15.

43. Pedersen, C. B., and Elberling, C. (1972): Temporal integration measured by brief-tone audiometry. *J. Auditory Res.,* 12:279–284.

44. Young, I. M., and Kanofsky, P. (1973): Significance of brief tone audiometry. *J. Auditory Res.,* 13:14–25.

45. Elliott, L. L. (1975): Temporal and masking phenomena in persons with sensorineural loss. *Audiology,* 14:336–353.

46. Jerger, J. F. (1955): Influence of stimulus duration of the pure tone threshold during recovery from auditory fatigue. *J. Acoust. Soc. Am.,* 27:121–124.

47. Hamernik, R. P., Henderson, D., Crossley, J. J., and Salvi, R. J. (1973): Interaction of continuous and impulse noise: audiometric and histological effects. *J. Acoust. Soc. Am.,* 55:117–121.

48. Henderson, D., Hamernik, R. P., and Sitler, R. W. (1974): Audiometric and histological correlates of exposure to 1-msec noise impulses in the chinchilla. *J. Acoust. Soc. Am.,* 56:1210–1221.

49. Henderson, D., Hamernik, R. P., and Sitler, R. W. (1974): Audiometric and anatomical correlates of impulse noise exposure. *Arch. Otolaryngol.,* 99:62–66.

50. Henderson, D., Hamernik, R. P., and Crossley, J. (1974): New data for noise standards. *Laryngoscope,* 84:714–721.

51. Ades, H. W., Trahiotis, C., Kokko-Cunningham, A., and Averbuch, A. (1974): Comparison of hearing thresholds and morphological changes in the chinchilla after exposure to 4 kHz tones. *Acta Otolaryngol. (Stockh.),* 78:192–206.

52. Parker, D. E., and Tubbs, R. L. (1975): Influence of intense noise exposure on masked pure tone thresholds. Paper presented at the 89th meeting of the acoustical society of America, Austin, Texas.

53. Viemeister, N. F. (1972): Intensity discrimination of pulsed sinusoids: The effects of filtered noise. *J. Acoust. Soc. Am.,* 51:1265–1269.

54. deBoer, E., and Bouwmeester, J. (1974): Critical bands and sensorineural loss. *Audiology,* 13:236–259.

55. Pal'gov, V. I., and Tereshchenko, V. N. (1973): Effectiveness of critical bands as indicator of the damage to the auditory system. *Biofizika,* 18:724–730.

56. Simon, G. R. (1963): The critical bandwidth level in recruiting ears and its relation to temporal summation. *J. Auditory Res.,* 3:109–119.

57. Salvi, R. J., Henderson, D., and Hamernik, R. P. (1973): Differential response of

neurons in the cochlear nucleus to TTS-producing tones. Paper presented at the 89th meeting of the Acoustical Society of America at Los Angeles, Calif.

58. Babighian, G., Moushegian, G., and Rupert, A. L. (1975): Central auditory fatigue. *Audiology*, 14:72–83.
59. Kiang, N. Y. S., Moxon, E. C., and Levine, R. A. (1970): Auditory-nerve activity in cats with normal and abnormal cochleas. In: *Ciba Foundation Symposium on Sensorineural Hearing Loss*, edited by G. E. W. Wolstenholme and J. Knight, pp. 241–273. Churchill, London.
60. Jauhiainen, T., Kohonen, A., and Jauhiainen, M. (1972): Combined effect of noise and neomycin on the cochlea. *Acta Otolaryngol. (Stockh.)*, 73:387–390.
61. Kellerhals, B. (1972): Pathogenesis of inner ear lesions in acute acoustic trauma. *Acta Otolaryngol. (Stockh.)*, 73:249–253.
62. Drescher, D. G., and Eldredge, D. H. (1974): Species differences in cochlear fatigue related to acoustic of outer and middle ear of guinea pig and chinchilla. *J. Acoust. Soc. Am.*, 56:929–934.

DISCUSSION

D. Henderson: Although it is true that we see good agreement between inner hair cell (IHC) losses and AER thresholds, we also have behavioral data that show normal, quiet thresholds with large lesions of outer hair cells (OHC). Figure 1 is from J. Hans, D. Henderson, and R. P. Hamernik [*J. Acoust. Soc. Am.* (1975), 57:S41(A)]. The chinchilla was exposed to 50 impulses, 1/min, and we measured its quiet thresholds with 500-msec and 20-msec signals. The middle turn has a loss of both IHC and OHC, while the basal turn is devoid of OHC. The audiogram shows elevated hearing levels in the 1–3 kHz region and normal hearing for high frequencies. The region of shifted thresholds correspond (using the CID map) to areas of the cochlea with missing IHC. We have heard from Spoendlin that, typically, with losses of OHC, there is an accompanying malformation of the IHC stereocilia. The exception to these observations comes from exposure to impulse noise, where he reports OHC lesions with normal IHC.

D. Lipscomb: The question arises as to the audiogram's ability to project to us what has happened in the cochlea. Many of you have seen individuals who report difficulty understanding speech, and yet they have trivial hearing losses and relatively normal discrimination. I submit, that our traditional interpretation of a limited high-frequency loss implying a limited loss in the basal end, may not work in every case. Because we do see enough examples of relatively normal hearing with a good deal of cell damage, there must be some kind of threshold for this effect, and when you reach that threshold, there must be a severe reduction in the ear's ability to handle complex situations, i.e., signal to noise.

D. Johnson: The one thing that I see when I look at animal data for establishing damage risk criteria (DRC) is that there is not enough information to even map the behavioral data of the chinchilla to the human. Unless you can do that, you cannot talk about absolutes and you are limited to generalities.

All animal data neglect taking into account presbycusis, they never worry about the age of the animal.

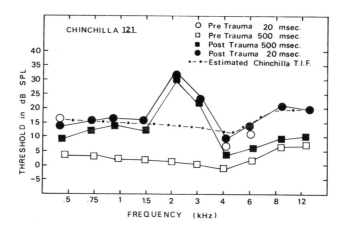

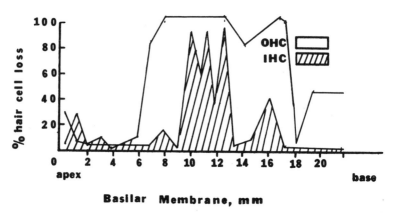

FIG. 1. Pre- and postexposure audiograms and cochleograms for a chinchilla exposed to 50 1-msec A-duration impulses at the rate of 1/min. The thresholds were obtained using shock avoidance technique.

J. Miller: That is one of the reasons for choosing the chinchilla, because it is a long-lived animal, so we don't have to worry about it. But don't think we don't think about it.

C. Trahiotis: Let me respond to the first part. I tend to agree with you, I don't think we should ask for quantitative relationships. Henderson [*J. Acoust. Soc. Am.* (1969), 46:474–475] has shown that temporal integration may be altered in the chinchilla during TTS, as Jerger [*J. Acoust. Soc. Am.* (1955), 27:121–124] also has shown that it may be altered in humans under TTS. What we can get from animal studies is an appreciation of phenomena that are not readily studied in humans and we should not ask for quantitative relations.

D. Johnson: How do you include them in criteria considerations if you don't have accurate numbers?

C. Trahiotis: For one thing, Jerger's data show that we do not want to add together the audiogram industrially obtained using long- and short-duration signals; because it seems clear that, when you use a short-duration signal, you underestimate the threshold shift. This is the type of principle that we can learn from animal data.

W. Ward: What is the alternative to the animal experimentation? We don't have very good data on the effects of noise on people. You don't know what the noise exposure was because you can't control their environment.

G. Price: Certainly one of the great factors regarding the variability between human and animal data is the conductive characteristics of the external and middle ears. Because the main component of impedance in the cochlea is resistive, there is not likely to be a great discrepancy between species in that domain. Consequently, if we paid more attention to what is getting into the cochlea, then I think a lot of the difference between animals and humans will be erased.

C. Trahiotis: If we want to look at data across the species, then it is best that we don't look at only one point. Instead, we look at the data in their totality, i.e., if we cut the data at one point, we can come to one conclusion, if we cut them at another, we can come to a totally different conclusion.

Part V
Epidemiological and Analytical Studies of Noise-Induced Hearing Loss
Introduction

One of the major problems is assessing the effects of noise on human hearing is that there is an infinite variety of possible exposures. Therefore, it becomes impossible to study scientifically each of the possible exposures that people might encounter. It follows that the principal goal of scientific research might be to build a model that will allow us to understand the infinite variety of exposures that can occur. A second fact of the effects of noise on human hearing is the tremendous variability that is observed, with small effects occurring in some people, and large effects occurring in others. It seems to me that many of the chapters in this volume are addressed to one or the other, or to both, of these questions. What kind of a model, however crude, must we have to incorporate the wide variety of exposures that can occur? Why is there such variation in the response to noise in human hearing? What may be some of the causes of that?

Effects of Noise on Hearing, edited by Donald Henderson,
Roger P. Hamernik, Darshan S. Dosanjh, and John H. Mills.
Raven Press, New York © 1976.

Models for Noise-Induced Hearing Loss

J. S. Keeler

University of Waterloo, Waterloo, Ontario, Canada

The principal objective in devising models of noise-induced hearing loss
(NIHL) is to simulate mathematically the hearing loss that a statistically
representative human subject is likely to experience when exposed to noise
of any arbitrary description. In other words, from a description of a noise—
simple or complex, pure-tone or broadband, continuous, intermittent or impulsive, of any duration—the models should generate a list of numbers or a
picture of how an exposed person's hearing loss would develop during exposure and (hopefully) disappear during recovery. It is also desirable to be
able to supply additional data on the subject's noise exposure and hearing
history and to get a prediction of the hearing loss which would be produced
by several years of habitual exposure. Numerous attempts have been made at
solving this difficult problem and revisions and refinements are going on almost
continuously.

The behavior of NIHL models can conveniently be divided into 3 parts:

1. Dependence on the physical parameters of the sound such as sound
   pressure level and spectrum
2. Dependence on the method of measuring the NIHL of the subject
3. Dependence on the temporal pattern of exposure and recovery

This chapter deals almost exclusively with 3, the time-dependent functions.

TYPES OF MODELS

Most of the time-dependent models proposed to date fall into one of 3
categories:

1. A power series in which time and other variables appear in linear,
   quadratic, and higher powered terms
2. Logarithmic expressions where hearing loss is a linear function of
   logarithmic time
3. Exponential expressions in which hearing loss is simulated by the sum
   of two or more exponential terms whose exponents are proportional to
   time

Some excellent examples of power series models have been derived by
Schneider et al. (1), in which hearing loss is stated as a function of "first

measured hearing loss" (FMHL), "time since first audiogram" (TSFA), and the subject's age. Equation (1) is an example of one of the power series models for a "quiet job within a noisy department."

$$\text{HL} = \text{FMHL} + 0.00051134(\text{TSFA})(\text{age})^2 + 1.678(\text{TSFA})(\text{age})/(\text{FMHL})^2$$
$$- 0.036014(\text{TSFA})^2(\text{age})(\text{FMHL}) \tag{1}$$

Logarithmic models have been in use for some time and have proven to be the most popular of the 3 types. An early example, if not the first, proposed by Ward et al. (2), is shown in Eq. (2)

$$\text{TTS}_2 = K[\log(t/1.7)] \tag{2}$$

where TTS_2 is the temporary threshold shift at 4 KHz 2 min after the cessation of t min of exposure. K is a constant that is dependent on the properties of the noise. A great many other models have been devised in which the time dependence is simulated by a factor containing the logarithm of time.

Exponential models were proposed by Keeler (3) to simulate the time dependence of hearing loss during both exposure and recovery conditions. An example appears in Eq. (3)

$$\text{TTS}(t) = \text{TTS}_1(\infty)[1 - e^{-t/\tau_1}] + \text{TTS}_2(\infty)[1 - e^{-t/\tau_2}] \tag{3}$$

where $\text{TTS}(t)$ is the total TTS after t minutes of exposure to noise; $\text{TTS}_1(\infty)$ and $\text{TTS}_2(\infty)$ are 2 constants which depend upon the physical parameters of the noise and the frequency at which hearing loss is measured; and τ_1 and τ_2 are two unequal time constants.

Each of these 3 types of models have strengths and weaknesses, advantages and disadvantages, and it is the primary objective of this chapter to discuss the problems in modeling and to assess the effectiveness of each type of model in handling those problems.

CHARACTERISTICS OF NIHL MODELS

Before discussing the 3 temporal models in detail consider the attributes which a perfect model will possess.

1. First and foremost, it will simulate the buildup of hearing loss during exposure to continuous noise from the inception to the cessation of the noise.

2. It must also simulate the decrease in hearing loss with time during recovery in a quiet environment.

3. The effects of the physical parameters of the noise, such as sound pressure level and spectrum, should be included in a general model in the form of adjustable factors which are functions of these parameters.

4. Because observed hearing loss depends on the frequency at which it is measured the ideal model will also be adaptable to this variable.

5. The simulation must be applicable to changing and intermittent noise

as well as continuous noise. Ideally the model will perform accurately for any temporal pattern without the need for manipulation of parameters and factors.

6. Property 5 should apply for impulsive noise.

7. The model should be mathematically simple enough to be practicable in applications of damage risk criteria and to be helpful in developing an intuitive understanding of NIHL.

At first glance, meeting the requirements of this short list seems to be a relatively simple problem, but recalling some of the difficulties encountered in applying models to real situations illustrates some of the ramifications.

At one time, a fairly popular hypothesis was that exposure to "equal energy" would produce equal hearing loss. This idea, if valid, would simplify the model quite considerably because it would require only that the noise be averaged (no matter what its temporal pattern) and applied to a very simple graph or list or algebraic function to translate it into hearing loss. It has been shown by a number of researchers that the "equal energy" rule is not valid. McRobert and Ward (4,5) showed that the "equal energy" did not apply for impulses, and Ward (6) indicated that it was not valid for intermittent noise when he concluded that there is a cumulative effect which delays recovery when the ear is repeatedly exposed. Rintelman's evidence (7) also refutes the "equal energy" rule when he concludes that continuous exposure produces significantly more TTS than does intermittent exposure. As a consequence of this strong evidence against "equal energy," the NIHL model, to be general, must take into account the effects of discontinuous exposure in some other way. As we shall see this requirement has far-reaching consequences on the choice of the model functions.

A number of other aspects of the experimental work on hearing loss must be kept in mind. For example, the majority of researchers have used sound pressure level (SPL) to describe the noise, but recently Cohen et al. (8) and Flugrath (9) have shown that A-weighted sound level [dB(A)] would be better. Realizing that dB(A) is a crude simulation of loudness, that the perception of loudness is a function of hair cell activity, and that hearing loss is related to hair cell damage caused by stimulation, one can easily conclude that hearing loss probably correlates better with sound level than with SPL.

The most important function of a model is to simulate the permanent loss (NIPTS) likely to be produced by a given exposure. Because well-documented data on NIPTS and the noise which caused it is sparse (and hopefully always will be) most models have been based on observations of temporary loss (NITTS). There is some doubt [Cohen (10) and Moller (11)] that the assumed equivalence of NIPTS after 10 years and NITTS after 1 day is valid, which implies that the model may have to be constructed in two sections —one for NITTS which is reversible, and the other for NIPTS which is irreversible. Perhaps this form of sectioning in the model will take account of the suggestions [e.g., Melnick (12)] that there are different mechanisms for threshold shift due to short loud exposures and for chronic exposures at lower levels. Another factor of which the model designer must be aware is the need for statistically representative data, because of the variability of observations. He must also adapt to the choice of test frequencies made by the experimenters —3 kHz, 4 kHz, or the average at 500, 1, and 2 kHz or whatever is used. Because preexisting hearing loss does have some effect on the development of additional loss, e.g., Ward (13), the model must either take this into account or it must be restricted to those cases with no previous loss.

Consistent with the objective that the model give some intuitive understanding of hearing loss to the otologist and acoustical scientist is a desire that the output be expressed in terms which the unfortunate layman who has the hearing loss can understand. Threshold shift in decibels has a very clear meaning to the specialist, but its meaning is obscure to the layman. It would be a simple matter to translate threshold shift in decibels into percent loss of loudness perception at threshold. That is, a 10-dB loss would become a 50% loss, 20 dB would be a 75% loss, and so on. Certainly it would give laymen a much better understanding of the serious consequences of excessive noise-exposure.

These then are the important specifications for a model and some of their ramifications which make the problem of modeling hearing loss so difficult. Consider how well each of the 3 types of models listed above satisfies the requirements.

ALGEBRAIC FUNCTIONS FOR MODELING NIHL

Power Series

Power series of the form shown in Eq. (1) are derived by multiple linear regression analysis from experimental data, a procedure which is relatively straightforward with numerical techniques on a digital computer. The series have the advantage that they can be made to fit almost any data to any degree of accuracy, simply by providing a large enough number of different terms in the relevant variables and computing the appropriate coefficients. The example chosen models hearing loss on a coarse time scale—years—and applies only to a particular class of noise environment—"quiet job within a noisy department." Other equations are needed for other environments. But the same technique could be used to generate models for finer time scales—minutes, for example—which include terms containing the physical and temporal properties of the noise.

Before devising such a model, first consider some of its shortcomings. Even with its restricted scope Eq. (1) is algebraically too complex to generate a qualitative image of the dependence of hearing loss on FMHL, age, or TSFA, nor does it contribute to the understanding of the physiological processes involved. If additional variables were added to make it more general —e.g., SPL, duration of exposure, duration of recovery, and test frequency— the descriptive meaning would be even more obscure, and its application would probably require the use of a computer.

Although the power series can be a very accurate model, its usefulness is restricted to situations where the number of variables can be limited, such as those where long service employees are exposed to a small number of different noise environments. Because of its complexity, the power series is not likely to be suitable for a general model of hearing loss as a function of time.

Logarithmic Functions

For scientists who have worked in the field of acoustics and noise the logarithmic function is an old friend appearing in the definition of SPL and the decibel,

$$\text{SPL} = 20 \log \left(\frac{p}{p_r}\right) \text{dB}$$

where p is the sound pressure and p_r is a reference sound pressure (approximately the threshold of normal hearing at 1,000 Hz). When used to model the hearing loss versus time relationship, the logarithmic function appears in the form shown in Eq. (2) or in some variation of that equation. One of the attractive features of the log function is the fact that it is a straight line when plotted on a logarithmic time scale, and the slope of the line is the constant K (see Fig. 1A). To take account of the effects of different levels of noise and different duty cycles, it is very convenient to be able to adjust the slope of the line (steeper slope for the more injurious exposures); and the log function appears to satisfy the requirement of being easy to apply.

But, attractive as these characteristics are, the logarithmic model has some very serious deficiencies. In the first place, what does "logarithmic time" mean? Logarithmic time has no intuitive meaning. A "50-hr" week is 50 linear hours not 1.7 (=log 50) logarithmic hours. And two "50-hr" weeks are twice as much, namely, 100 linear hours, not 2.0 (=log 100) logarithmic hours. Time is not perceived in logarithmic hours and to get around the problem linear hours or minutes are often added to the time scale in Fig. 1A. But this only creates a new difficulty because it distorts the picture the figure gives us of what is actually happening. Consider the graph of the logarithmic function against linear time (see Fig. 1B). This shows that the logarithmic function increases at a continuously decreasing rate. But the rate of increase never drops to zero; that is, the logarithmic function increases without limit as time goes on. In modeling hearing loss with a logarithmic function, this would imply that a subject exposed to continuous noise would lose his hearing without limit. Even when the loss makes the noise inaudible to him the loss still

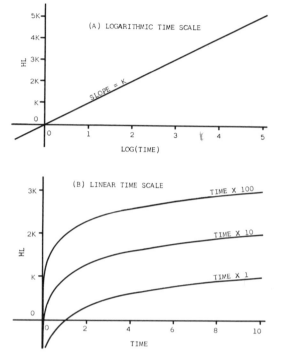

FIG. 1. Logarithmic model of hearing loss during exposure to noise. HL = K log (time).

continues to increase according to the model. However, a more serious shortcoming by far is the fact that the logarithmic function does not coincide with the starting point of hearing loss, i.e., hearing loss is zero after zero exposure. The logarithmic function is negative infinity at this point. One easy way to get around this anomaly is to add 1 unit to time and to change the function to

$$HL = K \log (t + 1)$$

Another way, the more prevalent way it turns out, is simply to ignore the anomaly. This is easy enough to justify for single-level exposures, but as we shall see it creates difficulties when the sound level is changing.

The logarithmic function also provides a deceptively simple model of the decrease in hearing loss during the recovery mode using an equation of the form

$$HL = -K \log (t) + C$$

Here C is a constant representing the hearing loss at the start of recovery [or more correctly when $\log(t) = 0$], and $-K$ represents a negative slope which many studies suggest is dependent on the way in which the original hearing loss was achieved. Figure 2A shows this function plotted on a

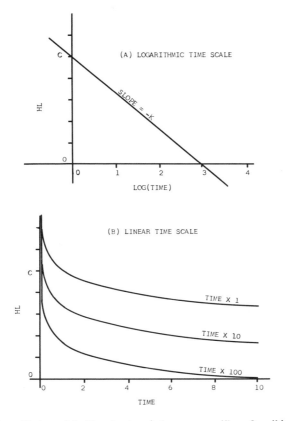

FIG. 2. Logarithmic model of hearing loss during recovery. HL = C — K log (time).

logarithmic time scale, and 2B on a linear time scale. The same strengths and weaknesses of the logarithmic function appear again in the recovery model. It cannot be made to coincide with the starting value C unless the time scale is arbitrarily adjusted by 1; and if recovery is allowed to continue arbitrarily long, any desired negative hearing loss can be produced. Nevertheless, the straight-line relationship in Fig. 2A is appealing because of its simplicity even if it is not (and cannot be) an accurate model for all values of time.

Now consider the application of the logarithmic model to hearing loss caused by alternating exposure and recovery periods that is intermittent noise. To give a pictorial result, the alternating periods are assumed to be 10 min long and the results are plotted on a linear time scale in Fig. 3A over 2 complete cycles. Note the discontinuities which occur at each change in exposure condition. Also note that if a logarithmic time scale had been used, the log time origin and scale would have to be reestablished at each change because

$$\log (t - 10) \neq \log (t) - \log (10)$$

Ward (6) showed that the log function predicts faster recovery from exposure to noise when a subject is exposed to additional noise than when the subject is placed in a quiet environment. The anomaly is partly due to the discontinuities at zero time, but it is also related to another deficiency of the logarithmic model. A number of studies have shown that recovery from hearing loss is dependent, not only on the amount of hearing loss, but also on the way in which it was produced—e.g., by continuous, intermittent, or impulsive noise. Threshold shift modeled by the logarithmic function contains no information about the exposure pattern, and even if it did, the logarithmic recovery function is not set up to handle it.

In summary the logarithmic function provides an excellent simulation of NIHL due to continuous noise except at very small and very large values of time; and with similar limitations it is also a good model for recovery. Because it can be represented graphically by straight lines on a logarithmic time scale it is easy to manipulate with pencil and straight edge. Qualitative comprehension of the model appears to be simple except for the problem in perceiving logarithmic time: however, microscopic physiological processes do not inherently lead to logarithmic functions of time and consequently the logarithmic model cannot assist a qualitative understanding of the mechanisms of hearing loss. But the most serious deficiency of the logarithmic

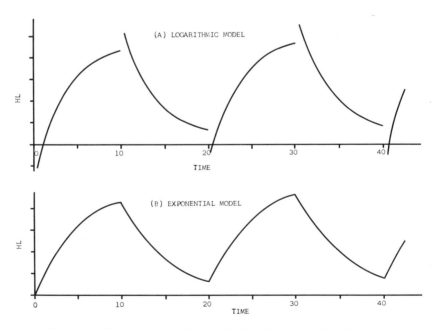

FIG. 3. Logarithmic and exponential models of hearing loss for intermittent noise.

model is its inability to cope with discontinuous and changing noise without the aid of adjustments to slopes and magnitudes by an expert operator. And as if these deficiencies were not enough, it is impossible to simulate a logarithmic function of time electrically except over a limited range. The logarithmic function is accurate and easy to use for simple exposure and recovery patterns, but not for more complex acoustic environments. Logarithmic time distorts the intuitive understanding of hearing loss and generates absurd results under some conditions.

Exponential Functions

In the field of acoustics the most familiar exponential function of time is the relationship describing the decay of sound pressure in a reverberant room,

$$p(t) = p(0)e^{-6.9t/RT}$$

where $p(t)$ is the sound pressure at time t seconds after the sound source is turned off and RT is the reverberation time in seconds. It is not a coincidence that this should be an exponential because wherever the rate of change of a variable is proportional to the variable (or its difference from a constant) the variable follows an exponential function of time. That is, if

$$\frac{dy}{dt} = ky$$

then

$$y(t) = Ce^{kt}$$

where C is the initial value and k is a constant which is negative in a degenerative, unexcited system. k has the dimensions of inverse time and, because it is negative, it is usually replaced by

$$k = -\frac{1}{\tau}$$

where τ is a time constant; i.e.,

$$y(t) = Ce^{-t/\tau}$$

Figure 4A shows this function graphically. Its similarity to the recovery curve for hearing loss is evident, and perhaps this suggests that the rate of recovery of hair cell activity is proportional to the number of unrecovered hair cells remaining—a not unreasonable postulate.

Plotted in this way, with both variables on a linear scale, the exponential does not have the apparent linear simplicity of the logarithmic function; however, if the dependent variable y were plotted on a logarithmic scale the function would become a straight line. Because this distorts the picture which the graph provides and complicates its application to all but very simple NIHL problems (just as it does for the logarithmic function) it is not recommended that a logarithmic scale be used.

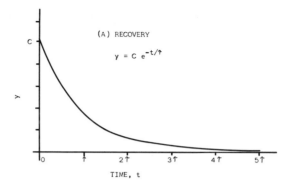

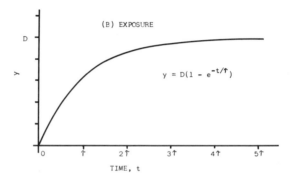

FIG. 4. Exponential recovery and exposure functions.

Compare some other properties of Fig. 4A with the logarithmic function. At the starting point $(t = 0)$ the exponential is finite $(y = C)$. In other words the exponential can be made to fit the hearing loss curve from the start of recovery. Also note that the exponential approaches zero for large values of time; it does not go negative.

The exponential function can also be used for increasing asymptotic functions as well, such as the growth of hearing loss during exposure. In this case the rate of change of the variable is proportional to its difference from a constant, i.e.,

$$\frac{dy}{dt} = k(D - y)$$

where D is the asymptote. This gives the function

$$y(t) = D[1 - e^{-t/\tau}]$$

which is shown graphically in Fig. 4B.

Characteristics corresponding to those for the recovery function also appear in the exposure function. In particular it starts at the starting point ($y = 0$) and it approaches a limiting value for large t.

To compare the behavior of exponential and logarithmic functions apply the exponentials in Fig. 4 to the cycled exposures in Fig. 3 (10 min on, 10 min off). Although the exponential and the logarithmic are equally suitable over most of the range, the exponential has the important advantage of being continuous no matter what the exposure pattern. The logarithmic function, on the other hand, has a discontinuity each time the exposure conditions are changed. This may not be serious if the analysis using mathematical models is done manually where the operator can make an appropriate adjustment (i.e., omission) of data after each change; but where the analysis or simulation is done automatically (for example, in a noise dose meter or in a computer) the discontinuities make the logarithmic functions impractical.

To complete the comparison of logarithms and exponentials consider the 3 functions shown in Fig. 5A on a log(time) scale and in Fig. 5B on a linear time scale. The 3 functions are: A, a linear function; B, an exponential function; and C, a logarithmic function. From Fig. 5A one could incorrectly conclude that (i) the linear function increases at an increasing rate; (ii) the exponential is not asymptotic; and (iii) the logarithmic function is finite for

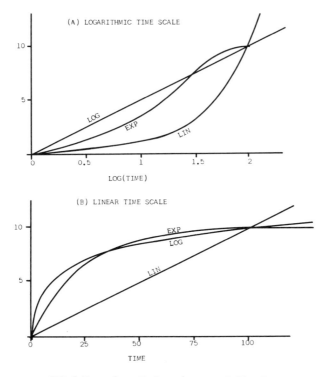

FIG. 5. Linear, logarithmic, and exponential functions.

all finite values of time. None of these conclusions would be correct as is evident in Fig. 5B where the time scale is linear. For this reason, logarithmic time scales must be avoided whenever the data are to be interpreted descriptively. Because exponential functions are finite and continuous for all values of time, and because they are used with a linear time scale which does not need to be changed with each switch from exposure to recovery mode or vice versa, they can simulate hearing loss continuously for constant steady exposure or for intermittent cycled exposure.

Two important questions about exponential functions remain to be answered. Can they be made to fit experimental data? Does the model of the exposure mode carry any information about the way in which hearing loss was produced which would affect the functioning of the recovery mode? The first question has been partly answered by Keeler (3,14) and by Botsford (15) who were able to fit exponential functions to a variety of exposure and recovery data for continuous noise. For other noise environments, including intermittent noise, further supporting evidence is given in the next section. To answer the second question consider Eq. (3), which is an exponential model of the exposure function. It contains 2 terms each of which is an exponential function. The 2 terms cannot be combined into 1 except for specific values of t, because the time constants τ_1 and τ_2 are not equal, and consequently the terms will develop at different rates. As a result the values of the 2 terms will depend on the stimulating noise and also on its temporal pattern. The same total hearing loss can be produced by any number of combinations of the 2 component parts, and, by preserving the value of the parts, information about the temporal pattern of the noise as well as its level and duration is carried over to the recovery phase. Examples of this aspect of exponential models are given in the next section.

In summary, exponential models have the disadvantage of being slightly more difficult to apply to simple exposure–recovery patterns but they overcome the many weaknesses in the logarithmic models. In particular they are finite for all values of t and do not have discontinuities at changes in exposure conditions. As will be seen they automatically fit a wide variety of exposure patterns by retaining information in two or more components which do not combine. The exponential is a commonly occurring relationship in natural phenomena and an exponential model could give some insight into the physiological processes involved in hearing loss.

EXPONENTIAL MODELS FOR NIHL

In the original exponential models (3,14) the dependent variable used was $TTS_2(t)$, the temporary threshold shift 2 min after the cessation of t min of exposure. This is the variable most frequently measured by experimenters and seemed like a logical choice. However, $TTS_2(t)$ does not exist during exposure, it only appears after 2 min of recovery, and for this reason it is not

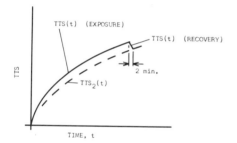

FIG. 6. Relationship between TTS (*t*) and TTS₂(*t*).

suitable for a general exposure model. Instead, TTS(t) is used in the model, which, although it may not take on the exact value of TTS after t min of exposure, it does take on values which decay to the correct value of TTS₂ after 2 min of recovery. Figure 6 shows the revision.

Also it has become apparent that 2 components are not sufficient to model the long-term effects or the response to intermittent noise. Accordingly, the models proposed are as follows:

$$\text{TTS}(t) = \text{TTS}_f(\infty)[1 - e^{-t/\tau_{ef}}] + \text{TTS}_m(\infty)[1 - e^{-t/\tau_{em}}]$$
$$+\text{TTS}_s(\infty)[1 - e^{-t/\tau_{es}}] \quad (4)$$

for exposure starting at $t = 0$, and

$$\text{TTS}(t) = \text{TTS}_f(0)e^{-t/\tau_{rf}} + \text{TTS}_m(0)e^{-t/\tau_{rm}} + \text{TTS}_s(0)e^{-t/\tau_{rs}} \quad (5)$$

for recovery starting at $t = 0$.

The meaning of the various symbols is as follows:

TTS(t) is the temporary threshold shift after t min of exposure in Eq. (4) or after t min of recovery of Eq. (5)
The subscripts "e" and "r" refer to "exposure" and "recovery," while "f," "m," and "s" refer to the "fast," "medium," and "slow" components
The TTS(∞) factors are the limiting values of the 3 components during exposure—their actual values depend upon the characteristics of the noise and the frequency at which TTS is measured
The τ factors are the time constants where $\tau_{ef} < \tau_{em} < \tau_{es}$ and $\tau_{rf} < \tau_{rm} < \tau_{rs}$
The TTS(0) factors represent the TTS at the beginning of recovery

Written algebraically the models give the impression of being more complex than they really are, but shown graphically (see Fig. 7) the significance of the various terms becomes apparent. The "fast" term reaches its limiting value very quickly during exposure. Similarly, the "medium" term changes more slowly and the "slow" term even more slowly. By keeping the three terms separate the shape of the recovery curve depends not only on the TTS at the end of exposure, but also on the way in which the TTS was produced, a necessary attribute in modeling intermittent exposure.

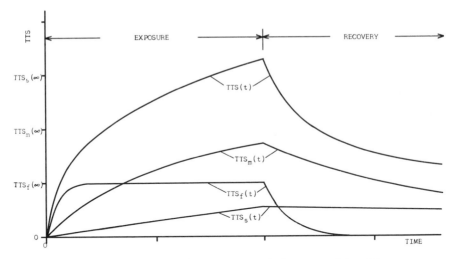

FIG. 7. Fast, medium, and slow components in the exponential model.

If a subject is exposed to a noise for T_e min, returns to a quiet environment for T_r min, then returns to the noise for T_e min, and so on, alternating exposure and recovery, it can be shown that after k cycles of exposure and recovery the "fast" component of TTS derived from repeated applications of Eqs. (4) and (5) is given by

$$TTS_f = \frac{TTS_f(\infty)[1 - e^{-T_e/\tau_{ef}}]e^{-T_r/\tau_{rf}}[e^{-k(T_e/\tau_{ef} + T_r/\tau_{rf})} - 1]}{[e^{(T_e/\tau_{ef} + T_r/\tau_{rf})} - 1]} \quad (6)$$

Corresponding expressions exist for the "medium" and "slow" components where the subscripts "f" in Eq. (6) are replaced by "m" or "s." As before, the total TTS is the sum of the three components TTS_f, TTS_m, and TTS_s. This appears to be a very formidable relationship, but in fact, once the values of all the parameters are known, the calculation of TTS for any number of cycles becomes simple arithmetic.

The key to the success of the exponential model is the choice of the values of the parameters which gives the best fit to experimental data. The 6 time constants are characteristics of the ear. They are independent of the noise environment causing the TTS, whether it is continuous, changing, or intermittent. However, the values of the time constants may be dependent upon the frequency or frequencies at which TTS is measured. On the other hand, the 3 limiting TTS values, $TTS_f(\infty)$, $TTS_m(\infty)$, and $TTS_s(\infty)$, depend on the physical parameters of the noise and also on the frequency at which TTS is measured.

On the basis of existing data it is unlikely that values for the parameters, or even relationships from which these values can be computed, can be devised for all possible conditions. Some experimenters measure TTS at several frequencies and take the average, while others do their measurements at only 1 frequency. Some experimenters use sound pressure level, in dB, and others use A-weighted sound level in dBA to describe the broadband noise used to induce hearing loss. Whether it is practical or even desirable to take into account all the possible variations in noise parameters and measuring conditions remains to be seen. In any event the models proposed do simulate the time dependence of TTS for any exposure pattern, steady and continuous, or intermittent and changing. They conform to the concept of asymptotic TTS and could be made to simulate permanent loss by the inclusion of an irreversible term with large time constant in the exposure equation only.

Application of the Exponential Models

To test the validity of Eqs. (4), (5), and (6) they may be compared with observed hearing loss under a variety of conditions reported in the literature. Some very useful data for this purpose are given by Ward (6). He exposed subjects to a variety of continuous and intermittent sounds and observed the buildup of TTS_2 during exposure and the decrease during recovery. In one series, subjects were exposed to "half-octave" noise in the 1,400 to 2,000 Hz band and TTS_2 was measured at 3 kHz. To simulate subjective response to 3 kHz the time constants in the exponential models are set at the following values:

$\tau_{ef} = 5$ min, $\tau_{rf} = 10$ min, $\tau_{em} = 47$ min, $\tau_{rm} = 100$ min, $\tau_{es} = 1,000$ min, $\tau_{rs} = 1,000$ min.

Sound pressure levels of 85 and 95 dB were used by Ward and the model parameters which correspond are:

$TTS_f(\infty) = 4.63$, $TTS_m(\infty) = 9.15$, and $TTS_s(\infty) = 15.30$ for 85 dB; and
$TTS_f(\infty) = 7.26$, $TTS_m(\infty) = 14.36$, and $TTS_s(\infty) = 24.0$ for 95 dB.

It is worth noting in passing first that the ratios of the fast, medium, and slow components are all the same for both levels; and second that the limiting values will be zero for a sound pressure level of 67.4 dB if the relationship is linear.

In 1 experiment subjects were exposed to 85 dB continuous sound for 8 hr. For these conditions the exponential models in Eqs. (4) and (5) take the following form:

$$TTS(t) = 4.63[1 - e^{-t/5}] + 9.15[1 - e^{-t/47}] + 15.30[1 - e^{-t/1,000}] \quad (7)$$

and

$$TTS_2(t) = 4.63[1 - e^{-t/5}]e^{-2/10} + 9.15[1 - e^{-t/47}]e^{-2/100}$$
$$+ 15.30[1 - e^{-t/1,000}]e^{-2/1,000} \quad (8)$$

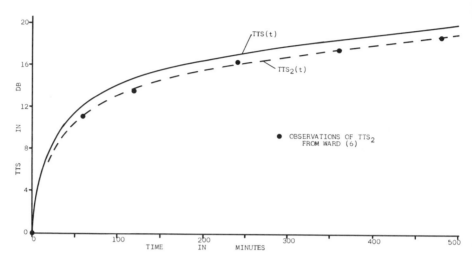

FIG. 8. Exponential model of exposure to 85 dB continuous noise.

To compare the model with the observations, Eqs. (7) and (8) and the measured values of TTS$_2$ are plotted in Fig. 8. Good agreement is apparent.

In another experiment the 85 dB noise was cycled 5 sec on and 5 sec off for 8 hr. Here the model for cycled exposure, Eq. (6), becomes

$$TTS = 3.10[1 - e^{-0.025k}] + 6.23[1 - e^{-0.00261k}] + 7.65[1 - e^{-0.000167k}] \quad (9)$$

for k cycles of exposure. This equation, the corresponding equation for TTS$_2$ and experimental observations are shown in Fig. 9. Again the agreement is good.

Some experiments were done with the louder sound, 95 dB, at various duty cycles. The predictions of the model and the experimental observations

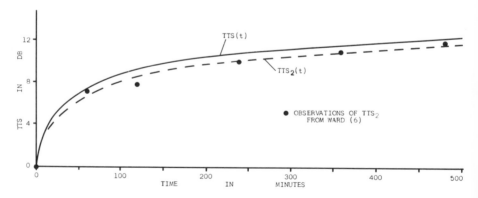

FIG. 9. Exponential model of exposure to 85 dB intermittent noise (5 sec on, 5 sec off).

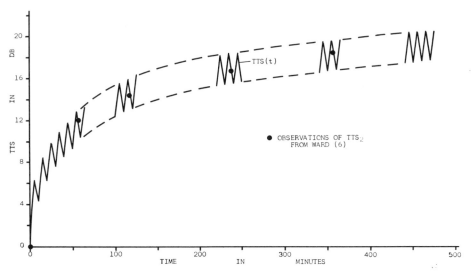

FIG. 10. Exponential model of exposure to 95 dB intermittent noise (5 min on, 5 min off).

for a 5-min on–5-min off pattern are shown in Fig. 10, whereas Fig. 11 shows results for a 10-min on–5-min off pattern.

It is interesting and perhaps informative to observe how fast, medium, and slow components develop during cycled exposure. Figure 12 shows the 3

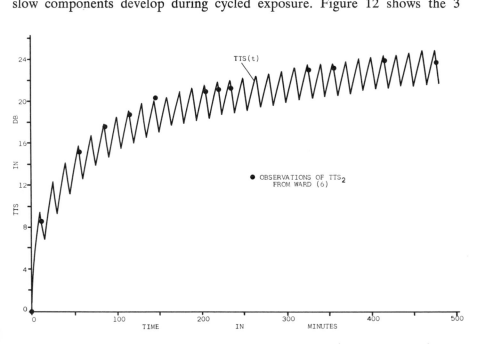

FIG. 11. Exponential model of exposure to 95 dB intermittent noise (10 min on, 5 min off).

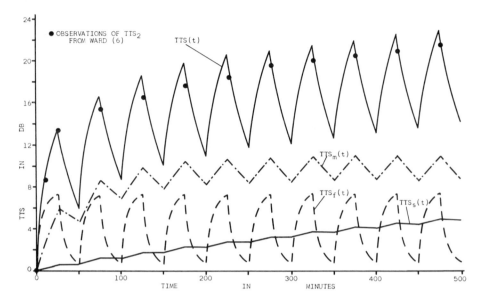

FIG. 12. Exponential model of exposure to 95 dB intermittent noise (25 min on, 25 min off).

components and the total TTS for a 25-min on–250-min off pattern, as well as Ward's experimental observations. Notice how the fast component very quickly takes on a regular pattern while the pattern of the medium component does not stabilize for about 25 min of exposure. By comparison

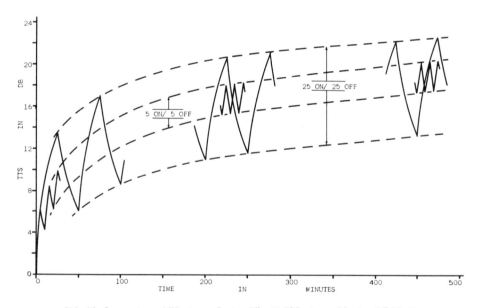

FIG. 13. Comparison of "5 min on, 5 min off" with "25 min on, 25 min off," 95 dB.

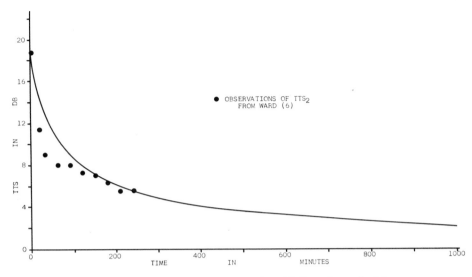

FIG. 14. Exponential model of recovery from 85 dB continuous for 8 hr.

the slow component continues to increase even after 8 hr of exposure and at this point accounts for the continuing upward drift of the total TTS.

Figure 10 (5-min on–5-min off) and Fig. 12 (25-min on–25-min off) each represents a 50% duty cycle for the same noise, and it is interesting to compare the curves for total TTS. This appears in Fig. 13. The maximum

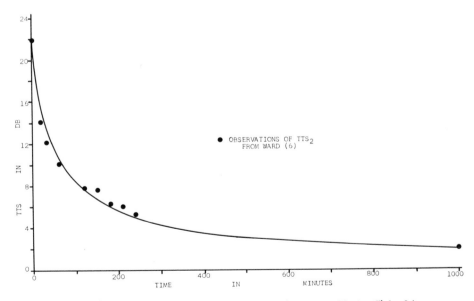

FIG. 15. Exponential model of recovery from 95 dB (25 min on, 25 min off) for 8 hr.

TTS and TTS$_2$ are both higher for the 25-min pattern, which agrees with experimental observations. But the average TTS (which is controlled largely by the slow component) is less for the 25-min pattern than it is for the 10-min pattern. Since the fast and medium components decay more quickly in recovery this raises the question of whether or not the short cycle is a greater hazard rather than the other way around as TTS$_2$ would predict. It would be interesting experimentally to compare residual TTS's after a recovery period greater than $4\tau_{rm}$ (400 min) when nearly all the fast and medium components would have disappeared.

In a sense comparison with observations for cycled exposure does test the model's validity for recovery as well as for exposure, because each contains a recovery period; however, it would be well to test it for long recovery periods as well. Two comparisons, shown in Figs. 14 and 15 confirm the validity of the model for long recovery.

CONCLUSIONS

Three types of models for noise-induced hearing loss have been examined—power series, logarithmic and exponential functions. No one of them is unequivocally the best for all applications—each has advantages and disadvantages.

Power series can be made to fit experimental data very accurately. They are most suitable for applications where the number and range of variables is limited, but not for a general model. They are of little value in explaining NIHL in qualitative terms.

On the other hand logarithmic functions can provide more general models easily applied to simple noise patterns. Graphically, they can give an intuitive understanding of the growth and decay of hearing loss, but subjective conclusions based on graphs employing logarithmic time are often incorrect. Serious weaknesses of the logarithmic models are their discontinuities for changing noise environments and their inability to retain information on the temporal patterns of exposure which affect the recovery process.

Exponential models are the most accurate and the most versatile for general applications. Notation is more complex than for logarithmic functions and graphical application to simple exposure patterns is more tedious. But the exponential function is fundamental to organic processes as a result of which exponential models can give some insight into the physiological processes involved in NIHL. In addition they have been shown to simulate accurately response to complex exposure patterns and it is unlikely they can be manipulated to generate absurd results.

REFERENCES

1. Schneider, E. J., Mutchler, J. E., Hoyle, H. R., Ode, E. H., and Holder, B. B. (1970): Progression of hearing loss from industrial noise exposures. *J. Am. Ind. Hyg. Assoc.*, 31(3):368–376.

2. Ward, W. D., Glorig, A., and Sklar, D. L. (1958): Dependence of temporary threshold shift at 4 Kc on intensity and time. *J. Acoust. Soc. Am.,* 30:944–954.
3. Keeler, J. S. (1968): Compatible exposure and recovery functions for temporary threshold shift—Mechanical and electrical models. *J. Sound Vib.,* 7(2):220–235.
4. McRobert, H., and Ward, W. D. (1972): Temporary threshold shift from impulses. *J. Acoust. Soc. Am.,* 52:130.
5. McRobert, H., and Ward, W. D. (1973): Damage-risk criteria: The trading relation between intensity and the number of nonreverberant impulses. *J. Acoust. Soc. Am.,* 53(5):1297–1300.
6. Ward, W. D. (1970): Temporary threshold shift and damage-risk criteria for intermittent noise exposures. *J. Acoust. Soc. Am.,* 48(2):561–574.
7. Rintelmann, W. F., Lindberg, R. F., and Smitley, E. K. (1972): Temporary threshold shift and recovery patterns from two types of rock and roll music presentation. *J. Acoust. Soc. Am.,* 51(4):1249–1255.
8. Cohen, A., Anticaglia, J. R., and Carpenter, P. L. (1972): Temporary threshold shift in hearing from exposure to different noise spectra at equal dBA levels. *J. Acoust. Soc. Am.,* 51(2):503–507.
9. Flugrath, J. M. (1972): Temporary threshold shift and permanent threshold shift due to rock and roll music. *J. Acoust. Soc. Am.,* 51:151.
10. Cohen, A. (1973): Some general reactions to Kryter's paper "Impairment to Hearing from Exposure to Noise." *J. Acoust. Soc. Am.,* 53(5):1235–1236.
11. Moller, A. R. (1975): Noise as a Health Hazard. *Ambio.,* 4(1):6–13.
12. Melnick, W. (1974): Human temporary threshold shift from 16-hour noise exposures. *Arch. Otolaryngol,* 100:180–189.
13. Ward, W. D. (1971): Presbycusis, sociocusis and occupational noise-induced hearing loss. *Proc. R. Soc. Med.,* 64:200–203.
14. Keeler, J. S. (1967): Predicting temporary threshold shift. Audiology Symposium, Inst. Sound and Vibration Research, Southampton, England, July 1967.
15. Botsford, J. H. (1968): Theory of TTS. Invited Paper, 75th meeting, *Acoust. Soc. Am.,* in Ottawa, Ontario, Canada.

DISCUSSION

J. Saunders: Let's take, for example, the ATS growth that was reported today by Jack Mills. If we applied your exponential model to these curves, and assuming we came up with three components indicating a fast, slow, and medium process, is the implication that there are three biological mechanisms that underlie the empirically obtained growth function?

J. Keeler: I don't know enough about the biology to say whether or not it is true, but I suggest that it may be. One more comment on Mills' data; these models that I have shown you have the same terms for both recovery and growth, which implies, of course, that the process is temporary. One way that one could model permanent threshold shift is to include a term in the exponential functions that does not correspond to the recovery functions.

J. Botsford: Does the time constant of these three exponential components change with noise level or pattern, or is it the same time constant for each always, indicating it is always the same process?

J. Keeler: I expect the time constant will be the same for a given species, provided you use the same technique for measuring the hearing loss.

Effects of Noise on Hearing, edited by Donald Henderson, Roger P. Hamernik, Darshan S. Dosanjh, and John H. Mills. Raven Press, New York © 1976.

Characteristics of Occupational Noise-Induced Hearing Loss

D. W. Robinson

National Physical Laboratory, Teddington, England

To examine the characteristics of this induced phenomenon we must consider 3 aspects—the biological effect itself, the physical agents producing it, and the relations between the two. The relevant physical parameters are easy to identify, namely, the spectral and temporal character of the noise, its absolute level, and its gross duration. On the biological side, the only accessible measure is the audiogram; but here, in addition to the noise, numerous intervening factors also operate, all of which tend to obscure the principal relationships. In an industrial context, should we assume that all the significant noise is of occupational origin and that, if it is not, the remainder is not the responsibility of the industry and should somehow be subtracted out? General acoustic wear and tear on the organs of the internal ear, or sociocusis, in greater or lesser degree is a reality of modern life. As far as can be gauged, the ear has no means of discriminating between one sort of sound and another as regards physiological damage, so that neglect of nonoccupational noise is tantamount to a straightforward underestimation of the accumulated noise dose. Here, then, at the simplest level of consideration is the possibility of quantitative error, perhaps significant at the lower end of the occupational noise range. The uncertainty is clearly greater if, in addition, there has been a history of exposure to specific acoustic episodes, such as the use of firearms. The difficulty in both these cases is that one does not know the quantity of noise involved, a practical rather than an intrinsic limitation but no less intractable for that. We can circumvent it only by declining to study persons who have had a significant history of extraneous noise exposure, and hope that the statistics are not distorted thereby.

With other intervening factors we are in still greater difficulty. Audiometric changes due to age, chronic disease, or the side effects of drugs, are simply not knowable in isolation, since a person cannot live his life twice over with and without these incidents. There is no way round this difficulty save recourse to hypothesis. Otherwise, we must abandon the possibility of describing in any degree of specificity the causal relationships between noise exposure and threshold shift, and rely simply on observational data.

Individual susceptibility to the audiometric effects of age, noise, and the combination, not to mention the extraneous factors, is well known to vary.

One could say, with justification, that the most striking characteristic is indeed this very variability and it is this which arouses difficulties and controversy when we resort, of necessity, to hypothesis. Thus, it would be quite simple to test whether presbycutic and noise-induced permanent threshold shifts (NIPTS) were additive if all ears responded more or less equally to similar treatment, but they do not. Nevertheless, the variability is not wholly haphazard, but may be described as well-structured with highly variable parameters in such a way that the processes can be rather precisely formulated in a statistical framework while being quite unpredictable in individual cases. This, at any rate, seems to be the picture for noise-induced hearing loss (NIHL) and age effects. The same cannot, unfortunately, be said for the incidental factors, or pathological overlay, which represent "noise in the system," transmission loss, and various distortions. Study of cause–effect relations in the occupational context is therefore made more explicit by eliminating subjects whose medical history is suspect. There is, of course, a legitimate question as to whether or not the results then tell the whole story.

A similar question arises with the index used to characterize hearing loss. Audiometry provides a measurement comparable in scientific precision with noise measurement, permitting the successful derivation of relationships to noise exposure. But these are held by some authorities, such as Atherley and Noble (1), to miss the vital point. Direct determination of the effect of noise on hearing in terms of capability for speech communication, or by a quantitative assessment of social handicap, has a relevance that the audibility of pure tones clearly has not. Unfortunately, this is not matched by precision of measurement, and the relation to noise exposure becomes more tenuous and less useful as a practical tool of hearing conservation.

PRINCIPLES OF INVESTIGATION

In approaching these questions, investigators should declare their interest, for identity of results cannot be expected if the aims are dissimilar, and misinterpretations can arise. At one pole of methodology, the characteristics of NIHL could be stated simply by its incidence, by counting heads in various industries and noting the proportions of employed persons having certain levels of hearing, as a function of the length of their employment. The predictive power of the results outside the particular industry studied is virtually nil. A more general approach recognizes that it is the noise which is implicated rather than the industry or process. Scope for controversy remains, however, as to whether investigation should be pursued in a clean form, with overlaying factors ruthlessly eliminated, or by taking subjects more or less as one finds them.

Burns and I (2) adopted the parametric approach to obtain a data field covering a wide range of exposure times, noise levels, and frequency spectra, with rigid subject selection, and it paid handsome dividends in revealing structured relationships. The results have been misunderstood in some quarters, because their undiscerning application suggests smaller threshold shifts than those reported elsewhere. Quite naturally so, because we went to great trouble to weed out other hearing loss where it was known or suspected to exist, but the discrepancies are more apparent than real. Also, the discovery of the structure, which was difficult enough anyway, would probably have been impossible if we had allowed other hearing imperfections to remain in the system. Others following us, for example, Scheiblechner (3), with the benefit of hindsight, have criticized the particular treatment of the data we adopted. Elsewhere I have been accused of conjuring mathematical functions out of thin air but this stems from a misunderstanding of the curve-fitting task. Anyone who does a linear regression is doing a simple version of the same thing, and where the facts will not submit to linear analysis, one has to do something more recondite. In this connection one also meets with a rather curious attitude about NIHL, absent from other branches of scientific inquiry, that things must be wrapped in a cocoon of empiricism; they are biological, so they cannot possibly be neat, tidy, and straightforward! Johnson (4) finds it difficult to believe that a particular mathematical function can be a best approximation to NIHL for all frequencies, implying that he does not find it unacceptable at some frequency. Most auditory phenomena behave regularly, so why not the processes in question? Naturally, one could not sustain the principle of economy of hypothesis if the facts were clearly against it, but careful investigation suggests that this is not so. It is as though electric current could not be simply proportional to voltage except in Ohm's laboratory, and for sure if one tries hard enough one will indeed find violations. It is a pretty good rule for practical purposes, nonetheless. This metaphor will serve again when comparing NIHL due to steady and unsteady noise: under alternating conditions, the constant in Ohm's law may change; what does not change is the direct proportionality between current and voltage. Be this as it may, the results obtained by Burns and me do allow succinct phrasing in a mathematical format, and one has only to attempt the task of critical comparison between studies where the parameters have all kinds of different values to appreciate the enormous advantage of it. The calculations can be done on a pocket electronic slide rule without pencil or paper. And to make it still easier for the user, Shipton and I have published complete sets of tables (5) connecting the key variables (noise level, duration, sex, age, percentage of exposed population, and threshold shift).

BASELINES OF COMPARISON

We must, however, return to the question of what the NIPTS data signify, which turns on the selection of test subjects and on assumptions concerning the interaction of threshold shifts due to noise and age. Each study has assumed a different base line for comparison, in the shape of a non-noise-exposed population presumed to resemble the noise-exposed. A glance at Kryter's 1973 paper (6), where he illustrates the percentage of nonexposed persons supposed to attain the "low fence" of 25 dB HL ISO (average of 0.5, 1, and 2 kHz) at various ages according to different authorities, is illuminating. At the age of 60 years, the data range from 10.2 through 37%. Other reports even extend the range below 10.2. This, one might think, was a very poor basis for standardization; yet it is a fact that the values that found their way into the international recommendation ISO R1999 (7) are those at the extreme upper boundary. It is clear that data of this type are quite unsuitable as a reference yardstick to evaluate particular research results; yet this is precisely what one finds being attempted, for example, by Sataloff et al. (8) seeking to show that intermittent noise is less damaging than an equivalent amount of steady noise. This may be so, but this is not a suitable way to prove it.

If these large differences occur among "control" populations, they surely also occur, but are hidden, among the noise-exposed populations and the differences, unless we are careful, will be falsely attributed to noise. Big differences are found in the literature, and it does not help much to speculate whether they are mainly due to the selection criteria of the controls, sociocusis, pathological overlay perhaps associated with differing standards of aural hygiene, or a combination. Even if one knew the principal cause, what use would it be as a basis for comparison of NIHL data unless these incidental factors could be quantified?

Imperfect separation of noise-induced and other threshold shift lies at the root of apparent discrepancies between different investigations. How then is one to estimate the effects of noise per se? The key is to look for a lower bound. The Burns–Robinson results are already on the low side, but if someone came up with another investigation of comparable scope which showed smaller NIPTS, I should be inclined to believe him—provided that this was not produced by some artifact of selection. This means that the test population should be free from temporary threshold shift (TTS); screened on its otological history, otoscopic and general health status at the time of test, on extraneous noise history (gunfire, military service, chronic addiction to pop music, perhaps), concussion and head injuries; and have a clean bill with regard to diseases likely to have been treated by ototoxic drugs; but not, in principle, selected on the results of the audiometry. We have, incidentally, been criticized on the last score by Passchier-Vermeer (9) for it is true that we made a number of rejections a posteriori when audiograms were inconsistent with personal data. We defend this practice, however, because the operative criterion was gross discordance, and one can never be sure by anamnesis that the full medical and personal history has been disclosed. This way of investigation will cut out a great deal of irrelevant material and produce a better chance of data bearing on the specific question of NIHL. Nothing in it selects out this type of hearing loss as such, but it does result in a larger proportion of long-exposure cases being eliminated. The losses are made up by scouring industry to obtain large enough numbers for statistical security.

This discussion will perhaps appear to be laboring the philosophy of investigation, but these preliminaries, and one more, are nevertheless necessary if we are to make a rational quantitative approach to topical questions concerning intermittency, equal-energy principle, impulse noises, and so on.

The additional factor concerns the relative magnitude of the errors and effects in question. Discrepancies in the baseline data for controls are of the order 12 dB in audiometric equivalent (10). Intersubject variance in a typical population of noise-exposed persons may be 100 dB² or more, and this sets an irreducible limit to the reliability of comparisons, even if the data were purged of systematic and experimental errors completely. Against this, ratings of fluctuating noise by equal-energy and 5 dB tradeoff rules differ relatively little. Attempts to sidestep the difficulties of working with noise-exposed human subjects only compound the uncertainties. Experimental work on TTS begs the question of the connection between this and NIPTS, and work with animals, however painstaking, cannot be done on a big enough scale and leaves wide open the question of transferability.

PRACTICAL CONSIDERATIONS

To summarize, the characteristics which can profitably be examined are those of the noise (spectrum, temporal pattern, gross duration, and intensity) and the audiometric correlates freed so far as possible from extraneous effects, in a context of preventive measures on a population basis. Those who are familiar with the work of Burns and my other collaborators in the 1960s will know that our main motivation was the feasibility of compensation under UK Industrial Injuries legislation. This has now been introduced (11), albeit in a circumscribed way, and the initiative has passed in this context to the otological profession for the assessment of individual cases. Meanwhile, our attention has turned to the preventive aspect, including monitoring audiometry, and the establishment of environmental standards. In these circumstances it is necessary to have full regard to the practicability of technical specifications, for the best may well be the enemy of the good. Technicians will not be concerned with the finer points of research nicety. This does not imply any disregard for scientific propriety, but rather a correct balance between ultimate fidelity and practical utility, and the desirability of setting standards that will stand the test of time. It is fortunate that the known characteristics of NIPTS are wholly compatible with this objective, and the realization is spelled out in the UK Code of Practice for Reducing the Exposure of Employed Persons to Noise (12). With the recent setting up of the UK Health and Safety Commission, moves are already being made toward taking over the technical content of this code into legislation.

STEADY-STATE NOISE

The published data on steady-state noise and hearing loss have been subjected to a number of reviews in recent years (2,4,13) and little would be gained from repeating the process here. Certain imperfections in these treatments have been pointed out, for example, by Guignard (14), and there are others that are less well known. One of these is the neglect, in the use of the Burns–Robinson data, of the sex-linked correction which is explicitly referred to in our book (add 1.5 dB to noise-immission level when calculating for males). This is a small matter, but the handling of age corrections is more troublesome. Among the criticisms leveled at our work, aside from predicting smaller NIPTS, is that we refer to presbycutic data (15) which are also smaller than most. The reason is fully documented in our report but 2 points may be restated. First, these presbycutic corrections were not selected arbitrarily, but were demonstrably those which suited the data (on the assumption of additivity). We tried corrections which were both larger and smaller, and both ways the result was less satisfactory by the test of accounting for variance in groups of similar noise exposure but different ages. I know of no other investigation where this has been done and it seems more logical than taking ad hoc control data. Second, our NIHL formula would be quite insensitive to the use of alternative values, because whatever had been subtracted would be added in again at the end of the calculation. The numerical coefficients in the formula giving what we termed the "age-corrected hearing level" or "presumed NIPTS" would have been marginally altered to compensate. It is perhaps not generally appreciated that our procedure was devised to predict the statistical distribution of hearing levels in exposed populations at a given age, not to identify the components of threshold shift separately. The correction for age was only an intermediate process. In fact, we subtracted a constant value for a given age, and that is manifestly imperfect. Against this, Passchier-Vermeer (13) and others have subtracted centile presbycusis correction from corresponding centile hearing level, and labeled the result as NIPTS at the same centile. This is plausible but illogical. If the 2 components are additive—and let us grant that hypothesis for want of another—finding the distribution of one component when one is given the distributions of the other component and of their sum is not a matter of subtraction, but of deconvolution. Because there is no way of knowing whether or not there is a correlation between the size of the components, the deconvolution cannot be performed. It may be that a presbycutically sensitive ear is also a noise-sensitive ear, in which case each element of the distribution transforms to a corresponding position in the deconvolved distribution. If there is no correlation, the elements of the distributions do not stand in this 1:1 correspondence. It is even possible that the correlation is negative if NIPTS is a kind of accelerated aging. Thus, one form of correction is as arbitrary as another.

The field data are discrepant, very much so in terms of original hearing levels, and rather less when artificially age-corrected, and numerical manipulation cannot paper over the differences. Passchier-Vermeer's approach to reducing the data from 8 investigations, not including ours, was to fit straight lines piecewise to arbitrarily chosen segments and average them. She thereby performed a useful service in extracting a resumé of these diverse studies. Without disrespect to the considerable labor entailed in this work, it seems doubtful whether the result gives insight into the true relationships, since data as discordant as those she blithely averaged cannot all be telling the same tale.

More revealing are those reviews in which data fields are compared as a whole. The first attempt to do this was by Baughn (*unpublished*) using his own results on 6,835 subjects (16), and the Burns–Robinson "presumed NIPTS" predictions. Agreement is far from perfect, but it turns out to be remarkably well ordered. In fact, a numerical shift of one data field by a nearly constant amount (12 ± 1.5 dB) brings the two into alignment over a considerable range of the parameters. This cannot be coincidence. Shipton and I have discussed this comparison (5), and it has been ventilated at more than one conference. No one has satisfactorily explained the difference, although a number of possibilities have been discussed by Guignard (14). It is interesting to note that Baughn's published results (17) are in terms of "percentage risk," that is, the percentage of persons in a given exposure and age group exceeding a specified hearing level minus the corresponding percentage in the control group. In this form the agreement with our data is exceedingly poor. The similarity is only brought out when one reverts to the quantities actually measured, hearing levels in decibels. "Percentage risk" is a useful device for describing NIHL to nontechnical people, but it is a very bad parameter for scientific comparisons. In view of the strictures I have already made on this in regard to nonexposed controls, it seems unfortunate that ISO R1999 also quotes the effect of noise in these terms. My justification of this rather severe criticism is that the numerical values for the document came from my own pen in 1967. Later events have convinced me that they are pitched far too high (18,19).

Johnson (4) has presented another facet of the comparison of data fields with a tabulation at selected noise levels and exposure durations. Here he has taken our data and illegitimately, although not unreasonably, represented our NIPTS distributions by subtracting the normal distribution for non-exposed young persons (in the manner of Passchier-Vermeer). Set alongside the data of Baughn corrected by Baughn–Glorig data for controls for various ages, the agreement is quite fair. The quasi-constant 12 dB difference for the 0.5, 1, and 2 kHz average results almost disappears, and this must mean that the hearing levels of the Baughn–Glorig controls were elevated relative to ours by about the same amount as that of the various noise-exposed groups. Johnson includes the data from Passchier-Vermeer's review as well, and considering all 3 data fields, he is able to conclude that there are not large differences, that is, few cases exceed 10 dB. This analysis seems to take the matter of interinvestigation comparisons about as far as the data will bear. It still does not help us much to go beyond qualitative observations on the characteristics.

GENERAL CHARACTERISTICS OF NOISE-INDUCED PERMANENT THRESHOLD SHIFTS

Experimental work on steady-state noise has established the following facts beyond doubt.

1. Hearing levels of exposed persons increase rapidly at first, then progressively slower; those of nonexposed persons rise slowly at first on an accelerating function; therefore, the gap starts from zero, rises to a maximum, and then declines.

2. NIPTS is nearly always greatest at 4 kHz, and less either side of this frequency, whereas for nonexposed persons the threshold shift increases progressively with frequency.

3. The dispersion of hearing levels increases with time in both groups, but more so in the case of exposed persons.

Let us examine these statements before attempting more precise formulations. First, the audiometric picture which they embody is invariant to the type of noise: a dip in the average audiogram at 4 kHz is always the first feature to appear (we may nevertheless recognize individual deviations with dips at 3 or 6 kHz). This dip at first deepens and later flattens off due to the decelerating function; thereafter, the hearing levels at other frequencies begin to catch up, beginning with 6 kHz because that is rising fastest with age. The dip then smears out or turns into a shape increasing progressively with frequency, distinguishable from that of nonexposed persons only by the increased levels at lower frequencies. The same pattern is found by investigators who have taken different views of subject selection, and two conclusions can be drawn from this. First, incidental hearing losses (the "pathological overlay") behave as extra attenuation in the auditory system and not, for instance, as though an already noise-damaged ear is protected. One can state this the other way round and say that an ear which is defective from some cause other than noise is not protected against the effects of noise. It is interesting to note that this does not hold for the combined effects of TTS and NIPTS. A corollary appears to be that sociocusis does not exhibit the decelerating characteristic with time (otherwise some of the nonexposed groups would show it); therefore, the acoustic element in sociocusis seems not to be significant compared to aging and incidental deficits.

Noise-exposed groups show much greater intersubject variability than controls, whether unpurged or "clean," which must mean that noise susceptibility is itself variable. To evaluate this variability leads us back to the separability question, but some evidence can be adduced from serial audiometry. For example, Burns and I found cases where the rate of deterioration corresponded to noise levels as much as 20 dB(A) below or above average.

ANALYTICAL FORMULATION

The above characteristics, supplemented by one important finding which is not immediately apparent from the data, namely, the rule of composition of exposure time and noise level, were precisely those which I sought to incorporate in an analytical format. The law of composition was suggested by the fact that the hearing levels of subgroups increase in a similar way with noise level and with the logarithm of exposure duration. This indicates that the quantity mediating NIPTS must be of the form $I \times T^n$, I being the sound intensity and T the duration. Regression analysis showed that n was pretty nearly equal to unity, hence the "equal-energy rule," for $I \times T$ is a measure of total acoustic energy. The decelerating trend of NIPTS with time could be well represented by a logistic function with (log time) as argument; and since the mediating quantity contained sound level plus ten times the logarithm of time (which we termed "noise-immission level"), the argument of the function could be generalized to the form $E_A = L_A + 10 \log (T/T_0)$. The T_0 is introduced only to make the equation dimensionally correct and is of no consequence. I will not recapitulate here the reason why we chose A-weighted sound level L_A and not some other, save to say that this was no arbitrary choice. Various functions will serve, but the easiest to handle is $1/[1 + \exp(-x)]$, also written as $\frac{1}{2}(1 + \tanh \frac{1}{2}x)$. As soon as I began to submit the data to fitting by this function, with undetermined constants attached to the argument (additive) and outside the brackets (multiplicative), it became clear that a remarkable invariance was at work. One had only to alter the additive constant to represent with equal fidelity the data at all of the audiometric frequencies; the multiplying constant stayed the same. At this stage I was working with median values of the data partitioned into 20 cells of noise level and exposure duration, and the frequency relation meant that a normalized form of the logistic function would fit all data cells at all frequencies. Carrying the process a stage further, other points of the distributions besides the median were equally amenable to this treatment and, still more remarkable, the displacement constant required to pass from one centile to another was itself invariant over the whole data field. This meant that a further collapse on to a single normalized logistic curve would embrace the entire age-corrected data. Hence the final formulation for hearing level:

$$H'(p) = 27.5 [1 + \tanh (E_A - \lambda + u)/15] + u + F$$

E_A being the noise-immission level, λ a frequency-dependent parameter, u a parameter depending on the percentage point p of the distribution, and F

the age correction. Refinements of the form of the function *u* have been suggested, such as the Weibull distribution. The normal distribution serves well enough, however, and more esoteric expressions to accommodate the slight skewness observed in groups of normal-hearing subjects do not seem justified.

There are a number of implicit relationships in this expression. First, the age-corrected audiogram shape depends only on the noise-immission level and the individual susceptibility represented by *u*. Of course, this statistical formula can say nothing about the fine structure of individual audiograms. Second, if one considers an initially unexposed person whose hearing level lies somewhere off median, say on the side of acute hearing, then *u* is a negative number and also the NIPTS following exposure is smaller than for the median subject because E_A is reduced by *u* in the numerator of the argument of the hyperbolic expression. This means that, on balance, better ears are more resistant to noise: they start better and suffer less. It is this feature which causes the dispersion of NIPTS to get larger as exposure goes on (all the evidence is in agreement on this). There may be some deeper meaning to this, for it is flatly opposed to the alternative hypothesis that a better ear transmits more sound to the cochlea and should therefore be more easily damaged. If this were true, the dispersion of hearing levels of noise-exposed persons would tend to be narrower than before they were exposed, contrary to the facts. Intersubject variability, therefore, is not explainable on the basis of variable transmissibility of sound in the conductive pathways. No doubt anatomical differences do occur (we are not here considering clinically diagnosable conductive disorders), but if so the effect is swamped by something working strongly in the opposite direction.

Another implication of the formula is that differences of susceptibility are equivalent to multiplication, upward or downward by an individual factor, of the amount of noise energy which is required to mediate a given threshold elevation. The same applies to the difference between threshold shifts at one frequency and another, as though the spread of the effect along the cochlea either side of the place of maximum effect (4 kHz) is determined by a sharing out of the incident sound energy according to mechanical principles.

RECENT DATA ON STEADY-STATE NOISE AND HEARING LOSS

A paper published in 1975 by Martin et al. (20) provides illustrative material for comparison with predictions. Their steelworks study included three noise situations one of which (in cold mills) was as steady as most that one finds in heavy industry. This example was at 86 dB(A) for 68% of the time, 87 dB(A) for 16%, and between 84 and 94 dB(A) for the remainder. The equivalent continuous level L_{eq} works out at 0.8 dB above the predominant level, thus 86.8 dB(A). Mean values for the 4 age groups of Martin et al. (20), corrected according to the corresponding controls are given in Table 1, together with predictions by the Burns–Robinson formula to the nearest decibel. The latter include the adjustment for males, and for skewness (the mean is between 0 and 1.3 dB different from the median depending on the magnitude of the threshold shift). The agreement on average is pretty good (0.5 dB overprediction). It is not so good if hearing levels, uncorrected for age, are compared and this seems to be a case where pragmatic acceptance of differing baselines works tolerably well in practice, even if its logical basis is decidedly insecure.

It is worth asking whether one could reasonably expect better agreement than that illustrated, for, obviously, it is not perfect. Looking at the raw data of Martin et al. (columns M, Table 1) one is struck by the fact that the hearing levels are generally progressive with age through the 4 groups, but when

TABLE 1. Hearing loss in steady-state noise—comparison of data from Martin et al. with Burns–Robinson predictions

| Fre-quency (kHz) | Age group (years) | | | | | | | | | | | | | | | | | |
| | 18–29 | | | | 30–39 | | | | 40–49 | | | | 50–65 | | | | All | |
	M	C	D	B/R	M	C	D	B/R	M	C	D	B/R	M	C	D	B/R	D	B/R
0.5	7	7	0	1	11	9	2	1	13	10	3	1	9	10	−1	2	1	1
1	4	5	−1	1	9	7	2	2	12	10	2	2	11	8	3	3	2	2
2	4	5	−1	2	9	7	2	4	13	8	5	5	17	14	3	6	2	4
3	8	6	2	4	15	10	5	7	31	16	15	9	36	25	11	11	8	8
4	14	9	5	6	23	16	7	9	40	23	17	11	51	33	18	13	12	10
6	18	19	−1	4	25	22	3	6	40	31	9	8	47	41	6	10	4	7
Av			1	3			3.5	5			8.5	6			7	7.5	5	5.5

Key: M, Martin et al. hearing levels of noise-exposed groups; C, Martin et al. hearing level of controls; D, Difference (M − C); B/R, Burns–Robinson prediction, presumed NIPTS for males, mean of distributions.

corrected by the corresponding controls (columns D, Table 1) this is upset. The top age group comes out with smaller presumed NIPTS than the next lower age band, and the correction makes some values negative. There is no way of knowing if this jarring note is due to the controls being different from the noise groups in more respects than just the noise. It seems fairly typical of what one might expect due to simple sampling error for groups of the size tested. Thus, in the top age group there were 17 persons; in the corresponding control group 21. Intersubject standard deviations are not given by the authors, but it would be surprising if they were not of the order 8 and 6 dB, respectively. The reliability of a difference of means on these figures is ±4.6 dB [95% confidence limits (CL)] or ±6.2 dB (99% CL). In the light of this the figures in Table 1 are as close as can be expected.

Various other errors can also enter into comparisons of this kind. Although any constant audiometer calibration error cancels out when subtracting control from noise-exposed data, error in the audiometry is not cancelled but multiplied by $\sqrt{2}$. At NPL we have made elaborate studies of the incidence and magnitude of audiometric error in industrial conditions (21,22) and, whereas it is true that highly accurate and repeatable results are obtainable from the great majority of subjects, it takes some trouble to do it. The variance of a single audiometric datum at a first test is typically 10 dB^2 under good testing conditions. The replication reliability of the mean of 17 or 21 results differenced is thus likely to be around ± 3 dB (95% CL)—a smaller uncertainty than that of subject sampling, but not negligible. Then there is the question of noise measurement error which is in fact more critical than audiometric error. A general rule is that 1 dB of noise makes an incremental difference in NIPTS of 1–2 dB as NIPTS runs from 10 through 30 dB; thereafter, the rate falls again to about 1 dB; this applies at any audiometric frequency. Differences of noise measurement technique and calibration can easily entail errors of 1–2 dB(A) and hence somewhat greater uncertainties of threshold shift prediction. One may question whether this aspect always receives the attention which is due to it. The position with absolutely steady noises is simply a matter of instrument calibration, and good sound level meters should be accurate within about 1 dB for different noises (though strict conformity with the standards would not guarantee such a close figure). With noises which are not so steady, but might be classed as such, other errors can occur. Nowadays there is a means of direct measurement of equivalent continuous level but few are in possession of this relatively sophisticated equipment. In our studies, Burns and I made a statistical analysis of noise level and our findings, which embraced a wide assortment of industrial processes, may be of interest. We were trying to find steady noise, but also to cover a wide range of noise level. The 759 subjects were identified with 280 different noises with L_{A50} ranging from 75 to 110 dB(A). Of these, 196 subjects had rock-steady noise (constant within a decibel) and a further 130 had noise with $(L_{A2} - L_{A50})$ equal to 1 dB; 272 lay in the range 2–5 dB, 121 in the range 6–10 dB and 40 upward of 10 dB. As a rough rule, the standard deviation, s, of the fluctuations is about $\frac{1}{2}(L_{A2} - L_{A50})$, and the equivalent continuous level L_{eq} is of the order $(L_{A50} + s^2/9)$. Exactly how L_{eq} is related to the visual average read on a sound level meter for want of strict instrumentation, is conjectural; it depends on the nature of the excursions and the dynamic setting of the controls. There is scope here for a 2- or 3-dB discrepancy in the reporting of noise levels. Finally, there is the uncertainty of noise-immission level, for it is one thing to know the noise level at a monitoring position, and quite another to know that this is the actual noise level received at the ears of the test subjects 8 hr/day for many years without significant variation or interruption. Searching for cases in which this was as sure as may be was one of the major preoccupations in our experimental planning. Fortunately, exposure time enters in as the logarithm so that a bad estimate does not make as much difference as might appear. Nevertheless, there is bound to be further uncertainty here equivalent to a decibel or two. All these factors should be borne in mind when evaluating results from different sources.

SHAPE OF THE AUDIOGRAM

Observation of the "4-kHz dip" goes back many years, to the beginning of systematic study of noise-induced deafness. Later evidence permits one to postulate that the whole shape of the average audiogram is invariant with respect to the noise spectrum within quite wide limits. This is in sharp contrast to the accepted notion that an audiogram of TTS reflects the causative noise spectrum smeared out and shifted perhaps half an octave up the frequency scale. The question may legitimately be asked of NIPTS whether the invariance is absolute or, if it is only relative, whether one may nevertheless adopt this simplification for practical purposes. The range of different noises in the Burns–Robinson study permitted us to make a critical examination of this question, and it clearly supports invariance. By rank-ordering subjects according to the slope of the noise spectrum, the group was divided into two and the mean audiogram calculated for each. These [shown in Fig.10.24 of our report (2)] are so close as to be barely distinguishable (0.5 dB). We have been criticized by Scheiblechner (3) for averaging away what differences there might be in our original data by using this treatment and he points to another of our illustrations (ref. 2, Fig.10.22) in support. However, this figure relates to subject groups at a level of subdivision where sampling error produces a relatively ragged diagram, and even main trends begin to be blurred. For this reason, I much prefer to rely on the data for the larger numbers (over 700 subjects). Passchier-Vermeer (13) also finds the invariant relation in the 8 investigations she reviewed. Martin et al. (20) report audiograms of workers in 3 different noises, but, unfortunately, give no noise analyses. They state, however, that for one noise (cold mills) the band analysis is constant from 31.5 to 1,000 Hz, falling thereafter, whereas the other two (slinger floor and furnace) are heavily weighted at the low frequencies. There is a classical "4 kHz dip" in the mean audiograms for all age groups and all 3 noises, and by averaging the "presumed NIPTS" (hearing level minus control for corresponding age) across age groups, for the cold mills and the other 2 sites, respectively, it is possible to make a broad comparison of the effect of low frequencies. This is shown in Table 2 where each of the above averages is coupled with the corresponding prediction by the Burns–Robinson formula. There is no appreciable difference of shape between the cold mills data and the mean of the other two (low frequency) noises. Compared with the predictions, the 4 kHz dip and the recovery at 6 kHz are a little more pronounced, but these features are almost identical for both types of noise.

Depending on which way one chooses to read the data, then, they either point unequivocally toward shape invariance, or show a slight tendency for the audiogram to follow the spectrum of the noise. For those whose concern is with hearing conservation rather than the byways of research there can be little doubt which course to choose. Contrary evidence is far too slight as a basis for quantitative statement and, of course, even if this could be done,

TABLE 2. Comparison of the shape of mean audiograms for exposure to noises with different frequency spectra

Group	Presumed NIPTS (dB)					
	0.5 kHz	1 kHz	2 kHz	3 kHz	4 kHz	6 kHz
F/S—C	1.6	2.3	5.9	11.9	13.6	6.6
F/S (B/R)	1.8	2.9	6.2	10.9	13.1	9.9
Difference	−0.2	−0.6	−0.3	1.0	0.5	−3.3
M—C	0.9	1.8	2.4	8.4	11.8	4.1
M (B/R)	1.2	1.9	4.3	7.9	9.8	7.1
Difference	−0.3	−0.1	−1.9	0.5	2.0	−3.0

Key: F/S—C, Martin et al., furnace and slinger floor average, noise-exposed minus controls, average over all age bands; M—C, Martin et al., cold mills, noise-exposed minus controls, average over all age bands; (B/R), Burns–Robinson prediction, presumed NIPTS for males, mean of distributions, average over all age bands.

it would necessitate describing all noises by spectrum. Instead of a single noise-immission level one would have to substitute 8 or more numbers. What kind of a formula would it have to be to digest this input and come up with another set of numbers giving threshold shifts? The number of combinations of eight numbers, averaged, weighted, added logarithmically, and so on, is limitless, and to produce convincing answers would require innumerable repetitions in its entirety of the analysis which I performed with A-weighted sound level. In any case, the more constants one tries to determine by curve-fitting, the less stable they are, as Scheiblechner's (3) multivariate analysis shows.

NON-STEADY NOISE

This subject has to be discussed under the three subheads of fluctuating, intermittent, and impulsive noise. Fluctuating noise may be further subdivided into that which is piecewise steady, changing from time to time, but steady for significantly long periods, and that which is varying from moment to moment according to no easily described pattern; it is unnecessary to regard these cases as essentially different, however, for they can both be represented by a histogram of the level distribution over the workday. For completeness, one should perhaps add the case where the noise is different from one day to the next, but as there are no experimental data at all on this, one must resort to a working hypothesis.

Fluctuating noise has been encountered in a number of studies reviewed by Passchier-Vermeer (9), and the conclusion seems to be that it causes the same effect as if the noise had been continuous for the same total duration at a level L_{eq} given by the energy rule. For reasons which I will elaborate, the data on TTS are not considered relevant. Passchier-Vermeer, dealing with these studies, is forced to compare the results with steady-state data from other sources, namely, her own summary of the steady-state relations (13) and the Burns–Robinson formula. The uncertainties in such indirect comparisons have been discussed above, but she concludes that for noise-immission levels up to 110 (e.g., 95 dB(A) for 32 years) L_{eq} correctly rates fluctuating noise. To carry out this analysis she corrected the data by Spoor's (23) presbycusis values for comparison with her own steady-noise relations, and further manipulated them for comparison with the Burns–Robinson predictions. They cannot both be right and, as indicated earlier, the age-correction step is hazardous anyway. My interpretation of her review would be rather that there is no systematic evidence that use of L_{eq} either overpredicts or underpredicts—the scatter is quite considerable in both directions. One may turn again to the paper by Martin et al. (20) for further examples of fluctuating noise, in this case with the advantage that they stand alongside a case of steady, or nearly steady, noise. The furnace and slinger floor noises here have histograms with bimodal and unimodal character, respectively. Table 3 compares the results with Burns–Robinson predictions, using the calculated L_{eq} values, on the same basis as Table 1. It will be recalled that good agreement (average overprediction of 0.5 dB) was found in the case of the steady cold mills noise. Now we have the situation that there are both over- and under-

TABLE 3. Hearing loss in fluctuating noise—comparison of data from Martin et al. with Burns–Robinson predictions

Frequency (kHz)	Age group (years)									
	18–29		30–39		40–49		50–65		All	
	F—C	B/R	F—C	B/R	F—C	B/R	F—C	B/R	F—C	B/R
0.5	1	1	0	2	2	3	7	4	2.5	2.5
1	1	2	2	4	1	4	11	6	4	4
2	0	5	0	8	5	9	14	12	5	8.5
3	1	9	7	13	10	16	21	19	10	12
4	2	11	4	16	13	19	27	22	11.5	17
6	−1	8	1	12	−1	15	17	17	4	13
Av.	0.5	6	2.5	9	5	11	16	13.5	6	9.5
	S—C	B/R	S—C	B/R	S—C	B/R	S—C	B/R	S—C	B/R
0.5	2	1	−1	1	−1	1	3	2	1	1
1	1	1	−1	1	−1	2	4	3	1	2
2	3	2	3	4	4	5	18	6	7	4.5
3	8	4	12	7	12	9	22	10	13.5	7.5
4	10	5	15	8	15	10	22	13	15.5	9
6	1	4	11	6	5	8	18	9	9	7
Av.	4	3	6.5	4.5	5.5	6.5	14.5	7	7.5	5
Grand av									7	7.5

Key: F—C, Martin et al., furnace, noise-exposed minus controls; S—C, Martin et al., slinger floor, noise-exposed minus controls; B/R, Burns–Robinson prediction, presumed NIPTS for males, mean of distributions.

predictions. Across the whole data field of the 2 fluctuating noises, however, the discrepancy again averages a mere 0.5 dB (overprediction), and perhaps this is the best conclusion that can be drawn. Examining the detail, one again notes features typical of small data groups: thus there is the large jump between the third and fourth age groups (perhaps a legacy of World War II); also the existence of pronounced "4-kHz dips" where one would not expect them (slinger floor workers, lower two age bands). Taken as a whole, these data seem to be as good confirmation as a single study is likely to produce of the validity of L_{eq} rating for fluctuating noise.

Turning to intermittent noise, Passchier-Vermeer's digest of several studies is treated alongside fluctuating noise. In this case she concludes that L_{eq} rating is satisfactory for sound levels up to 100 dB(A). However, once again, I would generalize her conclusion, for the data points are intermingled over the whole field with those for the fluctuating noise and lie both above and below the prediction curves with considerable scatter.

Impulse noise has often been treated as though it is some kind of outcast from the acoustical fraternity—a different kind of radiation—and a quite unnecessary mystique has surrounded its measurement and description. In fact, it lends itself without any discontinuity to treatment in the same terms as steady noise, but it is obviously nonsensical to try measuring it with an instrument having a time constant longer than the event itself and expecting the peak reading to mean much. Therefore, one must turn away from the sound level meter as such and inquire as to the essential quantity that it measures. The answer is the integrated square of the instantaneous (A-weighted) sound pressure divided by elapsed time. Ten times the logarithm of this relative to 20 μPa simply defines the A-weighted sound level if the noise is steady, and L_{eq} if it is not. Impulse noise is one of the latter cases, and is thus a mere extension of fluctuating noise. It remains to show whether ear damage effects stay invariant along this temporal dimension, for, as we have just seen, the relatively small step from steady to fluctuating noise is evidenced by data that are somewhat woolly, so it is possible that other relations apply when the fluctuations become rapid and large, that is, impulsive. To make the necessary comparison one is constrained to utilize data for which the noise has been measured in the appropriate way, or can be converted thereto.

There are 2 important studies in this category. In one of these, by Guberan et al. (24), it was done by calculation from oscillograms, and adding in the continuous noise contribution. In the other, by Atherley and Martin (25), it was done both by this method and by direct measurement on an integrating meter in my laboratory with close agreement of results. Both studies were in the drop-forging industry, and both show audiometric results in excellent agreement with the Burns–Robinson predictions. This evidence was considered sufficiently decisive in the United Kingdom for the Code of Practice (12) to embrace impulse noise, rated as described above in terms of

A-weighted L_{eq}. The National Physical Laboratory sponsored the development of a direct-reading "noise average meter" with 80 dB dynamic range for this purpose. It will, of course, work equally well on steady, fluctuating, or intermittent noise, and it is now marketed commercially.

SOME REFLECTIONS ON THE RATING OF NONCONSTANT NOISE

In the preceding chapters we have traversed the gamut of the temporal dimension and the picture with which we are left is that at both extremities, namely, the continuous and the impulsive, the "energy" relations hold provided that the noise is expressed in the right way. For intermediate cases, the experimental data as a whole are not inconsistent with these relations, indeed for the fluctuating type of noise there is support for them. It is only in the case of the intermittent or single brief-occurrence type that there seems to be insufficient evidence to draw better than shaded conclusions. Experimental difficulties no doubt contribute to this gap, as situations of this type with the prerequisite of long exposure to an unchanged pattern are hard to find in industry.

In these circumstances, the likelihood that some underlying unity is at work appears strong and it would seem perverse to postulate a different mechanism in the middle of the temporal spectrum. The experimental evidence, at least, would have to be rather persuasive to justify it, and this is just where it happens to be weakest. The amount of debate and prejudice which the rating of intermittent noise has aroused, crystallizing into 2 schools of thought typified by the "equinocivity" and "equal-energy" principles is well-known, and heat rather than light has often been generated in the resulting disputations no doubt because these principles are not equally permissive in their practical application.

The "equinocivity" principle seems to have been invoked specially to handle the intermittency problem as a way of sidestepping the difficulty of proof through direct observation of NIPTS, by substituting an appeal to the related but nevertheless quite distinct phenomenon of TTS. To many who have found this a practical way forward to the management of intermittent noises in hearing conservation, the equivalence of the 2 phenomena either appears, or has been made to appear, plausible. I believe this to be quite irrational, but before seeking to prove it the alternatives need putting into numerical perspective, for without this there is a certain sterility in controversy over hypotheses, neither of which is susceptible of invincible proof.

Once again I turn to the study by Martin et al., because the common methodology permits critical comparisons. From the histograms of their 3 noises one can compute both L_{eq} and what I call $L_{``5"}$, the first according to equal-energy and the other by the 5 dB tradeoff rule. The defining equations are

$$L_{eq} = 10 \log_{10}\left\{(1/T) \sum_i 10^{L_i/10}\right\}$$

and

$$L_{``5"} = (5/\log_{10}2) \log_{10}\left\{(1/T) \sum_i 10^{(L_i \log_{10}2)/5}\right\}$$

These 2 forms of equivalent continuous level are equal for a steady noise, but L_{eq} is always the larger otherwise, and it is simple in the case of the data of Martin et al. (20) data to determine the audiometric equivalent of the difference, by inserting both into the Burns–Robinson formula. The noise level differences are 1.9 dB(A) for the (bimodal) furnace noise, 0.7 dB(A) for the slinger floor (unimodal) noise, and 0.2 dB(A) for the nearly steady cold mills noise. The differences and their audiometric correlates work out quite small in spite of the 25–26 dB(A) noise level range in the fluctuating cases. The effect is most easily summed up in terms of the prediction error over the data field comprised of the slinger floor and furnace men's hearing levels averaged over all age groups and frequencies. As shown in Table 3, the use of L_{eq} results in a mean overprediction of 0.5 dB; substitution of the $L_{``5"}$ value changes this to a mean underprediction of 0.5 dB. Clearly, if these are the kinds of noise about which the argument is being waged it is shown up as ridiculous in relation to other uncertainties.

The biggest difference between L_{eq} and $L_{``5"}$ will occur when $x\%$ of the time is occupied at one noise level, say L_1, and the remainder of the time $(100 - x)$ at another (higher) level, L_2. If there is any occupancy of the intermediate levels, the difference is always reduced. We can therefore put an upper bound on the size of the difference, by considering just L_1 and L_2. It is also obvious that if $x = 0$ or 100, the difference is zero. The upper bound, therefore, occurs for some definite value of x. The position of the maximum moves towards L_2 as $(L_2 - L_1)$ increases. This is illustrated in Fig. 1. The furnace noise of Martin et al. (20) ranged from 79 to 105 dB(A) with the two modal values occurring around 82 and 96, carrying about 75 and 25% time occupancy, respectively. This may be approximated with $x = 75$ and $(L_2 - L_1) = 14$, which, from the diagram, indicates a difference of 1.9 dB, exactly the same as the true value calculated from the whole distribution. The reader may judge for himself the area of the diagram that covers fluctuating noise situations in industry.

Another case occurs in the study of coalminers by Sataloff et al. (8) where bursts of drilling noise between 115 and 119 dB(A) occurred against a background of 84 and, occasionally, 95 dB(A). The high noise level occupied typically 3 hr/day. Thus, on a generous estimate $(L_2 - L_1) = 35$ dB(A) and $x = 62.5$. The diagram shows that the difference could not exceed 2.7 dB. This investigation has frequently been cited as holding the key to hearing loss from intermittent noise exposure, but even here, in spite of the wide interval

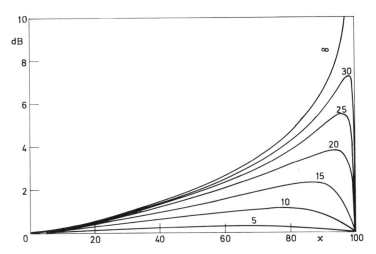

FIG. 1. Upper bounding value of the difference between equivalent continuous sound levels computed by the energy rule (L_{eq}) and 5-dB tradeoff (L''_5), respectively. x is the percentage of total time occupied at the lowest noise level L_1. The parameter is the difference between the highest and lowest noise levels ($L_2 - L_1$).

between noise and relative quiet, the on-time ratio is such as to make it quite an insensitive test of the 2 rules. The actual hearing levels reported appear to be out of line with prediction on either basis, both in magnitude and shape, and one does not know what to make of certain of their "control" data, for example, the otologically screened group of 25-year-old "new employees" with an average ISO hearing level of 35 dB at 4 kHz.

TEMPORARY THRESHOLD SHIFT

That this is a phenomenon closely related to PTS is indisputable; it is mediated by the same physical agency, is observed by the same kind of measurement, and operates in much the same arena of the anatomy. That the phenomenology is different is equally obvious; one is reversible and the other not. Some characteristics tend to highlight an association and others a dissimilarity. Thus there is a clear indication (2) that a person whose susceptibility is strong toward the one is also strong toward the other (individual correlation of PTS and TTS). On the other hand, TTS and PTS exhibit markedly different response patterns in the frequency domain, one depending on the spectrum of the stimulus and the other not. Another obvious dissimilarity is that, under continuous exposure, PTS goes on increasing whereas TTS settles down at a plateau value depending on the stimulus intensity.

These qualitative observations should immediately put us on our guard against assuming that some other characteristic will necessarily reflect the similarity rather than the difference, or the other way round. This question becomes acute when we turn to the quantitative characteristics—for it is in this mode that the protagonists of the "equinocivity" principle would have us place complete reliance on similarity. One statement that has always struck me as essentially trivial is that, for statistically large groups, the average TTS at 2 min after a day's exposure is numerically equal to the PTS after 10 years of repeated daily exposure to the same noise. Such an equation must necessarily exist, for, since the first term has a certain value, the other term can obviously be made equal to it by choosing the right number of years. This is a pseudoquantitative relation, albeit a handy mnemonic for the appreciation of threshold shift magnitudes. We are here concerned with a much more subtle use or misuse of quantitative equality, namely, that repeated daily exposure to a pattern of noise results in a PTS that is wholly characterized by TTS measured after 1 day's exposure to that pattern, independent of the pattern within the day. In particular, if steady noise and some arbitrarily nonconstant noise exposure produce the same TTS at the end of a day, they necessarily produce the same PTS at the end of so many years.

In spite of the advocacy which this principle has received, it rests on no surer foundation than superficial plausibility. By blatantly proclaiming it and then demonstrating that TTS does not follow "equal-energy" principles (which no one denies), some advocates of equinocivity commit the further error of asserting that therefore the equal-energy principle is false for PTS. Of course, this principle may be false (although the data I have reviewed do not make it look that way), but, if so, the proof of its falsity cannot be rested upon logic that is itself false. In proceeding to challenge the sanctity of "equinocivity," I recognize that I shall not thereby have proved the alternative: this must stand or fall by the evidence that is relevant to it.

A simple way to show that postexposure TTS is not a characterizing measure of noise dose is given in Fig. 2. Here noise A produces TTS equal to x dB. In case (i) this constitutes the whole daily exposure. In case (ii), noise A is as before, thus inducing the same TTS, but at its cessation noise B begins, the level of this being such that it just maintains the value x. There must be such a level, for if it were equal to that of A, TTS would continue to rise, whereas if it is sufficiently low, TTS decays. At the end of noise B, the TTS is the same as it was at the end of A, but the exposures are manifestly different. In case of protest that this is hypothetical, it must be acknowledged that equinocivity is at least dislodged: at best it is a pragmatic description of approximate reality. Next consider the model illustrated in Fig. 3. This is an abstraction, but it nevertheless reflects the cardinal facts that we know. The box labeled PTS is some kind of leakless integrator; the TTS box can have all the complicated rules with which this reversible process is endowed. The model incorporates the refinement that TTS diminishes as PTS advances. Supplied with the noise exposures illustrated, the PTS (measured as the reduced gain of the system compared with the initial state) is the same. The TTS is not the same. To confer some quantitative significance, let us assume, with Kryter,

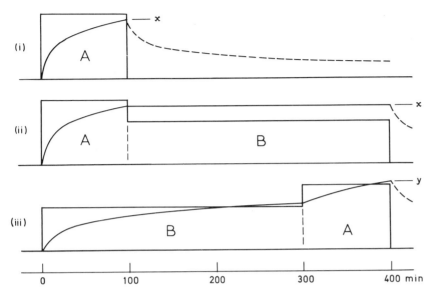

FIG. 2. Three patterns of noise and the resulting TTS. (i) Noise A produces TTS equal to x; (ii) noise A followed by noise B produce the same TTS, x; (iii) interchanging noises A and B alters the TTS to y(y ≠ x).

that TTS grows with 20 log (time) and decibel for decibel with sound level. The value of TTS_B is then up to 9 dB less than for the uninterrupted noise. Here I have demonstrated that a model exists in which equinocivity is violated. This, in itself, proves nothing except that the onus of proof should be laid on those who believe it is *not* violated. I have made repeated but fruitless attempts to find a converse model. Until someone can satisfactorily demonstrate that at least one such model exists I adhere to the view that this is one of the manifestations in which PTS and TTS, though clearly related, do not have a fixed quantitative relationship which is independent of the noise pattern.

More promising, as a means of utilizing TTS in a predictive capacity, may be some form of time integral. Exactly what form this should take, bearing in mind that TTS, though expressed in decibels, is not a physical quantity with rate-like properties which one normally visualizes as capable of meaningful time integration, is unclear, but it opens up possibilities and eliminates paradoxes. Kraak (26) proceeded by first demonstrating good correlation between TTS, integrated over the whole exposure and recovery, and the integral of the pth power of modulus of sound pressure during exposure. For steady and interrupted-steady sounds [up to 94 dB(A)] the exponent p comes out near unity. He next showed a correlation between this sound pressure integral, plus an "acoustic load" term equivalent to presbycusis, and the hearing levels of exposed populations. For this purpose Kraak used, among others, data from the studies reviewed by Passchier-Vermeer (13). Conjunction of the 2 correla-

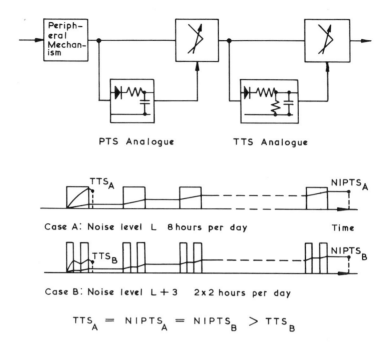

PTS Analogue   TTS Analogue

Case A: Noise level L   8 hours per day   Time

Case B: Noise level L + 3   2x2 hours per day

$$TTS_A = NIPTS_A = NIPTS_B > TTS_B$$

FIG. 3. Model of a system which violates the equinocivity principle but which reproduces the essential characteristics of TTS and PTS.

tions implies a close relation between NIHL and the TTS integral, but roughness in the data of the second correlation makes it difficult to assess the sensitivity of this predictive procedure.

REFERENCES

1. Atherley, G. R. C., and Noble, W. G. (1971): Clinical picture of occupational hearing loss obtained with the Hearing Measurement Scale. In: *Occupational Hearing Loss,* edited by D. W. Robinson, pp. 193–206. Academic Press, London and New York.
2. Burns, W., and Robinson, D. W. (1970): *Hearing and Noise in Industry,* Her Majesty's Stationery Office, London.
3. Scheiblechner, H. (1974): The validity of the 'energy principle' for noise-induced hearing loss. *Audiology,* 13:93–111.
4. Johnson, D. L. (1973): Prediction of NIPTS due to continuous noise exposure. AMRL-TR-73–91.
5. Robinson, D. W., and Shipton, M. S. (1973): Tables for the estimation of noise-induced hearing loss. National Physical Laboratory, Acoustics Report Ac 61.
7. International Organization for Standardization (1970): Assessment of noise exposure during work for hearing conservation purposes. ISO R1999. Geneva.
8. Sataloff, J., Vassallo, L., and Menduke, H. (1969): Hearing loss from exposure to interrupted noise. *Arch. Environ. Health,* 18:972–981.
9. Passchier-Vermeer, W. (1973): Noise-induced hearing loss from exposure to intermittent and varying noise. In: *Proc. Int. Cong. on Noise as a Public Health Problem,* pp. 169–200. EPA 550/9–73–008.

10. Robinson, D. W. (1970): Estimating the risk of hearing loss due to exposure to continuous noise. In: *Occupational Hearing Loss,* edited by D. W. Robinson, pp. 43–62. Academic Press, London and New York.
11. UK Department of Health and Social Security (1974): The National Insurance (industrial injuries) (prescribed diseases) Amendment Regulations 1974. Statutory Instrument No. 1414.
12. UK Department of Employment (1972): Code of Practice for reducing the exposure of employed persons to noise. Her Majesty's Stationery Office, London.
13. Passchier-Vermeer, W. (1968): Hearing loss due to exposure to steady-state broadband noise. Report 35, IG-TNO, Delft.
14. Guignard, J. C. (1973): A basis for limiting noise exposure for hearing conservation. AMRL-TR-73-90.
15. Hinchcliffe, R. (1959): The threshold of hearing as a function of age. *Acustica,* 9:303–308.
16. Baughn, W. L. (1968): Unpublished report dated 29 February, Medical Arts Research Corporation Inc., Anderson, Ind.
17. Baughn, W. L. (1966): Noise control: per cent of population protected. *Int. Audiol.,* 9:331–338.
18. Raber, A. (1973): The incidence of impaired hearing in relation to years of exposure and continuous sound level. In: *Proc. Int. Cong. on Noise as a Public Health Problem,* pp. 115–138. EPA 550/9-73-008.
19. Kryter, K. D. (1973): A critique of some procedures for evaluating damage risk from exposure to noise. In: *Proc. Int. Cong. on Noise as a Public Health Problem,* pp. 103–114. EPA 550/9-73-008.
20. Martin, R. H., Gibson, E. S., and Lockington, J. N. (1975): Occupational hearing loss between 85 and 90 dBA. *J. Occup. Med.,* 17:13–18.
21. Robinson, D. W., Shipton, M. S., and Whittle, L. S. (1973): Audiometry in industrial hearing conservation—I. National Physical Laboratory, Acoustics Report Ac 64.
22. Robinson, D. W., Shipton, M. S., and Whittle, L. S. (1975): Audiometry in industrial hearing conservation—II. National Physical Laboratory, Acoustics Report Ac 71.
23. Spoor, A. (1967): Presbyacusis values in relation to noise-induced hearing loss. *Int. Audiol.,* 6:48–57.
24. Guberan, E., Fernandez, J., Cardinet, J., and Terrier, G. (1971): Hazardous exposure to industrial impact noise: persistent effect on hearing. *Ann. Occup. Hyg.,* 14:345–350.
25. Atherley, G. R. C., and Martin, A. M. (1971): Equivalent continuous noise level as a measure of injury from impact and impulse noise. *Ann. Occup. Hyg.,* 14:1–23.

DISCUSSION

C. Trahiotis: You showed some individual data points relating initial hearing level and hearing loss level. Looking at those data, it appeared that there would be very low correlation; is that the proper way of looking at those data?

D. Robinson: I understand the question, but it's rather hard to answer briefly. First, because the results are so dispersed between people, i.e., the range between tough to tender ears being the dominant factor, all true correlations against a single curve or median or whatever, are bound to be poor. But if you do a more sophisticated correlation, I think we can get someone to show that was a rather good fit.

Effects of Noise on Hearing, edited by Donald Henderson, Roger P. Hamernik, Darshan S. Dosanjh, and John H. Mills. Raven Press, New York © 1976.

A Comparison of the Effects of Continuous, Intermittent, and Impulse Noise

W. Dixon Ward

Hearing Research Laboratory, University of Minnesota, Minneapolis, Minnesota 55455

Up to this point in this volume, the main emphasis has been upon the physiological effects of noise exposure on the auditory mechanism. Unfortunately, however, these direct effects, except for electrical potentials, are not observable in the intact unanesthetized organism. While it would be desirable to be able to specify the noise exposure that would just produce irreversible damage to some fixed number of hair cells, such exposures can be determined only in experimental animals. For practical purposes, therefore, some indirect means of assessing cochlear (or more central) damage must be found. The traditional solution, of course, has been to use the behavioral auditory threshold as the indicator. There have been numerous objections to this indicator, usually based on the fact that correlations are low between such threshold sensitivity and either hair-cell damage (1,2) or the ability to understand ordinary conversation, presumably the most important use of the auditory mechanism (3). Nevertheless, it will continue to be used for a long time, first, because as yet there are only dim prospects of agreement on how to measure the ability to hear everyday speech, and second, because even though the correlation between pure-tone thresholds and some measure of speech perception may be low, large changes in auditory sensitivity are nevertheless required before the individual is aware of any difficulty. Although auditory threshold may not be as sensitive an indicator of damage as is direct inspection of hair cells, it is more sensitive than any other known index that can be extracted from the intact organism. Although computer-assisted electrophysiological measurements may eventually be refined to the point that they are equivalent to measures of behavioral threshold, that day has not yet arrived.

The practical question, then, is this: "What noise exposures will lead to a particular change in auditory threshold in a specified fraction of those exposed?" The question may appear perfectly straightforward at first glance, but we know from half a century of trying to answer it that it is anything but that. The problem is not in the measurement of the auditory threshold as operationally defined, despite some inherent variability, nor therefore in determining a change in this threshold. True, in both before- and after-exposure measurements of threshold, we must keep constant or equivalent the audiometric apparatus, the testing environment, the instructions to the subject, and the specific procedure. But with care, these objectives can be attained. That is, it is at least possible to determine to any desired level of precision that between times T_1 and T_2 a given change in auditory sensitivity at a particular test frequency has occurred; whether this threshold shift (TS) at time T_2 is temporary (TTS) or permanent (PTS) can be inferred from a measurement at some subsequent time T_3.

The difficulty, we all realize, has to do with the imprecise term "noise exposure." Actually, there are 2 difficulties: first, in making sure that the only cause of a change in threshold between times T_1 and T_2 was exposure to noise (or to only industrial noise, if that is the agent whose action we are interested in), and second, and perhaps more importantly, in *defining* the noise exposure.

Now by definition of the noise exposure I do not mean measurement of the noise. Again, measurement is relatively straightforward, provided one follows accepted practices. A noise exposure can theoretically be specified rather precisely by a record of the instantaneous value of the acoustic pressure at the ear of the individual in question. But such a record—a history from T_1 to T_2 of the instantaneous pressure—has much too much information to be of value. Even if one accepts Fourier analysis as a valid method for analyzing sound, so that the short-term acoustic wave can be represented by the energy in a series of critical bands, such a spectrum can change from time to time, and furthermore the root-mean-square (rms) level—both overall and in each band—may also vary in an infinite number of patterns. So although we could express any given noise exposure as a three-dimensional matrix of frequency, level, and time, further simplification obviously is necessary.

One way out of the dilemma, of course, is to work only with noises having a constant spectrum, 1 or 2 levels, and a regular temporal pattern, hoping that by hard work or good fortune one will come upon a simplifying principle. This is what some of us have been doing for longer than I like to be reminded of. As a result, we know a great deal about the temporary shifts associated with exposures varying over a large range in spectrum, duration, and temporal pattern (4). The unifying principles, however, can hardly be said to exist in profusion. As far as permanent shifts are concerned, only one seems somehow to have survived—the total-energy theory, which postulates that all we have to do to define a noise exposure in a single number is to integrate over time the acoustic power entering the ear. It has survived not because of any extensive compelling evidence, but because of its seductive simplicity. That is, it would be so wonderful if it were true that it is hard to keep from pretending that it *is* true.

More than 20 years ago, though, Subcommittee Z24-X-2 of the American Standards Association mentioned the principle and found it wanting:

> It is not sufficient to record the amount of sound energy that has been absorbed by the ear during a period of exposure to noise. Although 2 exposures to

the same noise—1 for 1 hr/day for 10,000 days, the other for 10,000 continuous hours—may supply the same amount of energy to the ear, experience has shown that these 2 exposures are not equally effective in producing hearing loss.

Since the parameters of noise, exposure, and hearing loss are all complex, the relation of hearing loss to noise exposure is clearly not a "single-number" problem. No single magic number, such as over-all sound pressure level, separates safe from unsafe exposures. There is no escaping the conclusion that the relations of hearing loss to noise exposure are multidimensional in the way that situations not under experimental control so often are.

Have things changed much?

Even its most enthusiastic advocates admit one limitation of the total-energy theory—the dependence of effect on frequency. It has been obvious for decades that low-frequency energy is less hazardous than high-frequency energy, by almost any definition of "hazard." So it was obviously necessary to apply some sort of weighting factor to the spectrum of sounds—preferably one that would strongly deemphasize low frequencies in accordance with hazard, and completely reject frequencies outside the auditory range—before integrating the result. On the standard sound-level meter, the A-weighting scale—one designed originally to simulate the action of the auditory mechanism in judging *loudness* of *weak* sounds—gives the most deemphasis to low frequencies, so it has become fashionable to express sounds in terms of their A-weighted level, and the integral over time of the A-weighted power, converted for some reason back to decibels, is called the "immission level" (5). I expect that we will hear some words in its behalf in the next paper.

If the evidence for its validity were convincing, this volume would not have been prepared, as the problem would be solved. Nevertheless, the insistence of the most ardent proponents of total A-weighted energy has resulted in its acceptance by ISO (6) and by the Environmental Protection Agency (7), so it is likely to be used more and more in the future, despite its shortcomings. Therefore, it may prove instructive to examine noise exposures from the viewpoint of how correction factors may be adduced that, when applied to the immission level or $L_{eq(t)}$, will give approximately correct results (e.g., like the 5-dB penalty that was at one time attached to pronounced pure-tone components of a noise).

Let me turn now to the second problem I mentioned earlier: determining that the only cause of a threshold shift was in fact the intervening noise exposure. In TTS studies, one can control conditions sufficiently over the short time period usually involved to exclude extraneous causes of threshold shift. In studies of PTS, however, except for those involving acoustic trauma (shifts associated with a single severe exposure) in experimental animals, such control has simply not been possible. Nor, in man, is it evermore likely to *be* possible, especially since our government now requires ear protection in noise levels of 90 dB(A) or more. Our knowledge of the permanent effects of noise on man must be based on studies done before the advent of government paternalism in this area.

Nearly all of these studies of PTS from industrial noise (INIPTS) suffer from a variety of ills. One of the more significant is that the thresholds at the time the worker first entered the noisy environment are not known, and so must be assumed to have been normal. In addition, all too often the testing environment or the audiometric technique did not permit measurement of 0 dB hearing levels. Temporary threshold shifts may have existed because of failure to test hearing before the beginning of the day's work. The worst problem, however, besides that of determining what the industrial noise exposure over a period of years actually was, is how to exclude, or compensate for, changes in hearing caused by the aging process (presbycusis), by diseases, industrial chemicals, ototoxic drugs, and blows to the head (nosoacusis), and by intense sound experienced outside the work situation—sounds to which the individual exposes himself willingly, if not eagerly, such as motorcycle noise, loud music, or sports gunfire (sociocusis).

Since nobody is exempt from exposure to these 3 factors, it is in my opinion quite futile to attempt to find a sample of industrial workers whose hearing is free of presbycusis, sociocusis, and nosoacusis. Yet strangely enough, most studies of industrial NIPTS still seek this Holy Grail by frantically eliminating subjects from the experimental group instead of simply trying to obtain a control (comparison) group matched in all these factors. As a result, we still really do not know just where an industrial noise exposure becomes hazardous, even if we restrict ourselves to the most constant of noise environments. Although Fig. 1 shows what I consider (8) to be the most reasonable estimate at the moment of the growth of the median INIPTS after 10 years of daily 8-hr exposure as a function of A-weighted level for various frequencies, curves based on a synthesis by Passchier-Vermeer (9) of extant survey data, errors as large as 10 dB could easily exist. However, if these figures are eventually substantiated, then for a steady industrial noise having an "average" spectrum (whatever that might be), there is no hazard from 80-dB(A) noise, a barely measurable effect at 85 dB(A), and a significant high-frequency hearing loss at 90 dB(A), the level that seems to just fail to affect hearing at 2,000 Hz and below.

The situation with intermittent or time-varying noises is even worse. Individuals with intermittent exposures are usually excluded from audiometric surveys, so even less data is available, and of course in order to combine what few results there are, one must first make a decision about how to characterize the noise exposures. Thus, although the lack of hearing loss in air crew members, musicians, and its relatively low occurrence in miners seems to indicate that the hazard associated with intermittent noise is much less than what one would predict if the same daily dose of acoustic energy were experienced in a single burst, the exact relation remains unknown. Whereas

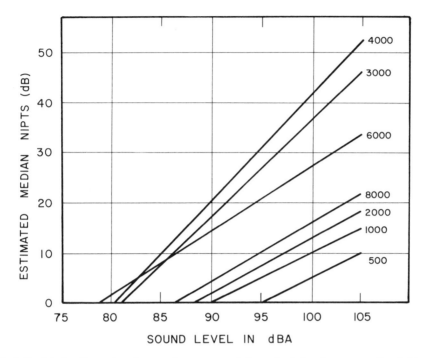

FIG. 1. Straight-line fits to data from various sources relating noise-induced permanent threshold shifts (HLs corrected for presbycusis and sociocusis) to exposures of 10 years or more to noise levels indicated on the abscissa. (Adapted from ref. 9.)

attempts have been made to "account for" intermittency by such devices as allowing a 5-dB increase in level for a reduction of 50% in exposure time, as in the present American standard, it is fair to say that such guesses have not found universal acclaim.

Since we know practically nothing about NIPTS, either industrial or sociocusic, it has always seemed reasonable to study TTS instead, with the hope that at least an ordinal relation exists between the TTS and NIPTS produced by a given noise. If so, then when, some time in the future, even a single reliable NIPTS-producing daily exposure is established, we may be able to tie a TTS grid to this point, giving a scale that would accurately reflect the hazard of all types of exposures—to steady, interrupted, and impulse noises. This assumption may or may not be correct, but I shall proceed as if it were.

A corollary of the above assumption is that if two noise exposures produce the same temporary effects, they will eventually lead to the same NIPTS, and hence are equally hazardous. Unfortunately, however, truly identical temporary effects are not generally produced by different noise exposures: they may be the same in some respects but not others. So the use of TTS in development of risk criteria is not a simple matter either. Let us nevertheless see what generalizations about the growth and recovery of TTS can be found.

The recovery process should be considered first, although this may seem paradoxical. This is so because the process of testing the threshold occupies a finite amount of time, during which recovery is of course proceeding. After a single uninterrupted moderate exposure to steady noise, recovery usually follows an exponential course, so that if TTS in dB is plotted against the logarithm of time, a reasonably straight line usually is found, one that indicates full recovery after at most 16 hours. This so-called "physiological fatigue" has in the past usually been characterized by its value 2 min after cessation exposure, TTS_2, that is, the TTS remaining after at least 2 shorter-lived types of auditory adaptation have run their course. The course of recovery is independent of whether the TTS_2 of say 20 dB is at 500 Hz or at 4,000 Hz, or whether the fatiguing noise dose was a long exposure at a relatively low level, or a short exposure at a high level, within limits of course.

In "pathological fatigue," on the other hand, recovery requires more than 16 hr. Practically speaking, this dividing line may be an important one, demarking the boundary between a TTS that is probably innocuous from one that may well eventually lead to a permanent loss. That is, in the ordinary work pattern of today, 8 hr of industrial noise exposure is followed by 16 hr of recovery. If the ear has recovered to normal by the time the next workday begins, then it is not very likely that repeated exposures will ever lead to permanent damage—assuming, of course, that the *same* noise dose is experienced each day. But if, instead, there is still some residual TTS as the new exposure begins, then the probability of gradually cumulative permanent effects would seem to be considerably higher.

However, the 16-hr dividing line is more than a capricious limit that depends on the particular work–rest pattern of our society and the 24-hr cyclicity imposed by the period of rotation of the earth. It has been found (4) that if full recovery requires more than 16 hr, then its course will *not* be linear in the logarithm of time, but linear in time. That is, in pathological fatigue, little change in TTS will be observed in the first few hours of recovery, so that this may be termed "delayed" recovery, and the threshold will improve by the same number of decibels each day. In short, the practical importance of incomplete recovery after 16 hr of rest lies in the fact that it is accompanied by a change in the pattern of recovery.

As mentioned before, if the exposure is to a continuous noise, then as long as TTS_2 is less than 25 dB, the recovery will proceed normally (linear in log time). If, therefore, all industrial noise exposures were to be continuous noise, it would be necessary only to restrict permissible exposures to those producing 20 dB of TTS_2 or less, and we could be confident that no permanent losses would develop. However, intermittent exposures at high levels (over 100 dB SPL or so) may produce a TTS_2 of less than 25 dB that nevertheless displays delayed recovery. Exposure to repeated impulse noise may also give delayed recovery. Therefore TTS_2 alone is not an unfailing index of the hazardousness of the noise dose that produced it.

This is an unfortunate state of affairs, because TTS_2, or at least the TTS shortly after cessation of exposure, is easy to measure, and is fairly predictable from the characteristics of the noise dose that produces it. Let me briefly review (4) some of the characteristics of TTS_2s of 10–30 dB.

1. The maximum TTS is produced at a frequency somewhat higher than the exposure frequency. Thus a pure-tone fatiguer will generate a TTS whose maximum lies about half an octave above; bands of noise of reasonably constant spectrum level will produce maximum TTSs half an octave above their respective upper filter cutoff frequencies.

2. For purposes of predicting TTS, it is necessary only to measure octave-band levels of noise; a finer analysis is only a waste of time, since the size of the "critical band" increases to about an octave at high levels. Although a pure-tone component of a real-life noise is more annoying than an equivalent amount of energy spread over an octave, it does not appear to be enough more hazardous, if any, to merit separate consideration.

3. The TTS_2 produced by a noise that is steady or fluctuates rapidly but regularly in time is proportional to the logarithm of exposure time, up to about 10 or 12 hr, at which time it has reached an asymptote. Although extending an exposure beyond 10 hr will not produce any greater TTS_2, the hazard that repeated daily exposures of more than 10 hr will eventually produce permanent damage probably is increased, if the daily TTS_2 is large, because the ear is not allowed to recover before the next noise exposure begins. The actual effect of maintaining such "asymptotic TTS" over a period of many days is not known; careful animal experimentation is still needed to establish the degree of increase in risk associated with say a 1-week continuous exposure relative to a 12-hr one, as they both produce the same initial TTS_2. We have found, however, that for moderate TTS_2s, the course of recovery after a 24-hr exposure is no slower than after an 8-hr one.

4. Other things being equal, TTS_2 is roughly proportional to the number of decibels by which the noise level exceeds a certain "base" value, SPL_0. Thus if an exposure for a certain time to a given noise at 90 dB produces 10 dB of TTS_2, and an exposure at 95 dB generates 14 dB, one can predict with some confidence that 100 dB will produce 18 dB.

5. Intermittent noise will not produce as much TTS as the same total energy of continuous noise. That is, a noise that is on half the time will generate less TTS_2 than the same noise, on continuously at a level 3 dB lower, even though the total acoustic energy presented to the ear is the same. If the noise bursts are of 3 to 4 min duration or less, the reduction

in TTS is considerable. For high-frequency noises, the reduction due to intermittency is approximately equal to the on-fraction of the noise: if the noise is on one-fourth of the time, it will generate only about ¼ as much TTS_2.

For low-frequency noises, the reduction due to intermittency is even greater; although an 8-hr exposure to a 250-Hz octave band of noise (i.e., 350–700 Hz) at 95 dB SPL will produce a TTS_2 of about 10 dB at 500 Hz, if the noise is made intermittent with an on-fraction of ½, the level may be raised to 115 dB SPL without generating more than 8 dB of TTS_2. Increasing the duration of noise bursts (and, of course, of the periods of quiet in between them) leads to a lesser "saving" of TTS_2.

For longer bursts of noise, however, the saving is not as great, and becomes practically negligible, at least at 4,000 Hz, when the bursts are as long as 20 min. Tables 1–3 and Figs. 2–4 illustrate the above principles. Ten normal-hearing listeners were exposed for 8 hr to octave-band noises at various levels with several on-fractions R (1, 0.5, 0.25, and 0.125) and cycle durations T of 1.5, 9, and 40 min. The resultant TTS_2s at the frequencies showing the most effect are listed in the tables and portrayed in the figures. It is clear that the longer pulses produce more TTS for a given total energy.

Figure 2 indicates that a trading relation of 5 dB for each halving of the exposure time is approximately correct for even this worst frequency, 4,000 Hz. That is, each time the on-fraction is cut in half, the level may be increased by 5 dB without increasing the TTS_2. Figure 3 shows that with 1,000-Hz octave-band noise, halving the on-fraction and raising the SPL by 5 dB results in even smaller TTSs; finally, Fig. 4 demonstrates that if the

TABLE 1. TTS_2 produced by 8-hr exposures to 4,000-Hz octave-band noise with various on-fractions R and on–off periods T (in minutes) at selected SPLs[a]

R	T	4,000-Hz Octave Band (2,800–5,600 Hz) Sound Pressure Level (dB)					
		75	80	85	90	95	100
1	Cont.	6.4	14.5	23.3	—	—	—
0.5	1.5	—	—	8.6	14.0	—	—
0.5	9	—	—	15.2	—	—	—
0.5	40	—	—	18.1	—	—	—
0.25	1.5	—	—	—	8.5	13.3	—
0.25	9	—	—	—	14.7	—	—
0.25	40	—	(3.5)	—	18.8	—	—
0.125	1.5	—	—	—	—	8.6	19.7
0.125	9	—	—	—	—	10.5	—
0.125	40	—	—	—	12.5	(>20)	—

[a] Average of 20 ears (10 normal-hearing test subjects) and 2 test frequencies (4,000 and 5,600 Hz).

TABLE 2. TTS_2 produced by 8-hr exposures to 1,000-Hz octave-band noise with various on-fractions R and on–off periods T at selected SPLs[a]

		1,000-Hz Octave Band (700–1,400 Hz) Sound Pressure Level (dB)				
R	T	85	90	95	100	105
1	Cont.	9.1	16.8	—	—	—
0.5	1.5	—	4.3	8.4	—	—
0.5	9	—	—	10.1	—	—
0.5	40	—	—	15.0	—	—
0.25	1.5	—	—	—	5.6	8.1
0.25	9	—	—	—	8.2	13.4
0.25	40	—	—	—	11.4	—
0.125	1.5	—	—	—	—	4.8
0.125	9	—	—	—	—	6.7
0.125	40	—	—	—	8.4	11.9

[a] Average of 20 ears (10 normal-hearing test subjects) and 2 test frequencies (2,000 and 2,800 Hz).

noise is on only half the time, levels of 250-Hz noise as high as 115 dB SPL will not generate more than 10 dB of TTS_2.

Because the 4,000-Hz data comes closest to supporting the total-energy hypothesis, it might be worthwhile to construct a table showing the "saving" effected by intermittency in this frequency range. For example, 85 dB, on half the time with a 1.5-min period (i.e., 45 sec on, 45 sec off), generates the same TTS as perhaps 77 dB of continuous noise. Since the energy of the intermittent exposure is the same as a continuous 82-dB noise, the "saving"

TABLE 3. TTS_2 produced by 8-hr exposures to 250-Hz octave-band noise with various on-fractions R and on–off periods T and selected SPLs[a]

		250-Hz Octave Band (175–350 Hz) Sound Pressure Level (dB)						
R	T	90	95	100	105	110	115	120
1	Cont.	5.1	8.0	—	—	—	—	—
0.75	1.5	—	—	7.9	—	—	—	—
0.75	9	—	—	8.0	—	—	—	—
0.75	40	—	—	9.3	—	—	—	—
0.5	1.5	—	(3.7)	(6.0)	4.7	5.4	7.5	—
0.5	9	—	—	—	—	—	9.5	—
0.5	40	—	—	—	—	—	—	—
0.25	1.5	—	—	—	3.3	4.9	5.4	5.6
0.25	9	—	—	—	—	—	5.5	—
0.25	40	—	—	—	—	—	6.6	—

[a] Average of 20 ears (10 normal-hearing test subjects) and 2 test frequencies (500 and 700 Hz).

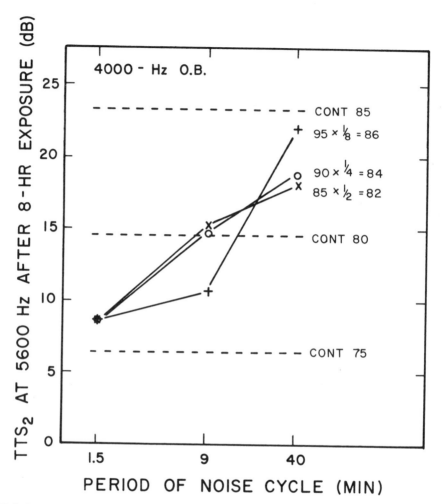

FIG. 2. Data from Table 1, plotted to show change in TTS$_2$ associated with the period of the noise cycle. Lines connect points corresponding to a constant on-fraction; L_{eq} is indicated at the left. 4,000 Hz.

here is 5 dB. For a 9-min cycle, however, the difference is only 2 dB, and for the 40-min cycle (20-min noise bursts) the saving appears to be nil, as the TTS is just about what would be expected from 82 dB continuous.

Table 4 shows the savings (the error in effective level that would exist if the total-energy theory were applied) for all 3 on-fractions. Similar tables for 1,000 and 250 Hz are shown in Tables 5 and 6; these show even larger "savings"—for example, there is a 3-dB saving at 1,000 Hz even for the 20-min-burst condition. However, if one grants that exposure standards should be based on the worst conditions, we should keep our attention on the 4,000-Hz data.

As I look at Table 4, I cannot see any simple way to correct total energy

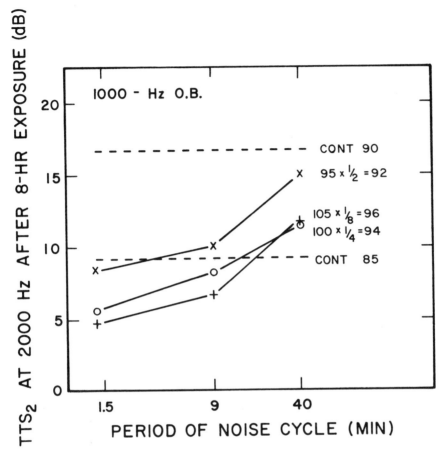

FIG. 3. Data from Table 2, plotted to show change in TTS$_2$ associated with the period of the noise cycle. Lines connect points corresponding to a constant on-fraction; L$_{eq}$ is indicated at the left. 1,000 Hz.

for intermittency. The correction depends on both the on-fraction and the burst duration. A 5-dB-per halving time rule will be better than the 3 dB of the total-energy procedure, but even it underemphasizes the reduction in effect in going from continuous noise to one on half the time if the bursts are short.

I submit, therefore, that at the present time there is insufficient evidence to justify changing the present American standard for noise exposure: viz., 8 hr at 90 dBA with a 5-dB (per halving exposure time) trading relation. If the equal-energy theory were accepted and used, we would have to develop such complicated correction factors that the basic simplicity of the equal-energy theory would be quite lost. It should be clear that *any* simple rule relating level, duration, and hazard is an oversimplification; which oversimplification gives the least error is still to be determined.

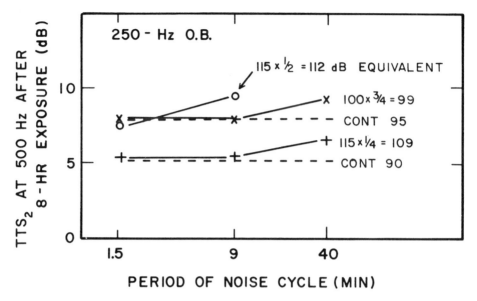

FIG. 4. Data from Table 3, plotted to show change in TTS$_2$ associated with the period of the noise cycle. Lines connect points corresponding to a constant on-fraction; L_{eq} is indicated at the left. 250 Hz.

TABLE 4. *Reduction in effective level, in dB, caused by breaking up a 4,000-Hz exposure through interjection of rest periods, for different on-fractions R*

			Period of noise cycle (min)		
SPL	R	L_{eq}	1.5	9	40
$85 \times \frac{1}{2} = 82$			5	2	0
$90 \times \frac{1}{4} = 84$			7	4	2
$95 \times \frac{1}{8} = 86$			9	9	2

TABLE 5. *Reduction in effective level, in dB, caused by breaking up a 1,000-Hz exposure through interjection of rest periods, for different on-fractions R*

			Period of noise cycle (min)		
SPL	R	L_{eq}	1.5	9	40
$95 \times \frac{1}{2} = 92$			7	6	3
$100 \times \frac{1}{4} = 94$			12	10	7
$105 \times \frac{1}{8} = 96$			14	13	9

TABLE 6. Reduction in effective level, in dB, caused by breaking up a 250-Hz exposure through interjection of rest periods, for different on-fractions R

			Period of noise cycle (min)		
SPL	R	L_{eq}	1.5	9	40
100 × ¾ = 99			4	4	1
115 × ½ = 112			17	14	—
115 × ¼ = 109			19	19	16

ACKNOWLEDGMENTS

The research reported herein was supported by a grant from the National Institute of Occupational Safety and Health of the Public Health Service, Department of Health, Education, and Welfare (Grant 5 R01 OH 00350).

REFERENCES

1. Bredberg, G. (1968): Cellular pattern and nerve supply of the human organ of Corti. *Acta Otolaryngol.* [*Suppl.*] (*Stockh.*), 236.
2. Eldredge, D. H., and Miller, J. D. (1969): Acceptable noise exposures—Damage risk criteria. *Noise as a Public Health Hazard,* edited by W. D. Ward and J. E. Fricke, pp. 110–120. ASHA Reports No. 4.
3. Ward, W. D. (1975): Effects of noise on oral communication. *Proceedings L'Uomo e il Rumore, Torino, Italy, 1975.*
4. Ward, W. D. (1973): Adaptation and Fatigue. In: *Modern Developments in Audiology,* edited by J. Jerger, pp. 301–344. Academic Press, New York.
5. Robinson, D. W. (1968): The Relationships between Hearing Loss and Noise Exposure, National Physical Laboratory Aero Report Ac 32, Teddington, England.
6. Anon., International Standards Organization, Technical Group 43.
7. Anon., Information on Levels of Environmental Noise Requisite to Protect Public Health and Welfare with an Adequate Margin of Safety, *U.S. Environmental Protection Agency Report No. 550/9–74–004.* U.S. Govt. Printing Office, Washington, D.C.
8. Ward, W. D. (1974): Noise Levels Are Not Noise Exposures. A Critical Look at the Levels Document, *Proceedings NOISEXOP Conference, Chicago, Illinois, 1974,* pp. 170–175.
9. Passchier-Vermeer, W. (1968): Hearing Loss Due to Exposure to Steady-state Broadband Noise, IG-TNO Report 35. Delft, Netherlands.

DISCUSSION

J. Keeler: You have correctly predicted that I was going to talk about exponential models this afternoon. You showed some data plotted against linear time. It pleases me to see you use linear time. But you showed that the decay was linear, therefore not exponential; you realize, I'm sure, that if you take a large enough time constant in your exponential, it looks linear.

J. Botsford: On those graphs, a vertical scale was logarithmic (dB) and the horizontal scale was linear, therefore it comes out to be a line which is exponential.

G. Price: If you monitor recovery with CM we find that uninterrupted CM recovers linearly in log time. However, interruption in the recovery process, particularly early in the recovery phase, can lead to serious long-term effects. When we understand this data, perhaps we can apply it to humans. Apparently there are processes within the ear which are very important to the recovery process. We've established this with the cat ear. Perhaps we should look at this in the human ear, then the problem which looks like a maze at the moment in the human ear, would make some sense.

Effects of Noise on Hearing, edited by Donald Henderson,
Roger P. Hamernik, Darshan S. Dosanjh, and John H. Mills.
Raven Press, New York © 1976.

The Equal Energy Concept Applied to Impulse Noise

Alan Martin

Institute of Sound and Vibration Research, University of Southampton, Southampton, England

Although it has been known since the work of Holt (1) and Barr (2) among boilermakers in the 19th century that excessive industrial impulse noise causes impairment of hearing, little quantitative research was carried out on the subject until about 15 years ago. Because the effects of impulse noise on hearing are less well documented than for steady-state noise, there is as yet no internationally agreed or accepted method for assessing the hazard to hearing from it. The problem is further confused by the relatively complex and large number of physical parameters which may be used to describe such noise, and the difficulties of obtaining a relationship between these parameters and noise-induced hearing loss (NIHL). Furthermore, methods of measuring impulse noise have, in the past, involved specialized and somewhat complex instrumentation, whereas the requirement in industry is for a relatively simple system of measurement which may be used by the "nonexpert."

At the present time there are 2 methods available for the assessment of hazard to hearing from impulse noise. One is the damage risk criteria (DRC) recommended by the American Natl. Research Council Committee on Hearing Biacoustics and Biomechanics (CHABA)(3) in 1968, which are based mainly on the work of Coles et al. (4). These DRC have been based mainly on temporary threshold shift (TTS) studies and were proposed for the assessment of gunfire noise, although attempts have been made to extend them to include industrial impact noise. A second approach has recently been made by Martin (5), Guberan et al. (6), Ceypek et al. (7) and others, who carried out retrospective studies in industry of permanent NIHLs in workers exposed to industrial impact noise, notably that caused by drop-forging. They showed that such NIHLs caused by long-term exposure may be related to impact noise in terms of the "equal-energy" concept, the latter being quantified in 1970 by Burns and Robinson (8) for exposure to steady-state industrial noise. This extension of the energy concept is an important step, as it presents the possibility of a unified and relatively simple system for the assessment of hazard to hearing from the majority of industrial noises.

This chapter reviews and compares available relevant information on the effects of impulse noise on hearing in light of the energy concept.

421

IMPULSE AND IMPACT NOISE

There are a number of different physical processes which act as sources of noise characterized by sharp initial transients. They may be divided into 2 main categories: those processes which produce a high initial sound pressure peak by the collision of 2 or more masses, such as drop-forging and hammering; and those which produce a high initial sound pressure peak by the sudden compression or rarefaction of gas, such as gunfire and explosions. Noise generated by mechanical impact is generally characterized

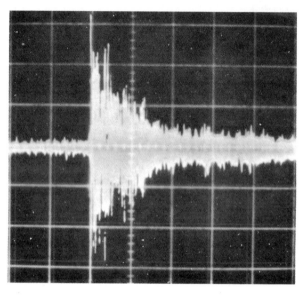

FIG. 1. Example of impulse noise waveform generated by the collision of two masses: drop-forging.

by a pressure amplitude–time waveform having a high initial peak which is followed by an approximately exponentially decaying envelope as the "ringing" of the objects involved in the impact is attenuated by the damping forces within them. An example of this type of waveform is illustrated in Fig. 1. On the other hand, impulse noise produced by explosive sources under free-field conditions is typified by a sound pressure waveform having an "N" configuration, as shown in Fig. 2. Under reverberant or semireverberant conditions, however, this type of noise assumes the exponentially decaying waveform shown in Fig. 1.

In general, therefore, the majority of impulse noises have sound pressure waveforms of the type shown in Fig. 1, while those generated mainly in free-field in the military sphere follow the example in Fig. 2. In general,

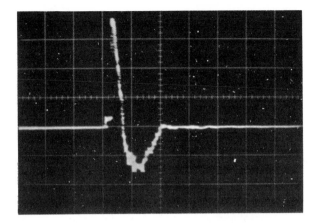

FIG. 2. Example of impulse noise waveform generated by a sudden expansion of gas under anechoic conditions: starting pistol shot.

those noises having exponentially decaying waveforms will be considered in this chapter.

THE ENERGY CONCEPT FOR HEARING DAMAGE

The ultimate objective of any scheme for rating the hazard to hearing from noise is to specify the maximum acceptable noise exposure in terms of noise level, frequency characteristics, and exposure duration. Owing to the physical nature of impulse noise, however, the specification of these quantities is complex, whereas the method of assessment should be simple. As Botsford (9) has stated: "Methods for estimating the hazard to hearing of noise exposure must be made as simple as possible in order to encourage the application of the information for preventing occupational hearing loss." A concept that fulfils these requirements is an energy concept.

A "constant energy" principle was proposed in 1955 by Eldred et al. (10), who suggested that the sound intensity multiplied by the exposure duration determines the amount of damage to hearing. This principle served as the basis for one of the first DRC formally established in America in 1956 (11).

The current energy concept for hearing damage may be summarized in terms of the following 3 hypotheses:

1. Equal amounts of A-weighted sound energy cause equal amounts of damage to hearing.
2. Hearing damage is proportional to some function of the acoustical energy received, although this function may not necessarily be a linear one.
3. A trading relationship exists between exposure time and noise level,

the product of the two being a measure of the total acoustical energy received.

These hypotheses define the principal elements which form the basis of a conceptual relationship between noise and damage to hearing.

The most convincing evidence that an energy concept is valid in the case of permanent NIHL from steady-state noise has come from the work of Burns and Robinson (8). Their research involved surveys of the hearing levels of a large number of noise-exposed subjects together with their noise histories and details of noise levels and spectra. A group of nonexposed control subjects was also investigated. The data from 759 rigorously screened noise-exposed subjects and 97 control subjects were corrected for age, using curves based on the presbycusis data of Hinchcliffe (36). An expression was derived by empirical methods relating "presumed noise-induced hearing-loss," H, to the A-weighted noise immission level, E_A

$$H = 27.5' [1 + \tanh (E_A + U_n - \lambda_f - b)/15] + U_n \qquad (1)$$

Where λ_f is a constant depending upon audiometric frequency, U_n is a correction parameter for the centile of the exposed population and b is a correction factor for the sex of the subjects. The immission level of the noise is given by the relation

$$E_A = L_A + 10 \log (T/T_0) \qquad (2)$$

Where L_A is the A-weighted sound level of the noise, T is the exposure time in months or years, on the basis of 8 hr/day 5 days a week, and T_0 is a reference duration equal to the unit in which T is reckoned.

These findings give strong support to the energy concept. Equation (2) indicates that a trading relationship exists between time and level and shows that their product is an appropriate measure of total sound energy. Furthermore Eq. (1) establishes the existence of a functional relationship between permanent NIHL and total incident sound energy, this being of a hyperbolic form.

The work of Burns and Robinson also produced a daily measure of noise exposure in terms of incident sound energy for fluctuating noise levels. This may be defined as the equivalent continuous sound level, L_{eq}, which in the course of a nominal working day would cause the same A-weighted sound energy to be received as that due to the actual sound over the actual working day. This is given by the expression

$$L_{eq} = 10 \log \frac{1}{T_R} \int_0^{T_S} \frac{[P_A(t)]^2}{P_0^2} dt \qquad (3)$$

Where T_R is the duration of the nominal working day, usually 8 hr, T_S is the total daily exposure time, P_A is the instantaneous A-weighted sound pressure in pascals (N/m²) and P_0 is the reference rms sound pressure of 2×10^{-5} pascals.

Thus the expression for immission level given in Eq. (2) may also be expressed as

$$E_A = L_{eq} + 10 \log \left(\frac{T}{T_0}\right) \tag{4}$$

So that immission level may be deduced in terms of L_{eq} and the number of years of exposure. From this the NIHL at different audiometric frequencies may be predicted for a particular percentage of an exposed population for a specific exposure period using Eq. (1).

The concept of L_{eq} is an important one, as it represents a measure of *noise dose,* itself a concept familiar to many other branches of medicine, but comparatively new to the field of acoustics.

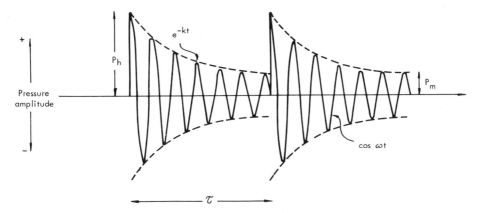

FIG. 3. Idealized representation of repetitive industrial impulse noise waveforms with relevant physical parameters.

So far in this discussion only steady-state noise has been considered. To examine the validity of the energy concept for impulse noise, it is first of all necessary to obtain a measure of L_{eq} in terms of the parameters of impulse noise.

The type of impulse noise waveform shown in Fig. 1 may be represented by a series of idealized pressure-time envelopes as depicted in Fig. 3. Martin (5) has shown that these may be adequately described in terms of the peak sound pressure, P_h in pascals, the decay constant k in reciprocal seconds (equal to $1/t_e$, where t_e is the decay time: the time in seconds taken for the pressure envelope to decay to $1/e$ (i.e., 0.37) of its initial peak height P_h) and the repetition rate, N in pulses/sec. Atherley and Martin (12) have shown that the equivalent continuous A-weighted sound level of such a noise is given by the expression

$$L_{eq} = 85.4 + 20 \log (P_h) + 10 \log (N_a) - 10 \log (k) + 10 \log (1 - e^{-2k/N}) \tag{5}$$

where N_a is the average repetition rate for a working day. The function has been verified experimentally using simulated impulse noise having variable waveform parameters (12). Thus by measuring typical values for the impulse waveform parameters P_h, k, and N_a, L_{eq} may be deduced for noises of this type. Consequently, a complex noise-exposure pattern such as this may be represented by a single number in terms of equivalent continuous sound level.

If it can be shown that L_{eq} is an appropriate measure of daily exposure to impulse noise and that, by deducing the immission level of the noise, the resulting NIHL may be adequately predicted by Eq. (1) from Burns and Robinson, this system may form the basis of a simple method for assessing hazard to hearing from impulse noise.

It is of interest at this stage to compare DRC for industrial impulse noise based on the energy principle with those proposed for gunfire noise by Coles et al. (4), CHABA (3), and the corrections to these by Coles and Rice (13) for larger numbers of impulses. This comparison is shown in Fig. 4. As these authors describe the duration of exponentially decaying impulses in terms of the time taken for the waveform envelope to decay by 20 dB from the initial peak (called the "B"-duration), it is necessary to relate this measure of duration with the decay time, t_e, mentioned above for Eq. (5). Thus: decay time, $t_e = 4.6$ ("B"-duration). Furthermore, an energy concept for impulse noise assumes a trading relationship between impulse duration and repetition rate (or total number of impulses received per day). Consequently a more useful representation of Eq. (5) may be obtained by

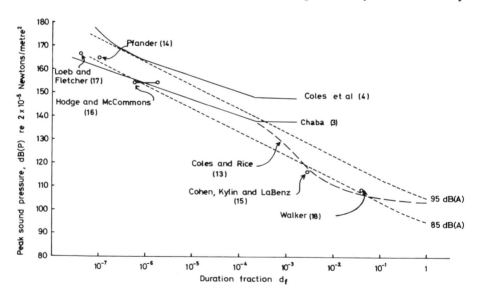

FIG. 4. Comparison of various DRC for impulse noise with equal energy curves for L_{eq} = 85 and 95 dB(A). [After Atherley and Martin (12).]

combining repetition rate and decay time into a composite parameter called the "duration fraction," d_f. Hence, $d_f = N_a.t_e$, where d_f represents the fraction of 1 sec that the peak sound pressure of the noise is at or greater than a level 8.7 dB beneath the peak sound pressure, P_h. By substituting for N_a and k $(= 1/t_e)$ in Eq. (5), the following expression is obtained

$$L_{eq} = 85.4 + 20 \log (P_h) + 10 \log (d_f) + 10 \log (1 - e^{-2/d_f}) \qquad (6)$$

This relationship forms the basis of a practical method for measuring L_{eq} for impulse noise and also allows the comparison of different DRC to be made.

Equation (6) has been used to compute the 2 equal energy curves for L_{eq}s of 85 and 95 dB(A), shown in Fig. 4, in terms of peak height, P_h, and duration fraction, d_f. Also shown in terms of these parameters are the DRC proposed by Coles et al. (4), CHABA (3), and the corrections of Coles and Rice (13), together with single point "criteria" derived from studies of impulse noise by Pfander (14), Cohen et al. (15), Hodge and McCommons (16), Loeb et al. (17), and Walker (18). These criteria have in common their basis on the results of TTS studies on human subjects and the implicit assumption that the limitation of TTS ensures the limitation of permanent NIHL.

As can be seen from Fig. 4, comparison of these various DRC with the equal energy curves indicates a general similarity between them. It would appear that these observations and recommendations are not in general conflict with an energy principle for impulse noise.

EXPERIMENTAL EVIDENCE

So far in this discussion an energy concept for impulse noise has been considered mainly from a theoretical viewpoint. It is now appropriate to examine it in the light of available experimental evidence. Furthermore, no direct distinction has yet been made between its application to temporary or persistent damage to hearing, nor has the influence of the acoustic reflex so far been considered.

The energy concept assumes that the temporal characteristics of noise exposure do not affect the resulting hearing loss, only the total A-weighted sound energy is important. However, the distribution of acoustical energy with time may be a material factor in the relationship between noise and hearing damage, whether temporary or permanent, as the recuperative and protective processes of the ear may be favored in some cases by particular temporal distributions of energy, and vice versa.

Available experimental evidence for an energy rule will be reviewed, first, in terms of TTS data, second, in the case of permanent NIHL, and finally, the possible protective influence of the acoustic reflex will be considered.

Temporary Threshold Shift

Quite a large number of studies of TTS produced by exposure to impulse noise have been carried out, and they are in general agreement that the energy concept does not adequately describe or predict TTS from this type of noise.

Investigations by Ward et al. (19), Ward (20,21), Fletcher and Loeb (22,23), Walker (18), and others have demonstrated that, not only does TTS from impulse noise fail to follow an energy rule, but also that no general clear relationships can be ascertained between the parameters of the noise, particularly its temporal distribution, and the degree of TTS produced.

The situation in this case is also complicated by the possible elicitation of the acoustic reflex, which may provide some degree of temporary protection under certain circumstances.

Martin (5) compared TTSs produced in 11 normally hearing subjects by impulse noises having equal sound energies but different temporal patterns. The envelopes of the noise waveforms were exponentially decaying. In one experiment, the subjects were exposed to repetitive impulses with peak sound pressures of 95, 100, 108, 115, and 120 dB(P) at a constant repetition rate of 50 pulses/sec. In a second experiment, the peak value was kept constant at 120 dB(P) and the repetition rates were 1, 2, 5, 10, 20, 50, 100, and

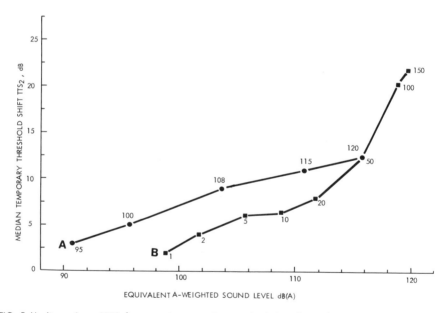

FIG. 5. Median values of TTS$_2$ (averaged over test frequencies 4, 6, and 8 kHz) plotted against A-weighted sound energy for variations in peak sound level (*curve A*) and variations in repetition rate (*curve B*), after Martin (5). Values of individual peak sound levels and repetition rates are shown for appropriate individual experimental points.

150 pulses/sec. The impulse waveform decay constant was 100 sec^{-1} in both cases. The median values of TTS$_2$ (TTS measured 2 min after cessation of the noise) averaged over audiometric test frequencies 4, 6, and 8 kHz are compared for the 2 experiments in Fig. 5 in terms of the A-weighted sound energy of the noise.

As can be seen from Fig. 5, equal amounts of sound energy do not cause equal amounts of TTS. The growth of TTS$_2$ with increasing peak sound pressure (curve A) is dissimilar to the growth of TTS$_2$ with increasing repetition rate (curve B), the 2 functions being significantly different (p < 0.005). The influence of the acoustic reflex may also be inferred from the plateau in function B for repetition rates of 5 and 10 pulses/sec, where the period of the impulses is of the same order as the reflex latency for these particular impulse noises.

These results may also be compared with those of other workers in terms of the total energy received by the ears. Figure 6 shows the average maximum TTS induced in 14 subjects by 1-min exposures to impulse noises having variable peak sound levels between 130 and 148 dB(P) reported by Ward et al. (19). Similar TTSs reported by Walker (18), who exposed 10 subjects to impulses having a peak level of 127 dB(P) for periods between 5 and 80 min are shown, as are the maximum TTSs found by Martin (5). It can be seen from Fig. 6 that not only does an energy rule not apply in this case, but also that there is no general agreement between the results of the different studies.

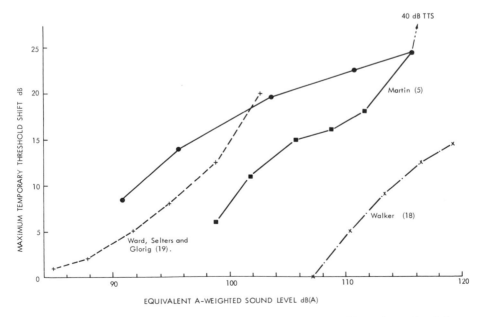

FIG. 6. Comparison of maximum TTS from exposure to impulse noise reported by various authors in terms of equivalent A-weighted sound energy.

McRobert and Ward (24) investigated the degree of TTS$_2$ induced in 7 normally hearing subjects. These were exposed on separate occasions to "nonreverberant" impulses (i.e., having an approximate "N"-wave configuration) presented at various peak levels for various durations. During each exposure the total energy presented to the ear remained constant. The results indicated that longer exposures to this type of impulse noise can be tolerated by a given decrease in peak level than is predicted by the energy concept.

Similar findings have been reported in animals. For example, Hamernik et al. (25) exposed groups of chinchillas to continuous noise, impulse noise, and a combination of both. They found that, whereas the TTSs incurred from the first 2 types of exposure were relatively mild and recovered to approximately normal hearing, the combination exposure produced about twice as much TTS, which did not recover and left sizeable amounts of permanent threshold shift (PTS). This degree of hearing loss is not predicted by an energy rule, as the combination of continuous and impulse noise added less than 1 dB to the impulse noise, whereas the hearing loss incurred was much more severe. Hamernik et al. attempted to explain this finding in terms of the metabolic processes in the cochlea.

Permanent Noise-Induced Hearing Loss

Relevant experimental data regarding persistent damage to hearing from impulse noise are rather hard to come by, being restricted to retrospective studies of permanent NIHL in man incurred during occupation, and to laboratory studies of PTS in animals. In addition to the usual difficulties of establishing previous noise exposure accurately, the former approach is further complicated by the increasingly widespread use of hearing protectors at the present time. This factor may tend to confound the estimation of noise exposure in future studies in industry where such hearing conservation measures are being undertaken.

Furthermore, results of animal experiments are difficult to interpret with accuracy because of species differences and the problems of extrapolation to man. In addition, histological studies have indicated that damage to the hair cells of the cochlea may occur from exposure to noise even though behavioral "audiograms" appear normal, thus bringing into question TTS as a measure of hearing loss.

Evidence for an equal energy hypothesis will be examined first, from experiments on impulse-noise-induced PTS in animals, and second from retrospective studies in NIHL in industry.

Experimentation on the effects of noise on the hearing of animals has become increasingly important within the last decade as new electrophysiological and histological techniques have been applied, in addition to the more classical behavioral methods of determining hearing threshold. However, comparatively little quantitative information is yet available on the effects of impulse noise on the hearing mechanism, particularly with regard to currently available DRC for impulse noise. Henderson and Hamernik (26) and their coworkers have carried out a series of experiments on the chinchilla to evaluate the effectiveness of the DRC proposed by Coles et al. (4). The parameters of the impulse noises used are compared in Fig. 7 with the Coles et al. DRC curve, together with those of impulse noises studied by Poche et al. (27) and Majeau-Chargois (28). Also shown are the DRC proposed by CHABA (3) and the equal-energy curve for an L_{eq} of 90 dB(A). The results of Henderson and Hamernik indicate that exposure to the highest peak sound pressure levels shown in Fig. 7 at each impulse duration produced both PTS (measured behaviorally) and hair cell losses in several experimental animals. The lower levels tended to produce little or no PTS, particularly at 158 and 140 dB(P), although the animals sustained losses of outer hair cells in the middle turn of the cochlea. Poche et al. (27) and Majeau-Chargois (28) exposed guinea pigs to numbers of impulses of different durations and peak sound levels and, although they did not carry out audiometry on the animals, they also reported considerable hair cell damage. Although complicated by species differences, these results tend to show that the CHABA and equal-energy DRC are apparently nearer the true estimate than the higher curve of Coles et al.

Henderson and Hamernik (29), in a review of animal experiments on this

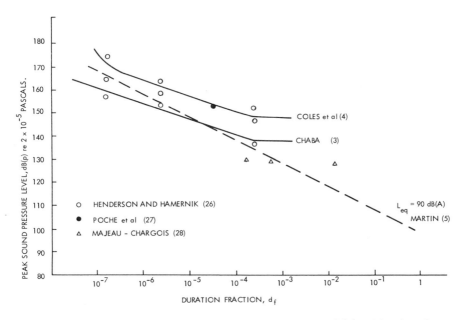

FIG. 7. Comparison of gunfire DRC and equal-energy curve for L_{eq} = 90 dB(A) with impulse noises employed in animal studies by Henderson and Hamernik (26), Poche et al. (27), and Majeau-Chargois (28).

topic, came to a similar conclusion. They considered that "several investigations have produced extensive cochlear damage in chinchilla and guinea pigs with impulses at least 25 dB below the Coles et al. (30) DRC curve for humans (27,28,31,32), although both chinchilla and guinea pig auditory thresholds are less sensitive than man's over a wide frequency range (Miller,33)."

Retrospective studies of impulse NIHL in man provide the most convincing evidence about the validity of the energy concept. They are concerned directly with long-term noise exposure and the resulting persistent loss of hearing, and do not rely upon investigations of "intermediary" factors such as TTS or animal studies.

In 1970 Martin (5,12) examined the hearing of 97 men exposed to drop-forge noise and investigated the relationships between the observed hearing losses and the parameters of the noise. Tests of hearing were made in the frequency range of 1–6 kHz 16 hr after the last exposure to noise and detailed noise histories were obtained. All men were examined otoscopically for abnormalities of the ear canal and eardrum. The results of 20 men were rejected because of auditory abnormalities or recent previous exposure to high-intensity noise other than drop-forging.

The noise parameters: peak sound pressure, decay time, and repetition rate were measured with a ¼-in. condenser microphone, wide-band amplifier, storage oscilloscope and Polaroid camera (Martin et al., 34). The average results for 2 factories are shown in Table 1, together with values of L_{eq} calculated using Eqs. (5) and (6). Each man's immission level, E_A, was then calculated from Eq. (4).

TABLE 1. Measured parameters of drop-forging noise

Factory	Peak height P_h (pascals)	Decay time t_e (sec)	Repetition rate, N (sec^{-1})	L_{eq} [dB(A)]
1	448	0.045	0.2	118
2	65	0.1	0.7	110

The hearing level of each man was corrected for age with the presbycusis corrections of Robinson (35) and these individual data are plotted against immission level for each of the 5 audiometric test frequencies in Fig. 8A-E. Also shown in the figure are curves of the 25, 50, and 75 percentiles of the presumed NIHL predicted by Burns and Robinson (8) from Eq. (1) over a range of immission levels between 100 and 140 dB. As can be seen from this figure, the agreement between the predicted curves and observed data is good. At each test frequency ~50% of the observed points lie between the predicted 25 and 75 percentile curves.

Cumulative distribution curves of these NIHL data are shown in Fig. 9 for

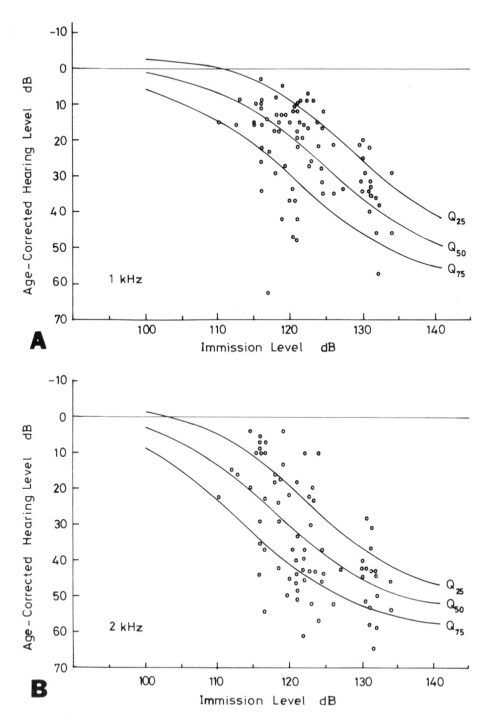

FIG. 8. (A–E) Individual age-corrected hearing levels of 77 drop-forgers plotted against noise immission level for audiometric test frequencies 1 to 6 kHz, after Martin (5). Also shown are median and quartile values (*solid curves*) predicted by Burns and Robinson (8). (C–E on pp. 434–435.)

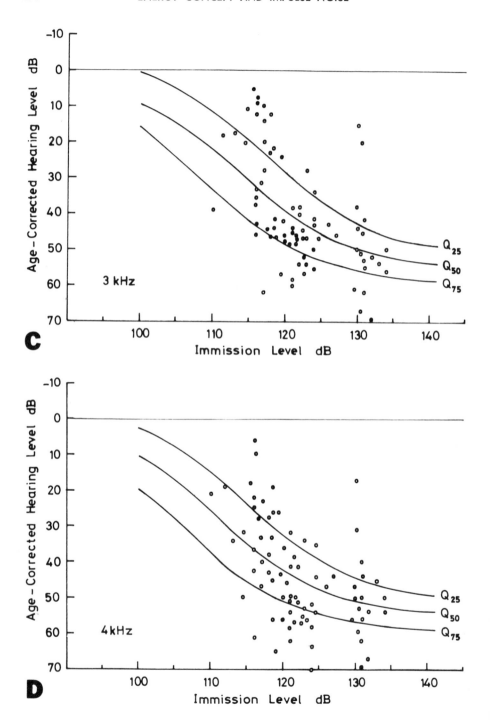

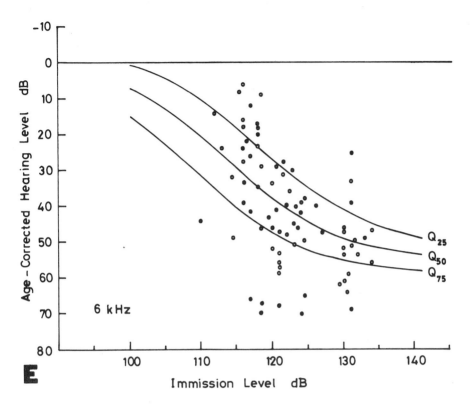

immission levels between 115 and 125 dB. Although the distributions are non-Gaussian, it can be seen that the shapes of the distribution curves at the different frequencies are similar to one another. Burns and Robinson, studying continuous noise, also reported cumulative distributions of this configuration, and they deduced values of the "normalizing" correction factors required to shift the curves at each test frequency along the hearing level axis so that they were superimposed upon the curve for 4 kHz. These correction factors are in fact the basis of the constant λ_f used in Eq. (1). Average values of these normalizing factors for impulse noise exposure have been deduced from the data in Fig. 9, and these are compared with Burns and Robinson's values in Table 2. Considering the relatively small number of data (55 subjects) used in this analysis of impulse noise exposure, the agreement between the two sets of data is surprisingly good. It indicates that the values of λ_f, the audiometric frequency correction parameter used in Eq. (1) reported by Burns and Robinson, are also applicable in the case of impulse NIHL.

The normalizing shifts of Burns and Robinson have therefore been applied to the data in Fig. 9 and the mean curve for an immission level of 120 dB is shown in Fig. 10. Also shown is the corresponding curve derived by Burns and Robinson in the case of steady-state noise. The agreement between the 2 curves

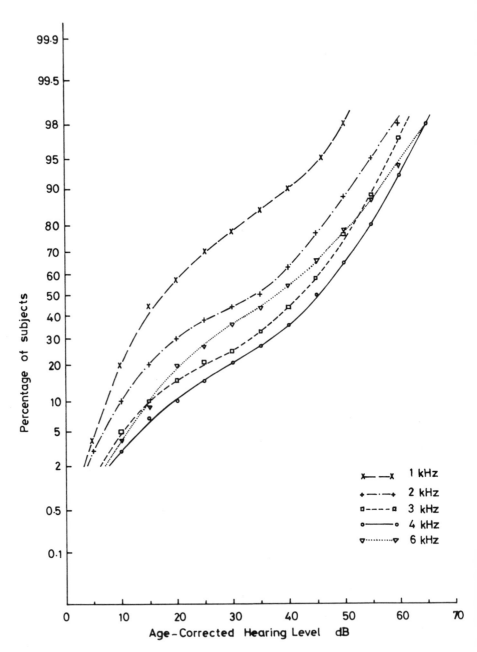

FIG. 9. Cumulative distributions of age-corrected hearing levels of 55 drop-forgers, at different audio-metric test frequencies, for immission levels between 115 and 125 dB. After Martin (5).

is good, and their shapes are similar to one another. As the shape of this trend curve governs U_n, the correction parameter for the centile of the population considered used in Eq. (1), the values of this parameter reported by Burns and Robinson should also apply to impulse NIHL. Thus, it is apparent that the constants of the predictive equation derived by Burns and Robinson in the case of steady-state noise may also be applied in the case of impulse noise produced by drop-forges.

A direct comparison between median and quartile values of observed and predicted age-corrected NIHLs is made in Fig. 11 for an immission level of 120 dB. As can be seen in the figure, agreement between the 2 sets of data is good, Eq. (1) tending to underpredict the observed hearing losses by an average of about 1 dB for median and quartile values across the test frequency range. A further comparison may also be made in terms of hearing levels not

TABLE 2. Normalizing shifts in decibels, for hearing-loss trend curves at different test frequencies

Audiometric frequency (kHz)		1	2	3	4	6
Axis	Martin (5)	18.5	9.5	2.7	0	4.3
Shifts	Burns and Robinson	14.0	7.5	2.0	0	3.0
(dB)	(8)					

corrected for presbycusis, as a check upon the applicability of the age corrections used by Burns and Robinson in their predictive system. Table 3 compares observed and predicted median hearing levels for a group of men exposed to impulse noise having an L_{eq} of 118 dB(A) for a median duration of 18.5 years, so that the immission level E_A is 130.7 dB. As in the previous comparison, the predicted data are an average of about 1 dB less than the measured hearing levels for the 5 test frequencies. Hence, the agreement between them may be considered to be excellent.

It is apparent from the above comparisons that there is close agreement between observed impulse NIHLs and those predicted by Eq. (1) for the range of immission levels so far considered. Furthermore, the shapes of the cumulative distribution curves indicate that the values of the parameters λ_t and U_n used to predict hearing loss from steady-state noise are also valid for exposure to impulse noise. Hence, Eq. (1) may be used to predict impulse NIHLs and, although it tends to underpredict the observed data by a small amount in this case, such discrepancies may be considered negligible compared with the variations usually associated with measurements of this type.

This study provides strong evidence that the energy concept, as embodied in Eq. (1), is a valid means of assessing the hazard to hearing from impulse noise of this type.

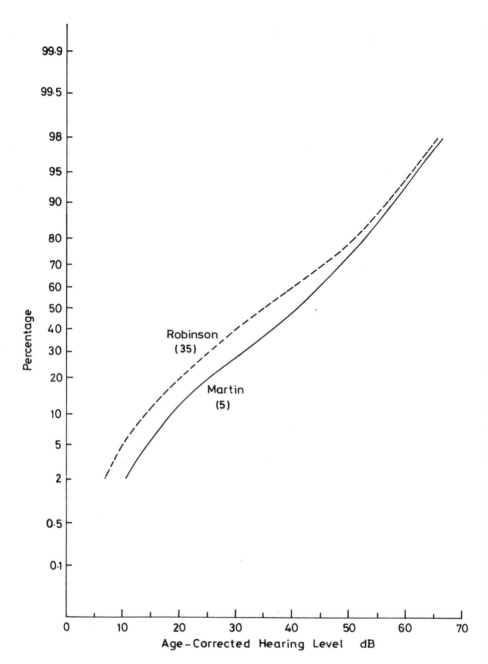

FIG. 10. Comparison of average cumulative distributions of frequency-normalized hearing levels reported by Robinson (35) and Martin (5) for similar immission levels.

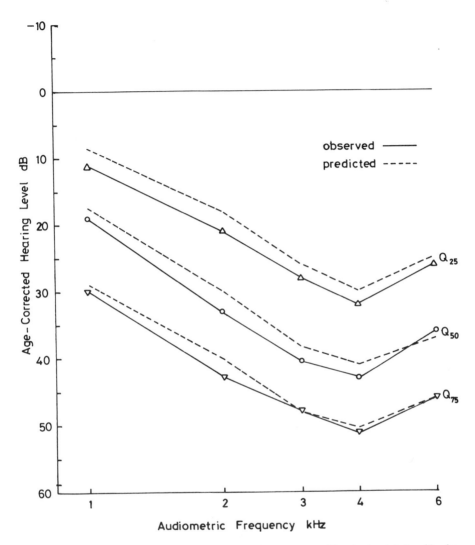

FIG. 11. Direct comparison of observed median and quartile age-corrected hearing levels induced by drop-forging noise with an immission level of 120 dB (Martin, 5) and predicted values (Burns and Robinson, 8).

Further evidence that hazard from impulse noise may be predicted by the energy concept comes from the work of Guberan et al. (6). They studied the hearing of 70 workers in 11 workshops in the drop-forging industry and 61 nonexposed controls, and measured the L_{eq}s of the impulse noises involved. The subjects were rigorously screened with otological examinations and noise histories and those having abnormalities rejected. The hearing levels of the exposed group were measured on Monday mornings.

The results were divided into 6 groups according to immission level. The ob-

TABLE 3. Median hearing levels, dB re BS 2497

Audiometric test frequency (kHz)	1	2	3	4	6
Observed	37.0	48.0	57.0	60.5	60.0
Predicted	41.3	48.5	55.3	58.7	58.6

From ref. 37.

served group mean hearing levels relative to the nonexposed controls are plotted against immission level in Fig. 12 for test frequencies 3, 4, and 6 kHz. Also shown are the hearing levels of 581 subjects in 20 groups reported by Robinson and Cook (38) for a range of steady-state noise immission levels between 95 and 130 dB. These latter data formed part of the basis for Eq. (1). It can be seen that there is reasonable agreement between the 2 sets of data for the 3 test frequencies.

Ceypek et al. (7) investigated the hearing levels of 213 drop-forge operators who were exposed to the noise for up to 30 years. Hearing tests were carried out at least 16 hr after the last noise exposure. The subjects were examined otoscopically and those with abnormalities or previous exposures to other types of noise excluded. Measurements of the impulse noise waveform parameters were made with a storage oscilloscope and ancillary equipment according to

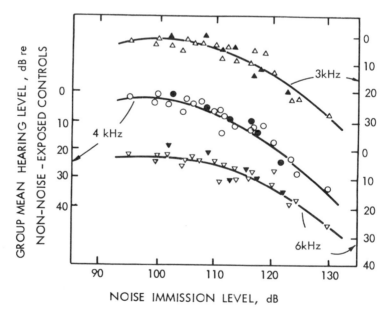

FIG. 12. Comparison of group mean hearing levels induced by drop-forging noise relative to non-noise-exposed controls reported by Guberan et al. (6) (*black circles and triangles*), with data of Robinson and Cook (38) for 581 subjects exposed to continuous noise.

the method of Martin and Atherley (3). The mean L_{eq} of the noise is calculated here from the data of Ceypek et al. to be 116 dB(A).

The thresholds of hearing data were divided into 8 groups according to exposure time and corrected for presbycusis with the data of Glorig and Nixon (40). These NIHLs are shown in Fig. 13A and B in the form of median au-

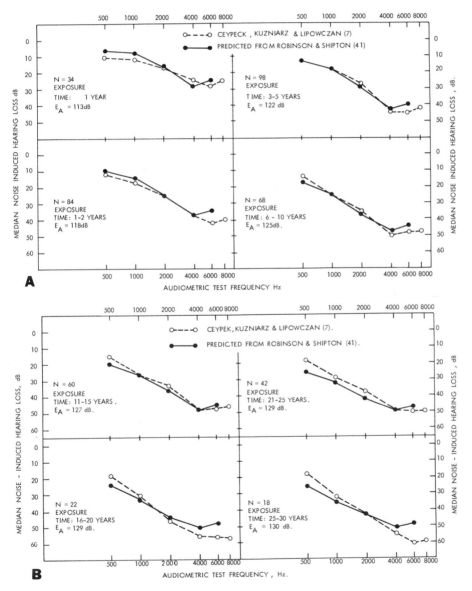

FIG. 13. (A and B) Comparison of median NIHL's reported by Ceypek et al. (7) in the case of drop forging noise with values predicted by Robinson and Shipton (41) for continuous noise, for 8 groups of subjects exposed for various periods of time.

diograms for each range of exposure time. Also shown in this figure are the median NIHLs predicted by the energy concept with the data reported by Robinson and Shipton (41) for immission levels between 113 and 130 dB. The number of ears tested, exposure time, and immission level are given in the figures for each group.

It can be seen from these comparisons that there is good agreement between observed and predicted NIHLs, in spite of the fact that Ceypek et al. used different presbycusis corrections from those employed by Robinson and his colleagues. The main discrepancy between the 2 sets of data occurs at 6 kHz, where the energy concept tends to underpredict the observed NIHLs by an average of about 4 dB. The average underprediction at 4 kHz for the 8 groups is less than 1 dB, while the overall difference between the 2 sets of data for the 5 test frequencies and 8 groups is an underprediction by the energy concept of less than 0.2 dB. This indicates the ability of the energy concept to predict NIHLs from impulse noises of this type with a high degree of accuracy.

A further comparison of these data is shown in Fig. 14, where the median NIHLs are plotted against exposure time for test frequencies 2 and 4 kHz. Also shown are the values predicted for these frequencies from the data of Robinson and Shipton. The abscissa is graduated in both exposure time and immission level, assuming an average L_{eq} of 116 dB(A). Here it can be seen

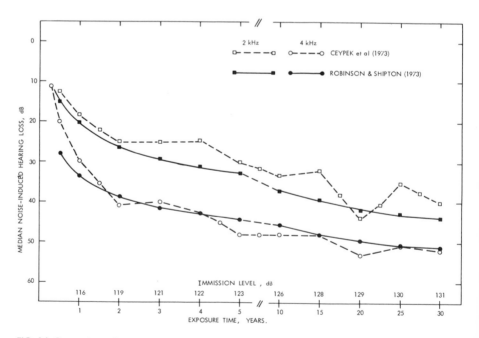

FIG. 14. Comparison of time course of median NIHLs reported by Ceypek et al. (7) for drop-forgers with data predicted by Robinson and Shipton (41) for test frequencies 2 and 4 kHz. The abscissa is graduated in both exposure time and noise immission level.

that the time course of the observed median NIHLs may be described adequately by the energy concept predictions. Kuzniarz (42) stated ". . . the measured and predicted median hearing losses were very close (to) each other. . . . There is a similar 'time-pattern' of the development of hearing loss induced both by continuous noise and industrial impulse noise of L_{eq} near 115 dB."

Atherley (43) examined the hearing levels of 71 men exposed to repetitive impulse noise produced by pneumatic chisels. This type of noise is generally produced in an interrupted manner. The subjects were rigorously screened as discussed above and consisted of 50 trimmers who use pneumatic chisels on manganese bronze castings. Their median age was 47 years and they were exposed to immission levels in the range 117–127 dB. The cumulative distribution of their hearing levels (re BS2497,37) averaged across test frequencies 1, 2, 3, 4, and 6 kHz is shown in Fig. 15 together with the cumulative distribution predicted by Eq. (1) for an immission level of 125 dB and age 47 years. This comparison shows good agreement between observed and predicted data, even

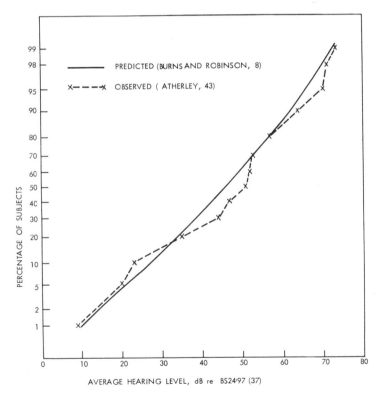

FIG. 15. Comparison of observed and predicted cumulative distributions of hearing levels (averaged over test frequencies between 1–6 kHz) for subjects (trimmers) exposed to interrupted repetitive impulse noise. Immission level 125 dB at age 47 years. [After Atherley (43).]

close to the extremes of the distribution at the 1 and 99 percentiles where such data are often less accurate. It provides evidence that an energy rule may also be applied to NIHL from exposure to interrupted bursts of repetitive impulse noise.

The investigations discussed above provide ample proof that the energy concept may be extended to include exposures to industrial impulse noises having peak sound pressures up to at least 150 dB(P). This extension includes noises having immission levels up to at least 135 dB and L_{eq}s of at least 125 dB(A).

It has been shown that, within the limits of the impulse noises considered, TTS does not follow an energy rule, whereas permanent NIHL does. Furthermore, the frequency at which maximum TTS occurs is strongly dependent upon the spectral content of the fatiguing stimulus, while maximum permanent NIHL is commonly found (8) in the region of 4 kHz, irrespective of the frequency characteristics of the noise. These factors may reflect a difference between the response of the ear to brief exposure and its response to habitual long-term exposure. In any event, the quantitative predictions of permanent NIHL from measurements of TTS would seem a procedure of doubtful validity. However, this is not to deny the principle underlying some DRC: namely, that noise insufficient to cause TTS will probably also be insufficient to cause much NIHL from habitual exposure to the same noise.

Action of the Acoustic Reflex

The elicitation of the acoustic reflex (AR) by an impulse noise and mixtures of this with continuous noise must be considered as a possible factor influencing an energy rule for impulse NIHL, as reflex contractions may affect the transmission of sound energy through the middle ear under certain circumstances. This subject has recently been extensively reviewed by Lutman and Martin (44).

There are 2 facets of this topic to be evaluated: the acoustic, temporal, and other conditions under which the middle ear muscles contract, and the effect that these contractions may have upon the transmission of sound through the ear. It is now generally accepted that, of the two middle ear muscles, the stapedius contracts as a reflex to acoustic stimuli at sound levels of about 80 dB and above and thus forms the major part of the AR of interest here, whereas the tensor tympani tends to react more as a startle response to sudden stimuli (Lutman and Martin, 44). However, the function of these muscles is still not fully understood, and there is as yet little direct evidence regarding the protective action of the AR during long-term exposures to noise producing permanent NIHL in man.

It has been shown by a number of workers that the AR may be elicited by wide-band noise having sound pressure levels above about 80 dB and pure tones above ~90 dB. Consequently, the AR certainly is elicited in the industrial environment where noise is a hazard to hearing. However, it has also been shown by Dallos (45), Djupesland et al. (46), and others that the reflex response tends to decline with time, mainly due to adaptation processes and particularly in the case of continuous stimuli. Thus the AR tends to adapt completely in 2 min or so in the case of high-frequency pure tones, and in 10 min or so in the case of low-frequency tones and random noise. However, it has also been shown by Gjaevenes and Sohoel (47) and others that the AR may easily be reelicited by a representation of the stimulus or a change in the stimulus frequency or level characteristics. Such changes in noise characteristics are common in the industrial environment.

In the cases of impulse noise and mixtures of impulse and continuous noises, the situation is more complicated. Slowly repetitive impulses of repetition rates less than about 1/sec will not be significantly affected by the AR due to its latent period. For repetition rates above about 5/sec, however, the effect of the latency is overcome and the AR response is elicited in an effective way. This is illustrated by the plateau in curve B in Fig. 5 and has been inferred by Cohen et al. (15) and Martin et al. (66) in the case of TTS studies, and illustrated directly by Corcoran (48) and Lutman (49) in the case of acoustic impedance measurements of the AR responses. These latter 2 workers have also shown that the AR response does not appear to adapt to any great degree to repetitive impulses of this type, and indeed may even grow under certain circumstances. The response of the AR to mixtures of steady-state and impulse noise has also been inferred from TTS studies by Cohen et al. (15) and Walker (18) and measured directly by Lutman (49). The AR response has been shown to be similar to steady-state noise and appears to adapt with time (49).

These findings indicate that in the majority of industrial environments, where noise characteristics usually vary somewhat with time, and mixtures of impulse and continuous noises are common, the AR may be active to a certain degree for much of the exposure time.

It now remains to examine the effect of this activity on the transmission of sound to the cochlea. Experiments on man by Fletcher and Riopelle (50), Chisman and Simon (51), Fletcher (52), and Ward (53,54) and on animals by Hilding (55) have shown that reductions in TTS of the order of 10 dB may be brought about by the acoustic elicitation of the AR prior to the oncoming impulses. However, it is not possible to infer a quantitative reduction in sound transmission through the middle ear from these somewhat oblique experiments, as the relationship between the effective reduction in stimulus level and the reduction in TTS in individual subjects is unknown.

The main work on this topic which indicates the probable effect on the transmission characteristics of the middle ear has been carried out by Borg (56,67) in rabbits. He has shown that the AR provides attenuation up to about 20 dB for frequencies below 1 kHz. Similar results have also been shown by Borg (68) in man, although giving less protection. Further, Lutman (49) has developed theoretical and analog models of the ear from which these transmission characteristics may be predicted. These agree with the data of Borg and show that the attenuation that does occur when the AR is elicited in man is at frequencies below about 1 kHz and is on average no greater than 10 dB.

Consequently, it is likely that, even if the AR were elicited 100% of a working day of hazardous noise exposure, the protection provided would be minimal. Predictions indicate (49) that this protection is likely to be of the order of 1 dB for broadband (pink) noise and therefore generally of no great consequence in the context of industrial hearing conservation.

Our present knowledge of the AR in this context may therefore be summarized as not generally providing sufficient attenuation to affect materially the degree of NIHL likely to result from exposure to hazardous noise. Consequently, it is also unlikely to affect the equal energy relationship between the parameters of noise exposure and permanent NIHL, and therefore no corrections need be made for it.

THE MEASUREMENT OF L_{eq} FOR IMPULSE NOISE

The acceptance of L_{eq} as a valid measure of the hazard to hearing from industrial impulse noise means that at long last a relatively simple method of measuring the noise is available to the "nonexpert." The measurement of the noise dose of an impulse noise requires merely the determination of the A-weighted sound energy of that noise, as defined in general terms by Eq. (3) and in particular by Eqs. (5) and (6). It is most conveniently achieved with long-term integration techniques.

The noise dosemeter is now generally available commercially which provides a direct and convenient measure of L_{eq} (69) according to an energy rule as defined by Eq. (3), for the majority of industrial impulse noises. The technical requirements of such devices in this case have been discussed by Martin (57). Suffice it to say here that the major limitations that may occur are usually associated with restricted dynamic range, where the fluctuations in sound level of certain impulse noise, of which drop-forging noise may be an example under certain circumstances, exceed the dynamic range of the measuring instrument. In such cases, or where a noise dosemeter is unavailable or inappropriate, the L_{eq} of the noise may be determined from oscillographs of the sound pressure—time waveforms of the impulses according to the method of Martin and Atherley (39). This method is based upon the relationship between L_{eq} and the impulse waveform parameters given in Eqs. (5) and (6). It divides impulse noise into 3 categories, according to repetition rate, and the technique employed varies according to category.

ANALYSIS

Some considerable experimental evidence has been presented which indicates the validity of extending an energy rule for NIHL to include industrial impulse noise.

That this is correct is not generally in doubt in the United Kingdom, where Government recommendations (Department of Employment, 58) apply the energy rule to all industrial noises whether continuous, fluctuating, or impulsive. Nevertheless, some limitation is placed on impulse noises by this document in the form of a maximum peak sound pressure level of 150 dB(P). Above this level it is stated no ear should be exposed unprotected, however short the duration. This limit is in force at the present time due to lack of experimental evidence regarding NIHL caused by impulse noises of greater peak levels. However, there is a considerable amount of circumstantial evidence available which indicates that the energy concept may be extended to include higher peak level impulses, such as gunfire noises.

Martin (5,12) compared the available DRC for gunfire noise with an energy concept limit of $L_{eq} = 90$ dB(A), as has already been illustrated in Figs. 4 and 7. It can be seen from these figures that there is broad agreement between the gunfire DRC proposed by CHABA (3) and the equal energy curve over the appropriate duration range.

Rice and Martin (59) recently examined in some detail the various methods for assessing hazard to hearing from impulse noise. Figure 16 shows their comparison of DRC proposed by CHABA (3), Forrest (60), and Coles and Rice (13) with the energy concept L_{eq} of 90 dB(A). The abscissa is graduated in terms of "B"-duration × number of impulses, and all curves have been corrected for 75% of population protected. It is apparent from the Fig. 16 that

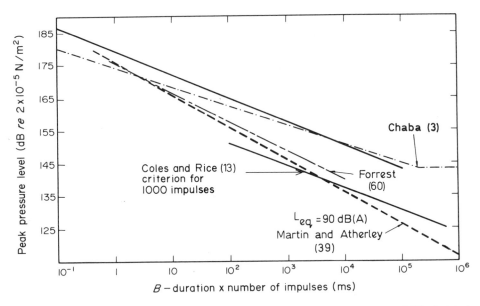

FIG. 16. Comparison of DRC for gunfire noise (3,13,60) with equal-energy curve $L_{eq} = 90$ dB(A) calculated following method of Martin and Atherley (39). All curves corrected for 75% protected, maximum number of impulses is 1,000 for gunfire criteria. [After Rice and Martin (59).]

the equivalent energy curve for 90 dB(A) is within about 5 dB of the other criteria in regions where these are conservative. Therefore the energy concept may be said to provide unification and simplification of them. Rice and Martin concluded that "The evidence currently available suggests that the equal-energy concept may be the unifying factor in the formulation of a method for the assessment of hearing damage risk for all types of noise exposure."

Forrest (61) reviewed the available methods for assessing hazard to hearing from impulse noise with particular reference to the military situation. He compared the "gunfire" DRC with the energy concept and concluded that they were similar and that the latter provides a particularly simple method of noise measurement. Forrest proposed the use of the impulse precision sound level meter (ISLM), conforming to DIN 45633 (62), to assess the hazard to hearing from gunfire noise in terms of total A-weighted sound energy. The ISLM has an integration time of 35 mm/sec which is apparently adequate for the majority of military impulse noises. Forrest carried out extensive theoretical and experimental validation of the technique and concluded that it was justified.

Coles et al. (63) considered the possibility of unifying current DRC for all types of impulse noise into 1 single system based on the equal-energy concept. They concluded that this was highly desirable, but required further experimental justification. However, as Rice and Martin (59) have pointed out, the current (and wholly admirable) trend toward efficient hearing conservation is likely to eliminate the possibility of obtaining such information in the future. Consequently, it may be possible that further advances in methods of assessing hazard to hearing from impulse noise will have to depend to a large extent upon already existing data on man and future data on experimental animals.

A possible temporary compromise between the different methods for assessing gunfire noise could be considered. Coles (64), in reporting the proceedings of an international specialist workshop held in 1974 on hazards from impulse noise, noted that "It was agreed that the 'energy concept' was a useful one for everyone as a unifying concept and first approach to evaluation of an impulse noise. If a particular noise was judged to be safe by (this) criterion, . . . then the noise almost certainly was safe. If hazardous by (this) criterion, this (result) could be the final answer for those countries where the energy concept was accepted by its Government. But, in countries where the law rested on the CHABA criterion for gunfire noises and the 5 dB per doubling OSHA (U.S. Occupational Safety and Hygeine Act) criteria for steady-state noises, further analysis would be needed for application of these criteria."

It should be apparent from these discussions that there is a basis for extending the application of the energy concept not only to industrial impulse noise but also to gunfire noise as well. The use of such a single and simple system of assessment would greatly facilitate the ultimate aim of reducing the general prevalence of noise-induced deafness from all types of noise.

CONCLUSIONS

The experimental evidence discussed in this chapter indicates most strongly that the equal energy concept should be extended from steady-state noise exposure to include industrial impulse noise, at least up to peak sound levels of 150 dB(P). Circumstantial evidence exists to show that it may also be applied to higher peak sound levels, gunfire, and explosive noises.

The equal energy concept, as embodied in the equations described above, has a firm mathematical and experimental basis and consequently may be used, without fear of misinterpretation, to predict hearing loss incurred after exposure to noise. It provides a "self-contained" system of assessing hazard to hearing and has already encouraged the design and manufacture of specialized instrumentation for the measurement of the energy parameter equivalent continuous sound level.

It has already been adopted for the assessment of steady-state noise (65) by the majority of European countries and for the assessment of this and impulse noise by the United Kingdom (58). Such acceptance of the equal energy concept for impulse noise means that a unified and relatively simple system is available for the assessment of the hazard from industrial noise in general. Furthermore, with the advent of the noise dosementer, such assessments may be carried out simply and quickly by the "nonexpert."

It is somewhat surprising that, in the past and in the context of injury to hearing, impulse noise has been treated as a special type of noise having different properties than steady-state noise. It is now apparent from research, as perhaps has been from a logical viewpoint for some time, that it merely forms part of a "temporal" continuum of noise, and therefore should be treated in a similar manner to the rest of that continuum.

ACKNOWLEDGMENT

The author wishes to thank the Medical Research Council for their support during the preparation of this paper.

REFERENCES

1. Holt, E. E. (1882): Boilermaker's deafness and hearing in noise. *Trans. Am. Otol. Soc., Boston,* 3:34–44.
2. Barr, T. (1886): Enquiry into effects of loud sounds on the hearing of boilermakers and others who work amid noisy surroundings. *Proc. Glasgow Phil. Soc.,* 17:223–239.
3. National Academy of Science, National Research Council Committee on Hearing, Bioacoustics and Biomechanics (1968): Proposed Damage Risk Criterion for Impulse Noise (Gunfire). *Report of Working Group 57.*
4. Coles, R. R. A., Garinther, G. R., Hodge, D. C., and Rice, C. G. (1968): Hazardous exposure to impulse noise. *J. Acoust. Soc. Am.,* 43:336–346.

5. Martin, A. M. (1970): Industrial Impact Noise and Hearing. Ph.D. Thesis. Department of Pure and Applied Physics, University of Salford.
6. Guberan, E., Fernandez, J., Gardiner, J., and Terrier, G. (1971): Hazardous exposure to industrial impact noise: Persistent effect on hearing. *Ann. Occup. Hyg.,* 14:345–350.
7. Ceypek, T., Kuzniarz, J. J., and Lipowczan, A. (1973): Hearing loss due to impulse noise: A field study. *Proceedings of the International Congress on Noise as a Public Health Problem,* Dubrovnik, Yugoslavia. U.S. Environmental Protection Agency.
8. Burns, W., and Robinson, D. W. (1970): *Hearing and Noise in Industry.* Her Majesty's Stationary Office, London.
9. Botsford, J. H. (1967): Simple method for identifying acceptable noise exposure. *J. Acoust. Soc. Am.,* 42:810–819.
10. Eldred, F. E., Gannon, W. J., and von Gierke, H. (1955): Cited by Acton, W. I. (1967): A review of hearing damage risk criteria. *Ann. Occup. Hyg.,* 10:143–149.
11. Air Force Regulation 160-3 (1956): Hazardous Noise Exposure. Department of Air Force, Washington, D.C.
12. Atherley, G. R. C., and Martin, A. M. (1971): Equivalent continuous noise level as a measure of injury from impact and impulse noise. *Ann. Occup. Hyg.,* 14:11–28.
13. Coles, R. R. A., and Rice, C. G. (1970): Towards a criterion for impulse noise in industry. *Ann. Occup. Hyg.,* 13:43–50.
14. Pfander, F. (1965): Abstract No. 186. *Aerospace Med.,* 37:1234–1240.
15. Cohen, A., Kylin, B., and LaBenz, P. J. (1966): Temporary threshold shifts in hearing from exposure to combined impact/steady-state noise conditions. *J. Acoust. Soc. Am.,* 40:72–74.
16. Hodge, D. C., and McCommons, R. B. (1967): Growth of temporary threshold shift from impulse noise: A methodological study. U.S. Army. Tech. Memo. 10–67. Human Engineering Laboratories, Aberdeen Proving Ground, Aberdeen, Maryland.
17. Loeb, M., Fletcher, J. L., and Benson, R. (1965): Some preliminary studies of temporary threshold shift with an arc-discharge impulse noise generator. *J. Acoust. Soc. Am.,* 37:313–318.
18. Walker, J. G. (1970): Temporary threshold shift from impulse noise. *Ann Occup. Hyg.,* 13:51–58.
19. Ward, W. D., Selters, W., and Glorig, A. (1961): Exploratory studies in temporary threshold shift from impulses. *J. Acoust. Soc. Am.,* 33:781–793.
20. Ward, W. D. (1962): Effect of temporal spacing on temporary threshold shift from impulses. *J. Acoust. Soc. Am.,* 34:1230–1239.
21. Ward, W. D. (1963): Auditory fatigue and masking. In *Modern Developments in Audiology,* edited by J. Jerger. Academic Press, New York.
22. Fletcher, J. L., and Loeb, M. (1967): The effect of pulse duration on temporary threshold shift produced by impulses. *J. Audit. Res.,* 7:163–167.
23. Fletcher, J. L., and Loeb, M. (1968): Impulse duration and temporary threshold shift. *J. Acoust. Soc. Am.,* 44:1524–1528.
24. McRobert, H., and Ward, W. D. (1973): Damage-risk criteria: The trading relationship between intensity and the number of non-reverberant impulses. *J. Acoust. Soc. Am.,* 53:1297–1300.
25. Hamernik, R. P., Henderson, D., Crossley, J. J., and Salvi, R. J. (1974): Interaction of continuous and impulse noise: Audiometric and histological effects. *J. Acoust. Soc. Am.,* 55:117–121.
26. Henderson, D., and Hamernik, R. P. (1974): Impulse noise: The effects of intensity and duration on the production of hearing loss. *Proceedings of 8th International Congress on Acoustics,* London.
27. Poche, L. B., Stockwell, C. W., and Ades, H. W. (1969): Cochlear hair-cell damage in guinea pigs after exposure to impulse noise. *J. Acoust. Soc. Am.,* 46:947–952.
28. Majeau-Chargois, D. A. (1969): The effect of sonic boom exposure on the guinea pig cochlea. National Aeronautics and Space Administration, Report CR102401. NASA.
29. Henderson, D., and Hamernik, R. P. (1971): Effects of impulse noise on the

production of auditory threshold shift. Dissertation Proposal, Syracuse University, New York.

30. Coles, R. R. A., Garinther, G. R., Hodge, D. C., and Rice, C. G. (1967): Criteria for assessing hearing damage risk from impulse noise exposure. U.S. Army Tech. Memo. 13–67. Human Engineering Laboratories, Aberdeen Proving Ground, Aberdeen, Maryland.

31. Hamernik, R. P., Henderson, D., Dosanjh, D. S., and Sitler, R. W. (1971): Impulse noise: Some electrophysiological and anatomical effects. Proceedings of 7th *International Congress on Acoustics*. Budapest.

32. Luz, G. A., and Mosko, J. D. (1970): The susceptibility of the chinchilla ear to damage from impulse noise. *Traumatic Origins of Hearing Loss*. Work Unit No. 126 (1970). U.S. Army Medical Research Laboratory, Experimental Psychology Division, Fort Knox, Kentucky.

33. Miller, J. D. (1970): Audibility curve of the chinchilla. *J. Acoust. Soc. Am.,* 48:513–523.

34. Martin, A. M., Atherley, G. R. C., and Hempstock, T. I. (1970): Recurrent impact noise from pneumatic hammers. *Ann. Occup. Hyg.,* 13:59–67.

35. Robinson, D. W. (1968): The relationships between hearing loss and noise exposure. N.P.L. Aero Report Ac 32, National Physical Laboratory, Teddington, England.

36. Hinchcliffe, R. (1959): The threshold of hearing as a function of age. *Acoustica,* 9:303–307.

37. British Standard 2497 (1954): The Normal Threshold of Hearing for Pure Tone Listening. British Standards Institution, London.

38. Robinson, D. W., and Cook, J. P. (1968): The quantification of noise exposure. N.P.L. Aero Report Ac31. National Physical Laboratory, Teddington, England.

39. Martin, A. M., and Atherley, G. R. C. (1973): A method for the assessment of impact noise with respect to injury to hearing. *Ann. Occup. Hyg.,* 16:19–26.

40. Glorig, A., and Nixon, C. (1962): Hearing loss as a function of age. *Laryngoscope,* 72:1596–1611.

41. Robinson, D. W., and Shipton, M. S. (1973): Tables for the estimation of noise-induced hearing loss. *N.P.L. Acoustics Report* Ac 61, National Physical Laboratory, Teddington, England.

42. Kuzniarz, J. J. (1975): Personal Communication. Silesian Medical Academy. Katowice, Poland.

43. Atherley, G. R. C. (1973): Noise-induced hearing loss: The energy principle for recurrent impact noise and noise exposure close to the recommended limits. *Ann. Occup. Hyg.,* 16:183–192.

44. Lutman, M. E., and Martin, A. M. (1974): The middle-ear muscles: A general review. I.S.V.R. Technical Memo No. 503. Institute of Sound and Vibration Research, University of Southampton.

45. Dallos, P. J. (1964): Dynamics of the acoustic reflex: Phenomenological aspects. *J. Acoust. Soc. Am.,* 36:2175–2181.

46. Djupesland, G., Flottorp, G., and Winther, F. O. (1967): Size and duration of acoustically elicited impedance changes in man. *Acta Otolaryngol. [Suppl.] (Stockh.),* 224:220–228.

47. Gjaevenes, K., and Sohoel, T. (1966): Reactivating the acoustic stapedius muscle reflex by adding a second tone. *Acta Otolaryngol. (Stockh.),* 62:213–216.

48. Corcoran, A. L. (1974): An investigation into the effects of rapidly repeated noise pulses on the acoustic reflex in human subjects. Dissertation submitted for B.Sc. Hons., Department of Mechanical Engineering, University of Southampton.

49. Lutman, M. E. (1975): The Protective Action and Function of the Acoustic Reflex. Thesis in preparation. Institute of Sound and Vibration Research, University of Southampton.

50. Fletcher, J. L., and Riopelle, A. (1960): Protective effect of acoustic reflex for impulse noise. *J. Acoust. Soc. Am.,* 32:401–404.

51. Chisman, J. A., and Simon, J. R. (1961): Protection against impulse type industrial noise by utilizing the acoustic reflex. *J. Appl. Psychol.,* 45:402–407.

52. Fletcher, J. L. (1965): Protection from high intensities of impulse noise by way of preceding noise and click stimuli. *J. Audit. Res.*, 5:145–150.
53. Ward, W. D. (1962): Studies on the aural reflex II: Reduction of temporary threshold shift from intermittent noise by reflex activity; Implications for damage risk criteria. *J. Acoust. Soc. Am.*, 34:234–241.
54. Ward, W. D. (1962): Studies on the aural reflex III: Reflex latency threshold shift from impulses. *J. Acoust. Soc. Am.*, 34:1132–1137.
55. Hilding, D. A. (1961): The protective value of the stapedius reflex: An experimental study. *Trans. Am. Acad. Ophthalmol. Otol.*, 65:297–306.
56. Borg, E. (1972): Regulation of middle-ear sound transmission in the non-anesthetized rabbit. *Acta Physiol. Scand.*, 86:175–190.
57. Martin, A. M. (1973): The assessment of occupational noise exposure. *Ann. Occup. Hyg.*, 16:353–362.
58. Department of Employment (1972): *Code of Practice for Reducing the Exposure of Employed Persons to Noise*. Her Majesty's Stationery Office, London.
59. Rice, C. G., and Martin, A. M. (1973): Impulse noise damage risk criteria. *J. Sound. Vib.*, 28:359–367.
60. Forrest, M. R. (1967): The effects of high-intensity impulse noise on hearing. M.Sc. Dissertation. Institute of Sound and Vibration Research, University of Southampton.
61. Forrest, M. R. (1973): Evaluation of hazard to hearing from impulse noise. A.P.R.E. Report 23/73 (R), Ministry of Defence, Army Personnel Research Establishment, Farnborough.
62. *DIN 45633* (1968): Parts 1 and 2: Precision Sound Level Meter and Additional Requirements for the Extension of the Precision Sound Level Meter to an Impulse Sound Level Meter.
63. Coles, R. R. A., Rice, C. G., and Martin, A. M. (1973): Noise-induced hearing loss from impulse noise: Present status. *Proceedings of the International Congress on Noise as a Public Health Problem*. Dubrovnik, Yugoslavia. U.S. Environmental Protection Agency.
64. Coles, R. R. A. (1974): *Proceedings of an International Workshop on Auditory Hazards from Impulse Noise*. Institute of Sound and Vibration Research, University of Southampton. *To be published*.
65. International Organisation for Standardisation (1971): Assessment of Occupational Noise Exposure for Hearing Conservation Purposes. ISO Recommendation R1999.
66. Martin, A. M., Acton, W. I., Lutman, M. E., and Walker, J. G. (1973): Studies in hearing conservation. *J. Sound. Vib.*, 28:333–357.
67. Borg, E. (1972): Acoustic Middle Ear Reflexes: A sensory control system. *Acta Otolaryngol. [Suppl.] (Stockh.)*, 304.
68. Borg, E. (1968): A quantitative study of the effect of the acoustic stapedius reflex on sound transmission through the middle ear of man. *Acta Otolaryngol. (Stockh.)*, 66:461–472.
69. Martin, A. M., and Rood, G. M. (1974): Evaluation of four noise dosemeters for the measurement of occupational steady-state and impulse noise. ISVR Technical Memo No. 520. Institute of Sound and Vibration Research, University of Southampton.

DISCUSSION

W. Ward: In talking with Kuzniarz in Poland, he made the statement that the background noise was 115 dB(A). If that is the case, then the agreement isn't so astounding with the other industrial data, because the impact noise raises the L_{eq} by only 3 dB.

K. Kryter: I like your idea that impulse noise is just one special case of sound. It seems to be generally accepted that the spectrum is an important feature of noise bands. I wonder if you would comment on how your method of measurement would take the spectrum of the impulse into account. Also, most of your examples tended to have impulse delivered at a very rapid rate, I wonder if you could generalize the Equal Energy Concept at this time to impulse noise with any interpulse interval.

A. Martin: Concerning the spectrum of the noise, it is an industrial impact noise and has a general broad band profile, just like any other industrial impact noise. Regarding the repetition rate we dealt with, it varied from 400 to 2,000 impulses per day. The 400 appears to be a very low rate to me. These were forging machines that would only hit the work once, cause a very loud noise, and then repeat in a random fashion.

General Discussion

C. Rice: I would like to raise one of the critical issues. Eldred was the first to bring up the 3–5 dB trading relationship. In listening to the arguments, I will go from this meeting feeling that the equal energy rule has distinct advantage over the 5 dB rule. I know that data can just as well be interpreted by the 5 dB rule. Moreover, there are distinct economic advantages to the 5 dB rule. Before leaving, I would like some more support for the 5 dB/doubling rule.

K. Kryter: I would like to comment on the 5 dB-vs-3 dB issue. With respect to the data presented here, they have been very good data, although somewhat restricted. I don't think that this audience is in a position to evaluate whether it should be 3 dB or 5 dB. I would resist our going on record in any way. Also, these other formulae have not been tried out with the impulse data, and I am not sure that these fits that we have seen cannot also be achieved by the 5 dB rule, as well as by the 3 dB rule. This may not be the critical problem that I think is being faced in the EPA–OSHA evaluation. On the other hand, I would like to underline how important the Burns and Robinson (*Hearing and Noise Industry,* 1970, H.M.S.O., London) study is, and also to point out that it is supported by a large mass of data that have not been mentioned at all in this symposium. I am referring to the data of Baughn (AMRL-TR-F3-53). This has to be qualified in some extent, but the facts are, if you consider the sample that Baughn took, some 6,000 men unscreened, and compare it with a random sample of the United States population, you find that the NIPTS relationship as a function of noise exposure is very similar to what Burns and Robinson found, and it comes out somewhat on the order of 75 dB, perhaps a little lower for the higher frequencies. At this time, it can be argued that the Baughn data cannot be accepted, because it is contaminated with PTS. This is a straw man and should be broken down.

W. Ward: Well, there is the Austrian data. A study of the Austrian textile workers with the objective of comparing results with the textile workers in England, the Austrian workers have smaller hearing loss than their English counterparts, moreover, there is no relation between level and loss at all until you get up above 95 dB(A). Also, the equal energy hypothesis does not predict the data at all. So I don't think you have an open-and-shut case one way or another. To reiterate, you don't know what the causes are of a man's hearing loss; if you don't know what his hearing was when he began, then there is a lot of room for different interpretations.

Part VI

Scientific, Medical, and Legal Considerations for Establishing A Damage Risk Criteria

Introduction

The construction of damage risk criteria involves scientific as well as economic, medical, and legal concerns. D. H. Eldredge (chapter 1) explains these considerations, and K. L. Eldred (chapter 2) presents some of the economic facts. Attention is now drawn to the scientific, medical, and legal concepts, especially in regard to hearing conservation problems and the behavioral measurement of hearing loss, hearing impairment, hearing handicap, and payment of Workmen's Compensation. During the entire conference, perhaps nothing provoked as much discussion as the issue of hearing impairment and handicap and the question of what constitutes a significant hearing loss. Of course, an attempt at reaching a consensus was not even contemplated, let alone attempted.

Another area with a history of substantial disagreement is the nonauditory effects of noise as discussed by Karl Kryter. The lack of a discussion for his chapter does not reflect agreement between conferees. Rather, it reflects the fact that the conference was behind schedule.

Effects of Noise on Hearing, edited by Donald Henderson, Roger P. Hamernik, Darshan S. Dosanjh, and John H. Mills. Raven Press, New York © 1976.

The Audiometric Profile of Noise-Induced Hearing Loss

Robert C. Bilger

Bioacoustics Laboratory, Department of Otolaryngology, Eye and Ear Hospital, Pittsburgh, Pennsylvania 15213

The task of describing the audiometric profile of noise-induced hearing loss is a formidable one, because the state of the art in audiology does not permit us to identify the eitiology or exact nature of sensorineural hearing losses solely on the basis of auditory test results. Many factors have contributed to our inability to classify sensorineural hearing losses as to their exact nature on the basis of hearing tests. The upshot of these factors is that we do not know enough about human hearing, about the relationship of anatomical structure to hearing, or about the disease processes that affect hearing, to be able to generate meaningful audiometric profiles.

Foremost on my list of the impediments to our understanding of normal and disordered hearing is the fact that we tend to study hearing in order to solve practical problems, such as the effects of noise on hearing, rather than to learn more about hearing. This point should have become clear to you when Eldredge (1) points out that the immediacy of the need for criteria for noise exposure forces us to deal with the problem in terms of the sensitivity to pure tones, because we do not know enough about speech perception to use the hearing of speech as the relevant measure of hearing. Perhaps it is well that some of us study hearing and not just the effects of noise on hearing.

Another impediment to our understanding of human hearing lies in the wide range of academic disciplines that necessarily are involved in trying to unravel the mysteries of human hearing. That is, as an experimental psychologist, I am not able to deal with the anatomy, biochemistry, or neurophysiology of hearing in a manner that is satisfactory to specialists in those areas. But, neither is their treatment of my specialty satisfactory to me. (Perhaps most of us can deal adequately with two of the relevant disciplines.) The need to deal with one another's specialties in terms of simple generalizations has forced us here to deal with hearing in terms of the pure-tone audiogram, with an occasional allusion to the recruitment of loudness. These simplifications are not sufficient to provide the basis of an audiometric profile of noise-induced hearing loss. Obviously, we will need to consider other measures of hearing.

The contribution of psychoacousticians and audiologists to our ignorance of human hearing also must be acknowledged. As a group, we tend to be insensitive to the need to study individuals and prefer to deal with the average ear. Two factors contribute to our reluctance to study the individual. One factor is that, dealing with individual's data, although highly desirable, tends to be a frustrating and messy business, as Robinson (2) has so aptly demonstrated. Further, the conventional statistical techniques for dealing with individual differences do not offer the pat answers afforded by tests for statistical significance and are less accepted by many of us. The other factor is that, as graduate students, most audiologists and experimental psychologists are forced to take courses that are concerned with "the design of experiments." Because the theoretical basis for these statistical designs involves complicated mathematics, too many of us learn our statistics in cookbook fashion. From the standpoint of individual differences, I am concerned by the need to assume that one's group of subjects is a random sample from the population in order to generalize to that population; and I think the consequence of this assumption is to discard all information about individual differences, except for obtaining an estimate of the variance of that population.

Finally, I would like to remind you of the remarks made by Møeller (3) in his summarization of the section of this book dealing with the electrophysiology of hearing. He noted that those of us who study human hearing have failed to make profitable use of the clinical material available to us. I would like to amplify his remarks. Too few psychoacousticians have shown any interest in the effects of hearing loss upon the complicated phenomena that they explore. Their interest would benefit all of us. Audiologists, as those most directly concerned with disorders of human hearing, are far too prone to average data across subjects within a group of patients. For example, it is typical to see averaged data for a group of subjects with sensorineural hearing loss. Our present problem is to determine how to unaverage their data in order to ascertain whether or not there is a unique audiometric profile for that subset of sensorineural hearing loss that we call "noise-induced hearing loss." Another characteristic of audiological research, related to test standardization and, thus, to individual differences, is the absence of cross-validation studies in the audiological literature. That is, audiological tests have been standardized retrospectively (using subjects categorized on nonauditory bases) and reported in terms of the average differences among groups; but no one has subsequently cross-validated his work by testing an unselected group of patients to ascertain that the mean difference between 2 groups allow accurate classification of individuals.

If, for the moment, we accept the fact that noise-induced hearing loss will tend to give audiometric results commonly associated with undifferentiated sensorineural hearing loss, then we can proceed with a state of the art description of noise-induced hearing loss. First, the person with noise-induced hearing loss will usually show a high-frequency hearing loss for air- and bone-conducted sound. Thus, although it is reasonable to assume that one can infer the spectrum of the exposure sound from an audiogram showing a large component of temporary threshold shift (TTS), especially for experimental data, permanent threshold shift (PTS) resulting from real-life noise exposures tends to be independent of the spectrum of the exposure noise (4). This high-frequency loss, of course, is characterized by the 4,000-Hz dip discussed by Tonndorf (5). Here we should recognize that the amount of noise-induced hearing loss, as reflected by various averages (6), can vary greatly from person to person, even among those qualifying for compensation.

When the effects of noise upon hearing begin to involve the frequencies below 3,000 Hz, the person will begin to show a loss for the loudness of speech as measured by the threshold for spondaic words. As this speech-reception threshold, and the average hearing level for 500, 1,000, and 2,000 Hz, gets poorer, the person's word-recognition ability (PB word score) will begin to diminish.

The person with noise-induced hearing loss also can be expected to demonstrate positive results on the other auditory tests for sensorineural loss, if his noise-induced PTS (or combined TTS and PTS) is great enough at the test frequency. In my experience in reviewing audiological records and correlating various audiometric test results with one another, I think I have observed that these special audiometric tests for sensorineural hearing loss give consistently positive results only when the hearing level at the test frequency is equal to or greater than 40 dB (ANSI, 1969). Thus, for the frequencies at which the combination of TTS and PTS equals or exceeds 40 dB, the person with noise-induced hearing loss can be expected to show (i) a positive SISI score, (ii) tone decay that is consistent with sensorineural hearing loss, and (iii) recruitment of loudness for the bifrequency monaural loudness balance test. In addition, he can be expected to show a type II Békésy audiogram.

The audiological literature does reflect some lack of agreement on the above points. Jerger (7), for example, has reported that one-third (7 out of 22) of his subjects with noise-induced hearing loss failed to show a type II Békésy audiogram. Sorenson (8), however, reported that fewer than half of his subjects with mild sensorineural loss tend to give equivocal results. Concerning these apparent inconsistencies, I would like to conclude that any failure to find positive results on the special tests for sensorineural hearing loss is related to the degree of shift in hearing level and not to the etiology of the lesion to the system.

As you can see, this description of noise-induced hearing loss as a subset of sensorineural hearing loss does not tell us a great deal about how or why noise-induced hearing loss is different from other sensorineural hearing losses. In fact, the only unique feature of noise-induced hearing loss that we have considered is the 4,000-Hz dip. Let us proceed, therefore, to a wider range of psychoacoustic data that might provide us with insight into the nature of noise-induced hearing loss or even to hearing in general. Before dealing with the positive suggestions that I have in mind, let me deal briefly with some of the aspects of psychoacoustics and hearing loss that will not contribute to our understanding of either noise-induced hearing loss or normal hearing.

Most of this negative evidence can be summarized by stating that, when one performs experiments on subjects with sensorineural hearing loss, one must use more intense sounds than those typically presented to subjects with normal hearing. If one then compares the results obtained for subjects with normal hearing in terms of the sensation level at which the signals were presented, then he will find that subjects with sensorineural hearing loss have smaller than normal intensity difference limens (10), more than normal harmonic distortion (11), wider than normal critical bandwidths (12), etc. In fact, though, when normal-hearing subjects are required to listen to the intense sounds that are necessary to use when testing subjects with sensorineural hearing loss and when the comparison between normal hearing and sensorineural hearing loss is effected in terms of the absolute intensity level of the signal ensembles, one finds that subjects with normal hearing perform in the same manner as those with sensorineural hearing loss. That is, normal-hearing subjects have the same small difference limen for intensity that characterizes sensorineural subjects (13), the same abnormally wide critical bandwidths (14), the same upward spread of masking (15,16), and the same harmonic distortion (17,18). These data perhaps should lead us to suspect that one real handicap associated with sensorineural hearing loss is the frequent need to be tested with loud sounds. Put another way, the data suggest that sensation level might not be the appropriate intensive metric to use in comparing subjects with normal hearing to those with sensorineural hearing loss.

From the point of view that sensation level (i.e., matching subjects on the basis of absolute threshold) may be an inappropriate technique, it might be wise for us to question our dependence on the concept of loudness recruitment as both a descriptive and a theoretical construct. Those of us who deal clinically with people who have sensorineural hearing loss, for example, use the term "recruitment" routinely to describe the patient who complains that loud sounds cause discomfort. If recruitment of loudness is a normal phenomenon, then the clinician needs to use a more appropriate term, e.g., phonophobia, to describe the patient who cannot tolerate loud sounds and to ascertain whether or not the patient's phonophobia is a direct consequence of his hearing impairment. After all, one of the benefits of normal hearing is to be able to avoid listening to loud sounds and thus avoid the label "phonophobe." And, if recruitment is a normal phenomenon, then the electrophysiologist needs to eschew the metonymy implicit in describing an input–output function in terms of one aspect of that function.

Once we recognize that the comparison of subjects with sensorineural hearing loss to those with normal hearing may be distorted by the dimensions along which the comparison is made, we are ready to look further at the problems of comparing normal-hearing and hard-of-hearing subjects. Egan (19) has pointed out that a psychometric function has 2 parameters, a slope and an intercept. For all practical purposes, the intercept value of interest can be called threshold. Egan notes that a legitimate comparison of 2 thresholds can be effected only if the slopes of the 2 underlying psychometric functions are equal. Work done on subjects with sensorineural hearing loss, however, seldom if ever deals with the entire psychometric function, but is restricted to obtaining a point estimate of threshold. Because the slopes of the psychometric functions that underlie many of our comparisons between normal hearing and sensorineural hearing loss may indeed be systematically different for the two kinds of subjects, it is possible to err significantly in such comparisons.

For example, it is consistently reported in the audiological literature that listeners with sensorineural hearing loss suffer more in the presence of noise than do normal-hearing listeners when the signal is speech (20–22). In our own work, however, we (23) have found that listeners with sensorineural loss do as well in noise as they do in the quiet, at least until the speech-to-noise (S/N) ratio becomes so adverse that normal-hearing listeners perform more poorly for that S/N than the subject with sensorineural loss performs in the quiet. That is, if the hearing-impaired listener can hear only 50% of speech sounds in the quiet, then he is not affected adversely by the noise until the S/N is adverse enough to drive normal-hearing subjects below 50% correct identification. Going back through the literature from this point, we found that Elkins (24) reported comparable results for sensorineural and normal-hearing listeners for the modified rhyme test. Here we conclude that the 2 groups of listeners perform differently on an open-message set but perform comparably on closed message sets. We suspect that these data allow us to presume that the real difference here lies in the subjects' criteria for responding to speech in the open-message-set context. From their different criteria we further would presume that normal-hearing subjects clearly can operate on one psychometric function while hearing-impaired subjects, in a poorly controlled experimental situation, are operating on an entirely different psychometric function. This line of reasoning would lead me to ask if anyone has ever heard a person with noise-induced hearing loss complain about the difficulty of hearing speech while he is at work in the noise to which his hearing loss is attributable.

Up to this point, I have been rather negative in that I have discussed things that I do not think will contribute to our understanding of noise-induced hearing loss. Now I would like to discuss 2 experiments which I think can be interpreted positively in terms of furthering our understanding of hearing losses in general and of noise-induced hearing loss in particular. The 2 experiments deal with (i) the effects of signal duration upon temporary threshold shift, and (ii) remote masking in subjects with sensorineural hearing loss.

In 1955, Jerger (25) reported that TTS was inversely related to the duration of the test signal. On a sample of 12 normal-hearing subjects, he measured TTS for a 4,000-Hz signal following a 2-min exposure to broadband noise at a level of 110 dB sound pressure level (SPL). He found that the mean TTS_2 was 9.5 dB for a 500-msec test signal, 6.6 dB for a 50-msec test signal, and 3.3 dB for a 5-msec test signal. When these data are evaluated in terms of absolute threshold rather than threshold shift, however, we see that the initial thresholds vary inversely, as they should, with signal duration, so that the base thresholds for 500, 50, and 5 msec, respectively, were 15.0, 19.1, and 29.1 dB SPL. Therefore, absolute thresholds 2 min after cessation of the exposure were 24.5, 25.1, and 32.4 dB, respectively, for 500, 50, and 5 msec. Here we can note that, if the preexposure data are fitted to the model for temporal summation of acoustic power proposed by Plomp and Bouman (27), then the time constant for Jerger's preexposure data would be 110 msec, while that for his postexposure data would be only 30 msec. In other words, the effect of this moderate exposure includes a drastic disruption of the ear's ability to integrate acoustic power. Jerger's basic observation that TTS is dependent upon signal duration has been replicated successfully on at least 2 occasions.

In 1961, Bilger and Anderson (27), as part of their study of poststimulatory fatigue of masked thresholds also observed that less TTS was obtained for brief than for long-duration tones. Their exposure was a 1,000-Hz tone at 110 dB SPL for 2 min and their test tone was 1,400 Hz.

Henderson (28) also replicated this basic observation in 1969. He exposed 2 chinchillas to an octave band of noise centered on 2,000 Hz at 105 dB SPL for 3 hr and measured their thresholds for a 2,000-Hz tone. In Henderson's data (28, Fig. 2), it is interesting to note that, in essence, no temporal summation is obvious when TTS exceeds 20 dB, but that, as TTS becomes less than this, the threshold for a 25-msec tone approaches its preexposure value more quickly than thresholds for the longest duration tone, 750 msec, that he used.

Although the route may be tenuous, we nevertheless may use these results on temporal summation and auditory fatigue to suggest that the outer hair cells play a critical role in the process of temporal summation. From the above-cited experiments (25–28), it seems clear that the process of temporal integration is disrupted by even mild exposures to sound. Next, the anatomical evidence would seem to indicate that the outer hair cells are more susceptible than the inner hair cells to the effects of noise exposure (29–31). This leads me to suggest that the outer hair cells facilitate response of the auditory system by integrating the input to the system over time. This line of reasoning is consistent with the suggestion of Ryan and Dallos (32) that, if the outer and inner hair cells interact at all, then the effect is facilitatory rather than inhibitory as suggested by Zwislocki and Sokolich (33).

If indeed, temporal summation is related to the outer hair cells, then we may gain insight into the present equivocal status of audiological tests based on temporal summation. Whereas data averaged across subjects do show that subjects with sensorineural hearing loss have shorter "time constants" than do those with normal hearing, brief-tone audiometry has not proved to be a useable clinical test for sensorineural hearing loss because of wide individual differences among subjects (34). That is, if temporal summation is related to outer hair cells, then, perhaps in sensory lesions that do not involve hair-cell loss, such as salicylate intoxication (35), temporal summation might be relatively normal. If this is the case, then tests of temporal summation, such as those advocated by Wright (36), should not be considered as tests for undifferentiated sensorineural loss but as tests of outer hair cell function.

The second experiment that may shed light on noise-induced hearing loss involves remote masking. This phenomenon, which involves masking of low-frequency sounds by a band of noise that is more than an octave and a half above the test frequency, was first described by Bilger and Hirsh (37). In 1965, Bilger (38) reporting on remote masking in subjects who had no intra-aural muscles, noted that for his subjects who had a sensorineural component remote masking was essentially normal, and he suggested that this supported the notion that remote masking represented a form mechanical distribution within the cochlea. In 1969, however, Keith and Anderson (39) reported that remote masking was essentially absent in their hearing-impaired listeners. In our own subsequent work with remote masking in subjects with sensorineural loss (40), we found that remote masking was absent in most of our subjects. It was present and essentially normal in those subjects who reported having worked in a noisy environment and who felt that noise exposure had played a role in their hearing loss. It is not possible to extract from Keith and Anderson (39) any insight into this issue because they did not categorize their subjects according to etiology and they reported only data they averaged across subjects.

Here we should note that our earlier subjects with sensorineural hearing loss who had shown normal remote masking (38) had incurred that loss during middle-ear surgery (41), which is quite comparable to noise-induced hearing loss. That is, noise-induced hearing loss presumably represents acoustical trauma via the air-conduction pathway, while the loss incurred during middle-ear surgery represents acoustical trauma via a bone-conduction pathway.

There are 2 hypotheses that need to be considered in seeking an explanation for why our subjects with "noise-induced hearing loss" show normal remote masking while other kinds of sensorineural hearing loss do not. First, noise- and surgically induced hearing loss are basically external in origin. That is, any changes in the physiology of the sense organ are consequences of the trauma; while in other cases of sensorineural hearing loss, the hearing loss reflects changes in the internal milieu. The second hypothesis is the one already presented to deal with the effects of noise-induced hearing loss on temporal summation. That is, the differences seen in remote masking may be the result of differential sensitivity to internal and external hair cells. The simpliest way to differentiate between these 2 hypotheses would be to compare the subjects with confirmed noise-induced hearing loss to those having ototoxic hearing losses attributed to some drug like kanamycin. Were remote masking normal in these subjects, we would know that remote masking is mediated by internal hair cells.

My attempts to specify the audiometric profile of noise-induced hearing loss are admittedly sketchy. Most of the comments I have had to offer have been negative in nature and have indicated what of the repertoire of clinical audiology is not going to contribute to the differential of noise-induced hearing loss from other normal hearing losses. The use of tests of the temporal summation and of remote masking, however, should allow us to begin differentiating one kind of sensorineural loss from another.

REFERENCES

1. Eldredge, D. H. (1975): *This volume.*
2. Robinson, D. W. (1975): *This volume.*
3. Møeller, A. (1975): *This volume.*
4. Ward, W. D., Fleer, R. E., and Glorig, A. (1960): Characteristics of hearing losses produced by gunfire and by steady noise. *J. Auditory Res.,* 1:325–356.
5. Tonndorf, J. (1975): *This volume.*
6. Alberti, P. W., Morgan, R. P., Fria, T. J., and LeBlanc, J. C. (1975): *This volume.*
7. Jerger, J. (1960): Békésy audiometry in analysis of auditory disorders. *J. Speech Hear. Res.,* 3:275–287.
8. Sorensen, H. (1960): A threshold tone decay test. *Acta Otolaryngol.* [Suppl.] *(Stockh.),* 158:356–360.
9. Owens, E. (1964): Tone decay in VIIIth nerve cochlear lesions. *J. Speech Hear. Dis.* 29:14–22.
10. Jerger, J., Shedd, J. L., and Harford, E. (1959): On the detection of extremely small changes in sound intensity. *Arch. Otolaryngol.,* 69:200–211.
11. Lawrence, M., and Yantis, P. A. (1956): Thresholds of overload in normal and pathological ears. *Arch. Otolaryngol.,* 63:67–77.
12. DeBoer, E., and Bouwmeester, J. (1974): Critical bands and sensorineural hearing loss. *Audiology,* 13:236–259.
13. Swisher, L. P., Stevens, M. M., and Doehring, D. G. (1966): The effects of hearing level and normal variability on sensitivity to intensity change. *J. Auditory Res.,* 6:249–259.
14. Bilger, R. C., and Wolf, R. V. (1974): Level dependence in the two-tone masking experiment. *J. Acoust. Soc. Am.,* 56:S36 (A).
15. Martin, E. S., and Pickett, J. M. (1970): Sensorineural hearing loss and upward spread of masking. *J. Speech Hear. Res.,* 13:426–437.
16. Bilger, R. C., and Reed, C. M. (1975): The upward spread of masking in sensorineural hearing loss. Submitted to *J. Speech Hear. Res.*
17. Nelson, D. A., and Bilger, R. C. (1974): Pure-tone octave masking in normal-hearing listeners. *J. Speech Hear. Res.,* 17:223–251.
18. Nelson, D. A., and Bilger, R. C. (1974): Pure-tone octave masking in listeners with sensorineural hearing loss. *J. Speech Hear. Res.,* 17:252–269.
19. Egan, J. P. (1965): Masking-level differences as a function of interaural disparities in intensity of signal and of noise. *J. Acoust. Soc. Am.,* 38:1043–1049.
20. Ross, M., Huntington, D. A., Newby, H. A., and Dixon, R. F. (1965): Speech discrimination of hearing-impaired individuals in noise. *J. Auditory Res.,* 5:47–72.
21. Cooper, J. C., Jr., and Cutts, B. P. (1971): Speech discrimination in noise. *J. Speech Hear. Res.,* 14:332–337.
22. Keith, R. W., and Talis, H. P. (1972): The effects of white noise on PB scores of normal and hearing-impaired listeners. *Audiology,* 11:177–186.
23. Bilger, R. C., Stiegel, M. S., and Stenson, N. (1975): Effects of sensorineural loss on hearing speech in noise. *Trans. Am. Acad. Ophthalmol. Otolaryngol. (in press).*
24. Elkins, E. F. (1971): Evaluation of modified rhyme test results from impaired and normal-hearing listeners. *J. Speech Hear. Res.,* 14:589–595.

25. Jerger, J. F. (1955): Influence of stimulus duration on the pure-tone threshold during recovery from auditory fatigue. *J. Acoust. Soc. Am.*, 27:121–124.

26. Plomp, R., and Bouman, M. A. (1959): Relation between hearing threshold and duration of tone pulses. *J. Acoust. Soc. Am.*, 31:749–758.

27. Bilger, R. C., and Anderson, C. V. (1961): Post stimulatory fatigue of masked threshold. *J. Acoust. Soc. Am.*, 33:1656 (A).

28. Henderson, D. (1969): Temporal summation of acoustic signals by the chinchilla. *J. Acoust. Soc. Am.*, 46:474–475.

29. Moeller, A. R. (1975): Noise as a health hazard. *Ambio.*, 4:6–13.

30. Miller, J. D. (1974): Effects of noise on people. *J. Acoust. Soc. Am.*, 56:729–764.

31. Stockwell, C. W., Ades, H. W., and Engstrom, H. (1969): Patterns of hair cell damage after intense auditory stimulation. *Ann. Otol. Rhinol. Laryngol.*, 78:1144–1169.

32. Ryan, A., and Dallos, P. (1975): Effect of absence of cochlear outer hair cells on behavioral auditory threshold. *Nature*, 253:44–46.

33. Zwislocki, J. J., and Sokolich, W. G. (1974): Model of neuromechanical sound filtering in the cochlea. *J. Acoust. Soc. Am.*, 56:S21.

34. Gengel, R. W., and Watson, C. S. (1971): Temporal integration. I. Clinical implications of a laboratory study. II. Additional data from hearing-impaired subjects. *J. Speech Hear. Dis.*, 36:213–224.

35. Myers, E. N., and Bernstein, J. M. (1965): Salicylate ototoxicity. *Arch. Otolaryngol.*, 82:483–493.

36. Wright, H. N. (1968): Clinical measurement of temporal auditory summation. *J. Speech Hear. Res.*, 11:109–127.

37. Bilger, R. C., and Hirsh, I. J. (1956): Masking of tones by bands of noise. *J. Acoust. Soc. Am.*, 28:623–630.

38. Bilger, R. C. (1966): Remote masking in the absence on intra-aural muscles. *J. Acoust. Soc. Am.*, 39:103–108.

39. Keith, R. W., and Anderson, C. V. (1969): Remote masking for listeners with cochlear impairments. *J. Acoust. Soc. Am.*, 46:393–398.

40. Bilger, R. C., and Hopkinson, N. T. (1970): Masking of low-frequency tones by high-frequency bands of noise and frequency-modulated tones. *J. Acoust. Soc. Am.*, 47:107 (A).

41. Paparella, M. (1962): Acoustic trauma from the bone cutting ban. *Laryngoscope*, 72:116.

Effects of Noise on Hearing, edited by Donald Henderson, Roger P. Hamernik, Darshan S. Dosanjh, and John H. Mills. Raven Press, New York © 1976.

Otological Considerations in Noise-Induced Hearing Loss

James B. Snow, Jr.

Department of Otorhinolaryngology and Human Communication, University of Pennsylvania School of Medicine, Philadelphia, Pennsylvania 19104

Noise-induced hearing loss is a major cause of disability in mechanized societies. It is estimated by the United States Public Health Service that 10 million Americans in industrial work have hearing losses which may be related to noise exposure. In this symposium, we have witnessed precise definition of the structural, electrophysiological, and biochemical changes that intense sound produces in the auditory system and particularly in the inner ear. The clinical evidence for the loss of hearing induced by loud noise leaves little room for doubt of the magnitude of the medical and social problems that are created by intense sound.

The physician who participates in the care of patients with noise-induced hearing loss (NIHL) must consider, in addition to the diagnosis, prevention, occupational counseling, compensation for disability, and rehabilitation. In prevention, the physician should participate in the design and conduct of the hearing conservation program. Occupational counseling of the individual seeking employment in a high-noise industry, and of the individual who has already developed a loss of hearing in his field of work, is fraught with many uncertainties in our present state of knowledge. In compensation, he must determine the medical probability that the hearing loss is causally related or aggravated by noise exposure and establish a quantitative determination of the disability in terms of the hearing and of the whole person. Lacking medical or surgical therapy for NIHL, and seeing no immediate prospect for developments that are likely to alter NIHL once it has been established, rehabilitation now and for the future is of major concern.

PHYSICIAN PARTICIPATION IN HEARING CONSERVATION PROGRAMS

The Walsh-Healey Act of 1969 and the Occupational Safety and Health Act of 1971 require the development of hearing conservation programs in industry in which the noise level is 90 dB(A) or higher.

The responsibility for development of hearing conservation programs is placed on the company employing the worker. Although the requirement for medical supervision remains in doubt in the proposed regulations, the need for medical participation is clear cut. Because the compensation and legal aspects of NIHL are very good reasons for the development of a hearing conservation program, many firms had developed excellent programs prior to the legislation. Federal employees have had hearing conservation programs for a quarter of a century.

Emphasis in the new legislation is placed on the reduction of exposure by engineering methods where feasible, but ordinarily this approach is of limited effectiveness. Every place of business should make reasonable efforts to control noise at the source and to isolate the worker from the noise source (1). Likewise, administrative methods are emphasized, and administrative methods include rotation of workers between high- and low-noise areas and limiting the number of hours of exposure for each worker in noisy areas. Personal protection of workers with ear defenders, such as earplugs, earmuffs, and helmets, are advocated after engineering and administrative methods prove to be inadequate.

Audiometric Surveillance

Noise levels must be measured accurately where the workers are located, and records of the intensity and duration of exposure at the work places must be maintained. If the damage risk criteria are exceeded, preemployment audiometric and medical evaluation should be carried out. A medical diagnosis must be established in those with a loss of hearing. A decision regarding the advisability of noise exposure for the individual must be made. There is great individual variation in the susceptibility to NIHL. There are no reliable methods to predict which individuals are susceptible and which are not. The hope that determinations of the preemployment temporary threshold shift would serve as a useful predictor has not been fulfilled.

The first postemployment audiogram should be obtained not later than 90 days after initial noise exposure. Followup audiometric surveillance should occur as often as 3 to 6 months in individuals with a loss of hearing, but under no circumstances less frequently than every 12 months. Frequent measurement of hearing is the best way to determine if individual sound protection is being carried out effectively.

Audiometric equipment must be maintained in calibration. The testing must be done in adequately soundproofed test suite. Under the proposed regulations, the testing must be done by certified audiometric technicians or professionals such as audiologists or physicians. The audiometric and medical records must be carefully maintained. Each worker must be informed of the level of noise to which he is exposed and of his hearing level if there is a change from previous levels.

Medical Evaluation

Medical evaluation should be carried out on all individuals with pre-employment hearing loss. A medical diagnosis should be established employing the studies usually applied in the otologic evaluation of patients with a loss of hearing. A detailed history of the evolution of the hearing loss and related symptoms must be obtained, and the general medical background of the patient must be known. A careful otorhinolaryngologic physical examination and measurement of pure-tone air and bone conduction thresholds, speech reception thresholds, and discrimination should be performed. Tympanometry and special audiologic evaluation including tests for recruitment and tone decay at threshold and suprathreshold levels as well as determination of the short increment sensitivity index and Békésy audiometry should be carried out as indicated. Electronystagmography and caloric testing may be indicated, as well as radiographs of the mastoids and tomography of the temporal bone. In patients with sensorineural hearing losses, a metabolic workup, in addition to the neurotological evaluation, should be performed and include a fasting blood glucose, a glucose tolerance test, serum cholesterol and triglycerides, lipoprotein electrophoresis, and T_3 and T_4 levels. A serologic test for syphilis, particularly the FTA–ABS, is indicated. With the increased involvement of physicians in hearing conservation as proposed in the regulations, the evaluation of hearing-impaired individuals will be greatly enhanced. The presence of chronic otitis media, otosclerosis, and other middle ear abnormalities should be detected, the chance of overlooking pontine angle tumors, such as an acoustic neurinoma, should be greatly reduced, and establishing the etiology of cochlear hearing losses unrelated to noise exposure should be improved. The medical evaluation should be repeated in individuals who develop a loss of hearing during the period of employment.

Criteria for Exclusion of Individuals with Preexisting Hearing Loss from Employment in High-Noise Environments

It is generally recognized that conductive hearing losses tend to protect the inner ear from damage attributed to loud noise. Individuals with a conductive hearing loss have a built-in attenuation equal to the conductive component of the loss of hearing. This attenuation may be further augmented by the use of ear defenders of various types. Aside from the patient who has had a recent stapedectomy, the presence of a conductive hearing loss should not exclude an individual from employment in a high-noise environment.

On the other hand, a preexisting sensorineural hearing loss presents a problem. Although it is not clearly established that exposure to loud noise will regularly result in additional hearing loss in individuals who have developed a sensorineural hearing loss from causes other than noise exposure, there is experimental evidence that the simultaneous application of noise and other causes of hearing loss produce a greater loss of hearing than either alone. This additive effect has been most convincingly demonstrated with ototoxic drugs and noise, but may well occur with hereditary, traumatic, infectious, degenerative, and metabolic sensory hearing losses. Not infrequently, it has been observed clinically that the loss of hearing from noise exposure can be additive to the hearing loss of other cochlear lesions. The likelihood of aggravation of neural hearing losses is more speculative. The exclusion of all individuals with a sensory or neural hearing loss from employment in a high-noise environment is probably not necessary or enforceable. Certainly individuals with progressive sensorineural hearing losses should be excluded from work in noisy environments (2). Individuals with mild non-noise-induced sensory or neural hearing losses should be monitored particularly closely for progression of the hearing loss. Should progression be detected, such an individual should be excluded from further employment in a high-noise environment. Individuals with borderline serviceable hearing, either because of a speech reception threshold approaching 40 dB or a discrimination score of 80% or less, should be advised to seek work in which the residual hearing is not at risk. Individuals with sensorineural hearing losses who require a hearing aid for communication should not be placed in work in a high-noise environment.

A more difficult question arises in the individual with well-documented NIHL from previous employment. Should such an individual be permitted to begin or continue work in an environment in which further impairment of the hearing may occur. If we make the assumption that someone must do the work in the noisy environment for generally accepted societal needs, is it better to return or continue the individual with NIHL to further damage, or subject a new individual with normal hearing to the risk of developing a hearing loss? Is it better to produce a more severe loss in an individual who has already had his hearing damaged, or is it better to subject a normal-hearing individual to possible loss?

The individual variation in susceptibility to noise-induced hearing loss plays a role in this judgment. Is the individual who has already developed a loss unusually susceptible to noise-induced hearing loss or by virtue of long and intense exposure is this individual unusually resistant to noise-induced hearing loss? Will the individual with normal hearing who is the alternate possibility for the position be unusually susceptible or resistant?

An additional consideration is that the loss of hearing at 3,000 Hz and above tends to stabilize at 60–70 dB after several years even in very intense noise. The hearing loss at lower frequencies increases gradually. First, the threshold at 2,000 Hz slowly approaches 60–70 dB, and later, the threshold at 1,000 Hz slowly approaches 60–70 dB.

The evidence favors leaving workers who have already sustained a hearing loss in high-noise exposure work; however, in counseling individual patients, it is difficult to advise continued exposure once a significant loss has occurred. It has been my observation that, in the past, physicians have had very little influence on this decision in an individual patient. Those patients who had worked in high-noise exposure and had developed a loss of hearing tended to continue in such work until the loss of hearing became a major disability.

The military situation, in which patients are profiled and limitations of duty are strictly enforced, is the exception to the general lack of influence of medical advice in this problem. The new legislation may change this situation in the civilian population.

Certainly, compensation for hearing loss should influence management's attitude on this subject. Since the development of a hearing loss or the aggravation of a preexisting hearing loss are compensable, it would appear prudent to avoid employment of individuals with preexisting NIHL to work in a high-noise environment. On the other hand, too many of the skilled work force have a loss of hearing to exclude them. It is the most experienced and skillful worker that is most likely to have already sustained a loss of hearing. From a practical point of view, society simply cannot get along without these individuals working in noise. The individual worker, of course, wants to continue in the skilled position for which he has trained and for which his pay is the highest.

Sound Protection

Although it would seem that the regular and conscientious use of ear defenders would make such considerations unimportant, the facts are that effective means of individual protection have been available for more than 30 years and yet NIHL occurs in industrial establishments that have had well-developed and apparently well-enforced programs for the use of ear defenders.

There is ample evidence that ear defenders are capable of attenuating most industrial noise to nondamaging levels. The 35–40 dB of attenuation achieved is adequate for protection, but has been demonstrated not to interfere with communication in a high-noise environment in the laboratory and under actual working conditions.

The combination of earplugs and -muffs adds relatively little additional attenuation. The main problem is not in obtaining sufficient attenuation to be protective, but it is in obtaining regular and conscientious compliance on the part of workers.

Avoidance of Potentiating Factors

Part of a conservation of hearing program must be to inform workers in high-noise environments of what we do know of a practical nature about NIHL. In particular, it is important for them to understand that the various causes of sensory hearing loss are synergistic. They must know to avoid noise exposure under circumstances wherein they are exposed to another known etiologic factor in sensory hearing loss. They should be aware of what drugs are ototoxic. They should be informed of the potentiating effects of the aminoglycoside antibiotics, some diuretics, salicylates, and quinine and its derivatives, and synthetic analogs with noise.

COMPUTATION OF DISABILITY

The physician and audiologist are frequently called upon to determine the degree of disability that NIHL causes. In a patient with NIHL, it is difficult to select the appropriate criteria that adequately describe the hearing loss. Since the greatest loss occurs at 4,000 Hz, formulas that use lower frequencies do not reflect the area of greatest organic change in NIHL. Inclusion of 4,000 Hz in the computation of disability has not generally been considered appropriate, because of the limited effect that 4,000 Hz has on the intelligibility of speech.

In 1959, the *Guide for the Evaluation of Hearing Impairment, a Report of the Committee on Conservation of Hearing of the American Academy of Ophthalmology and Otolaryngology* established certain assumptions in the computation of hearing impairment that have persisted (3). One assumption is that the disability from conductive hearing losses and sensorineural hearing losses can be computed with the same formula. The frequencies of 500, 1,000, and 2,000 Hz were chosen, since they are the so-called speech frequencies, or the ones that are the most important for understanding speech. These frequencies serve very satisfactorily for the quantification of disability for conductive hearing losses where the loss at 500, 1,000, and 2,000 Hz are likely to be similar to one another and are likely to be similar to the thresholds at higher and lower frequencies. In other words, the loss of hearing in conductive hearing losses does not spare or favor the speech frequencies; and, therefore, the disability caused by a conductive hearing loss is easier to quantify. The frequencies of 500, 1,000, and 2,000 Hz serve very poorly for the quantification of sensorineural hearing loss, and particularly poorly for NIHL, in which the greatest damage is 4,000 Hz. Since the elevation in the thresholds for most sensorineural hearing losses increases with each higher frequency, the assumption that the 3 frequencies should receive equal weight is questionable. The lack of consideration in the computation for the age of the subject is another assumption that is debatable.

Computation of Monaural Hearing Impairment

The method of the American Academy of Ophthalmology and Otolaryngology for measuring and calculating hearing impairment was based on the American Standards Association Z 24, 5–1951 scale. Each ear is considered separately. This method estimates the hearing level for speech by averaging the hearing levels at the 3 frequencies, 500, 1,000, and 2,000 Hz. If the average hearing level at 500, 1,000, and 2,000 Hz was 15 dB or less, no impairment was considered to exist. This level has been spoken of as the low fence. For every decibel that the average of the speech frequencies exceeded 15 dB, 1.5% of monaural hearing impairment was considered to exist, up to a maximum of 100%. The maximum was reached at 81.7 dB. This determination of monaural hearing impairment is based on the assumption that impairment increases linearly with threshold at a predetermined percent per decibel.

Computation of Binaural Hearing Impairment

Monaural hearing impairments for each ear are converted to binaural hearing impairment according to the following equation:

$$\text{Binaural hearing impairment} = \frac{5 \times \% \text{ impairment of better ear} + \% \text{ impairment of worse ear}}{6}$$

This formula introduces the unsubstantiated assumption that the better ear is 5 times more important than the poorer ear.

Computation of Impairment of the Whole Person

The Committee on Medical Rating of Physical Impairment of the American Medical Association accepted this system and published a table for the Computation of Binaural Hearing Impairment in the *Journal of the American Medical Association* in 1961 (4). The Committee related the percentage of binaural hearing impairment to the whole-man impairment and published a table for determining the percentage of impairment of the whole man from the percentage of binaural hearing impairment (Table 1). The maximum impairment of the whole man for hearing is 35%. That is, 100% binaural hearing impairment yields a 35% impairment of the whole man. Impairment of other functions is additive to binaural hearing impairment in determining the impairment of the whole man. The percentage of impairment of the whole man is applied to the annual salary in determining disability compensation of federal employees and other workers.

This system has been widely used, although rarely officially accepted by the state governments. With the change in 1964 from the standard of the American Standards Association (ASA) to the standard of the International Organization for Standardization (ISO), a correction factor was used for each frequency to convert the ISO threshold to the ASA threshold, and the same procedure has been used since 1969 with the standard of the American National Standards Institute (ANSI).

It is of interest that some districts of the Bureau of Employees Compensation of the Department of Labor arbitrarily substitute 4,000 Hz for 500 Hz in the use of the Table for the Computation of Binaural Hearing Impairment during the mid-1960s for the determination of disability of federal employees.

In 1973, the American Academy of Ophthalmology and Otolaryngology published a revised system based on the ANSI standard of 1969 (5). The frequencies of 500 1,000, and 2,000 Hz are again used. The low fence is increased to 25 dB, and 1.5% of monaural hearing impairment is considered to exist for each decibel of estimated hearing level for speech above 25 dB. The maximum is reached at 92 dB. The Committee on Rating of Mental and Physical Impairment of the American Medical Association adopted the revision.

A Working Group of the Committee on Hearing, Bioacoustics, and Biomechanics (CHABA) of the National Academy of Sciences–National Research Council was asked by the Navy to provide a formula for converting the

TABLE 1. *Percent of binaural hearing impairment as related to whole-person impairment*

Binaural hearing impairment (%)	Whole-person impairment (%)	Binaural hearing impairment (%)	Whole-person impairment (%)
0 – 1.7	0	50.0– 53.1	18
1.8– 4.2	1	53.2– 55.7	19
4.3– 7.4	2	55.8– 58.8	20
7.5– 9.9	3	58.9– 61.4	21
10.0–13.1	4	61.5– 64.5	22
13.2–15.9	5	64.6– 67.1	23
16.0–18.8	6	67.2– 70.0	24
18.9–21.4	7	70.1– 72.8	25
21.5–24.5	8	72.9– 75.9	26
24.6–27.1	9	76.0– 78.5	27
27.2–30.0	10	78.6– 81.7	28
30.1–32.8	11	81.8– 84.2	29
32.9–35.9	12	84.3– 87.4	30
36.0–38.5	13	87.5– 89.9	31
38.6–41.7	14	90.0– 93.1	32
41.8–44.2	15	93.2– 95.7	33
44.3–47.4	16	95.8– 98.8	34
47.5–49.9	17	98.9–100.0	35

Data from: Guides to the Evaluation of Permanent Impairment, Ear, Nose, Throat and Related Structures, JAMA, 177: 489–501, 1961.

pure-tone thresholds of 1,000, 2,000, and 3,000 Hz into percentages of binaural hearing impairment for federal employees without substantially altering the monetary compensation due the employees (6). The first problem was what hearing threshold level for 1,000, 2,000, and 3,000 Hz is equivalent to the hearing threshold level of 25 dB for 500, 1,000, and 2,000 Hz. The Working Group limited their inquiry in this problem to sensory hearing losses and in particular to NIHL. The data of Burns and Robinson would indicate that an individual with NIHL who had a hearing threshold level for 500, 1,000, and 2,000 Hz of 25 dB would have a hearing threshold level for 1,000, 2,000, and 3,000 Hz of 34 dB (7). Likewise, von Lupke's (8) data would suggest a threshold level of 12 dB at 1,000 Hz, 33 dB at 2,000 Hz and 53 dB at 3,000 Hz or an average of 33 dB for such a person. The Working Group recommended that 35 dB be the low fence for hearing threshold levels at 1,000, 2,000, and 3,000 Hz. The recommendation on the high fence was to keep it at 92 dB; and, therefore, the rate of increase per decibel of hearing threshold level for 1,000, 2,000, and 3,000 Hz above 35 dB would be 1.75%. It was reasoned that the high fence should not be increased because the hearing threshold level for 3,000 Hz will have to reach 53 dB before any impairment is considered to exist, and only another 47 dB exist between 53 and 100 dB, the limit of most audiometers; and the hearing loss at 3,000 Hz tends to stabilize at 60–70 dB even after prolonged, intense noise exposure. No change in the formula for the computation of binaural hearing impairment was made. The Working Group did recommend that the American Academy of Ophthalmology and Otolaryngology reexamine the assumptions upon which the formula is based.

Hearing measurement for purposes of computation of the disability should be made only after the patient has been removed from noise exposure for a sufficient period of time to eliminate any temporary threshold shift, so that the measurement is of permanent threshold shift only. The Bureau of Employees Compensation recommends a 6-week period free of noise exposure before such testing is carried out.

Relationship to Preexisting or Concomitant Losses of Hearing

It is impossible to differentiate what part of a patient's sensorineural hearing loss is due to noise exposure, and what part is due to aging or preexisting or concomitantly developing hearing loss. Arbitrary decisions by physicians on the amount of hearing loss due to noise exposure and to other causes are unjustified and inappropriately reduce the amount of disability compensation to which the employee is entitled. The whole issue over the precise apportionment of the hearing loss to the possible etiologies disappears when it is recognized that the patient is entitled to compensation for the development of a hearing loss and for the aggravation of a preexisting hearing loss. In other words, if it has been established that the hearing has become worse during the period of employment, that the employee is exposed to damaging noise, that there has been no nonoccupational cause of the hearing loss and that the loss of hearing is compatible with the sensory loss that occurs with exposure to loud noise, the medical probability is that the loss of hearing has been aggravated by noise exposure, and the employee is entitled to compensation. Since industrial concerns are responsible for compensation for aggravation of preexisting conditions, the employment of an individual with a preexisting sensory hearing loss invites substantial compensation.

Rehabilitation

Auditory training and speech reading are valuable in the rehabilitation of the patient with NIHL. The importance of observing the speaker's face closely and gaining as much information as possible from nonauditory clues should be emphasized. Amplification is helpful to many patients with NIHL. These individuals require very careful hearing-aid evaluations to determine the most appropriate hearing-aid configuration. Recruitment and problems of tolerance often make accommodation to a hearing aid difficult. Vented ear molds are often of particular help to them. Subsequent counseling on the use of the aid to achieve the best possible accommodation to the amplification is an important part of their rehabilitation.

REFERENCES

1. Sataloff, J. (1974): Preventing hearing loss due to excessive noise exposure. *J. Occup. Med.*, 16:470–471.
2. Sataloff, J., and Vassallo, L. A. (1969): Hiring employees with nerve deafness. *J. Occup. Med.*, 11:319–321.
3. Anon. (1959): Guide for evaluation of hearing impairment: A report of the committee on conservation of hearing. *Trans. Am. Acad. Ophthalmol. Otol.*, 63:2.
4. Anon. (1961): Guides to the evaluation of permanent impairment of ear, nose, throat and related structures, *JAMA*, 177:489–501.
5. Anon. (1973): Guide for Conservation of Hearing in Noise, American Academy of Ophthalmology and Otolaryngology, Rochester, MN.
6. Anon. (1975): Compensation Formula for Hearing Loss, NAS-NRC Committee on Hearing, Bioacoustics and Biomechanics, Washington, D.C.
7. Burns, W., and Robinson, D. W. (1970): Hearing and Noise in Industry, Her Majesty's Stationery Office, London, 1970.
8. von Lupke, A. (1972): Audiometrie in Industriebetrieben Kampf dem Lärm 19:5.

DISCUSSION

W. Ward: Dr. Snow says that hearing losses are found to continue in industries that have apparently well-developed hearing conservation programs and use ear protection. I think it is important if you have evidence for that other than the occasional worker who comes in and who works in a place where there is noise and he allegedly wears ear protection and yet he has some hearing loss. *Health* just published a story on what is going on at Du Pont, and they show conclusively that their hearing conservation program works and the progression of loss is not greater than what you would expect from the passage of years. This (Dr. Snow's observation) is important data if you have some comments.

J. Snow: No, I don't have such data, the problem of course is noncompliance. I have seen workers who have claimed to use ear protection, but show a progressive loss of hearing over time. I believe such individuals are not using their protectors regularly or properly.

W. Ward: There is also the problem of outside noise exposure, i.e., they go to a rock concert and decide that this isn't noise, this is music and I don't have to wear protections. Unless you eliminate all these things, conclusions from individual cases can be misleading.

J. Snow: Yes, but don't you think that the average situation is more like the way I described it, rather than the report you mentioned?

W. Ward: No, recent surveys show very little increase of hearing loss in controlled programs. I wish the people that have done these surveys would show the proportion of people who actually wore the protection.

A. Feldman: I would think that a lot of that comes from the fact that the use of ear protection has not been mandated.

J. Snow: But the emphasis of the new program has been in the opposite direction, i.e., toward engineering solutions and administrative control, rather than individual ear protection. They are given a secondary role, only to be used when the others fail, and I think this is a general recognition of the failure of ear protectors as a solution of the problem.

W. Ward: Yes, it is a failure that is taken for granted without the evidence, except in the individual case. Dr. Alberti, do you have any evidence?

P. Alberti: Yes, the evidence is that hundreds of individuals have come in, where in certain industries they say it is "plain impossible" or so uncomfortable to wear ear protectors that they refuse to wear them. This is an ear protection program that doesn't work. I have a great deal of sympathy for the miner. I heard someone yesterday say that miners don't develop occupational hearing losses—I have miners who sure as hell do; they work underground in temperatures of 85° to 90°, high humidity, in hard hats and eye glasses. They are scared like hell that they won't hear the rock when it's going to come down. First thing they do is remove the muffs—they say (a) we are scared and (b) we just can't wear it in these conditions. There are many industries where an expanded hearing conservation program is inappropriate.

Two other points I would like to bring up with Dr. Snow: his comment that perhaps industries should exclude by preemployment audiogram those workers who are hard of hearing. This is a hell of a hard job in a one-horse town, or in a one-industry town or area. This is something we come across regularly in the mining industry. A mine closes—a miner is competent—he has been working for twenty years, he has another twenty years to work—he goes down to the next mine—he is perfectly fit, but the hearing test is unacceptable—sorry, Mac, no job. In northern Ontario, where there is a shortage of miners, it surely makes more sense to lift the liability of the employer.

The third point, you were careful not to give any opinion of which of the formulas you favor. Whether you are suggesting we return to AAOO, or go to the average 1, 2, and 3 with the appropriate gates. I would appreciate some comment on this problem, because I feel there are many workers with hearing relatively normal up to 2,000 Hz, who can indeed hear in quiet surroundings, but are totally socially handicapped in group speech or normal life, because of a high-frequency hearing loss. I personally feel that a rule should include the 3,000 Hz.

J. Snow: I didn't say that individuals with some hearing loss shouldn't be employed. I simply discussed some of the implications of their employment. In order for society to go on, we have to have these people working in noise, at least for the time being. I just discussed some of the implications of employing these people, if compensation really gets started in this country. (Aside from federal employees, hearing loss is not compensated in the U.S.—at least in the states I have lived.) Most of the state legislation (including New York) tends to prohibit individuals from making a claim for hearing compensation, and even for Federal employees it's not easy.

The thing that needs to be changed is this—not the description of the binaural impairment, but the description of what these disabilities amount to in terms of the impairment of the whole man. A person who is stone deaf is only 35% disabled; hearing impairment should be given greater value in terms of the impairment of the whole person.

Effects of Noise on Hearing, edited by Donald Henderson, Roger P. Hamernik, Darshan S. Dosanjh, and John H. Mills. Raven Press, New York © 1976.

Percentage Hearing Loss: Various Schema Applied to a Large Population with Noise-Induced Hearing Loss

P. W. Alberti, P. P. Morgan, T. J. Fria, and J. C. LeBlanc

Department of Otolaryngology, Mount Sinai Hospital, University of Toronto, Toronto, Ontario

Two philosophies underlie the many formulas currently in use to quantitate hearing loss for legal and compensation purposes. One attempts to measure percentage hearing loss, while the other attempts to measure percentage hearing handicap, with the implication that some hearing loss may be suffered without producing a significant hearing handicap. There is also a difference of opinion about which frequencies should be taken in account—the earlier formulas were produced when there was considerable conductive hearing loss, with its concomitant flat audiogram; some of the newer formulas are rather significantly weighted in favor of predominantly high-frequency hearing loss. Here again there is a fundamental difference in viewpoint between those who believe that all that need be considered are the so-called speech frequencies 500–2,000 Hz, and those who believe that hearing in the higher frequencies should also be taken into account for its less well defined, but nonetheless, important role in sound localization. In our opinion, many of the formulas now in use are empirical simplifications, popular more because they are readily applied than because of their scientific veracity.

As there is a considerable interest in many parts of the world in establishing criteria for equitable compensation of occupational hearing loss, we thought it would be of interest to compare several of the current and proposed formulae on a single population of workmen claiming compensation for hearing loss caused by noise. The differences that are demonstrated are attributable to differences in the formulas themselves, for the patient population used is identical in all cases.

MATERIAL AND METHODS

In the Province of Ontario, with a population of approximately 8,000,000, hearing loss from prolonged noise exposure has been compensable through the Workmen's Compensation Board since about 1952. The number of new claims has risen steadily and is now well over 1,000 per year, a tenfold increase in each of the past 2 decades.

The Workmen's Compensation Board of Ontario referred 964 patients to one of us (PWA) in the 5-year period 1970–1975, for assessment of occupational hearing loss. They underwent full audiological and otological evaluation at Mount Sinai Hospital. Portions of this group had been previously reported (1). For the purposes of this study it was decided to limit the group to those with pure but noise-induced permanent threshold shift (NIPTS). Patients were excluded from this study if their hearing loss was judged to be due to blast or head injury, if they had middle ear disease or unrelated inner ear disease (such as Menière's syndrome), if they were above the age of 68 (not many), or if their audiograms were judged to be unreliable. This chapter is based upon the results of the remaining 467 subjects, all of whom had worked in sufficient noise as judged by sound level measurements and had an occupational history of adequate length of exposure to warrant a claim for occupational hearing loss. The sound level measurements in the vast majority of cases were made by the Ontario Department of Health and are on file.

The group are representative of those making claims for NIPTS in the Province, and most were seen prior to a change in the law which now allows people to continue working in noise even after a claim has been adjudicated. Approximately 90% of the group had quit working in noise when seen, and all were away from noise for an adequate period before the evaluation was made.

The results of the clinical and audiometric investigation were coded, punched, computer-stored, and analyzed.

We have modeled the mean percentage and distribution of hearing loss of this group, and then modeled percentage hearing loss using some formula currently in use in the United States, in Canada, the United Kingdom and Australia (Table 1). We have chosen 3 examples from the United States; the widely used AAOO formula, the same formula using a presbycusis correction of ½ dB/year from age 40 onward, which is still applied in some states, and finally the Californian formula that includes 3 kHz on the average. The latter is of considerable current interest as it has been suggested as a model which takes into account the loss of high-frequency hearing from noise which may cause difficulty of listening to speech in a background of everyday sounds. We have used 4 sets of figures from Ontario as Canadian examples—a scheme used until 3 years ago averaging the same frequencies as the AAOO formula, but with a low fence 10 dB higher, i.e., 35 dB, and utilizing a nonlinear percentage rise with the percentage hearing loss per decibel dB increasing more rapidly at higher hearing losses. As this formula was applied with a ½ dB/year presbycusis correction from age 50 onward, this is also shown. About 3 years ago the Province of Ontario included 3 kHz in its average, retaining the same 34 dB gate, and adopted a presbycusis correction of ½ dB/year from age of 60; both are illustrated.

Recently the United Kingdom introduced a scheme for compensation purposes in which the frequencies averaged are 1, 2, and 3 kHz, quite noteably excluding 500 Hz, and using a low gate of 40.5 dB, with a 2% increment for each dB of hearing loss above this. This is modeled with and without the currently used presbycusis correction of 0.5% per year from the age 65 upward.

TABLE 1

Source	Frequencies averaged (kHz)	Low fence	Weighting for better ear	Presbycusis correction	Rise/dB above fence (%)
USA					
AAOO	½,1,2	25	5:1	None	1½
AAOO (p)	½,1,2	25	5:1	½ dB/year from age 40	1½
California	½,1,2,3	25	5:1	None	1½
Canada					
Ontario pre-1972	½,1,2	35	5:1	None	Nonlinear[a] 1–3
pre-1972 (p)	½,1,2	35	5:1	½ dB/year from age 50	1–3
post-1972	½,1,2,3	35		None	1–3
post-1972 (p)	½,1,2,3	35	5:1	½ dB/year from age 60	1–3
United Kingdom					
Current	1,2,3	40.5	4:1	—	2
Current (p)	1,2,3	40.5	4:1	½ dB/year from age 65	2
Australia	½,1,1½,2,3,4	∼ 20 dB	Complex	Not recommended	Nonlinear greatest rise for lower losses

[a] 8% minimum, then 1%/dB until 55 dB; 1.2%/dB to 65 dB; 1.5%/dB to 75 dB; 1.8%/dB to 89 dB; 3%/dB 90 dB and above.

Finally, we have modeled the most recently proposed Australian federal scheme (Appendix), which is very different from any of the above. Percentage ratings are given for hearing loss at each of the 6 frequencies, 500, 1,000, 1,500, 2,000, 3,000, and 4,000 Hz and added rather than averaged. The frequencies are weighted differently with the greatest weighting given to 1,000 Hz. The formula is, however, noteable in including 1.5, 3, and 4 kHz. Its low gate is significantly below any of the others, i.e., about 20 dB. It has complex weighting for the better ear, and the regulations do not recommend a presbycusis correction, although one is quoted if required by state law. The formula for determining percentage hearing loss is nonlinear, progressively decreasing in percentage rise for each decibel of hearing loss, with larger rises being given for lesser hearing losses.

Figure 1 depicts the rate of percentage hearing loss increase versus the increase in hearing loss for the British, American, and Canadian schemes. It demonstrates well the nonlinearity of the Canadian scheme, and, in particular, a minimum hearing loss of 8% at the gate with an approximate 1%/dB rise for the next 10-dB hearing loss, gradually increasing to 3%/dB at the higher levels, although the latter is illusory in its generosity, for few people with NIPTS have losses so severe. The Australian figures are not shown for they

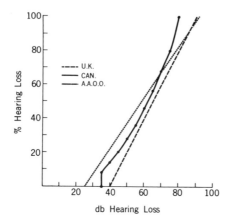

FIG. 1. Percentage hearing loss versus actual hearing loss according to British, American, and Canadian schemata. The Canadian quantitation of hearing loss is nonlinear, increasing with severe hearing losses (of a type which seldom occur with NIPTS). Because of the high fence, even the British method of quantitating with its constant 2%/dB increment does not overtake the Canadian or AAOO figures within a useable range.

are a family of curves varying both with the binaural differences in hearing, and frequency, although, in general terms, the curves have the reverse shape to the Canadian curve.

RESULTS

Table 2 demonstrates the occupation and mean age of the subjects. The predominant occupation represented was mining, although there are large num-

TABLE 2

Occupation	Mean age	Sample size
Miners	55	245
Heavy engineering	57	97
Papermakers	61	47
Others	56	78
Total:	56	467

bers of engineers and papermakers. The mean age at the time of making the claim was 56 years. In general, the papermakers had worked longer and were older than the miners making claims. This table is interesting for its omissions, as its content demonstrates that there are many occupations in the Province from whom claims have not yet been received—particularly the construction industry, perhaps due to its transient work force.

Pure-tone Audiogram

The pure-tone audiograms were compared for each of the groups of workers and is shown in Fig. 2. The audiograms are remarkably similar in shape

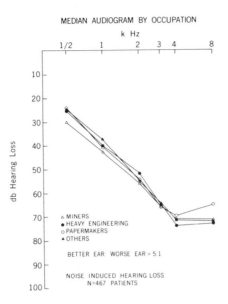

FIG. 2. Median audiograms for the various occupational groups included in this study. Note the similarity, even though the type of noise exposure varies widely.

in spite of the different type of noise exposure experienced by the workers. Papermakers work in a background of steady wide-band sound, the engineers included drop-forge operatives, and many hard rock miners using pneumatic drills with predominant impact exposure. Nevertheless, the audiometric configurations were almost identical, sufficiently so to be combined together for the rest of this paper. The audiometric data are based on a 5:1 weighting for the better ear, if there was a difference between the two, for all the American and Canadian formulae. Appropriate adjustments are made when the British formula is used, because of the 4:1 weighting in use in that country.

The group median audiogram is shown in Fig. 3, which also indicates the 5th, 25th, 75th, and 95th percentile distribution for each of the 6 frequencies tested. There is a considerable variation, but none so great as at 8 kHz, which perhaps fortunately is not used in any of the formulas. This illustration is of importance because it gives a picture of the hearing spectrum of claimants for noise-induced hearing loss in a region where this type of compensation claim is well established. Even the hardy 5th percentile of claimants have quite a significant hearing loss at the higher frequencies and the 25th percentile have an audiogram which is usually considered to indicate a fairly significant social handicap with its 30-dB average speech frequency loss and higher loss in the high frequencies.

It is noteworthy how linear the results are from 0.5 to 4 kHz.

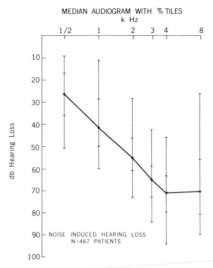

FIG. 3. Group median audiogram, together with 5th, 25th, 75th, and 95th percentile distribution for each of the 6 frequencies tested. Note the considerable variation, but also that even the 5th percentile group have a quite demonstrable hearing loss.

Mean Percentage Hearing Loss

These are shown in Table 3. It can be seen that the Australian figures are significantly more generous than any of the others, and that the old Canadian figures were particularly harsh. The new Ontario formula mean figure, due to

TABLE 3

Group	Mean loss in dB	Group with compensable hearing loss (%)
AAOO	23.9	85.1
AAOO (p)	13.8	71.7
California	31.2	94.6
Old Ontario	17.1	85.9
Old Ontario (p)	13.2	76.7
New Ontario	24.5	95.0
New Ontario (p)	23.3	94.0
United Kingdom	26.0	82.4
United Kingdom (p)	25.9	82.4
United Kingdom (with 20% rule)		70.2
Australia	41.1	0

Showing mean percent hearing loss in dB, and % of group who would have a compensable hearing loss, by the various formulas.

the inclusion of 3 kHz, even with its 35-dB gate, is virtually the same as the AAOO formula, as is the British mean percentage hearing loss because the higher gate compensates for lack of good low-frequency hearing. The California figure is, however, much more generous because of its low fence.

The introduction of a presbycusis correction of ½ dB/year from age 40 upward makes the AAOO figure about as harsh as the abandoned Ontario one; this will be dealt with more fully below.

Percentage of People Who Receive Compensation

Table 3 also shows the percentage of the total group who would receive some compensation under each of the schemes described. Note the difference that is made by the British "20%" rule, for, at present, no hearing is considered compensable until at 20% hearing loss, i.e., 50 dB loss, is incurred. Only about 70% of the population studied would receive any compensation under current British practice.

The Effect of Presbycusis Correction

It should be stated that in most American States in which ½ dB/year above the age of 40 is removed from the hearing loss prior to computing the percentage hearing loss, this rule is applied only for each year above the age of 40 in which the worker was not working in noise. For the sake of this paper it has been assumed that the men had stopped working in noise at the age of 40. Figure 4 shows the percentage hearing loss correction using the American formula, the discarded Canadian formula based upon the age of 50, the present Canadian formula based upon age 60, the present British formula based on age 65—which has a different slope because of the different methodology employed, plus the proposed Australian legislation based upon the work of Spoor (2), which is a synthesis of many previous other workers reports. This latter is the only formula which bears any relationship to actual presbycusis, and even it may not be as accurate as some more modern work. It does, however, serve to demonstrate how deplorable are arbitrary corrections made from age 40 to 50 onward. It is, however, the authors' belief that formulas for developing percentage hearing loss for compensation purposes should not include presbycusis corrections if they have low fences as high as used in the British, Canadian, and United States formulas. Even the Australian recommendations, with their lower low fence, strongly argue against the use of a presbycusis correction.

Spread of Percentage Hearing Loss with the Various Formulas

These results indicate enormous differences in derived percentage hearing loss between the various formulas used; they are shown in Tables 4, 5, 6, and

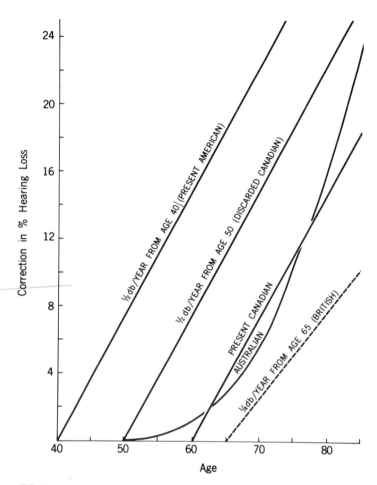

FIG. 4. Percentage hearing loss correction using various presbycusis formulas.

7. They demonstrate both the percentage of claimants who would not have a compensable percentage hearing loss, and also the percentage of claimants who fall into each 10% group of hearing loss.

The extreme presbycusis correction applied to the AAOO formula in certain states doubles the number of claimants who would fail to receive any compensation, and ensures that those with a compensable hearing loss of less than 20% or less make up 70% of the population as opposed to 40% of the population if the presbycusis correction is removed (Table 4).

By virtue of its higher gate and low initial percentage increment for each decibel of hearing loss, even the latest Canadian figures cluster at the low end of the scale (Table 5). This is in contradistinction to the Australian figures, which are the most generous (Table 6). Under the latest (and so far the most generous) Ontario formula, 63% of claimants have a hearing loss of 20% or

TABLE 4. *Frequency distributions of percent hearing loss according to American formulas*

Formula: 0% for index ≤ 25 dB, 1½%/dB > 25 dB
Better ear to worse ear weighting = 5:1

Frequencies involved in index (kHz)	0.5, 1, 2	0.5, 1, 2	0.5, 1, 2, 3
Presbycusis correction	None	½ dB/year from age 40	None
% Hearing Loss	% sample	% sample	% sample
0	14.1	28.3	5.4
0.1–10	11.1	18.3	5.0
10.1–20	15.4	24.1	8.6
20.1–30	30.9	16.5	36.9
30.1–40	14.8	8.9	17.2
40.1–50	7.0	2.2	14.0
50.1–60	5.2	1.1	11.8
60.1–70	0.7	0.2	1.1
70.1–80	0.2	0.4	0
80.1–90	0.4	0	0
90.1–100	0.2	0	0
Mean hearing loss (%)	23.9	13.8	31.2

Table 5. *Frequency distributions of percent hearing loss according to Canadian formulas*

Formula: 0% for index < 35, nonlinear increase for index ≥ 35
Better ear to worse ear weighting = 5:1

Frequencies involved in index (kHz)	0.5, 1, 2	0.5, 1, 2	0.5, 1, 2, 3
Presbycusis correction	None	½ dB/year from age 50	None
% Hearing Loss	% sample	% sample	% sample
0	14.1	23.3	5.0
0.1–10	28.3	29.1	12.9
10.1–20	21.7	23.3	28.0
20.1–30	20.9	15.9	23.7
30.1–40	8.5	5.9	16.8
40.1–50	3.9	1.3	9.0
50.1–60	1.3	0.7	3.6
60.1–70	0.4	0	1.1
70.1–80	0.2	0	0
80.1–90	0	0.2	0
90.1–100	0.7	0.4	0
Mean hearing loss (%)	17.1	13.2	24.5

TABLE 6. *Frequency distribution of hearing loss according to Australian formula*

Formula: Empirically derived nonlinear formula

% hearing loss	Without presbycusis correction
	% sample
0	0
0.1–10	1.6
10.1–20	4.5
20.1–30	16.0
30.1–40	25.4
40.1–50	26.6
50.1–60	14.8
60.1–70	9.4
70.1–80	1.6
80.1–90	0
90.1–100	0
Mean hearing loss (%)	41.1

less; 6.1% of the same population when assessed by the Australian formula would have a hearing loss of less than 20%.

The United Kingdom figures are shown both with and without the current British "20%" rule. If in Britain, their formula was applied without this rule,

TABLE 7. *Frequency distributions of percent hearing loss according to British formulas*

Formula: 0% for index $\leq$ 40 dB., 2%/dB $>$ 40 dB
Better ear to worse ear weighting = 4:1
Frequencies involved in index (kHz): 1, 2, 3

Hearing loss (%)	Without presbycusis correction % sample	With presbycusis correction: ½%/year from age 65 % sample
0	17.6	17.6
0.1–10	12.2	12.2
10.1–20	18.3	18.3
20.1–30	19.4	19.4
30.1–40	17.2	17.2
40.1–50	9.7	9.7
50.1–60	4.7	4.7
60.1–70	0.7	0.7
70.1–80	0.4	0.4
80.1–90	0	0
90.1–100	0	0
Mean hearing loss (%)	26.0	25.9

the distribution would be remarkably similar to the AAOO figures. As it is at present, they compensate only those with severe hearing losses who under their formula would make up only 70% of our total population. Inspection of the group audiogram shown in Fig. 3 demonstrate that an English working man must have a severe hearing loss, i.e., equivalent to the 30th percentile audiogram or worse (if their audiometric configurations resemble those found in Canada) to receive any compensation.

ANALYSIS

This chapter has dealt only with percentage hearing loss, and has demonstrated that a large and representative group of workmen with accepted NIPTS would have very different percentage hearing losses when computed by the different formulas described. This, however, is only the start; we have not yet attempted to discuss the question of disability or handicap rating which seems on many occasions to be only marginally related to hearing loss. There are so many variables used around the world that even with the same formulas for measuring hearing loss, the end results differ enormously. For example, 100% hearing loss in various jurisdictions may be equated with anything from 30–100% total disability, and this percentage may vary according to whether the injury is acute or chronic. In Ontario, the maximum equivalent total body disability pension payable for 100% chronic hearing loss is 30%, whereas it is 60% if the hearing loss is acute. In many of the United States federal agencies 100% hearing loss equates with 35% total body disability, while in the United Kingdom percentage hearing loss and percentage disability are identical. The length of time for which compensation is paid varies enormously; it may only be paid if a man does not continue to work in noise, it may only be paid for a limited period of time or it may continue for life. In Ontario, the law was recently changed to allow a man to continue working in noise even though he is receiving compensation for hearing loss. In certain American states, the percentage of hearing loss may be reduced by the amount of help given by a hearing aid, and it may be altered by the presence or absence of tinnitus. In Britain occupational deafness is a prescribed disease; only if one works in one of the prescribed industries can a claim be entertained, irrespective of whether there has been sufficient noise exposure in another industry. In Sweden, the amount of money paid varies according to the claimants' salary with no upper limit, as it does in certain American states. In most other jurisdictions, the monies paid are a percentage of the worker's salary, up to a basic maximum which is fixed irrespective of the man's previous occupation, and may indeed be much less than he previously earned.

There appears to be a rather major philosophical difference in various jurisdictions about what is being compensated for: Is it loss of ability to earn a living, or is it loss of ability to communicate? Is the handicap lack of earning power, or lack of enjoyment of life? The answer given by Compensation

Boards used to be lack of earning power, and this is the reason why some compensate for a limited period of time during which retraining may take place, and stop compensation thereafter, and why some stop payment at retirement age. However, in some countries and certainly in parts of Canada, compensation is frequently only paid when the man quits working in noise, usually on retirement at age 65, and then continues for life. These people are obviously being compensated for lack of ability to enjoy the remainder of their life. If this is the case, then it is suggested that the whole method of working out a percentage disability be re-evaluated to include factors in hearing other than the ability to hear pure tone, even high-frequency pure tones, in quiet surroundings, which may only be related indirectly to real-life-listening circumstances. The tenuous relationship between sound level, physical damage to the ear, hearing loss, and social handicap has recently been well reviewed by Coles (3).

CONCLUSION

It is the authors' strong belief that formulas used for assessing compensable hearing loss should include higher frequencies, i.e., at least 3 kHz, because what evidence exists seems to suggest that this is more closely related to speech discrimination than the so-called speech frequencies which are related merely to speech detection. In any complex listening circumstances with background noise, as is common in everyday life, there is a demonstrable handicap if hearing in frequencies above 2,000 Hz is impaired. The authors have previously suggested (1) that 500 Hz be dropped from formulas used to devise percentage hearing loss for those with sensorineural hearing loss and it remains our opinion that the theoretical basis of the British scheme is better (for NIPTS) than the formulas based upon averages of 500, 1,000, and 2,000 Hz, or even 500, 1,000, 2,000, and 3,000 Hz. The authors' experience with the Australian scheme is too limited to offer any opinion about its place in the hierarchy. We do feel, however, that the British scheme as presently applied is unduly harsh, and would qualify our liking for it by stating that all hearing loss above 40 dB should be compensated. Inspection of the median audiograms in this study would lend support to using an even lower gate; the 5th percentile have a mean hearing loss of 27 dB using the 1, 2, and 3 kHz average and even they frequently have a demonstrable hearing handicap. We would suggest a gate of 35 dB as a currently acceptable compromise.

Whereas relatively high "fences" are used for hearing loss assessment, and we feel all of the fences in this chapter, with the exception of the Australian, and perhaps the Californian are high, there is a good case for rapidly rising percentage hearing losses once the gate is passed—to use a figure of 1%/dB above 35 dB as is done in Ontario is very low, particularly when later scaled down in a ratio to total disability. We also feel there is no good basis for the

Ontario practice of increasing the percentage rating at higher levels in the current manner because in practice, the hearing losses have to be so high before the rise is instituted that the adjustment is virtually irrelevant in NIPTS.

This discussion has centered solely around noise-induced hearing loss, and our recommendations are for this injury only. There is a small but still significant number of workers whose hearing is injured by blast or direct trauma to the skull. Their pathology may be conductive, and their audiometric configuration flat or even rising. If they are to be appropriately assessed, then a scheme including lower frequencies would be more appropriate. The California, and current Ontario, practice has the advantage of accommodating this group.

The great variations evident among the schemes illustrated merely demonstrates, in our opinion, the lack of generally accepted philosophy of what is being attempted. Is it the compensation of any hearing loss as in the Australian proposals? Or is it the presence of a significant hearing handicap as in the Ontario and British schemes? To take an analogy from other areas, should a worker be compensated for loss of a finger in all circumstances, or only if it produces a "significant" handicap?

Even if one accepts that hearing handicap is being compensated, there seems to be no single acceptable method of determining what constitutes such a handicap nor how it should be measured. It should be emphasized that these differences exist before financial considerations enter the picture, and here further chaos reigns—to suggest in one part of the world that a 100% hearing loss is equivalent to a 30% total body disability and that the same loss in another part of the world merits a 100% disability, is illogical. In addition, the length of time for which compensation is paid varies enormously, from a maximum of 100 weeks in some states of the United States to life in Canada. These variations demonstrate the lack of an agreed rationale for the assessment of NIPTS.

ACKNOWLEDGMENT

This research was supported in part by a grant from the Workman's Compensation Board of Ontario.

REFERENCES

1. Alberti, P. W., Morgan, P. P., and LeBlanc, J. C. (1974): Occupational hearing loss—an otologists view of a long term study. *Laryngoscope*, 84:1822–1834.
2. Spoor, A. (1967): Presbycusis values in relation to noise induced hearing loss. *Int. Audiol.*, 6:48–57.
3. Coles, R. R. A. (1975): Relationships between noise induced threshold shifts, morphological change and social handicap. Proceedings of the Symposium on Sound Reception in Mammals, 21–22, March, 1974. Zoological Society of London and the British Society of Audiology. (In press.)

APPENDIX

PROCEDURE FOR DETERMINING PERCENT LOSS OF HEARING: NATIONAL ACOUSTIC LABORATORIES AUSTRALIAN DEPARTMENT OF HEALTH

Latest Recommendations*

October 31, 1974

It is recommended that the following procedure be used to assess the degree of hearing loss of claimants for compensation for loss of hearing under various Australian Compensation Acts, both Federal and State.

1. Measure the hearing levels (HLs) of the claimant at the audiometric frequencies 500, 1,000, 1,500, 2,000, 3,000, and 4,000 Hz with an audiometer calibrated to the reference specified in Australian Standard AS-Z43, Part 2, Reference Zero for the Calibration of Pure Tone Audiometers. This reference is commonly known as ISO-1964 or simply ISO.

2. Determine the better and worse ear at each of these frequencies. At a particular frequency, the better ear is the ear with the smaller HL. The better ear at one frequency may be the worse at another.

3. Using the HLs of the better and worse ears, read the percent loss of hearing (PLH) at each frequency from the appropriate table (Table I-500, I-1000, I-1500, I-2000, I-3000 or I-4000) and add these 6 values of PLH together to obtain the overall (binaural) PLH.

TABLE I—500. *Values of percent loss of hearing corresponding to given hearing levels in the better and worse ears at 500 Hz*

								HL — Better ear										
HL — Worse ear	≦15	20	25	30	35	40	45	50	55	60	65	70	75	80	85	90	≧95
≦15	0																
20	0.3	0.7															
25	0.6	1.1	1.5														
30	0.9	1.5	2.0	2.6													
35	1.3	1.9	2.5	3.3	4.1												
40	1.7	2.3	3.0	3.9	4.9	5.8											
45	2.0	2.7	3.3	4.3	5.4	6.5	7.4										
50	2.2	2.9	3.6	4.6	5.8	7.0	8.1	9.0									
55	2.5	3.2	3.9	4.9	6.1	7.3	8.6	9.7	10.6								
60	2.7	3.4	4.1	5.1	6.3	7.6	8.9	10.1	11.2	12.2							
65	2.9	3.6	4.3	5.3	6.5	7.8	9.1	10.4	11.7	12.8	13.7						
70	3.1	3.8	4.5	5.5	6.7	8.0	9.3	10.6	11.9	13.2	14.4	15.3					
75	3.2	3.9	4.6	5.6	6.8	8.1	9.4	10.7	12.1	13.4	14.7	15.9	16.7				
80	3.3	4.0	4.7	5.7	6.9	8.2	9.5	10.8	12.1	13.5	14.8	16.1	17.2	17.9			
85	3.3	4.0	4.7	5.7	6.9	8.2	9.5	10.8	12.1	13.5	14.8	16.2	17.4	18.3	18.9		
90	3.3	4.0	4.7	5.7	6.9	8.2	9.5	10.8	12.2	13.5	14.8	16.2	17.4	18.4	19.1	19.5	
≧95	3.3	4.0	4.7	5.7	6.9	8.2	9.5	10.8	12.2	13.5	14.8	16.2	17.4	18.4	19.2	19.7	20.0

* Information kindly provided by Dr. J. H. Sherrey, President of the Australian Otolaryngological Society, whose help is gratefully acknowledged.

TABLE I—1000. *Values of percent loss of hearing corresponding to given hearing levels in the better and worse ears at 1,000 Hz*

HL — Worse ear	HL — Better ear ≤15	20	25	30	35	40	45	50	55	60	65	70	75	80	85	90	≥95
≤15	0																
20	0.4	0.9															
25	0.7	1.3	1.9														
30	1.2	1.9	2.5	3.3													
35	1.6	2.4	3.2	4.1	5.2												
40	2.1	2.9	3.7	4.9	6.1	7.2											
45	2.5	3.3	4.2	5.4	6.8	8.1	9.2										
50	2.8	3.7	4.5	5.8	7.3	8.7	10.1	11.2									
55	3.1	4.0	4.8	6.1	7.6	9.2	10.7	12.1	13.2								
60	3.4	4.3	5.1	6.4	7.9	9.5	11.1	12.6	14.1	15.2							
65	3.6	4.5	5.4	6.6	8.2	9.8	11.4	13.0	14.6	16.0	17.2						
70	3.9	4.7	5.6	6.9	8.4	10.0	11.6	13.3	14.9	16.5	18.0	19.1					
75	4.0	4.9	5.8	7.0	8.5	10.1	11.8	13.4	15.1	16.7	18.4	19.8	20.9				
80	4.1	5.0	5.8	7.1	8.6	10.2	11.8	13.5	15.2	16.8	18.5	20.1	21.5	22.4			
85	4.1	5.0	5.9	7.1	8.6	10.2	11.9	13.5	15.2	16.9	18.5	20.2	21.7	22.9	23.6		
90	4.1	5.0	5.9	7.1	8.6	10.2	11.9	13.5	15.2	16.9	18.6	20.2	21.8	23.0	23.9	24.4	
≥95	4.1	5.0	5.9	7.1	8.6	10.2	11.9	13.5	15.2	16.9	18.6	20.3	21.8	23.0	24.0	24.7	25.0

TABLE I—1500. *Values of percent loss of hearing corresponding to given hearing levels in the better and worse ears at 1,500 Hz*

HL — Worse ear	HL — Better ear ≤15	20	25	30	35	40	45	50	55	60	65	70	75	80	85	90	≥95
≤15	0																
20	0.3	0.7															
25	0.6	1.1	1.5														
30	0.9	1.5	2.0	2.6													
35	1.3	1.9	2.5	3.3	4.1												
40	1.7	2.3	3.0	3.9	4.9	5.8											
45	2.0	2.7	3.3	4.3	5.4	6.5	7.4										
50	2.2	2.9	3.6	4.6	5.8	7.0	8.1	9.0									
55	2.5	3.2	3.9	4.9	6.1	7.3	8.6	9.7	10.6								
60	2.7	3.4	4.1	5.1	6.3	7.6	8.9	10.1	11.2	12.2							
65	2.9	3.6	4.3	5.3	6.5	7.8	9.1	10.4	11.7	12.8	13.7						
70	3.1	3.8	4.5	5.5	6.7	8.0	9.3	10.6	11.9	13.2	14.4	15.3					
75	3.2	3.9	4.6	5.6	6.8	8.1	9.4	10.7	12.1	13.4	14.7	15.9	16.7				
80	3.3	4.0	4.7	5.7	6.9	8.2	9.5	10.8	12.1	13.5	14.8	16.1	17.2	17.9			
85	3.3	4.0	4.7	5.7	6.9	8.2	9.5	10.8	12.1	13.5	14.8	16.2	17.4	18.3	18.9		
90	3.3	4.0	4.7	5.7	6.9	8.2	9.5	10.8	12.2	13.5	14.8	16.2	17.4	18.4	19.1	19.5	
≥95	3.3	4.0	4.7	5.7	6.9	8.2	9.5	10.8	12.2	13.5	14.8	16.2	17.4	18.4	19.2	19.7	20.0

TABLE I—2000. *Values of percent loss of hearing corresponding to given hearing levels in the better and worse ears at 2,000 Hz*

HL — Worse ear	≤15	20	25	30	35	40	45	50	55	60	65	70	75	80	85	90	≥95
≤15	0																
20	0.2	0.5															
25	0.4	0.8	1.1														
30	0.7	1.1	1.5	2.0													
35	1.0	1.5	1.9	2.5	3.1												
40	1.2	1.8	2.2	2.9	3.7	4.3											
45	1.5	2.0	2.5	3.2	4.1	4.9	5.5										
50	1.7	2.2	2.7	3.5	4.4	5.3	6.1	6.7									
55	1.9	2.4	2.9	3.7	4.6	5.5	6.4	7.3	7.9								
60	2.0	2.6	3.1	3.8	4.7	5.7	6.7	7.6	8.4	9.1							
65	2.2	2.7	3.2	4.0	4.9	5.9	6.8	7.8	8.8	9.6	10.3						
70	2.3	2.8	3.4	4.1	5.0	6.0	7.0	8.0	8.9	9.9	10.8	11.5					
75	2.4	2.9	3.5	4.2	5.1	6.1	7.1	8.1	9.1	10.0	11.0	11.9	12.5				
80	2.5	3.0	3.5	4.2	5.2	6.1	7.1	8.1	9.1	10.1	11.1	12.1	12.9	13.4			
85	2.5	3.0	3.5	4.3	5.2	6.1	7.1	8.1	9.1	10.1	11.1	12.1	13.0	13.7	14.1		
90	2.5	3.0	3.5	4.3	5.2	6.1	7.1	8.1	9.1	10.1	11.1	12.2	13.1	13.8	14.4	14.7	
≥95	2.5	3.0	3.5	4.3	5.2	6.1	7.1	8.1	9.1	10.1	11.1	12.2	13.1	13.8	14.4	14.8	15.0

TABLE I—3000. *Values of percent loss of hearing corresponding to given hearing levels in the better and worse ears at 3,000 Hz*

HL — Worse ear	≤15	20	25	30	35	40	45	50	55	60	65	70	75	80	85	90	≥95
≤15	0																
20	0.1	0.2															
25	0.3	0.5	0.7														
30	0.5	0.7	1.0	1.3													
35	0.7	1.0	1.3	1.7	2.1												
40	0.8	1.2	1.5	1.9	2.4	2.9											
45	1.0	1.3	1.7	2.2	2.7	3.2	3.7										
50	1.1	1.5	1.8	2.3	2.9	3.5	4.0	4.5									
55	1.2	1.6	1.9	2.4	3.0	3.7	4.3	4.8	5.3								
60	1.4	1.7	2.1	2.6	3.2	3.8	4.4	5.1	5.6	6.1							
65	1.5	1.8	2.2	2.7	3.3	3.9	4.6	5.2	5.8	6.4	6.9						
70	1.6	1.9	2.3	2.7	3.4	4.0	4.7	5.3	6.0	6.6	7.2	7.7					
75	1.6	2.0	2.3	2.8	3.4	4.1	4.7	5.4	6.0	6.7	7.3	7.9	8.4				
80	1.6	2.0	2.3	2.8	3.4	4.1	4.7	5.4	6.1	6.7	7.4	8.1	8.6	9.0			
85	1.7	2.0	2.3	2.8	3.5	4.1	4.7	5.4	6.1	6.7	7.4	8.1	8.7	9.1	9.4		
90	1.7	2.0	2.3	2.8	3.5	4.1	4.8	5.4	6.1	6.7	7.4	8.1	8.7	9.2	9.6	9.8	
≥95	1.7	2.0	2.3	2.8	3.5	4.1	4.8	5.4	6.1	6.7	7.4	8.1	8.7	9.2	9.6	9.9	10.0

TABLE I—4000. *Values of percent loss of hearing corresponding to given hearing levels in the better and worse ears at 4,000 Hz*

	HL — Better ear															
HL — Worse ear	≤20	25	30	35	40	45	50	55	60	65	70	75	80	85	90	≥95
≤20	0															
25	0.1	0.4														
30	0.3	0.6	0.8													
35	0.5	0.8	1.0	1.4												
40	0.6	1.0	1.3	1.7	2.2											
45	0.8	1.2	1.5	2.0	2.6	3.1										
50	1.0	1.3	1.7	2.2	2.8	3.4	3.9									
55	1.1	1.5	1.8	2.4	3.0	3.7	4.3	4.8								
60	1.2	1.6	2.0	2.5	3.2	3.9	4.6	5.2	5.7							
65	1.3	1.7	2.1	2.6	3.3	4.0	4.7	5.4	6.0	6.5						
70	1.4	1.8	2.2	2.7	3.4	4.1	4.8	5.6	6.3	6.9	7.4					
75	1.5	1.9	2.3	2.8	3.5	4.2	4.9	5.6	6.4	7.1	7.7	8.2				
80	1.5	1.9	2.3	2.8	3.5	4.2	4.9	5.7	6.4	7.1	7.9	8.5	8.9			
85	1.5	1.9	2.3	2.8	3.5	4.2	4.9	5.7	6.4	7.2	7.9	8.6	9.0	9.4		
90	1.5	1.9	2.3	2.8	3.5	4.2	4.9	5.7	6.4	7.2	7.9	8.6	9.1	9.5	9.7	
≥95	1.6	1.9	2.3	2.8	3.5	4.2	4.9	5.7	6.4	7.2	7.9	8.6	9.1	9.6	9.8	10.0

DISCUSSION

A. Martin: I'd like to make a comment in defense of the British. We don't pay any compensation until the hearing loss is 50 dB. This is not a policy based on moral reasons. It's not that we don't have the money to pay them. We just don't have the facilities which would be required to deal with a million or more men. I understand that the British scheme is going to be changed as our facilities are gradually developed.

W. Ward: I'd like to comment that in Poland they've adopted a little different slant. They age-correct the individual data, rather than put a correction on the disability. A recent proposal which I think has been adopted, is that they base the compensation on the low fence of 30 dB—average of 1, 2, and 4 kHz, with an age correction of the individual data, so that by the time you get to the age of 65, it's a pretty large number.

B. Lempert: Is it true that people with unilateral losses are included? If so, why?

P. Alberti: Included where? In our area people with unilateral hearing losses can get compensation, but it's very much less. I think the maximum is somewhere between 15 and 20% hearing loss. For the purpose of this paper, I chose to deal with the noise only group, and there are some people with noise differences between the ears, but by and large we've thrown them out to make the examples easier.

R. Willson: What's the source of funds for the payment of compensation? Is it the workman's contribution to the compensation fund? Is it the manufacturers' compensation, or is it the government funds? What's the percentages of these sources?

P. Alberti: The compensation for Ontario and most of the Canadian provinces, perhaps not all, is a government agency totally funded by levies on Industry. Industries are levied as a group, depending upon their risk. For example, if you are running an insurance company in downtown Toronto, the number of claims are low, so your levy as an industry will be low. If you're running mine industry, your levy is high. Within the industry there are high and low charges, depending upon your individual past experience, and these are reviewed every 3 years. As far as I can tell, the total cost is borne by the industries that are levied, and every industry must pay something if they employ more than 8 or 10 people. There are no deductions taken from the worker.

Effects of Noise on Hearing, edited by Donald Henderson,
Roger P. Hamernik, Darshan S. Dosanjh, and John H. Mills.
Raven Press, New York © 1976.

Presbycusis as a Complicating Factor in Evaluating Noise-Induced Hearing Loss

John F. Corso

State University of New York, Cortland, New York 13045

Nearly 2 decades ago, Corso (1) pointed out that "the increased interest in the effects of noise on hearing (2) has . . . focused attention on the American reference level of normal hearing. If the loss of sensitivity caused by prolonged or excessive noise exposure is to be separated from the loss which might be expected to accrue as the usual result of the process of aging, it is critical that normal hearing (zero reference) be appropriately defined" (p. 14). Since that time, considerable progress has been made and the current American standard of normal hearing is contained in the 1964 specifications of the International Organization for Standardization (ISO) for pure-tone audiometers (3).

These values, however, represent median threshold values for normal young adults and provide only part of the data relevant to the issue of noise exposure. As indicated by Corso (4) in 1959:

> Although . . . (new) data may lead to the re-establishment of the normal threshold values for the pure-tone hearing of young adults, the problem (will still remain) of validly assessing the effects of noise exposure on the auditory functions of older age groups. . . . In establishing the degree of hearing loss, the factor of primary importance is the reference standard against which a person's hearing is evaluated. If the loss of sensitivity due to noise exposure is to be assessed adequately, the normal (reference) standard must be defined to take into account the effects of presbycusis. . . . Thus, the loss of sensitivity produced by prolonged or excessive noise exposure will be, at least in part, separated from the loss which might be expected to accrue from the process of aging. (p. 498)

From these and other background sources, it is evident that concern for the valid assessment of the presbycusis component in occupational noise-induced hearing loss has been expressed for more than two decades. The task of this chapter is to focus directly on this problem and to determine the manner in which a data-based resolution of the problem may be attained.

In more precise terms, the problem under consideration may be defined by 4 specific questions. (*i*) Is the concept of presbycusis, i.e., age-related hearing loss, due to physiological changes in the auditory system, scientifically valid as an etiological basis for permanent threshold shifts? (*ii*) Given that presbycusis is a genuine phenomenon, what experimental data are to be used as normative values for establishing the relationship between aging and auditory deficits? (*iii*) Because noise-induced permanent threshold shifts (NIPTS) also show progressive changes over time, how is the loss of auditory sensitivity which is expected to occur as the normal process of aging to be separated from the effects of noise exposure or, stated in a different form, are the 2 factors (age and noise exposure) additive or multiplicative in producing their decremental effects on auditory sensitivity? (*iv*) What recommendations, if any, may be made as a tentative or proposed resolution to the problem of providing a correction factor for presbycusis in NIPTS?

PATHOLOGY IN NOISE EXPOSURE AND IN PRESBYCUSIS

In this section a brief review of some empirical evidence on the physiological correlates of occupational noise-induced hearing loss (ONIHL) and presbycusis will be presented. The material is intended only to substantiate the position that the physiological changes in the auditory system attributable to noise exposure appear to differ at least in some respects from those which accrue as a result of the aging process.

Normal Cochlear Structures

Because the hearing loss attributable to noise exposure primarily involves damage to the receptor elements in the organ of Corti, the normal structures of the human inner ear are presented in Fig. 1. This is a photograph taken by stereomicroscopy and shows the normal-appearing cochlea from a 25-year-old white woman (5). Specific references are made in Fig. 1 to the various structures contained in the organ of Corti.

The elements of primary significance in normal hearing are the hair cells which underlie the acoustic transductive process. These cells are arranged in parallel rows, with 3 rows of outer or external hair cells (OHC) lying away from the center of the spiral (arches of Corti) and a single row of inner or internal hair cells (IHC) located toward the center of the spiral. The human organ of Corti is about 34 mm in length with about 395 outer hair cells and 100 inner hair cells per millimeter, as reported by Bredberg (6). These total about 17,000.

Figure 2 presents a cross-sectional drawing of one coil of the cochlea (7), with a detailed identification of the elaborate structural elements in the organ of Corti. In later sections of this chapter, particular reference is made to the outer and inner hair cells, the stria vascularis, and the auditory (cochlear) nerve fibers.

Hair Cell Damage in Noise Exposure

Current evidence strongly supports the proposition that excessive noise exposure produces irreversible physiological damage in the structures of the

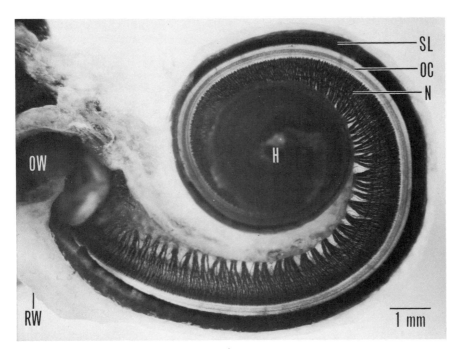

FIG. 1. Enlarged photograph of a dissection of a human cochlea showing the heliocotrema (H), the organ of Corti (OC), the spiral ligament (SL), the oval window (OW), and the auditory nerve fibers (N). (From ref. 5.)

organ of Corti (8). Figure 3 contains 3 photomicrographs of cross sections of the organ of Corti from postmortem human specimens for 3 different situations. In Fig. 3a, the organ of Corti is essentially normal and closely resembles the representation in Fig. 2. In Fig. 3b, the cross section is from a man who worked for a few years inside small compartments of boilers and was exposed to the noise of riveting machines for prolonged periods of time. Although the inner hair cell is present in this cross section, only 1 outer hair cell is present where 4 would normally have been expected. In Fig. 3c, the cross section is from a worker in a noisy steel factory. Here the organ of Corti has collapsed and the normal receptor cells are completely absent. It should be noted that the elements in Fig. 3 are from a selected limited location within the ear, not for the entire length of the organ of Corti where further damage may be expected.

It has also been found that for chinchillas exposed to impulse noise of 166 dB SPL (dB re 0.0002 μbar), the loss of outer hair cells may be observed up to 30 days after exposure. Furthermore, the outer hair cells are more susceptible than inner hair cells to acoustic trauma (9).

In rhesus macaque monkeys exposed to well-defined impulse noise [158-dB peak sound pressure level (SPL)], considerable variability was found in the severity and extent of cochlear damage (10). Along the initial segment of the basilar membrane, all ears showed destruction of the organ of Corti and

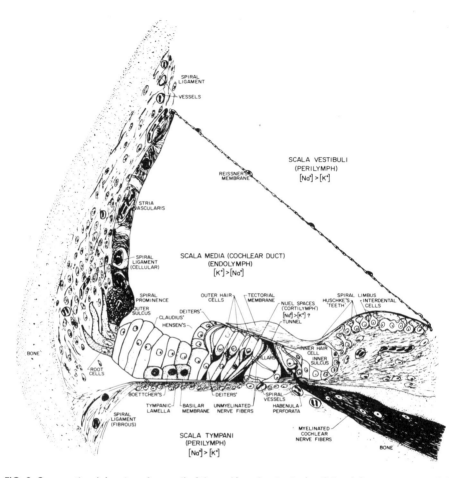

FIG. 2. Cross-sectional drawing of one coil of the cochlea, showing in detail the elaborate structure of the organ of Corti. (From ref. 7.)

myelinated nerve fibers. Further damage was limited mainly to the outer hair cells, with the greatest percentage of hair cell loss in the third or outermost row. Transitions between the damaged and normal areas were abrupt; in half of the experimental animals, Hensen's cells were split away from Deiter's cells in the lower (basal) turn of the cochlea.

Not all studies, however, have reported detectable damage to hair cells or ganglion cells in the presence of a permanent threshold shift (PTS), at least for squirrel monkeys exposed to pure-tone stimulation at high intensity levels (11). In this case, PTS of 10–20 dB failed to produce permanent damage to hair cells as observed by phase microscopy. The data appear at variance with the findings in other experiments in which intense noise exposure failed to alter the normal behavioral (absolute) threshold in chinchillas, but produced com-

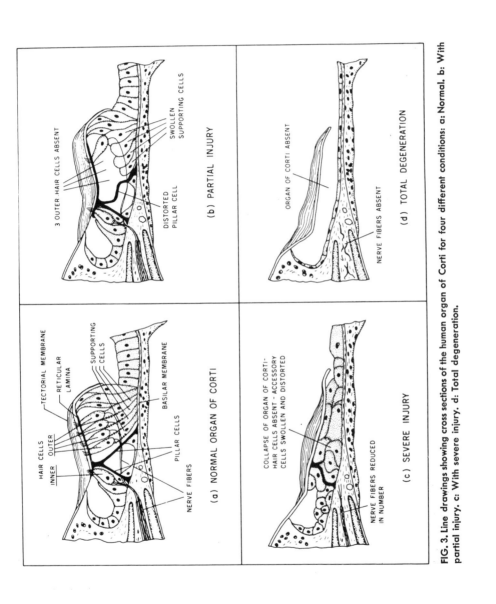

HAIR CELLS
INNER
OUTER
TECTORIAL MEMBRANE
RETICULAR LAMINA
SUPPORTING CELLS
BASILAR MEMBRANE
PILLAR CELLS
NERVE FIBERS

(a) NORMAL ORGAN OF CORTI

3 OUTER HAIR CELLS ABSENT
SWOLLEN SUPPORTING CELLS
DISTORTED PILLAR CELL

(b) PARTIAL INJURY

COLLAPSE OF ORGAN OF CORTI-
HAIR CELLS ABSENT - ACCESSORY
CELLS SWOLLEN AND DISTORTED
NERVE FIBERS REDUCED IN NUMBER

(c) SEVERE INJURY

ORGAN OF CORTI ABSENT
NERVE FIBERS ABSENT

(d) TOTAL DEGENERATION

FIG. 3. Line drawings showing cross sections of the human organ of Corti for four different conditions: a: Normal. b: With partial injury. c: With severe injury. d: Total degeneration.

plete loss of OHC in the first 1½ turns of the cochlea (12). These and other data suggest that only normal IHCs are needed for normal absolute thresholds of hearing; for intense exposure with pure tones or narrow-band noise, the extent of OHC and IHC damage is positively correlated with the amount of PTS (13). However, caution should be exercised in generalizing the results from animal studies to man; for example, differences in susceptibility to damage from impulse noise in the chinchilla versus man or monkey (14) or cat (13) have already been reported.

It should also be noted that the effects of acoustic trauma extend beyond the physiological changes in OHC and IHC. These changes are the most salient features of overstimulation of the organ of Corti, but are followed by later degeneration of nerve fibers and ganglion cells in those regions of the basilar membrane where all hair cells have been lost (5). Thus, the elimination of hair cells represents an extreme level of injury. In such cases, the morphological characteristics of cellular structures may also be altered in the organ of Corti (15) or biochemical changes may be produced in relation to oxygen metabolism, DNA, RNA, or other factors (16). However, the role of biochemical processes in noise-induced hearing loss is not well understood at present, and there appear to be no biochemical changes that directly reflect changes in sensitivity in temporary threshold shift (TTS) or PTS (17).

Hair Cells and Other Damage in Presbycusis

With age, unlike noise exposure, deterioration may occur in the neural structures at any level of the auditory nervous system, as well as in the peripheral components of the ear which are directly involved in the transmission of acoustic energy. However, inasmuch as the hearing deficits associated with aging are characteristically sensorineural and not conductive in nature, the present material will consider only those age-related changes which have been found to occur at or beyond the level of the inner ear.

In the inner ear, temporal bone histopathology has shown that at least 4 general classes of disorders may occur in the morphological structures of the cochlea as a function of age (18). These are: (*i*) sensory presbycusis, in which there is a loss of hair cells and supporting cells in the organ of Corti and at the basal end of the cochlea, with secondary neural degeneration where the degeneration process is severe enough to involve supporting cells; (*ii*) neural presbycusis, in which there is a loss of neuron population, particularly of first order neurons (cochlear nerve); (*iii*) metabolic presbycusis, in which there is a deficiency in the electric and biochemical properties of endolymph with associated atrophy of the stria vascularis; and (*iv*) mechanical presbycusis, in which the motion mechanics of the cochlear partition are disturbed, probably by the stiffening of the basilar membrane or atrophy of the spiral ligament.

Two additional categories of presbycusic auditory disorders have recently been delineated by Johnsson and Hawkins (5): (*i*) vascular presbycusis, which is characterized by a loss of the minute vessels that supply the spiral ligament, stria vascularis, and tympanic lip; and (*ii*) central presbycusis, in which there is a loss of neurons from the cochlear nucleus and other auditory centers of the brain. It should be emphasized that, whereas 6 main types of presbycusis have been identified, the various types of presbycusis rarely, if ever, occur separately.

The effects of noise exposure on cochlear pathology appear to be most similar to those found in sensory presbycusis, and perhaps to a lesser extent

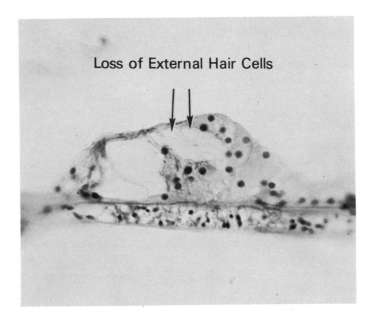

Loss of External Hair Cells

FIG. 4. High-power photomicrograph of the human organ of Corti in the lower basal turn in sensory presbycusis; hair cell loss is present, with only one external hair cell remaining. (From ref. 18.)

in neural presbycusis. The primary site of degeneration in sensory presbycusis, as in noise exposure, is the organ of Corti, with the loss of hair cells and supporting cells at the basal end of the cochlea. Where the degenerative processes are sufficiently severe and involve the supporting cells, secondary degeneration of auditory neurons also occurs.

Figure 4 is a high power photomicrograph of the organ of Corti of a 70-year-old male (18). Audiometric data obtained during hospitalization immediately before death indicated pathologies of sensory and neural presbycusis. In the basal turn of the cochlea from 3.3 to 12 mm, there was a loss of ~ 50% of the hair cells and ganglion cells. Missing hair cells were also found occasionally throughout the cochlea. In the cochlear region photographed in Fig. 4, there is only 1 external hair cell present. Comparison of Fig. 4 and Fig. 3b shows a remarkable degree of similarity in cochlear degeneration.

Although extensive empirical evidence exists for the major classifications of presbycusic disorders as described above, other age-related changes in the auditory system have been observed, but the findings in some cases are equivocal. It is not clear, for instance, whether or not there is a loss of neurons in the ventral cochlear nucleus (VCN) with advancing age. Some investigators (19,20) have observed the neuronal loss in VCN as well as other degenerative changes; others (21) have not. The latter investigators (21) did find a decrease in VCN volume from a maximum of 12.1 mm^3 at 50 years to 8.2 mm^3 at 90 years; however, the decrease was attributed to a decrease in the number of myelinated axons and not to a loss of auditory cells.

With increasing age, the ganglion cells of the medial geniculate body show a reduction in number and a shrinkage in size, with an accumulation of pigment. Beyond 68 years, the size of the ganglion cells is also reduced in the superior olivary nucleus. In the inferior colliculus, the medium-sized nerve cells become irregular in shape, and the small-sized cells show an increase in the ratio between the size of the nucleus and that of the cell body (22).

Beyond these studies, the literature dealing with the pathological and anatomical alterations in the central auditory pathways and brain of aged individuals is rather limited. Some evidence tends to show that both diffuse and localized changes occur in the brain as a consequence of arteriosclerosis, and that these alterations affect the cerebral pathways and auditory centers in the same way (23). Severe degeneration has also been reported in the glial part of the acoustic nerve, as well as in the white matter of the brainstem and auditory centers (20). The temporal lobes show normal stratification of the cortex, but there is a loss of ganglion cells; with the deterioration of cells, there is an accumulation of degeneration products in the cytoplasm. The alterations appear to be bilaterally symmetrical.

In the fundus of the internal auditory meatus, some changes have been observed in the region of the basal coil of the cochlea (24). With age, a bony substance accumulates at the entrance of the cochlear branch of the auditory artery, which seems to produce degenerative changes in the walls of the arterial vessels. However, since many other age-related factors may influence the blood supply in the inner ear structures, the functional significance of these changes remains unknown (25).

There is a general lack of evidence that arteriosclerosis may occur in the cochlea, but some investigators suggest that arteriosclerosis may be not only an essential concomitant of presbycusis, but a causative factor (26). According to another hypothesis on the pathogenesis of presbycusis, the progressive bone apposition produced in the fundus of the internal auditory canal gradually reduces the number of holes accommodating the nerve fibers of the spiral tract. It is estimated that from 2 to 26 years there are on the average 32,500 acoustic nerve fibers of which only 30,300 remain from 44 to 60 years. By 80 to 90 years, the channels for the nerve bundles are almost completely closed by osteoid, and contain few, if any, fibers (24).

Evaluative Comment

It may be concluded, therefore, that noise exposure and presbycusis do produce, at least to some degree, differential anatomical and morphological alterations in the auditory nervous system. In particular, the effects of noise may destroy or disrupt the outer and inner hair cells of the organ of Corti, with subsequent degeneration of corresponding nerve fibers and ganglion cells; presbycusis affects not only the hair cells, but also the first-order neurons of the cochlear nerve, the stria vascularis, the cochlear partition (basilar membrane and spiral ligament), the higher acoustic nerve centers, and the temporal lobes of the brain. In short, the pathology of presbycusis appears to extend over the entire auditory system and is not restricted to cochlear damage. Hence, the physiological evidence points to underlying differences in presbycusis and noise exposure, particularly in relation to the locus of lesions and the extent of damage throughout the auditory system; the two factors appear to be involved as separate causative agents, among others, in producing permanent hearing loss.

Current evidence on presbycusis appears to implicate vascular degeneration and atrophy in the inner ear as a primary destructive factor; this degeneration may be related to the general aging process and perhaps to arteriosclerosis. While changes in the homeostatic balance of the inner ear fluids due to devascularization may alter the physiology of the cochlea to produce hearing loss per se without hair cell loss, the evidence indicates that, with time, devascularization results in a secondary loss of hair cells (5).

Nevertheless, in studies using techniques of microdissection and surface specimens, it is essentially impossible to identify absolutely those cases which represent presbycusis, uncontaminated by noise damage, and those representing noise exposure alone. [Constriction of cochlear blood vessels has been observed in the guinea pig after sound exposure (27).] Nor can the age of the cochlea be defined or measured in terms of the number of missing hair cells or ganglion cells, or by the degree of atrophy in the stria vascularis; yet, the phenomenon of presbycusis as a physiological age-related process appears irrefutable. Hair cell loss has been observed in the extreme basal turn in newborns less than 1 day old and in infants, which suggests that the high-frequency losses usually associated with aging can begin soon after birth and may begin *in utero* (5). Phalangeal scars have even been reported in 2 fetuses (6). In addition, since atrophy of the stria vascularis is an important cause for sensorineural deafness in aging, the assertion that strial atrophy is probably of genetic etiology lends further support to the present position (28).

Finally, data on an animal model for presbycusis (29) provide rather convincing evidence that under conditions in which noise damage and otoxicity can be ruled out, albino rats (Sprague-Dawley strain) show functional hearing losses as expected from the normal aging process. These animals raised in quiet surroundings were measured for cochlear microphonics (CM) and for masked and unmasked 8th nerve action potentials (AP) at different age levels; both CM and AP were found to be age-dependent, with an augmentation up to 1 year of age, and a decline thereafter. Furthermore, the progressive decline of AP voltages was most pronounced for high-frequency components and resembles the descending audiometric curve found in mechanical presbycusis in man, due to alterations in the physical properties of the cochlear partition.

Despite the apparently overwhelming evidence in support of a purely physiological basis for presbycusis, this section must close with a word of caution. Abundant clinical and experimental findings have supported the view that atrophy of cochlear and neuronal elements of the auditory system can occur under a wide variety of circumstances other than noise exposure and presbycusis. Additional causal factors include, for example, hereditary deafness, ototoxic drugs, severe head injuries, barotrauma, infections, and disease. Furthermore, recent findings suggest the possibility of experimental postmortem artifacts which resemble the cellular and vascular changes attributed to drugs, noise, and aging. Cochlear animal specimens fixed at different time intervals after sacrifice show that the most rapid and severe changes occur within 20 min and are localized in the stria vascularis; also, the sensory cells are affected sooner than the supporting elements in the organ of Corti (30). Therefore, because postmortem alterations or artifacts can occur in surface preparations of the cochlea, it appears advisable to interpret the physiological evidence with caution and to examine additional forms of evidence in exploring the presbycusis–noise exposure problem.

AUDIOMETRIC EVIDENCE

The Audiogram in Noise Exposure

The pattern of onset of NIPTS and its subsequent development are now presumably well established in pure-tone audiometry, with a rather predictable sequence of events. The initial sign is typically a small depression in the audiogram between 3,000 and 6,000 Hz, commonly at 4,000 Hz. With continued noise exposure, the dip at 4,000 Hz deepens, but remains primarily in the same frequency region; later, the notch broadens to affect frequencies higher and lower than 4,000 Hz depending on the duration, intensity, and spectral characteristics of the noise exposure. At this stage, the 4,000-Hz dip shows little further deterioration.

A typical audiogram for a 34-year-old weaver after 20 years of service is shown in Fig. 5 (31). In this case, the NIPTS occurs mainly at 4,000 Hz and the notch has not yet spread to affect other frequencies outside this region to any great extent.

The overall pattern of NIPTS obtained from the audiograms of jute weavers after various durations of noise exposure is shown in Fig. 6, according to Taylor et al. (32). The curves in Fig. 6 show that the median hearing loss is in-

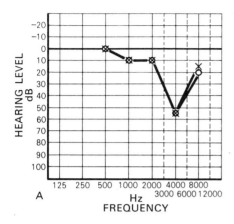

FIG. 5. Audiogram showing noise-induced permanent threshold shift for an industrial worker: age 34 years, 20 years' weaving. (From ref. 31.)

creased as a function of length of exposure, with greater losses occurring at the higher frequencies than at lower frequencies when exposure duration is held constant. It should be noted that the curves in Fig. 6 have been "corrected" for age.

The Audiogram in Presbycusis

Although the audiogram pattern in noise exposure has a fairly predictable form, the hearing deficits associated with presbycusis appear to vary according

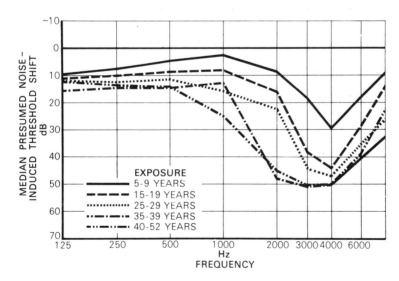

FIG. 6. Data on hearing of weavers (women) presented in the form of audiograms. Presumed noise-induced permanent threshold shifts are expressed as group medians with duration of noise exposure as the parameter; medians have been age-corrected for presbycusis. (From ref. 32.)

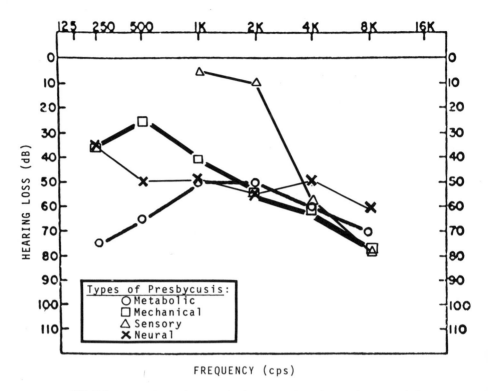

FIG. 7. Representative audiograms for four types of presbycusis. (After ref. 18.)

to the particular pathological correlates of these deficits (18). The audiograms associated with 4 kinds of presbycusis are taken from Gacek and Schuknecht (18) and are presented in Fig. 7. In each case, the audiograms are for a given patient; however, the curves are representative of the 4 classes of presbycusis: (*i*) abrupt high tone loss: sensory presbycusis; (*ii*) moderate or no audiometric loss, but a loss of speech discrimination: neural presbycusis; (*iii*) flat depressed audiometric curve: metabolic presbycusis; and (*iv*) descending audiometric curve: mechanical presbycusis.

While the physiological damage to the inner ear due to noise exposure most nearly resembles that of sensory presbycusis, the audiogram for sensory presbycusis in Fig. 7 shows no evidence of the typical noise exposure dip, as in Fig. 5. Thus, pure-tone audiograms obtained in noise exposure and in presbycusis appear at least in some cases to be qualitatively different, supporting the proposition that presbycusis and noise exposure at least to some degree affect the auditory system by means of different pathological processes. However, except for very limited data (29), it must be recognized that in all audiograms which purport to show NIPTS the age-related components of hearing loss are inherently present, unless some correction has been made.

The Relationship of Presbycusis and Noise Exposure

Since the effects of aging and of noise exposure on hearing are inextricably related in a given audiogram, assuming that both factors have exerted a significant influence on hearing, the question is raised concerning the manner in which pure-tone hearing may be expected to be altered by the joint effects of the 2 factors. Stated somewhat differently, the question is whether a particular noise exposure produces a specific degree and kind of PTS, regardless of the age of the listener's ear. If so, this would imply that the hearing losses from noise exposure and presbycusis are additive and that there is no interaction between the two.

In 1954, the American Standards Association (2), supported the additivity hypothesis since there was a lack of data showing that the presence of presbycusis served to protect the ear from further injury by noise, or that presbycusis made the ear more sensitive to noise damage. More recent data also support the additivity hypothesis. Mollica (33) found that when audiometric data from 200 workers were corrected for presbycusis, the loss from noise exposure (110–130 dB SPL) for the same number of working years (2 to 20) was independent of age.

More direct evidence was obtained in a longitudinal study by Macrae (34) in which the effect of aging was measured on the same subjects for normal 1,000-Hz thresholds and for 4,000 Hz with considerable hearing losses due to noise exposure. It was found that, on retesting some years later, threshold levels at both 1,000 and 4,000 Hz had increased by approximately the amounts predicted by presbycusis curves (35). The results thus support the hypothesis that presbycusis and noise-induced hearing loss are independent and additive at 4,000 Hz. Data from workers exposed to engine noise (~112 dB SPL) for about 30 years failed to show that chronic exposure produced any change in the pattern of presbycusis (26).

There are, however, some data which favor the interactive rather than the additive hypothesis of presbycusis and noise exposure (36,37). Nevertheless, the weight of evidence and opinion at the present time seems to favor the additive hypothesis.

RATIONALE FOR A PRESBYCUSIS CORRECTION FACTOR

This section highlights some of the major points that have been made in the preceding sections of this chapter and, in a summary manner, provides the primary basis for supporting a presbycusis correction factor in cases involving noise-induced hearing loss.

Physiological Evidence

The physiological data on presbycusis and noise exposure show that the structural damage in the auditory system differs for the two sources of pathology, particularly at the retrococholear levels. Evidence supports the view that either factor operating alone is sufficient to produce some degree of histopathological or pathophysiological disorder; the effects of noise exposure appear to be most similar to the variety of presbycusis called sensory presbycusis. Given a particular specimen, however, in which epithelial atrophy has occurred in the cochlea due to sensory presbycusis or noise exposure, or both, it is not possible by current techniques to determine which factor(s) produced the specific damage. The physiological evidence, however, clearly supports the operation of at least 2 factors in the etiology of hearing loss: presbycusis and noise exposure.

Audiometric Evidence

The major behavioral evidence for the differentiation between noise exposure and presbycusis arises from audiometry. The typical noise-exposure audiogram demonstrates a characteristic dip at 4,000 Hz; the audiogram in presbycusis yields a particular pattern contingent upon the form of disorder which is present, as shown in Fig. 7. It frequently occurs that various forms of presbycusis may occur together, or in combination with other factors such as acquired deafness, in a particular case. If, for example, strial atrophy (metabolic presbycusis) is combined with noise induced hearing loss, the audiometric pattern would exhibit the summed effect of the disorders, i.e., a flat loss accompanied by the typical 4,000-Hz dip (28).

In the assessment of hearing disorders in presbycusis, a variety of audiological tests in addition to the pure-tone audiogram have been found to be useful (37). These include speech discrimination, the short increment sensitivity index (SISI), loudness recruitment, the tone decay test, pitch discrimination, directional hearing, and the binaural filtered speech test. The use of these tests in conjunction with a pure-tone audiogram permits a more accurate assessment of the nature and locus of the pathology in the presbycusic patient.

For noise-induced hearing loss, the most commonly used method of diagnosis is the absolute threshold for pure tones as depicted in an audiogram. The suitability and adequacy of other audiological measures have been carefully considered, such as CM, tone decay, loudness recruitment, pitch shifts, and average evoked response ($\overline{A}$ER), but, according to Ward (38), it appears that in noise exposure there is at present "no better method of inferring cochlear damage than from pure-tone threshold shifts" (p. 384). Hence, in considering hearing dysfunctions due to noise and presbycusis, the use of the pure-tone audiogram seems to be a valid initial measure for attempting to assess the etiology of the dysfunction, the potential locus of the pathology, and the degree of functional impairment which may be present.

Presbycusis or Age Correction Factor?

In considering a correction factor for noise-induced hearing loss, some investigators (39) have proposed a distinction between presbycusis (as hearing loss due to the normal physiological processes of aging) and sociocusis (as hearing loss attributable to the conglomerate sounds of societal living). At a given point in time, the hearing level of an individual is said to represent the effects of purely physiological changes coupled with the effects of a variety of factors that are so common in our society that, although harmful to hearing, are accepted as routine hazards of modern life. The issue, as typically stated, is whether a correction factor should include only presbycusis or presbycusis + sociocusis, and regardless of which is used, whether to make the correction by simply subtracting decibels from the overall (raw) hearing levels of the noise-worker's audiogram.

The notion of sociocusis was originally based upon the results of audiometric surveys (39) in which it was found that even in individuals with a negative history of high-intensity noise exposure, gunfire, or head blows, hearing levels declined with age before 60 years. Thus, it was presumed that these average losses of hearing represented not presbycusis, but the effects of modern living in which everyday noises impinged upon and affected the hearing of the general public. This hypothesis has several weaknesses. (*i*) It now appears well-established that presbycusis exists as a separate entity and occurs to some degree well before 60 years; (*ii*) The effects of sociocusis have not been quantitatively established and the inclusion of a multitude of factors which can influence hearing ability under a single rubric seems to compound the issue, rather than to delineate significant parameters for further study; (*iii*) As will be shown in the next section of this paper, certain available data on presbycusis are essentially unbiased by factors which might tentatively be subsumed under the concept of sociocusis; (*iv*) Even within a fairly limited segment of a given society, there is little likelihood that all individuals in that segment will be exposed to a common core of circumstances so that the concept of a uniform sociocusis correction factor has potentially little empirical significance; and (*v*) While numerous debilitating factors on hearing are assumed under the classification of sociocusis, the most pervasive and universal is probably noise exposure, so that the meaning of presbycusis + sociocusis in practice might be interpreted as aging with some minimal level of noise bias. Therefore, it does not appear appropriate to consider implementing a separate sociocusis correction factor in NIPTS.

The value of the sociocusis concept is that it provides an awareness that influences other than occupational noise exposure may affect hearing acuity. This minimizes the probability that changes in hearing level will be attributed entirely to the noise factor and may lead to a search for other etiological factors in specific compensation cases.

In contrast, the phenomenon of presbycusis has now been adequately documented and, in those studies in which appropriate controls have been observed, little contamination due to noise exposure (or sociocusis) may be assumed to be present (40,41). Although different techniques have been used and different populations have been tested in a variety of studies, good agreement on behavioral thresholds and physiological changes provides convincing evidence that a universal phenomenon of aging occurs in the auditory system. Although it cannot be denied that factors other than noise exposure and aging may produce a loss of auditory sensitivity, these effects are usually unique within one's personal life history and should not be presumed to represent a commonality of detrimental agents to which all members of a given society are inherently exposed. Therefore, the position is taken that current presbycusis data represent a more valid basis from which to derive a correction factor in evaluating noise induced hearing loss than presbycusis + sociocusis (i.e., an age correction factor).

In summary, given that a person's auditory function reflects the joint influences of aging, occupational noise exposure, and a broad range of societal factors, the derivation of a correction formula to be used in cases of occupational hearing loss may ignore the inclusion of a general societal component without unduly biasing the correction value. Evidence of unique effects of factors within sociocusis should be expected to be resolved on an individual basis within the context of legal settlements in noise-induced damage suits.

Presbycusis, Additivity, or What?

Given that a presbycusis correction factor is justified on the basis of the foregoing arguments, the next question concerns the manner in which such a correction should be applied. Is there any evidence to support the hypothesis that sensory hearing losses are additive? The data are extremely limited, but a few studies do lend support to this view as already indicated (33,34). The primary result of any severe noise exposure is hair cell destruction followed in certain cases by secondary effects; diseases, drugs, aging, and other factors also affect the integrity of the hair cells. Thus, it is the total effect of these disturbances which is reflected in the behavioral form of audiological data.

A correction factor based strictly upon additivity, however, faces certain difficulties. There are 3 major considerations which argue against additivity: (i) TTSs are primarily end-organ phenomena and do not show strictly cumulative effects with successive noise exposures (42); (ii) TTSs do not summate with preexisting permanent losses to exceed the auditory fatigue that is evidenced in normal ears by similar exposure conditions (42); and (iii) in a constant work situation, noise-induced hearing loss over time increases, at least 4,000 Hz, in a negatively accelerated, nonlinear fashion, while presbycusis shows an increasing function with positive acceleration beyond ~35 years of age. Whether or not additivity is justified, these arguments tend to mitigate against a correction factor for presbycusis which increases uniformly (linearly) with time.

Furthermore, recent evidence has shown that after repeated exposures to pure tones separated by 3–4 weeks, neither the location nor the extent of the damaged area of sensory cells is changed from that obtained by a single exposure to the given frequency (43). These findings obviously do not support the hypothesis of additivity; they do, however, provide grounds for an alternative proposition. Specifically, additivity may or may not occur depending on the locus and extent of hair cell destruction following noise exposure of a given intensity and duration. When destruction of sensory cells following exposure is essentially complete in a given region of the basilar membrane, subsequent noise exposures, or the deleterious effects of aging, or the destructive effects of other etiological factors may not be expected to add further deficits in hearing functions unless new areas of injury are implicated.

As it is now fairly certain that particular agents can produce patterns of destruction in which virtually all outer hair cells of the basal half of the cochlear spiral are eliminated while the inner hair cells remain intact (44), it may be argued that all factors which in some way affect the displacement of the basilar membrane (and hence affect the potentials of the outer hair cells which dominate the response of the normal cochlea) operate in an additive fashion until a maximal level of degeneration is attained. Any further destructive effects capable of implicating the outer hair cells would be irrelevant, for an asymptotic level of damage would already have been attained at a particular locus; however, degeneration might occur in other regions with less damage as first order or second order effects. Restated, the effects of presbycusis and noise exposure may be additive in terms of anatomical destruction at the hair cell level, but the degree of impairment which can be added by noise after a given length of exposure may be limited and of smaller magnitude than that of presbycusis, since presbycusis continues throughout the lifetime of the individual.

Data from a study by Corso, Wright, and Valerio (45) on temporal summation in older subjects tends to support this proposition. As shown in Fig. 8, the threshold–duration function at 4,000 Hz is the same for older subjects (51 to 57 years) whether or not they have had a prior history of noise exposure; also, the functions do not differ from those for a young noise-exposed sample (mean age, 29.5 years) tested by Wright (46). Thus, the factor of noise exposure in the 51 to 57-year-old sample does not reduce the threshold–duration function below that for a comparable age group without noise exposure. Aging and noise exposure affect the threshold–duration function at 4,000 Hz, but noise alone in the younger group has sufficiently damaged the auditory system that an additional 25 years of aging cannot be detected by the temporal summation measure. The neurophysiological disturbances of presbycusis and noise exposure probably operate independently to affect auditory temporal summation; but, at least for the conditions of this experiment, the 2 factors do not appear to summate in their behavioral effects on the threshold–duration function.

These data, nevertheless, are not contradictory to the hypothesis that, at least to a certain level of destruction, the 2 factors may operate additively in anatomical terms; but, beyond this critical level the noise factor may cease to exert any further appreciable detrimental effect. In these terms, the noxious

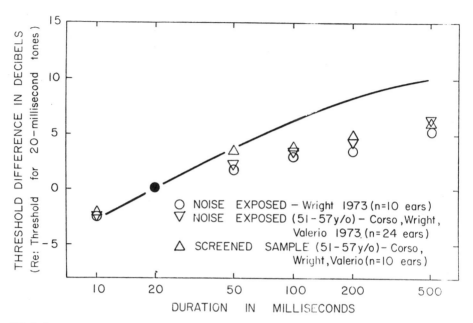

FIG. 8. Comparison of threshold–duration functions for combined right and left ears at 4,000 Hz for three different samples: a: Noise exposed young subjects (mean age 29.5 years). b: Noise exposed older subjects (51–57 years). c: Screened (non-noise-exposed) older subjects (51–57 years). (From ref. 45.)

effects of noise exposure on hearing may be considered to represent certain aspects of "premature presbycusis." The notion of acceleration of destructive effects appear reasonable when it is recognized, for example, that damage to the inner ear caused by the ototoxic side effects of an antibiotic (kanamycin) creates a predisposition to a more rapid development of hearing deficits due to industrial noise (47).

Furthermore, cochlear cell damage due to broadband noise stimulation may be widespread throughout the length of the basilar membrane, but pure-tone tests may not fully depict the status of the cochlear end organ, in that greater damage may exist than is apparent in audiometric findings (48). Such widespread damage may perhaps serve to sensitize the cochlear structures for additive damage through presbycusis.

When temporal integration is used as the measure of auditory efficiency, there is a descending ability to integrate acoustic energy with increasing hearing loss for the frequencies 2,000, 4,000, and 8,000 Hz, whether the losses are due to acoustic trauma or presbycusis; normal temporal integration for some frequencies and abnormal temporal integration for others occurs within the same ear and the relationships are almost identical for acoustic trauma and presbycusis (49). Thus, the histopathology of cochleas damaged by acoustic trauma and by presbycusis must be assumed to be essentially similar, lending additional support to the hypothesis that cumulative physiological effects are a potential reality. This view is consistent with the finding that hearing loss following exposure to noise above a critical level is related to a reduction in cochlear blood flow, which in turn impairs the potassium transport function of the stria vascularis (50); as previously noted, a metabolic breakdown involving the stria vascularis also occurs in presbycusis (18). It appears, therefore, that both audiometric and physiological findings support the concept of anatomic additivity of detrimental effects in noise exposure and presbycusis; however, while the general hypothesis appears to be correct, the specific manner in which additivity must be taken into account as a correction factor in the assessment of NIHL needs to be considered.

PRESBYCUSIS DATA BASE

In order to consider a possible correction factor for presbycusis in NIHL, careful consideration must be given to the basic data base from which an appropriate correction may be calculated. As arguments have already been advanced in earlier portions of this chapter that preclude special considerations of factors under the category of sociocusis, the major problem appears to be one of trying to obtain the best possible estimates of "pure" presbycusis as a starting point in resolving the current problem. Subsequently, the additivity hypothesis (with certain restrictive conditions) will be considered in an attempt to provide a somewhat more realistic solution to the presbycusis–noise exposure problem than has been available up to the present time.

The Corso Study and Confirming Data

The definition of a criterion of hearing impairment and the measurement of degrees of impairment, whether for speech or for pure tones, implies a valid specification of hearing ability in normal young adults. Furthermore, the valid specification of hearing in normal adults of all ages is critical for the definition of a criterion of damage risk for the general population and for the measurement of degrees of risk which exceed a given impairment criterion. Simply, the existence of presbycusis must be taken into consideration in establishing an appropriate population baseline for the assessment of NIHL.

Kryter (51) has considered this problem and has provided estimates, according to several studies, of the prevalence in the population of hearing losses exceeding 25 dB at 500, 1,000, and 2,000 Hz as a function of age. These data are presented in Fig. 9. After critically evaluating the appropriateness of each of the functions in Fig. 9 as a potential reference baseline, Kryter (52) has concluded that "Corso's data (41) are probably the best determination of pure presbycusis for the U.S. population because of the careful otological examination and screening applied to his subjects and because of the quiet living environment from which they were taken" (p. 119).

Support for the validity of Corso's data (41) has been found in a population

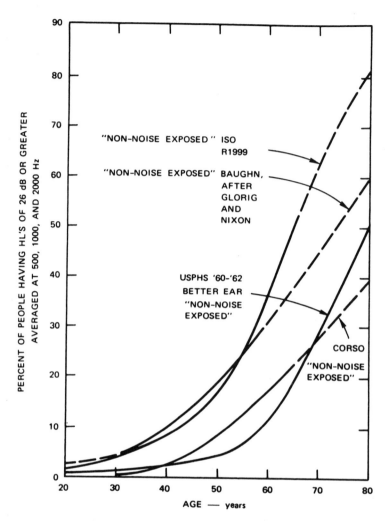

FIG. 9. Curves showing percentage of populations having greater than 25 dB HL, averaged at 500, 1,000, and 2,000 Hz. Dashed lines are extrapolations. (From ref. 51.)

study performed on the island of Westray in the extreme northwest of the Orkney group of islands off the northern coast of Scotland (53). At the time of the study, the population of Westray was 602 inhabitants over the age of 15 years, of which 93% were born in and 75% had not lived outside the Orkney island group. The economy of Westray is based wholly on agriculture and fishing, with no industry other than a shellfish processing factory opened in 1968.

The data of this study clearly show a gradual deterioration of hearing with age for both men and women, otologically normal and non-noise exposed. As in the Corso (41) study, the Westray males were found to have lower pres-

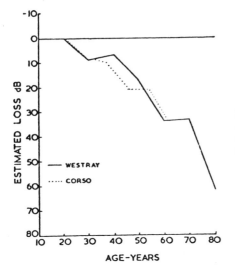

FIG. 10. Comparison of presbycusis values at 4,000 Hz for males, based upon data from island of Westray (53) and United States (41). (After ref. 53.)

bycusis values at 1,000 Hz and below, but higher values at 2,000 Hz and above than the Westray females. A comparison of the curves for presbycusis obtained in the Corso (41) and Westray (53) studies for males at 4,000 Hz is presented in Fig. 10. The data of the two studies appear to be in very good agreement and are representative of the findings in general.

The major conclusion to be drawn from the Westray study (53) is that the Corso (41) data may be considered to be relatively uncontaminated by noise exposure and otological abnormalities and that the data at the present time probably represent the most valid estimates of presbycusis in American men and women.

General Correction for Presbycusis

As of 1969 in medicolegal cases involving compensation claims in the 50 states and the District of Columbia, 23 states made no correction for aging relative to occupational hearing loss due to noise exposure; 12 states had no established policies on this matter; 4 states made corrections when recommended by medical examiners; in four other states age corrections were possible; and in the remaining 8 states, age corrections were routine. Of these eight, Maine, Mississippi, and Utah used a procedure in which a 0.5 dB correction was made for each year of age after 40 (54).

In an attempt to derive general curves for presbycusis which might be applied in Western countries of the world, Spoor (35) analyzed presbycusis data from 8 different sources: (*i*) Hinchcliffe (40); (*ii*) Corso (41); (*iii*) Jatho and Heck (55); (*iv*) Johansen (56); (*v*) Beasley (57); (*vi*) 1954 ASA Report (2); (*vii*) Glorig and Nixon (39); and (*viii*) Glorig et al. (58). Data from these studies were statistically manipulated to provide median

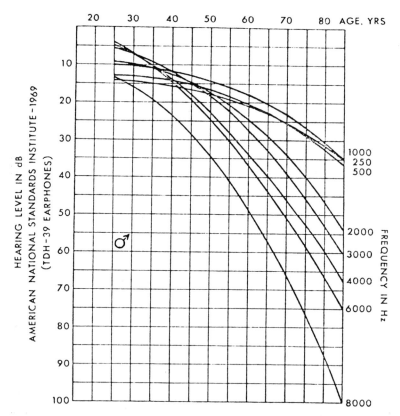

FIG. 11. Composite presbycusic curves for males, according to Spoor (35), modified to conform to ANSI-1969 standard. (From ref. 54.)

hearing loss values for both men and women for different age groups adjusted to a reference age level of 25 years.

Since Spoor's (35) data were based upon the ASA-1954 calibration values, Lebo and Reddell (54) have converted Spoor's general presbycusis curves to conform to the ANSI-1969 standard values. Figure 10 shows the composite male presbycusis curves, and Fig. 11 shows the composite female presbycusis curves based upon the ANSI-1969 standard.

Given the data of Figs. 10 and 11, Lebo and Reddell (54) then proceeded to derive and to plot age correction curves for men and for women for 2 groups of frequencies: (*i*) 500, 1,000, and 2,000 Hz; and (*ii*) 500, 1,000, 2,000, and 3,000 Hz. From alternatives, the formula preferred by Lebo and Reddell (54) for calculating a monaural age-corrected hearing impairment (M_2) is given as follows:

$$M_2 = m_1 \left(\frac{V - C}{V} \right) \tag{1}$$

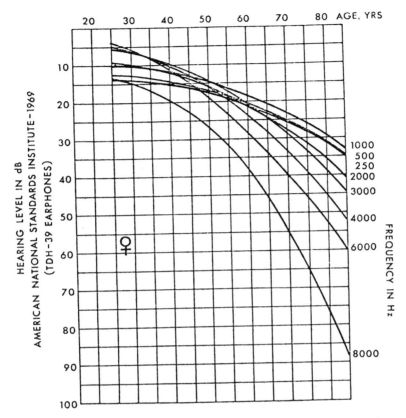

FIG. 12. Composite presbycusis curves for females, according to Spoor (35), modified to conform to ANSI-1969 standard. (From ref. 54.)

where m_1 is the monaural hearing impairment in percent (re ANSI-1969) and is calculated from the formula $m_1 = 1.5$ $(a_1 - 25)$ in which $a_1 = V/n$; V is the sum of hearing losses in dBHL (ANSI-1969) at the specified frequencies; n is the number of specified frequencies; and C is the sum of presbycusic hearing losses in dBHL (ANSI-1969) at the specified frequencies as taken from Fig. 10, or 11, depending upon the sex of the subject. Given a male subject, age 50, with $V = 130$ dB, $n = 4$, and $C = 75$, M_2 as calculated by Eq. (1) has a value of 4.74%.

PROPOSED REVISION OF CORRECTION FOR PRESBYCUSIS

Some Problems in Current Practice

The method of Lebo and Reddell (54), among others, is based on the rationale of averaging the effects of NIHL and presbycusis in patients with an established exposure to damaging sound pressure levels. Thus, Eq. (1) assumes the fundamental validity of additivity in terms of dB hearing loss which, as suggested earlier, does not appear justifiable over the entire life-span. Ward (42) has shown that unrestricted use of the additivity hypothesis with its dB interpretation may often lead to bizarre conclusions. Thus, the additivity (dB) hypothesis as currently applied seems to have certain limitations, particularly when presbycusis corrections are made at older age levels. Nevertheless, until a more acceptable technique becomes available for dealing with the presbycusis correction factor in occupational hearing losses, Eq. (1) appears to have some practical value.

General Recommendations for a Presbycusis Correction Factor in Noise-Induced Hearing Loss

On the basis of the totality of empirical evidence cited in this chapter, some tentative general recommendations for a presbycusis correction factor in NIPTSs appear to be warranted and may serve as guidelines for future developments in this area.

1. In the evaluation of occupational hearing losses, appropriate audiological measurements must be made to differentiate as far as possible noise effects from other types of ear pathology; this implies that audiometric tests must be administered early in the worker's life history, as the advanced effects of noise and aging combine to produce pure-tone threshold curves which tend to be nonspecific.

2. Since a person's total hearing disability is only partially dependent upon noise exposure and a significant portion may be due to presbycusis, a correction factor for presbycusis should be introduced in cases of NIPTS. The correction should be independently considered for men and women, and perhaps by ear; the most valid data from which to derive a general correction for presbycusis are those of Spoor (35), as recalculated by Lebo and Reddell (54) for ANSI-1969 standards. For the United States alone, the data of Corso (41) are probably the most appropriate.

3. A small, constant presbycusis correction factor should be introduced for men below 35 years of age and for women, below 40 years, since single frequencies from 250 through 3,000 Hz show a maximal hearing loss of only about 10 dB over this frequency range and age span. These losses are of no great practical significance, but occur at a time when noise exposure, whether due to occupational hazards or sociocusis, is quite likely to have produced some degree of permanent damage in cochlear structures.

4. Beyond 35 years for men and 40 years for women, the advisability of using pure-tone thresholds as the sole criterion for attempting to separate the effects of noise exposure and aging should be reexamined. As suggested earlier, the concept of additivity of effects attributable to these two factors may be appropriate in terms of anatomical considerations, but some qualifications

seem to be required for dB hearing losses. It is hypothesized that in early stages of noise exposure and at relatively young age levels, which differ for men and women, the effects of noise exposure and aging are physiologically or neuranatomically related and summative. Beyond this period, there may be some further limited damage due to continued noise exposure, but the primary detrimental effect is then believed to be that of presbycusis. On this assumption, it does not appear appropriate to apply a single formula for a presbycusis correction based upon linearity of additive effects throughout the entire lifespan of an individual. As a first approximation, the upper limit of additivity may be considered to be 60 years for men and 65 years for women, based upon the presbycusis curves of Lebo and Reddell (54) and other data.

5. If the assumption is correct that damage in the auditory system due to noise exposure reaches an asymptotic level, independent of aging, then estimates should be made of maximal values of hearing loss due to noise exposure and the number of years required to reach those values in different noise environments. It is suggested that the asymptotic level is attained when pure tone hearing losses are no longer adequate to explain decrements in speech intelligibility, i.e., presbycusis is evident. Jerger (59) has amply demonstrated that when hearing loss is held constant across age, there is a disproportionate loss in the understanding of speech (PB_{max}) with a progressive aging effect. The decremental effect is initially observed starting in the fifth decade ($PB_{max} = 90\%$) and declines steadily to the eighth decade ($PB_{max} = 59\%$). This phenomenon is not related to any substantial degree to the presence or absence of loudness recruitment and points, therefore, to a central rather than peripheral explanation of the effect. These data support the proposition that noise and aging effects are probably not additive beyond the fifth or sixth decade. It appears, therefore, that an additivity presbycusis correction may be appropriate for men from approximately 35 to 60 years and for women, from approximately 40 to 65 years.

6. Beyond approximately 60 years for men and 65 for women, the additivity hypothesis should be discarded. Nixon and Glorig (60) have shown that the NIPTS at 4,000 Hz, corrected for age, reaches its asymptotic level after approximately 20 years of exposure, with the absolute value determined by the noise SPL characteristics. For 2,000 Hz, however, NIPTS had not leveled off even after 40 years of exposure. These findings suggest that different frequencies require different durations of exposure before attaining an asymptotic level. Assuming that an individual starts his working life in industry at approximately 20 years, the data of Nixon and Glorig (60) suggest that the limits of 60 years for men and 65 for women may represent the upper bounds of additivity. Hence, beyond these limits presbycusis continues to accrue, but further damage due to continued noise exposure is expected to be negligible. Furthermore, at these older age levels, an individual's hearing ability can no longer be adequately assessed for practical purposes solely in terms of puretone thresholds; additional audiological measurements need to be made, in-

cluding speech discrimination, before the degree of auditory impairment can be adequately established.

SUMMARY STATEMENT

This chapter has considered the matter of presbycusis as a complicating factor in the objective appraisal of NIHL. Both physiological and audiometric evidence confirms the fact that excessive noise exposure and aging can produce permanent damage in the human auditory system; at a behavioral level, such damage is typically demonstrated in terms of increased pure tone thresholds or decreased speech discrimination. The effects of noise exposure occur primarily at the cochlear level, whereas aging produces physiological deterioration not only at the cochlear level but throughout the entire auditory system including the temporal lobes of the brain. The audiometric identification of a noise-induced hearing loss is possible only in early cases of exposure, because noise and aging at the cochlear level tend to affect similar structures, for example, hair cells.

The issue of additivity of hearing losses due to noise exposure and aging has been examined in detail. Additivity of deteriorating effects at the psysiological level due to these 2 factors appears reasonable, but additivity in behavioral terms, i.e., dB hearing loss, appears to have limited applicability. Current practices in evaluating occupational hearing losses based upon the assumption of additivity have been considered and some general recommendations for a presbycusis correction factor in noise induced hearing loss were proposed. The recommendations include: (*i*) a small constant correction for aging up to 35 years for men and 40 years for women; (*ii*) a variable aging correction factor by sex from 35 to 60 years for men and 40 to 65 years for women, based upon Spoor's (35) data as recalculated re ANSI-1969 by Lebo and Reddell (54); and (*iii*) a maximal constant noise correction factor by sex for all ages beyond these upper age limits. The advisability of using audiometric measurements other than pure tone thresholds for the assessment of hearing impairments due to noise exposure and aging has been suggested.

REFERENCES

1. Corso, J. F. (1958): Proposed laboratory standard of normal hearing. *J. Acoust. Soc. Am.,* 30:14–23.
2. Exploratory Subcommittee Z24–X–2. (1954): *The Relations of Hearing Loss to Noise Exposure,* pp. 5–55. American Standards Association, New York.
3. Davis, H., and Kranz, F. (1964): International audiometric zero. *J. Acoust. Soc. Am.,* 36:1450–1454.
4. Corso, J. F. (1959): Age and sex differences in pure-tone thresholds. *J. Acoust. Soc. Am.,* 31:498–507.
5. Johnsson, L. G., and Hawkins, J. E., Jr. (1972): Sensory and neural degeneration with aging, as seen in microdissections of the human inner ear. *Ann. Otol. Rhinol. Laryngol.,* 81:179–193.
6. Bredberg, G. (1968): Cellular pattern and supply of the human organ of Corti. *Acta Otolaryngol.* [Suppl.] (*Stockh.*), 236:135.

7. Hawkins, J. (1966): Hearing: Anatomy and acoustics. In: *The Physiological Basis of Medical Practice,* 8th ed., edited by C. H. Best and N. B. Taylor, pp. 375–394. Williams and Wilkins, Baltimore, Md.
8. Miller, J. D. (1974): Effects of noise on people. *J. Acoust. Soc. Am.,* 56:729–764.
9. Hamernik, R. P., Henderson, D., and Sitler, R. W. (1972): Cochlear degeneration following impulse noise exposure. Paper presented at the 83rd Annual Meeting of the Acoustical Society of America. Buffalo, N.Y.
10. Jordan, V. M., Pinheiro, M. L., Chiba, K., Jimenez, A., and Luz, G. A. (1972): Cochlear pathology in monkeys exposed to impulse noise. U.S. Army Med. Res. Lab., Fort Knox, Ky., Report No. 968, 1–24.
11. Hunter-Duvar, I. M., and Elliot, D. N. (1972): Effects of intense auditory stimulation: Hearing losses and inner ear changes in the squirrel monkey. *J. Acoust. Soc. Am.,* 52:1181–1192.
12. Ward, D. W., and Duvall, A. J. (1971): Behavioral and ultrastructural correlates of acoustic trauma. *Ann. Otol. Rhinol. Laryngol.,* 80:881–896.
13. Hunter-Duvar, I. M., and Bredberg, G. (1974): Effects of intense auditory stimulation: hearing losses and inner ear changes in the chinchilla. *J. Acoust. Soc. Am.,* 55:795–801.
14. Luz, G. A., and Lipscomb, D. M. (1973): Susceptibility to damage from impulse noise: chinchilla versus man or monkey. *J. Acoust. Soc. Am.,* 54:1750–1753.
15. Eldredge, D. H., Bilger, R. C., and Davis, H. (1961): Factor analysis of cochlear injuries and changes in electrophysiological potentials following acoustic trauma in the guinea pig. *J. Acoust. Soc. Am.,* 33:152–159.
16. Nakamura, S. (1964): Some of the basic problems in noise trauma. *Jap. Otol.,* 67:1669–1684.
17. Ward, W. D. (1970): Biochemical implications in auditory fatigue and noise-induced hearing loss. In: *Biochemical Mechanisms in Hearing and Deafness,* edited by M. M. Paparella, pp. 103–113. C. C Thomas, Springfield, Ill.
18. Gacek, R. R., and Schuknecht, H. F. (1969): Pathology of presbycusis. *Int. Audiol.,* 8:199–209.
19. Kirikae, I., and Shitara, T. (1961): Recent advances in the study on presbycusis. *Ronenbyo,* 5:18.
20. Hansen, C. C., and Reske-Nielsen, E. (1965): Pathological studies in presbycusis. *Arch. Otolaryngol.,* 82:115–132.
21. Konigsmark, B., and Murphy, E. A. (1972): Volume of the ventral cochlear nucleus in man: Its relationship to neuronal population and age. *J. Neuropathol. Exp. Neurol.,* 31:304–316.
22. Kirikae, I., Sato, T., and Shitara, T. (1964): A study of hearing in advanced age. *Laryngoscope,* 74:205–220.
23. Scheidegger, S. (1963): Präsenile spongiose gehirnatrophie schweiz. *Arch. Neurol. Psychiat.,* 91:211.
24. Krmpotic-Nemanic, J. (1969): Presbycusis and retrocochlear structures. *Int. Audiol.,* 8:210–220.
25. Fritsch, V., Dabozi, M., and Grieg, D. (1972): Degenerative changes of the arterial vessels of the internal auditory meatus during the process of aging. *Acta Otolaryngol. (Stockh.),* 73:259–266.
26. Bochenek, Z., and Jachowska, A. (1969): Atherosclerosis, accelerated presbycusis and acoustic trauma. *Int. Audiol.,* 8:312–316.
27. Hawkins, J. E., Jr. (1971): The role of vasoconstriction in noise induced hearing loss. *Ann. Otol. Rhinol. Laryngol.,* 80:903–913.
28. Schuknecht, J. F., Watanuki, K., Takahashi, T., Belal, A. A. Jr., Kimura, R. S., Jones, D. D., and Ota, C. Y. (1974): Atrophy of the stria vascularis, a common cause for hearing loss. *Laryngoscope,* 84:1777–1821.
29. Crowley, D. E., Schramm, V. L., Swain, R. E., Maisel, R. H., Rauchbach, E., and Swanson, S. N. (1972): An animal model for presbycusis. *Laryngoscope,* 82:2079–2091.
30. Jordan, V. M., Pinheiro, M. L., Chiba, K., and Jimenez, A. (1973): Postmortem changes in surface preparations of the cochlea. *Ann. Otol. Rhinol. Laryngol.,* 82:111–125.

31. Littler, T. S. (1958): Noise measurement, analysis and evaluation of harmful effects. *Ann. Occup. Hyg.,* 1:11.
32. Taylor, W., Pearson, J., Maier, A., and Burns, W. (1965): Study of noise and hearing in jute weaving. *J. Acoust. Soc. Am.,* 38:113–120.
33. Mollica, V. (1969): Acoustic trauma and presbyacusis. *Int. Audiol.,* 8:305–311.
34. Macrae, J. H. (1971): Noise induced hearing loss and presbycusis. *Audiology,* 10:323–333.
35. Spoor, A. (1967): Presbycusis values in relation to noise induced hearing loss. *Int. Audiol.,* 6:48–57.
36. Goldner, A. J. (1953): Deafness in shipyard workers. *Arch. Otolaryngol.,* 57:287–309.
37. Schmidt, P. H. (1967): Presbycusis. *Int. Audiol.,* 6:Suppl. 1, 1–36.
38. Ward, W. D. (1973): Noise-induced hearing damage. In: *Otolaryngology,* Vol. 2, edited by M. M. Paparella and D. A. Shumrick, pp. 377–390. Saunders, Philadelphia, Pa.
39. Glorig, A., and Nixon, J. (1962): Hearing losses as a function of age. *Laryngoscope,* 72:1596–1610.
40. Hinchcliffe, R. (1959): The threshold of hearing as a function of age. *Acustica,* 9:303–308.
41. Corso, J. F. (1963): Age and sex differences in pure-tone thresholds. *Arch. Otolaryngol.,* 77:385–405.
42. Ward, W. D. (1971): Presbycusis, sociocusis, and occupational noise-induced hearing loss. *Proc. Roy. Soc. Med.,* 64:200–203.
43. Pye, A. (1974): Acoustic trauma after double exposure in mammals. *Audiology,* 13:320–325.
44. Dallos, P., Billone, M. C., Durant, J. D., Wang, C. Y., and Raynor, S. (1972): Cochlear inner and outer hair cells: Functional differences: *Science,* 177:356–358.
45. Corso, J. F., Wright, H. N., and Valerio, M. (1975): Auditory temporal summation in presbycusis and noise exposure. *J. Gerontol. (in press).*
46. Wright, H. N. (1973): Unpublished data, included in Ref. 45.
47. Krochmalska, E. (1974): Effect of industrial noise and ototoxic antibiotics on cochlear functions. *Acta Otolaryngol.,* 77:44–50.
48. Lipscomb, D. M. (1972): Noise exposure and its effects. *Oticongress,* 2:3–8.
49. Pedersen, C. B. (1973): Brief tone audiometry in patients with acoustic trauma. *Acta Otolaryngol.,* 75:332–333.
50. Schneider, E. A. (1974): A contribution to the physiology of perilymph. Part III: On the origin of noise-induced hearing loss. *Ann. Otol. Rhinol. Laryngol.,* 83:406–412.
51. Kryter, K. D. (1973): Impairment to hearing from exposure to noise. *J. Acoust. Soc. Am.,* 53:1211–1234.
52. Kryter, K. D. (1970): *The Effects of Noise on Man.* Academic Press, New York.
53. Kell, R. L., Pearson, J. C. G., and Taylor, W. (1970): Hearing thresholds of an island population in North Scotland. *Int. Audiol.,* 9:334–349.
54. Lebo, C. P., and Reddell, R. C. (1972): The presbycusis component in occupational noise-induced hearing loss. *Laryngoscope,* 82:1399–1409.
55. Jatho, K., and Heck, K. H. (1959): Schwellen audiometrische Untersuchungen über die Progredienz und Charakteristik der Alterschwerhörigkeit in den verschiedenen Lebensabschnitten. *Z. Laryngol., Rhinol., Otol. Grennzgbiete,* 38:72.
56. Johansen, H. (1943): *Den Aldersbetingede Tunghored.* Munksgaard, Copenhagen.
57. Beasley, W. C. (1938): *National Health Survey (1935–1936) Preliminary Reports, Hearing Study Series,* Bulletins 1–7. *U.S. Public Health Service,* Washington, D.C.
58. Glorig, A., Wheeler, D., Quiggle, R., Grings, W., and Summerfield, A. (1957): *Wisconsin State Fair Hearing Survey 1954.* Subcommittee on Noise in Industry of the American Academy of Ophthalmology and Otolaryngology, Los Angeles.
59. Jerger, J. (1973): Audiological findings in aging. *Adv. Otorhinolaryngol.,* 20:115–124.
60. Nixon, J. C., and Glorig, A. (1961): Noise-induced permanent threshold shift at 2000 cps and 4000 cps. *J. Acoust. Soc. Am.,* 33:904–908.

Effects of Noise on Hearing, edited by Donald Henderson, Roger P. Hamernik, Darshan S. Dosanjh, and John H. Mills. Raven Press, New York © 1976.

Industrial Hearing Conservation Programs

Alan S. Feldman

State University of New York, Upstate Medical Center, Department of Otolaryngology, Communication Disorder Unit, Syracuse, New York 13210

The impetus for hearing conservation programs in industry can hardly be presumed to originate from industry's moral concern for the worker's health. The damaging effects of noise on hearing cannot be viewed as a recent discovery and the existence of excessive noise levels in industrial settings is commonplace knowledge. While there is concern on the part of nonindustrial groups that the noise levels in industry do impair hearing, it has been difficult to enlist the support of industry to voluntarily develop hearing conservation programs. Rather, the impetus for hearing conservation programs arises from legal pressures which stipulate that the work environment cause "no material impairment of health or functional capacity" (1). It is indeed interesting that other legal pressures, primarily those relating to workmen's compensation have been in existence considerably longer on a statewide basis than has the federal regulation for industrial noise control, and yet it is the federal regulation that is providing the primary stimulus for the development of hearing conservation programs within industry. In some respects, workmen's compensation claims constitute a far greater potential cost to industry than does noncompliance with the federal regulation. However, workmen's compensation seems to have had almost no impact in the development of hearing conservation programs and in fact, the fear of alerting the older worker to the fact that he has a compensable problem has probably been a major deterrent to the development of programs.

Federal regulations (OSHA), as we are all aware, have stimulated the development of standards for Occupational Noise Exposure (2). A considerable amount of time and debate has ensued over such factors as damage risk criteria and the minimum noise level to which employees might be exposed. Much of the dispute appears to relate to the fact that the primary means of compliance with the federal standard relates to the specification that noise control first be approached from an engineering standpoint. That is, when engineering technology is feasible, the noise should be engineered out. However, that concept of feasibility is really disputed by industry from an economic standpoint and the use of ear protection is advanced as a viable option rather than an intermediate step.

The intent of federal regulation, being one of prevention, has resulted in a series of regulations for many areas of health and safety. When it comes to the effects of noise, primary attention has focused upon the damaging effect of noise on hearing. Nonauditory effects have been generally ignored. With respect to the effects of noise on hearing, the proposed regulations specify that employees who are exposed to potentially damaging levels of noise must either be provided with sufficient nonexposure periods or alternative plans must be developed and implemented for the reduction of noise in order to achieve compliance with the regulations. Presently, the latter option is the first mandated choice. When noise exposure of employees occurs, a hearing conservation program must be established.

The process industry may use to determine whether or not it is in compliance with federal regulations is demonstrated in Fig. 1. This flow chart naturally begins with a review of the Occupational Health and Safety Guidelines on Industrial Noise and proceeds through the various stages available to achieve compliance with the regulations. Hearing conservation programs are an integral part of programs when exposure exists. In addition to the federal guidelines, other regulations may be introduced at the state level and may, in fact, be more stringent. Consequently, an industry must not only evaluate its program in terms of the federal guidelines, but when existing state guidelines exist, they must be considered as well.

In any event, the first step in achieving compliance with occupational noise guidelines and determining the need for a hearing conservation program is to conduct a noise survey. This will demonstrate either (i) the noise level in the workplace is below 85 dB(A), or (ii) in excess of 85 dB, presuming a 90 dB(A) damage risk criteria and a 5 dB doubling rule that would mandate implementation of a hearing conservation program at 85 dB(A) exposure. If the noise survey verifies that noise does not exceed that level then the program is automatically in compliance and a hearing conservation program is not necessary. However, if the noise level exceeds 85 dB(A), the next question is to establish whether or not there is personnel exposure. If employees are not exposed to noise then the noise level itself is inconsequential (3) and the company is still in compliance. On the other hand, if personnel are exposed a determination of the extent of individual exposure must be carried out. With this in hand, it is possible to determine whether or not the individual exposure exceeds the guidelines which, at the present time, specify a daily noise dose equal to or exceeding 0.5 (85 dB(A) for 8 hr). If exposures do not reach this level this material is then documented and the company is in compliance and without the need for a hearing conservation program.

Should exposure exceed the damage risk criteria, a comprehensive sound survey is necessary in order to begin to determine whether engineering controls which can reduce noise levels are feasible. If they are, they should be implemented and the track returns to a repeat noise survey which would establish

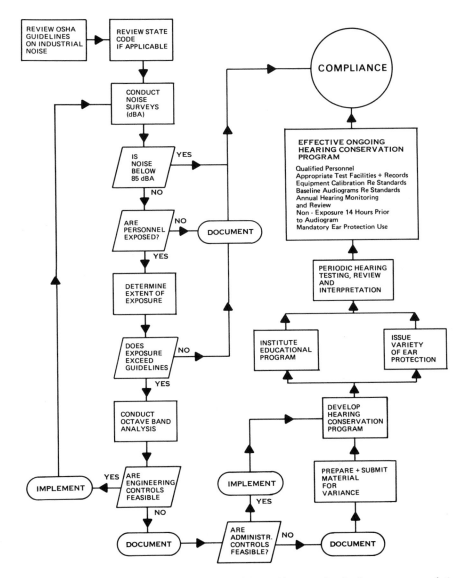

FIG. 1. Flow chart to be followed to determine compliance with occupational noise exposure regulations and determining the need for a hearing conservation program. (Reproduced by courtesy of Environmental Hearing and Vision Consultants, Ltd.)

whether or not the level of noise has been reduced to a point of compliance. If engineering controls are not feasible or still result in potentially damaging exposure, this material must be documented and the feasibility of administrative controls such as work schedule modification and machinery on time modification must be reviewed and, if feasible, implemented.

Administrative and engineering controls may not prove to be feasible and employee exposure may still persist. For example, a weaving mill noise level will generally be well in excess of 100 dB and administrative controls such as employee rotation and intermittent equipment on time are not feasible. In addition, there is both economical and technological lack of feasibility for engineering a significant noise reduction. These facts must be documented and the company could prepare an application for a variance. In any event, whether engineering controls are or are not feasible and whether administrative controls are or are not feasible, as long as the exposure time exceeds the guidelines a hearing conservation program must be established.

The hearing conservation program may be viewed as multifaceted. It should include an educational program which provides personnel education for both management and labor as to the effects of noise on hearing and the prevention of impairment. In addition to this a variety of ear protection should be made available for exposed employees. Hearing protection is presently viewed as a temporary substitute in lieu of feasible engineering and administrative controls. The ear protection issued to the employee in conjunction with the educational program would be presumed to reduce the effective exposure to levels below those cited in the damage risk criteria. The effectiveness of the program in achieving this goal is then validated by a periodic hearing testing program with professional review and interpretation. This package would then provide the company with an effective ongoing hearing conservation program leading to compliance with the federal occupational noise exposure guidelines. Compliance then, means either the elimination of (i) potentially hazardous noise; (ii) the effective reduction of exposure to existing hazardous noise; and (iii) audiometric monitoring of the overall effectiveness of the noise control program.

The detailed components of an effective hearing conservation program are:

1. Qualified personnel and professional surveillance
2. Appropriate test facilities and records
3. Equipment calibration policies
4. Baseline audiograms
5. Annual hearing monitoring and review
6. A 14-hr nonexposure period prior to audiometry
7. Mandatory ear protection use

These components are specified in the occupational noise-exposure standard (2). There are, of course, several approaches that industry may elect to follow in order to establish the hearing conservation program. A major criticism by industry of the requirement for such a program involves its expense. It is indeed costly to train personnel, obtain equipment, and test all employees on a regular schedule. However, hearing impairment is also costly. In order to establish that hearing impairment is not occurring as a consequence of employee exposure to potentially hazardous noise levels, the companies have the option of either internally organizing, equipping, and training personnel to carry out an effective hearing conservation program, or employing outside professional consultants to establish and run the program. The former instance would include the training of someone within the company to function as an industrial hearing conservationist. This would provide the company with someone who can test, issue, and fit ear protection and cooperate with the educational program. Administration of the hearing conservation program itself could be in any number of channels. This could be a program that is coordinated under the medical department or, as is more common in smaller plants, under safety personnel or some other administration structure. What would be important would be that the people involved in the program are appropriately trained and credentialled professionals.

The audiometric data which is obtained provides only a baseline audiogram which serves as a reference audiogram against which future hearing tests are checked for a significant shift as stipulated by law. Should the company wish to go further, the audiogram may serve as a potential health screening device, and employees may be referred for additional and more elaborate investigation of their apparent hearing problem. This latter, however, is not currently mandated, and consequently, is not a stipulated requirement of the hearing conservation program. All that is mandated is that a baseline audiogram be established and that the testing be carried out on at least an annual basis. The employee is to be notified when a significant change in hearing occurs. Hopefully, additional followup beyond reinstruction in the use of ear protection will be incorporated into the program.

An effective hearing conservation program would be one which goes beyond the identification of shifts in hearing level and monitoring of ear protection use and effectiveness. It should also encourage evaluation of significant hearing losses which are detected by the hearing screening program. Whether companies elect to develop internal programs or contract out to consulting firms, the technical and professional aspects of the hearing conservation program should be the responsibility of appropriately credentialled professionals.

SUMMARY

Hearing conservation programs are the mechanism for monitoring hearing health of the employee who is exposed to potentially hazardous noise levels. These programs are necessary when the workplace noise levels and exposures cannot be reduced below hazardous levels. The programs minimally provide valid threshold audiograms in specified test environments with calibrated instrumentation generated by appropriately trained personnel. This audiometric data serves as the means of validating that noise control and ear protection are effective in preventing noise-induced hearing loss. The additional dimension of identification of other kinds of hearing loss and referring for appropriate evaluations is an as yet optional but desirable feature of many programs.

REFERENCES

1. Public Law 91–596 (1970): Occupational Safety and Health Act.
2. Occupational Noise Exposure: Proposed rules, Dept. of Labor, Occupational Safety and Health Administration Federal Register 39, 207, Oct. 24, 1974.
3. Ward, W. D. (1974): Noise levels are not noise exposures. Proceedings of the Noise Expo National Noise and Vibration Control Conference, Chicago, Ill. June 1974.

Effects of Noise on Hearing, edited by Donald Henderson,
Roger P. Hamernik, Darshan S. Dosanjh, and John H. Mills.
Raven Press, New York © 1976.

Extraauditory Effects of Noise

K. D. Kryter

Stanford Research Institute, Menlo Park, California 94025

The major extraauditory effects of noise to be discussed in this chapter
will be responses of the cardiovascular, vegetative, glandular, and muscular
systems of the body that are controlled primarily by the autonomic nervous
system, and which conceivably may contribute to a state of ill-health in persons exposed to noise. Also, mention will be made of some mental and motor
behavior in response to noise that is not necessarily mediated by the autonomic nervous system.

Noise can cause activation of the autonomic nervous system through 3
rather different mechanisms or neural processes: (i) unconditioned defense
or startle reflex responses of the body to sound above a certain level of
intensity because, perhaps, of direct mid- or lower-brain connections of the
auditory nervous system with the spiral ganglia of the autonomic system;
(ii) higher brain center connections to the autonomic system that can serve
to elicit these extraauditory system responses due to cognitive meanings, such
as fear of injury from the presence of the source (e.g., an oncoming vehicle)
which is connoted by the sound or noise; and (iii) activation of the autonomic
nervous system by higher brain centers as the result of a psychological state
of annoyance, fear, or anger, because a noise has interfered with, or is believed to have interfered with, some desired activity such as communications
or sleep.

It should be mentioned that besides the usual airborne path of the external
ear, acoustic energy can enter the body through the skin or other tissues. In
the present chapter we are to be concerned only with extraauditory system
responses that result from normal (airborne) stimulation of the auditory
system by the part of the acoustic spectrum that is called audible (i.e., is
perceived as having, as a minimum, subjective pitch and loudness). The effect of stimulations of the auditory system by frequencies falling below or
above these limits (so-called infra- and ultrasound) will not be discussed.

DISCUSSION

Orienting and Defense Responses

Research on the responses of extraauditory systems to noise, and the interpretation of the results thereto, has been focused on 2 major schools of

thinking. The one school has attempted to explain its research findings in terms of the mechanistic, neural-learning models of Pavlov (23) and Sokolov (24)—that is, innate reflexive responses become conditioned into patterns of behavior which depend on reinforcement of some sort. Some of the research on these concepts has been rather recently reviewd by Graham (10), Jackson (13), and Ginsberg and Furedy (8). This reinforcement, or lack

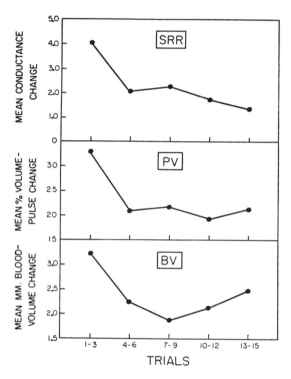

FIG. 1. Showing mean skin resistance response (SRR), peripheral pulse volume (PV) and peripheral blood volume (BV) responses to stimulus repetition (80 dB; 200 Hz tones, or bright light). [From Ginsberg and Furedy (8).]

thereof, will cause the responses to be modified, habituated, or inhibited in a way that best adapts the organism to its environment.

This reflexive-learning concept of extraauditory responses to noise, or meaningless sound, appears to be best formulated by Sokolov, who postulated 2 reflexive types of responses that are built into man. One Sokolov calls the orienting response (OR), wherein the autonomic nervous system responds to any sound stimulus in order to alert and make ready the organism for the purposes of receiving and responding, as appropriate, to this stimulus situation. This OR, it is postulated, would tend to get larger as the noise stimuli became weaker, because the organism would require more effort to react to weaker than to more readily observed stimuli. The second reflex response of the autonomic system to noise postulated by Sokolov is a defensive response (DR) that prepares the organism for flight or fight. This DR, unlike the OR, becomes stronger as the strength of the noise is increased.

The reader is reminded that these OR and DR responses occur to meaningless sounds or noises, but that as the meaning becomes, through repetition of the noises, established (e.g., the noise does not warrant either an orienting or a defensive response) the response becomes inhibited or habituated. The

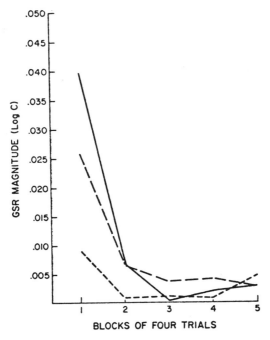

FIG. 2. Galvanic skin response (GSR) to repetition of 2-sec, 1,000 Hz tones of (---) 40, (– –) 70, or (—) 100 dB. [From Harper (12) after Graham (10).]

complex constructs that have been developed from this basic conditioned-response theory to explain the many varieties of data that have been obtained need not concern us here, nor will the number of unresolved theoretical questions as well as apparent inconsistencies in the data (i.e., sometimes one particular measure of autonomic activation, such as peripheral blood volume, will appear to be a more sensitive measure of autonomic activation than another, for example, peripheral pulse volume, and sometimes the reverse).

Figures 1, 2, and 3 show the rather rapid habituation of responsiveness to the meaningless sounds or noises typically found in these types of investigations. It is clear that, while initial responsiveness increases with increases in stimulus intensity, habituation seemingly always becomes nearly complete.

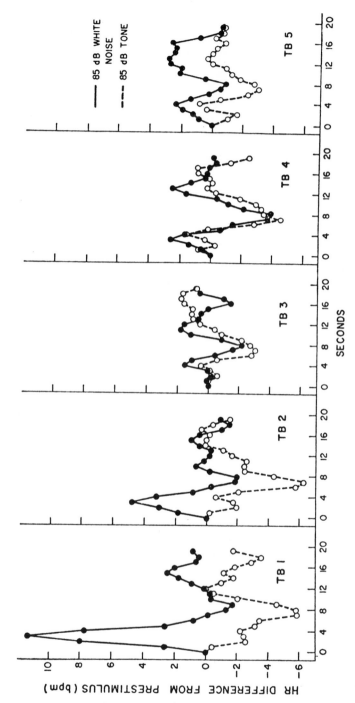

FIG. 3. Heart rate (HR) response to white noise and 1,000 Hz tone of 5 sec duration 85 dB, on 5 trial blocks (TB) of 2 trials each. [From Graham and Slaby [11].]

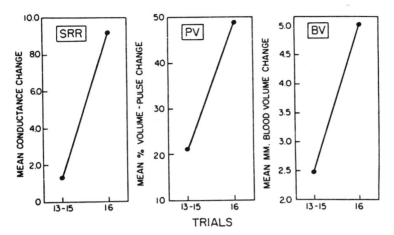

FIG. 4. Mean skin resistance response (SRR), peripheral pulse volume (PV), and peripheral blood volume (BV) responses to repeated (13–15) trials and change (16) trials. [From Ginsberg and Furedy (8).]

That this reduction in response with stimulus repetition is not due to a fatiguing of the mechanism is shown in Fig. 4 from the study by Ginsberg and Furedy. It is seen in Fig. 4 that following 15 repetitions (trials) of an 80 dB, 200 Hz tone, or a bright light (increase from 2.9 to 4.7 ft lumens) the autonomic responses were much less than to the 16th trial when the stimulus was changed from the tone to light stimulus (for half the Ss) or from light to tone stimulus (for the other Ss).

It is also worth noting here that these particular psychophysiological researchers and theorists never suggest or consider the possibility that these extraauditory responses of the autonomic system represent any undue stress or health-threatening phenomena; partly, perhaps, because these responses tended in most of their studies to show such rapid adaptation or habituation, and partly, perhaps, because the magnitude of the physiological changes that are associated with these responses are rather small in comparison to the range of physiological conditions or states observed in the human organism during homeostatic operations of the autonomic system normal to daily living. For example, in regard to this point, the greatest heart rate change shown in Fig. 3 is about 11 beats/min, from 75 to 86, and this for only 1 or 2 beats, and the peripheral blood volume changes last but for 10–20 sec or so. Consider that changes much greater than these occur from mild exercise, fright, sudden changes in air temperature, laughter, etc.

Health Effects

We now turn to the data and theories of a second school of researchers—persons interested in public and industrial health. The findings of this group are controversial in many respects. Perhaps Jansen's writings (14–17) give

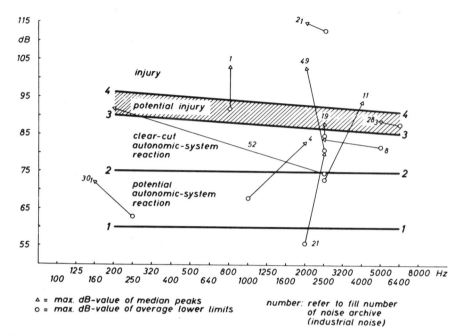

Δ = max. dB-value of median peaks
o = max. dB-value of average lower limits

number: refer to fill number
of noise archive
(industrial noise)

FIG. 5. Limits for the assessment of autonomic-system reactions produced by noise. Note: The terms "clear-cut autonomic-system reaction" and "potential autonomic-system reaction" must be understood in the context of the present working hypothesis, ie., that preventive medicine, until there is evidence to the contrary, should assume that "suprathreshold" noise exposures, either frequently repeated or lasting for long periods, may eventually produce damage. [From Jansen (16, 17).]

the clearest picture of the notion that noise somehow directly stimulates or causes activation of the autonomic nervous system so as to be a threat to the physical health of people. Indeed, as shown in Fig. 5, Jansen sets up limits for noise exposure that must not be exceeded in order to maintain this health. I quote briefly from Jansen's monograph (16) of 1967, positions which he essentially repeats in other papers (15,17).

> The results reported by a number of authors, including those obtained in this laboratory . . . have demonstrated that the human body undergoes a sympathicotonic reaction upon exposure to sounds of higher intensity. This effect is independent of the psychological responses to the noise. There are no indications thus far that the physiological reactions are suppressed or altered in any manner due to "habituation." The psychological responses, admittedly, have fairly wide tolerance limits which vary among individuals and may change with habituation in a given individual. Nevertheless, the autonomic nervous system does not appear to adapt to "supra-threshold" sound levels. . . . Suffice it to say that the first changes in the balance of the autonomic nervous system

that are statistically significant occur, as a rule, at about 75 dB SPL, i.e., at intensity levels which in a "physiological" environment subserve signal transmission, carry warning sounds, or are encountered in human utterances. (Pages 43–44, Belton Translation, 16.)

. . . In contrast to the stimulation of other sense modalities, which were only followed by transitory vasoconstrictions, auditory stimulation was seen to cause vasoconstrictions lasting for the full durations of the exposure. (Page 16, Beltone Translation, 16.)

Jansen bases the above concepts on 2 sets of data. One is shown in Fig. 6 from work of Meyer-Delius (22). Figure 6 shows that indeed there is little adaptation or habituation to the bursts of noise. But, also note after 30 min in the test room the nonnoise control subjects (lowest panel on Fig. 6) had as great a reduced peripheral blood flow (showing constriction of the blood vessels and a presumed condition of "stress" according to this general theory) as did the test subjects at the end of the 30-min test session. It can at least be questioned from these data that the noise during the session had a more lasting "stress" effect on the subjects than that which resulted from merely sitting in the test room, in the quiet, for a similar length of time.

Further, Jansen (16) maintains, on the basis of other data, that this noise-induced stress lasts as long as the noise is on or above a certain level;

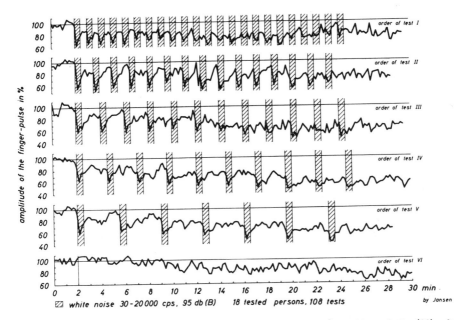

FIG. 6. Autonomic-system reactions during a series of noise exposures. [From Meyer-Delius (22), after Jansen (16).]

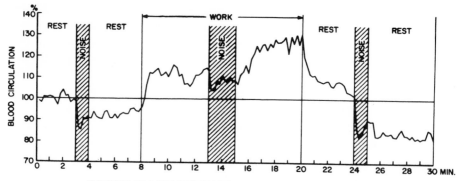

INFLUENCE OF A TWO MINUTE NOISE EFFECT DURING A TWELVE MINUTE WORK PERIOD.
NOISE: WIDE-BAND 95 DIN-PHON; WORK: 5 MCP/SEC. BICYCLE ERGOMETER; 53
TESTS, 7 SUBJECTS.

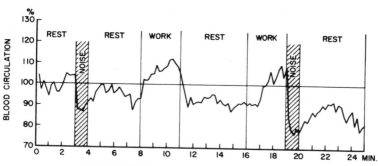

INFLUENCE OF NOISE AFTER TERMINATION OF NOISELESS MANUAL
WORK. NOISE: WIDE-BAND 95 DIN-PHON; WORK: 5 MCP/SEC. BICYCLE
ERGOMETER; 45 TESTS, 7 SUBJECTS.

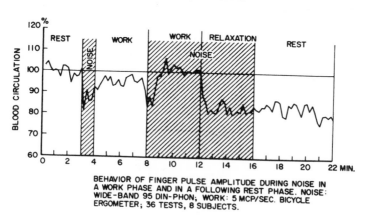

BEHAVIOR OF FINGER PULSE AMPLITUDE DURING NOISE IN
A WORK PHASE AND IN A FOLLOWING REST PHASE. NOISE:
WIDE-BAND 95 DIN-PHON; WORK: 5 MCP/SEC. BICYCLE
ERGOMETER; 36 TESTS, 8 SUBJECTS.

FIG. 7. Showing effects of combinations of work, rest, and noise on blood circulation: A reduced percentage indicates vasoconstriction of the peripheral blood vessels. [From Jansen (15).]

i.e., steady-state noise. However, there is no consistency in Jansen's published data (15), that I could find, to support this conclusion. Figure 7, for example, indicates that, as the noise continues, the peripheral blood circulation takes, following an initial constraint to the noise, a state apparently appropriate for either the work or rest phase of activity.

It seems clear that the data presented earlier on the ORs and DRs to tones and noise do not support Jansen's generalizations. Also, in our own labora-

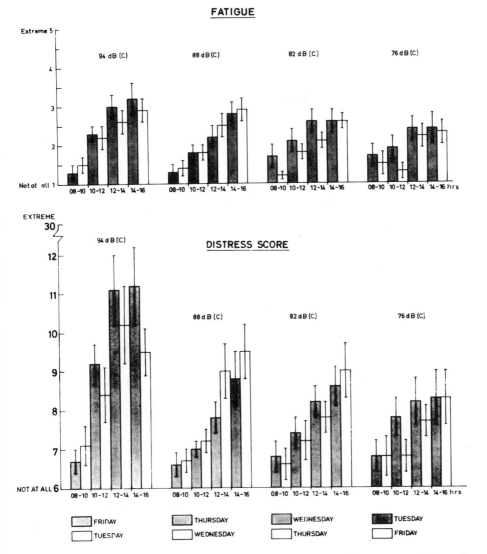

FIG. 8. Self-rated "fatigue" of office machine (IBM) operators (*upper graph*) and self-rated "distress" under different noise conditions and during different times (*abscissa*) of the day. [From Carlestam et al. (4).]

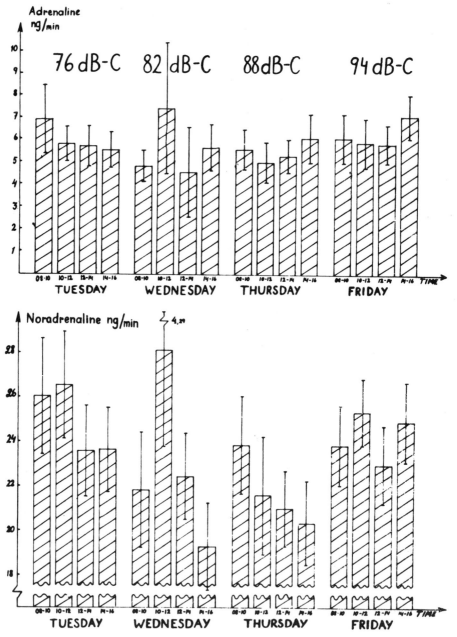

FIG. 9. Urinary excretion of epinephrine (adrenaline) and norepinephrine (noradrenaline) of office machine (IBM) operators during 4 consecutive days with increasing noise level. [From Carlestam et al. (4).]

tory we have been unable to date to obtain continued autonomic system responses of subjects exposed to noise in experiments aimed at replicating some of Jansen's studies. I believe, at the time of this writing, that the psychological set of the subjects and their concept as to what stimuli in the experimental situation they are supposed to respond to, or that some inadvertent conditioning of the subjects to the noises in experiments of this sort, may explain these apparent discrepancies in experimental findings. For example, we found (Kryter, 20), that the average heart rate and freedom of peripheral blood flow were as much, if not more, related to the experimental

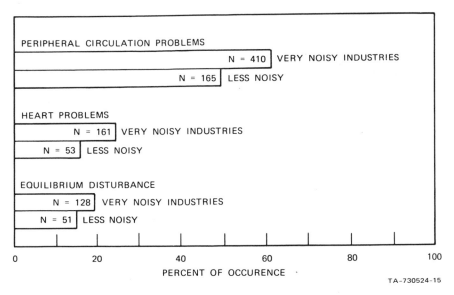

FIG. 10. Showing differences in percent of occurrence of health problems in 1,005 industrial workers. [After Jansen (14).]

sequencing of the test sessions than to the presence of quiet and noise per se.

In any event, I think it fair to say that Jansen's contentions of: (i) no habituation in stress responses to repeated noises at levels above 75 dB(A) or so, and (ii) continued stress throughout the duration of an intense noise are resting on meager, if not contrary, experimental grounds.

Levi (21) and his colleagues at the Karolinska Institute have also espoused the notion that autonomic nervous system activation constitutes a stress condition that can be harmful. However, Carlestam, Karlsson, and Levi (4) have expressed doubts as to whether autonomic systems response to noise may be adequate to explain such results as shown in Fig. 8. Figure 8 shows that there was progressive apparent increase in psychological feelings of distress and fatigue with increased noise levels present in an office (IBM operators) work situation; however, as shown in Fig. 9, there was no apparent parallel increase in autonomic system "stress" reaction as measured by adrenal gland excretions found in the urine of the workers.

The second set of data on which Jansen builds his theory is shown in Fig. 10. Figure 10 shows a clear-cut increase in health problems in men working in noisy industries as compared to men in less noisy industries. Somewhat similar findings have been reported in other European studies (Andrukian, 1). Figure 11 shows data reported by Cohen (5) from a study conducted in two U.S. industries with both high-noise [above 95 dB(A)] and low-noise [below 80 dB(A)] work areas. We see in the upper graphs in Fig. 11 that in Plant A the number of medical problems was significantly higher in the high-noise group in Plant A but not in Plant B. Also, the

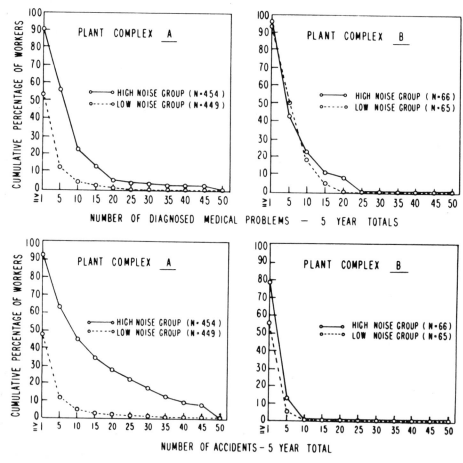

FIG. 11. Cumulative percent frequency distributions of workers in high [above 95 dB(A)] and low [below 80 dB(A)] noise groups in Plant Complexes A and B with a specifiable number of diagnosed medical disorders (*upper graphs*) and specifiable number of accidents (*lower graphs*) over the 5-year period 1966–1970 [From Cohen (5).]

lower curves in Fig. 11 show the number of accidents in Plant A to be much greater than in Plant B, particularly in high noise.

Cohen suggests that the differential risk of injury in the high-noise job areas (boiler factory) in Plant A may have been much greater than in Plant B (electronics and missile parts plant) and that it was the anxiety over danger of injury or accidents and not the high-noise level per se that could have been the cause of increased medical problems in the workers in high noise in Plant A. These problems included digestive, respiratory, urological, glandular, cardiovascular disorders—all suggestive of possible autonomic system stress effects. The question of the existence of extraauditory health problems in industry because of noise must, I believe, remain open until studies are completed in which personnel selection procedures, socioeconomic status and other factors (such as differential bodily injury hazards in different quiet versus noisy work situations) related to the general health conditions of the workers before and during employment are more fully understood and controlled.

Mental and Motor Task Performance

So much for autonomic controlled vegetative reactions *per se*. Research on the effects of noise on work performance, both mental and psychomotor tasks, that does not involve auditory inputs for completion continues, by and large, to show mostly negative results—i.e., noise has negligible, if any, adverse effects. A few studies involving so-called "watch" and complex memory tasks [Broadbent (3), Cohen (6), and others] occasionally show some adverse effects, but other studies do not. Again, as with autonomic nervous system reactivity, the psychological factors present in the experiment [what Azrin (2) called stimulus and response contingencies or knowledge] appear to play a more major role in the performance of nonauditory mental and psychomotor tasks than does the noise. This is perhaps well illustrated by Fig. 12 from a study of Glass and Singer (9). Here we see that the number of insoluble puzzles attempted for solution in the presence of noise was not nearly as much influenced by noise level (108 dB for loud vs 50 dB(A) for soft), as it was by whether the subjects expected or did not expect the noises to occur.

Other Extraauditory Effects

Extraauditory effects can be defined so as to include other areas of research, especially if one includes such matters as the annoyance and possibly correlated health problems of people living in noisy communities. I have attempted to delimit the studies discussed largely to those which were aimed, or supposedly aimed, at elucidating the direct "nonpsychologically controlled" extraauditory effects of noise on man.

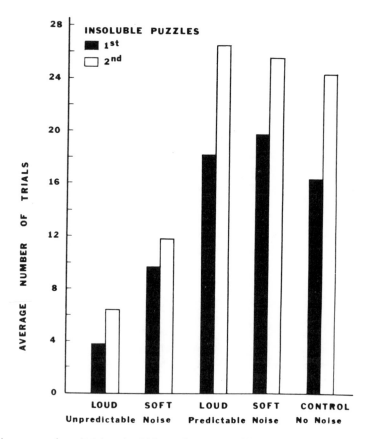

FIG. 12. Average number of trials on insoluble puzzles attempted by groups in different noise conditions and no noise. From [Glass and Singer (9).]

Perhaps, however, brief mention should be made of autonomic system responses (which are herein classed as extraauditory) that are related to feelings of annoyance that occur, when they do, indirectly from exposures to noise. Setting aside the annoyance felt by people because they fear the source (such as an airplane) of a noise rather than the noise per se, it appears that noise in the general living environment causes annoyance and anger because the noise interferes with speech and other forms of auditory communications and arouses people from, or prevents, sleep. These auditory effects of noise may elicit feelings of annoyance or anger which, in turn, cause activation of the autonomic system responses that are possibly sufficiently physiologically stressful in some persons, when oft repeated, to cause or contribute to ill health.

The prevailing approach of controlling community noise down to exposures that provide generally acceptable amounts of annoyance from speech interference and sleep should provide ample protection against these indirectly noise-induced stresses upon the body. The limits generally set for noise in order to avoid significant annoyance because of interference with speech communication and sleep are of the order of 35 to 75 dB(A) at the position of the listener, depending upon the duration of the noise (7,18). These levels are less than even those suggested by Jansen as the levels of noise capable of causing a reflexive autonomic system stress response in man (see Fig. 5). Accordingly, it would appear that these noise limits would avoid the directly (reflex) elicited stress responses (the persistent existence of which is very debatable), as well as stress responses that may be indirectly elicited because of annoyance from direct auditory effects of the noise.

CONCLUSIONS

In spite of the very large gaps in our knowledge and the existence of some apparently conflicting research results, the following conclusions are put forth, with, of course, the usual admonition that more research is needed before they can be accepted with great confidence.

1. There is no likely damage risk to a person from the possible unconditioned stress responses to noise that are mediated by the autonomic system.

2. Noise may often be concomitant with danger and adverse social–environmental factors that are more important than the noise itself as a cause of apparent greater incidences of various physical and psychological disease and accidents in industry.

3. Autonomic system stress responses could conceivably be a contributing factor to ill health in some persons as the result of noise in their living environment directly interfering with auditory communications and sleep, and, thereby, creating the feelings of annoyance and anger that serve as the direct cause of the stress responses.

4. It would appear that controlling meaningless noise to levels that permit auditory communication and sleep behavior adequate for a given work or living environment would obviate the occurrence of any extraauditory responses in the body of a stressful nature.

ACKNOWLEDGMENT

This paper was prepared in part under Contract 68–01–2273 with the U.S. Environmental Protection Agency.

REFERENCES

1. Andrukian, A. A. (1961): Influence of sound stimulation on the development of hypertension, clinical and experimental results. *Cor. Vassa*, 3:285–293.
2. Azrin, N. H. (1958): Some effects of noise on human behavior. *J. Exp. Anal. Behav.*, 1:183–200.
3. Broadbent, D. (1971): *Decision and Stress*. Academic Press, London.

4. Carlestam, G., Karlsson, C., and Levi, L. (1973): Stress and disease in response to exposure to noise: A review. *Proceedings of International Congress on Noise as a Public Health Problem,* U.S. Environmental Protection Agency, Washington, D.C. 479–486.

5. Cohen, A. (1973): Industrial noise and medical absence, and accident record data on exposed workers. *Proceedings of International Congress on Noise as a Public Health Problem,* U.S. Environmental Protection Agency, Washington, D.C. 441–453.

6. Cohen, H. H., Conrad, D. W., O'Brien, J. F., and Pearson, R. G. (1973): Noise effects, arousal, and human information processing task difficulty and performance. Dept. of Psychology and Industrial Engineering, North Carolina State Univ., Raleigh, N.C.

7. Environmental Protection Agency (1974): Information on levels of environmental noise requisite to protect public health and welfare with an adequate margin of safety, U.S. Environmental Protection Agency, Washington, D.C.

8. Ginsberg, S., and Furedy, J. J. (1974): Repetition, change, and assessments of sensitivities of and relationships among an electrodermal and two plethysmographic components of the orienting reflex. *Psychobiology,* 11:35–43.

9. Glass, D. C., and Singer, J. E. (1973): Behavioral effects and after-effects of noise. *Proceedings of International Congress on Noise as a Public Health Problem,* U.S. Environmental Protection Agency, Washington, D.C. 409–416.

10. Graham, F. K. (1973): Habituation and dishabituation of responses innervated by the autonomic nervous system, Chap. 5 in *Habituation,* H. Peeke and M. Herz, Eds. Academic Press, New York and London.

11. Graham, F. K., and Slaby, D. A. (1973): Differential heart rate changes to equally intense white noise and tone. *Psychophysiology,* 10:347–362.

12. Harper, M. M. (1968): The effects of signal property and stimulus intensity on the skin resistence response to repetition of auditory stimuli. Unpublished M. A. Thesis, Univ. of Wisconsin, Madison.

13. Jackson, J. C. (1974): Amplitude and habituation of the orienting reflex as a function of stimulus intensity. *Psychophysiology,* 11:647–659.

14. Jansen, G. (1961): Adverse effects of noise on iron and steel workers, *Stahl. Eisen.* 81:217–220. (In German).

15. Jansen, G. (1964): The influence of noise at manual work. *Int. Z. Angew. Physiol.,* 20:233–239. (In German).

16. Jansen, G. (1967): Extra auditory effects of noise. *Zentr. Arbeitsmed. Arbeitsschutz, Suppl. 9, 1967.* (In German; translation No. 26, Beltone Institute for Hearing Research, Chicago, 1972).

17. Jansen, G. (1973): Non-auditory effects of noise, physiological and psychological reactions in man. *Proceedings of International Congress on Noise as a Public Health Problem,* U.S. Environmental Protection Agency, Washington, D.C. 431–439.

18. Kryter, K. D. (1970): *The Effects of Noise on Man,* Academic Press, New York.

19. Kryter, K. D. (1972): Non-auditory effects of environmental noise. *Am. J. Public Health,* March, 389–398.

20. Kryter, K. D. (1973): Some laboratory tests of heart rate and blood volume in noise. *Proceedings of International Congress on Noise as a Public Health Problem,* U.S. Environmental Protection Agency, Washington, D.C. 487–497.

21. Levi, L. (1973): Stress, Distress and Psychosocial Stimuli. *Occup. Mental Health,* 3,3:2–10.

22. Meyer-Delius, J. (1957): Die Schallein-Wirkung auf den Menschen. *Automobiltechn. Z.,* 10.

23. Pavlov, I. P. (1927): *Conditioned Reflexes: An Investigation of the Physiological Activity of the Cerebral Cortex.* Oxford Univ. Press, London and New York.

24. Sokolov, E. N. (1963): *Perception and the Conditioned Reflex.* Macmillan, New York.

Effects of Noise on Hearing, edited by Donald Henderson,
Roger P. Hamernik, Darshan S. Dosanjh, and John H. Mills.
Raven Press, New York © 1976.

Summary of Present Damage Risk Criteria

H. E. von Gierke and Daniel L. Johnson

Aerospace Medical Research Laboratory, Wright-Patterson Air Force Base, Ohio 45433

Damage risk criteria should describe the relationship between the probability of incurring noise-induced hearing impairment and the exposure environment. They should not be confused with industrial or environmental
exposure standards, permissible exposure limits, or the identification of
safe/protective limits which are based on additional nonbiological factors
such as social values, definition of handicap and compensability, economic
factors, feasibility of noise control, and legal and political considerations.
This summary maintains that in spite of uncertainties and open scientific
questions, the available data base is consistent enough to predict for preven-
tive/protective purposes the amount of noise-induced permanent threshold
shift to be expected in a population as a result of habitual noise exposure.
For noise exposure levels to have no effect on a population's hearing after
40 years of daily exposure, a "safe" level of approximately 75 dB(A) is
derived following the arguments advanced in the EPA "Levels Document."

WHAT ARE DAMAGE RISK CRITERIA?

The current state of damage risk criteria is confusing, in some respects, as
evidenced by the heated public debate in the United States on permissible
occupational noise exposure limits. In part, this problem is the fault of the
scientific community. Unfortunately, from the original introduction of the
concept of Damage Risk Criteria by Parrack and the first CHABA Working
Group (1), damage risk has always been set equal to compensable hearing
loss. However, today damage risk criteria are usually defined as the relationship between noise exposure and hearing loss. Obviously, compensable hearing loss is not the same as hearing loss per se. Any future attempt to demonstrate the validity of criteria should take this distinction into account, because
what constitutes a compensable hearing loss may change with legal interpretation, with the economic situation, with social changes, and so on, even
though the relationship between hearing loss and noise exposure does not
change.

Good damage risk criteria that are based on the relation of hearing loss
to noise exposure are essential. Compensation should be a later consideration, and should be left out of the definition of scientific damage risk criteria.
Based on such scientific criteria, one can select and recommend a protective

noise exposure level not to be exceeded in daily life. This certainly requires that in accordance with good preventive medicine practices, the protective level selected be set below the level that would lead to a compensable hearing loss. Unfortunately, the compensable hearing loss concept was used in the derivation of many damage risk criteria. One worried about the compensable hearing loss, that is, the handicap acquired by the time of retirement, but one did not worry about the amount of hearing loss between the level of normal hearing and the level of compensable hearing handicap which also occurred during this time period. Exposure type standards implemented by regulations are usually derived from criteria for which compensation is the basis. In addition to hearing risk, these regulations must also consider politics, feasibility, economics, etc. As a consequence of these additional factors, one usually arrives at more lenient standards that differ basically from the protective, preventive type standard. (To make it clear to foreign participants in this meeting, the term "standard," which has been used in U.S. legislation, has a completely different meaning from an ISO standard or an American National Standard. Certainly, ANSI or ISO could put out standardized damage risk criteria, but they are not to be confused with standards like the OSHA standard, which includes legally binding limits.)

CRITERIA FOR NOISE-INDUCED HEARING LOSS

About 2 years ago our laboratory was asked by the EPA to identify safe levels of noise exposure, as required by the Noise Control Act of 1972. On the basis of evidence accumulated over almost 6 years of deliberation, the U.S. Congress decided, not the scientific community, that safe levels could be identified below which one does not have to worry about hearing loss. Congress also set a time limit that was very short, so by the time our laboratory received the assignment, only 6 months remained to do the investigation. We solicited the help of a few experts, who perhaps might not like to be listed in this connection, but we would like to list them if only just to spread the blame. Seriously, these experts were some of the best in the country and were (1) as follows:

Dr. W. L. Baughn
Guide Lamp Div.
General Motors Corporation
Anderson, Indiana

Dr. Alexander Cohen
Dept. of Health, Education and Welfare
Public Health Service/NIOSH
Cincinnati, Ohio

Dr. John L. Fletcher
Department of Psychology
Memphis State University
Memphis, Tennessee

Dr. Aram Glorig
Callier Hearing and Speech Center
Dallas, Texas

Dr. Terry Henderson
Dept. of Health, Education and Welfare
Public Health Service/NIOSH
Cincinnati, Ohio

Dr. Karl K. Kryter
Stanford Research Institute
Menlo Park, California

Mr. Barry Lempert
Dept. of Health, Education and Welfare
Public Health Service/NIOSH
Cincinnati, Ohio

Dr. J. H. Mills
Central Institute for the Deaf
St. Louis, Missouri

Dr. W. Dixon Ward
University of Minnesota
Minneapolis, Minnesota

From our laboratory, Drs. Nixon, Johnson, and von Gierke were involved. Dr. Guignard, who worked at the University of Dayton at that time, was the compiler of the information and of the inputs received from all these distinguished experts. As far as possible, an effort was made to get all relevant information and arrive at a consensus on the issues of concern, but, as you know, for some of us, that is not possible.

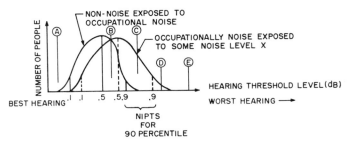

FIG. 1. Hypothetical changes of the statistical distribution of hearing threshold levels of a typical population due to some noise exposure. (From ref. 2)

The first step was to publish scientific damage risk criteria defined in accordance with the introduction as the cause–effect relationship between noise exposure and hearing loss. The identification of "safe levels" was not even considered at this point in time. The first step was to define unambiguously what was meant by hearing loss due to noise. Examination of Fig. 1 shows how we resolved this problem. The hearing risk concept of defining hearing loss is derived from the statistical distribution of hearing levels between occupationally exposed and nonoccupationally exposed populations. Depending on where you put the "fence," you get a large hearing risk or a small hearing risk. If you put the fence at locations either A or E, the hearing risk values will be small, whereas, if you put it at B, the hearing risk for exactly the same noise-exposed population will be very great. Now more likely the fence, of 25 dB (re ISO) determined by compensation considerations, is somewhere between location C and D, and this is the hearing risk to which most of our industrial data relate. The large discrepancy in the risk values from many studies occurs because we don't know where the median of the distribution is located and it is this location that influences the risk. This fact explains why in the current OSHA controversy (14) the values of risk from the various experts who testify vary from 2% to 29% for the 90 dB(A) exposure limit. As stated earlier, we placed ourselves in this predicament by applying the fence concept too broadly. As an alternative to the fence concept, the Noise-Induced Permanent Threshold Shift (NIPTS) concept (2) was adopted. Using this concept, we look at the differences between the 2 distributions at various percentiles. The difference in decibels between the same point for each distribution is called NIPTS, and it is shown in Fig. 1 for the 90th percentile level.

Using this NIPTS concept, we used the average (3) of the data bases of Passchier-Vermeer (4), Burns and Robinson (5), and Baughn (6). As part of this exercise, Baughn's data were published for the first time. It really doesn't make too much difference in the final result if you throw away 1, or even 2, of the data sets; and if only Robinson's data remain, which we hear today from Robinson are the most accurate. But, if you take all 3, it gives you a good average that normally differs at the most from any of the 3 individual methods by less than 5 dB. Thus, it doesn't make too much sense to say that there is not a good data base just because you dislike 1 or 2 of these studies. Certainly, these differences are not enough to confuse the whole world and especially the nonscientific public. It is interesting and de-

TABLE 1

SUMMARY OF THE PERMANENT HEARING DAMAGE EFFECTS
EXPECTED FOR CONTINUOUS NOISE EXPOSURE AT
VARIOUS VALUES OF THE A-WEIGHTED AVERAGE
SOUND LEVEL

75 dB for 8 hrs.

	av. .5, 1, 2 kHz	av. .5, 1, 2, 4 kHz	4 kHz
Max NIPTS 90th percentile NIPTS at 10 yrs. 90th percentile	1 dB	2 dB	6 dB
Average NIPTS	0	1	5
Max NIPTS 10th percentile	0	0	1
	0	0	0

80 dB for 8 hrs.

	av. .5, 1, 2 kHz	av. .5, 1, 2, 4 kHz	4 kHz
Max NIPTS 90th percentile NIPTS at 10 yrs. 90th percentile	1 dB	4 dB	11 dB
Average NIPTS	1	3	9
Max NIPTS 10th percentile	0	1	4
	0	0	2

85 dB for 8 hrs.

	av. .5, 1, 2 kHz	av. .5, 1, 2, 4 kHz	4 kHz
Max NIPTS 90th percentile	4 dB	7 dB	19 dB
NIPTS at 10 yrs. 90th percentile	2	6	16
Average NIPTS	1	3	9
Max NIPTS 10th percentile	1	2	5

90 dB for 8 hrs.

	av. .5, 1, 2 kHz	av. .5, 1, 2, 4 kHz	4 kHz
Max NIPTS 90th percentile	7 dB	12 dB	28 dB
NIPTS at 10 yrs. 90 percentile	4	9	24
Average NIPTS	3	6	15
Max NIPTS 10th percentile	2	4	11

sirable in scientific circles to discuss the "perfect study," but it is clear that even today without such a study there is adequate information available to predict with reasonable confidence the hearing impairment produced in the general population by a lifetime's exposure to continuous noise.

The NIPTS for different exposures and audiometric frequencies, taken from this average of 3 studies, is obtained as seen in Table 1, which provides true scientifically defined damage risk criteria.

DEVELOPMENT OF "SAFE" LEVELS

Using this information as a basis, the next step was to identify safe levels which were defined by law as those levels "requisite to protect the public health and welfare with an adequate margin of safety" (7). With respect to hearing, there was agreement between most of us that this should not involve any acknowledgment of an arbitrary fence. At this symposium we have also heard statements to the effect that pure-tone audiometry does not allow us to evaluate the effect of hearing loss. Perhaps pure-tone audiometry does not allow us to evaluate the functional problems once we have a hearing loss, but I think it is all we need to prevent hearing loss due to noise exposure from occurring. The next step, then, was to identify the noise exposure levels at which no significant pure-tone hearing changes occur so that potentially the total population is 100% protected. What we really mean by protection of 100% of the population is that we will attempt to find that noise level at which the 2 statistical distributions depicted in Fig. 1 do not differ by more than a prescribed amount, regardless of which percentile we decide to protect. Note that we have drawn Fig. 1 to show more NIPTS for the higher percentiles. This conclusion is directly the result of Table 1. For a constant NIPTS, the relation between percentile protected and exposure level can be drawn as shown in Fig. 2 (8). In this figure is also included the curve from the U.S. Public Health Service (9) data which shows the hearing level at various percentiles at age 60. We evoke the concept that by the time one has had 40 years of noise exposure, the part of the population that has, for instance, a 60-dB hearing level, is not going to be affected by a 60-dB noise because, certainly, it is hard to believe that a noise that you cannot hear can hurt your hearing. Therefore, we came up with the conclusion that the constant NIPTS curve cannot continue on as shown in Fig. 2 but, instead, had to approach the Public Health Service data curve. Thus, we get one minimum level which turns out for 4,000 Hz to be at 73 dB at which point you protect, at least theoretically, 100% of the population distribution against more than 5 dB NIPTS. Some might intuitively disagree with this argument, but, for all practical purposes, there is no reason to think it is not valid. Therefore, based on this concept, we derived the results for other frequencies and NIPTS values as depicted in Fig. 3 (8). Through the construction of these minimum levels in each case for various values of NIPTS, you get the rela-

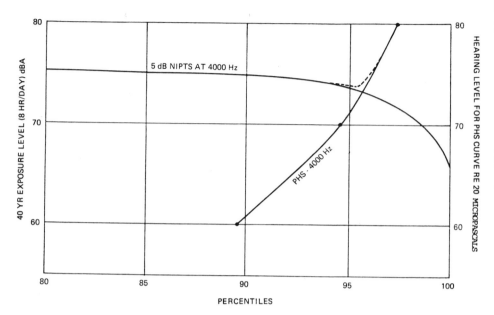

FIG. 2. Exposure level and hearing level as a function of population percentile, showing the 5-dB NIPTS curve merging with the PHS 4,000 Hz curve. (From ref. 8)

tionships shown in Fig. 4, which, as a reminder, are again for 40 years' exposure and a constant exposure level.

Having obtained this final curve, one is now in a position to identify a safe level. This step is based on an answer to the following 3 questions: (i) What is meant by "hearing"?, (ii) What are "significant effects"?, and (iii)

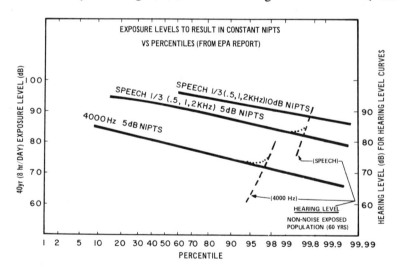

FIG. 3. Exposure level and hearing level as a function of population percent, showing merging of different NIPTS curves with Public Health Service curves. (From ref. 8)

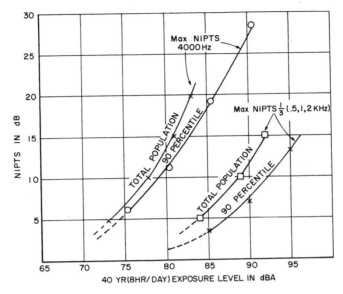

FIG. 4. NIPTS as a function of exposure level for the 90th percentile and the total population. Values are for 4,000 Hz and the traditional speech frequencies (0.5, 1, and 2 kHz). For the total population curves, the assumption that a noise that cannot be heard cannot damage hearing is invoked.

What population is considered? These decisions are always, to some extent, arbitrary and must be answered differently if one discusses population averages and an application to preventive-medical purposes, or individual cases and an application to compensation purposes.

These questions were answered in the EPA "levels document" (8) by first considering "hearing" to include all normally measured audiometric frequencies. Thus, in order to say a noise has no effect on hearing, one must look at the most sensitive audiometric frequency, namely 4,000 Hz. Therefore, the derivation of safe levels was based on the avoidance of any significant effects at 4 kHz.

Second, as a definition of a significant effect on hearing, a 5-dB NIPTS was selected somewhat arbitrarily as the smallest change that can be reliably measured and verified in an individual and yet can still be significant in cross-sectional studies. Finally, the population considered by the EPA was the total population.

At this point, it is informative to look at alternatives to these 3 decisions made in the levels document. If you do not want to accept the arguments used in the development of protection of the total population, a concept primarily appealing to politicians and the legal profession, one can always protect an arbitrary percentile; e.g. the 90th percentile. NIPTS values for the 90th percentile are more accurate; at least they require fewer assumptions, but then the argument is, why didn't you protect the 95th or higher percentiles instead of the 90th percentile. It really does not make too much difference, with respect to the final values obtained, whether you protect the 90th percentile or the total population, but legally this is a very touchy point. So, it is much more appealing to show protection of the total population. With respect to the 5-dB NIPTS, some have claimed that even a 10-dB shift at 4,000 Hz would not be sensed by an individual. We certainly hope that this is true, because remember, only the statistical populations are being protected from a 5-dB shift, not individuals. As pointed out clearly in the levels document, some sensitive individuals may have more than a 5-dB PTS due to a 73 dB(A) noise exposure. We have done work (10) that does indicate that, for any likely true statistical distribution of hearing loss in individuals, it would be unlikely for an individual to have more than a 10-dB NIPTS from the 73 dB(A) noise exposure. If one only protects the total population distribution against a 10-dB NIPTS, however, certain sensitive individuals might be expected to develop individual NIPTS as high as 20 dB. Hence, we certainly believe that protecting the total population distribution against more than 5 dB NIPTS is not overly conservative.

If one selects the traditional speech frequencies instead of the most sensitive 4 kHz frequency, total protection from 5 dB NIPTS requires an exposure level below 84 dB and protection of the 90th percentile requires a level of 87 dB. We have the curve also for the average of 500, 1,000, 2,000, and 3,000, and for the average of 2,000, 3,000, and 4,000 Hz, but they all fall between the two sets of curves of Fig. 4, that is, between the 4,000 Hz curves and the traditional speech frequency curves. So, even if one defines hearing conservation to protect only the speech frequencies (depending on how you interpret what frequency range is required for speech), one will get different answers anywhere between about 75 and 85 dB. But clearly, the data shown in Fig. 4 do define the range of levels which can be interpreted as having no effect on hearing. It is certainly hard to conceive how levels above 85 dB can be considered to have no effect on hearing.

THE EXPOSURE TIME-INTENSITY TRADE-OFF

The only reliable data points relating occupational hearing loss to noise exposure are for daily exposures to a nominal 8-hr day. All safe, as well as protective, exposure limits are anchored on these data. To allow for shorter exposure times to higher levels, a condition particularly frequent in military operations, for example, aircraft maintenance, the Air Force introduced in 1956, after extensive study by a CHABA Committee, the "equal-energy rule" (11). This rule allows a 3-dB increase in level for halving of exposure time (1). This equal energy concept was also used in the EPA levels document. The meager evidence available based on temporary threshold shift data (TTS) indicated that this rule might be rather overprotective instead of underprotective, a desirable asset of any preventive approach. The 17-year experience with this rule incorporated into the Air Force Regulations on hazardous noise exposures did not show any evidence to the contrary. TTS data accumulated afterward in laboratory experiments clearly indicate that no simple TTS-vs-time relationship fits the data perfectly. However, the TTS-vs-exposure time data for 4 kHz are fitted better by the equal energy rule than by the 5-dB increase of level per halving of time relationship.

The 5-dB rule might fit the data in the conventional speech range better. In the final analysis, the arguments in favor of the equal energy rule were never based so much on its exact scientific validity, but on the basis that it is certainly more protective and, therefore, safer than the less conservative 5 dB per doubling rule.

The 5-dB rule for halving of exposure time (13) was an attempt to correct for intermittency. For some types of evenly interrupted noises, in which the level is not extremely high, the 5-dB rule does better predict TTS even for 4,000 Hz. However, the sad facts of life are that not all interrupted noise is evenly spaced or at relatively low levels. Thus, the 5-dB rule can be misused and allow exposures for which its use was not originally intended. Such misuse would be an uninterrupted exposure to 115 dB for 15 min per day. This dose, allowable according to the OSHA rule (13), is definitely judged as too high by most experts. If you start with 85 dB(A) as the 8-hour anchor point and use equal energy, you arrive at 115 dB for approximately 20 sec as allowable exposure time. A 115-dB exposure for 20 sec is certainly more reasonable than the 15-min exposure time. The very short exposure time of 15–20 sec is definitely more in the safe range with respect to what was presented at this symposium by Dr. Spoendlin. If you remember, he discussed possible transitions in the type of hearing damage observed for amplitudes in the 115–125 dB range. Finally, if the 5-dB rule is argued on the basis of intermittency, then the rule should be made foolproof. A preventive measure should not only protect against the most probable daily exposure pattern, it should be protective for all possible practical situations.

In summary, the 3-dB rule is more conservative, as well as more protective. The 5-dB rule leads with the anchor point at 90 dB(A) definitely to levels too high for short durations, namely, 115 dB(A) for 15 min. A further point in favor of the 3-dB rule is its incorporation into the ISO Standard R1999 (12). The United States voted in favor of this standard in 1970. The basis for this vote was that of all the technical, industry, government, and interest group representatives in the United States, 26 voted affirmative on this standard, 5 negative, and 1 abstained.

PRACTICAL CONSIDERATIONS FOR NOISE EXPOSURE STANDARDS

The establishment of noise exposure limits short of levels completely safe for 100% of the population is a social, economical, legal, and in short, administrative decision. Scientific data can be used to rationalize the decision by predicting its consequences but, no matter how good and complete they are, they cannot be used to justify the result of the decision. It is highly misleading to hide the real issues and consequences behind scientific arguments or excuses stating that scientific data are not good enough to make the decision.

The largest differences of opinion between experts in the field of noise-induced hearing loss comes about, not because of variability of the basic data, but because many researchers add their interpretations of feasibility and significance to the interpretation of the data. This is why the work done in the "levels" document is unique. For the first time that we know of, an attempt was made to define a "safe" level that did not have this bias.

From the earlier discussion of safe levels (Fig. 4), it is clear that neither 85 nor 90 dB(A) is a truly safe level. They might be the practical levels we must settle on based on feasibility determined at this instant in time. But we must keep in mind that feasibility changes, whereas true "safe" levels do not. No scientific argument will ever prove that the practical level selected is safe by invoking the argument that only a few workers will suffer hearing losses requiring compensation. It is inconceivable to us how some experts try to "prove" this.

The OSHA law states that "material impairment of hearing" is to be prevented. It is obvious that the requirement to prevent any "material impairment of hearing" is not necessarily the same as the prevention of any significant hearing loss, which would be achieved by "safe" levels. Although at what point a "material impairment of hearing" begins is debatable, we believe it is certainly present if hearing for conversational speech is affected by 5 dB or more. The requirement is clear that material impairment is to be prevented and not material handicap. Figure 4 shows that prevention of a 5-dB average NIPTS at the traditional speech frequencies (0.5, 1 and 2 kHz) in the 90th percentile of the population requires levels to be kept below 87 dB(A). To protect practically the total population would require levels below 84 dB(A). Taking 3,000 or 4,000 Hz into consideration as important to the speech frequency range, as most experts admit these days, reduces this level further. In summary, the unequivocal fact that emerges is that an 8-hour, 90 dB(A) standard does not prevent "material impairment of hearing."

THE PRACTICAL STUDIES NEEDED TO IMPROVE DAMAGE RISK CRITERIA

We do not want to imply that we now have scientific damage risk criteria so accurate that there is no room for improvement. We have always expressed the possibility of an error of as much as ± 5 dB and certainly this shows room for improvement. Six general areas of study are proposed.

First, in keeping with Dr. Henderson's opening remarks, we agree that of most practical importance are more field studies of the actual hearing loss occurring in various industrial situations.

Second, hearing level strictly as a function of sociocusis needs to be better defined.

Third, the long-term effectiveness of hearing protectors must be better defined. Do hearing protectors, indeed, provide the hearing protection predicted by their attenuation characteristics?

Fourth, the only way to address individual susceptibility will be to do longitudinal studies. These studies need to be done for both the occupationally noise-exposed and the nonoccupationally noise-exposed populations. Perhaps we can learn why boys at the age of 17 to 18 years start to lose hearing at frequencies above 2,000 Hz faster than girls.

Fifth, we need to keep working on the development of nonauditory criteria. Certainly, noise can cause stress effects, but are these stress effects important in comparison with the other life stresses?

Sixth, what are the combined effects of noise with other environmental factors such as heat, fatigue, diet, etc.? It is possible that by eliminating one of these factors, the auditory tolerance to noise could be increased? Animal studies are certainly a necessity here.

In summary, we think that adequate damage risk criteria are available now, and "safe" levels can be established. Nevertheless, there are good reasons for not only continuing, but increasing our research effort.

ACKNOWLEDGMENTS

This research was sponsored by Aerospace Medical Research Laboratory, Aerospace Medical Division, Air Force Systems Command, Wright-Patterson Air Force Base, Ohio 45433. This paper has been identified by Aerospace Medical Research Laboratory as AMRL-TR-75-58. Further reproduction is authorized to satisfy needs of the U.S. Government.

REFERENCES

1. Guignard, J. C. (1973): A basis for limiting noise exposure for hearing conservation. EPA 550/9-73-001-A or AMRL-TR-73-90.
2. Guignard, J. C., and Johnson, D. L. (1975): The relation of noise exposure to noise induced hearing damage. *Sound Vibration,* 9(1):18–23.
3. Johnson, D. L. (1973): Prediction of NIPTS due to continuous noise exposure. U.S. Environmental Protection Agency and U.S. Air Force Aerospace Medical Research Laboratory, AMRL-TR-73-91, EPA-550/9-73-001-B.
4. Passchier-Vermeer, W. (1968): Hearing loss due to exposure to steady-state broad band noise. Report 35. Institut voor Gezondheidstechniek, Delft, Netherlands.
5. Robinson, D. W. (1968): The relationships between hearing loss and noise exposure. National Physical Laboratory, Aero Report AC32, Teddington, England.
6. Baughn, W. L. (1973): Relation between daily noise exposure and hearing loss

based on the evaluation of 6,835 industrial noise exposure cases. U.S. Environmental Protection Agency and U.S. Air Force Aerospace Medical Research Laboratory, AMRL-TR-73-53.

7. Noise Control Act of 1972, Public Law 92-574, 92 Congress, HR 11021, October 27, 1972.
8. U.S. Environmental Protection Agency (1974): Information on levels of environmental noise requisite to protect public health and welfare with an adequate margin of safety. EPA Document 550/9-74-004.
9. National Center for Health Statistics (1965): Hearing levels of adults by age and sex, United States, 1960–1972. Vital and Health Statistics, PHS Pub. No. 1000-Series 11—No. 11. Public Health Service, Washington, D.C., U.S. Government Printing Office.
10. Johnson, D. L. (1975): Effect of imposing various skewed distributions of hearing loss on a normally distributed population. Paper presented at the 89th meeting of the Acoustical Society of America, Austin, Texas.
11. Department of the Air Force, Medical Service (1956): Hazardous noise exposure, AF Regulation 160–3.
12. Assessment of occupational noise exposure for hearing conservation purposes. ISO Recommendation ISO/R1999. Geneva:ISO (1971).
13. Occupational Safety and Health Act of 1972, Section 6(b)(5).
14. Proposed OSHA Occupational Noise Exposure Regulation, Environmental Protection Agency, Federal Register, Vol. 39, No. 244, pages 43802–43809, Dec. 18, 1974.

DISCUSSION

Editors' Note: There was not time for discussion of the von Gierke–Johnson manuscript, but because of its relevance, the editors have included comments submitted by J. Botsford after the presentations.

J. Botsford: In establishing limits on occupational noise exposure, it is necessary to decide (1) what is the effect that is to be prevented, (2) what duration of exposure is to be considered, and (3) what fraction of the population is to be protected from this effect.

We heard from Dr. von Gierke on the second day that his goal was to prevent any change in any audiogram exceeding 5 dB at 4 kHz. This is essentially saying that there should not be any change in any audiogram whatsoever.

Dr. von Gierke went on to say that this injury should be prevented in the total population after 40 years of exposure. There is no quarrel with this view as a social goal. But I know of no precedent for such a stringent view when it is to be the basis for public health standards as Dr. von Gierke recommends. So I think we must examine Dr. von Gierke's recommendations rather closely.

The slide he presented on the second day showing a 90th percentile curve and another curve labeled "total population" is misleading. The "total population" referred to in that figure was all the people exposed to the same noise for 40 years. This is an extremely small group, much less than 1% of the working population. The curves do not apply to the total population of the country, or even to the total working population as one might conclude from the labeling of the slide.

Now Dr. von Gierke is telling us the truth, but not the whole truth. He is basing his arguments on a "worst case" example.

We do not have the exact statistics needed to put this matter in perspective, but what we do have serves fairly well. Of the 72 million in the United States civilian labor force at the beginning of 1966, those in the age range 55 to 64, who would conceivably be in Dr. von Gierke's "total population," accounted for only 13½ % of the work force. They had held their jobs nowhere near 40 years, as the median time on the job was about 9 years. Labor statistics also show that those who had the same employer and therefore might have had the same noise exposure for 30 years or more accounted for only 3.8% of the working population.

Closer to the point are some actual employment data obtained from a major steel company. Records were examined to learn how many of those hired 40 years ago were still employed. Of the number hired during a 12-month period 40 years earlier, only 0.9% were still employed. Only ½% of those hired 30 years earlier remained. And it was very surprising to find that only 15% of those hired 2 years earlier were still working.

Although we would like to have statistics coming even closer to the point, that must be a matter of future research. But from the statistics we do have, it is clear that the group Dr. von Gierke has singled out is extremely small and not typical of the working population.

When the entire working population is considered, quite a different picture is seen. One analysis brought out this difference by multiplying the fraction of the labor force at each age by the fraction impaired at each age to obtain the fraction of the working population impaired at each age. These fractions were then summed over the 18- to 65-year age range to give the fraction of the total working population afflicted with impaired hearing.

Results of this analysis showed that, for sound levels at work of 81 dB(A) or less 9.4% had impaired hearing due to causes other than noise exposure at work. At 85 dB(A), 12.8% showed impaired hearing, an increase of 34 cases of impaired hearing per thousand exposed workers due to occupational noise. At 90 dB(A), 16.6% showed impaired hearing for a total of 72 cases of hearing loss induced by occupational noise per thousand exposed. This analysis demonstrates that only a small portion of the working population will suffer occupational hearing loss at 90 dB(A). It also shows that lowering exposure limits from 90 to 85 dB(A) would benefit only 38 out of every 1,000 persons employed in those levels.

Regarding the controversy over whether the national standard should be set at 85 or 90 dB(A), no one has pointed out that the Department of Labor has proposed an 85 dB(A) standard. It provides that those exposed to levels of 85–90 dB(A) must have annual audiograms. For those few individuals whose examinations show hearing damage resulting from noise exposure, ear protection is to be furnished and worn. Audiometric monitoring is to continue. This means was selected as an economical one for protecting the relatively few persons who might be affected by exposure to these low levels.

von Gierke/Johnson reply to Botsford: We are glad to see that Mr. Botsford has no quarrel with the view that as a social goal, injury from noise to the hearing organ in the total population after 40 years of exposure should be prevented. But if Botsford is willing to accept this as a social goal, we find it difficult to understand why it must be automatically rejected as a basis for public health standards. Now we certainly agree that when setting a public health standard that will be enforced by law, factors such as technical feasibility and economic feasibility are important. These considerations may require such a public health standard (for example the OSHA standard) to be different from longer range social goals. But as we said in our paper, you select the social goals as a baseline from which to temporarily depart for technical and economic reasons.

Most of Botsford's critique now revolves around how to make the tradeoff between the level set by a legal standard and technical and economic consideration. In such an analysis, it is important to consider the number of persons that are being exposed to different levels for different periods of time. But it is even more important to consider the costs of implementing any standard to the benefits gained. We, of course did not do this, since the purpose of the paper was not to propose legally enforceable standards but to derive "safe" levels, that is, levels below which noise-induced hearing loss is negligible for essentially the total population. On the other hand, neither does Botsford's reasoning in support of the OSHA standard use such as economic analysis. Who knows? Maybe a good analysis would suggest that the OSHA level for an 8-hour day might be lower than 85 dB(A) or even higher than 90 dB(A). We do not see how such an occupational exposure limit can be set by simply saying that lowering the exposure levels from 90 to 85 dB would benefit only 38 out of every 1,000 persons. First, it is not really obvious that 3.8% is such a small number. Furthermore, this number comes from use of the hearing risk concept discussed in our paper and as such, neglects the changes in hearing occurring in the exposed population below the 25-dB fence that defines handicap. Likewise it also ignores what happens to the exposed population above the fence, which in this case is over 10% of the exposed population. Finally, it ignores any loss to audiometric frequencies above 2,000 Hz. How can one make such an important decision as what the OSHA standard should be on such a small part of the data? We are sorry that Botsford feels that the "total population" in Fig. 4 does not tell the whole truth, but the basic idea was to look at all the people exposed to a specific exposure condition, not just those near the fence that defines handicap. So by "total population" we mean we consider the change in the statistical distribution of hearing levels that results from some noise exposure for all hearing level percentiles. From this, we obtain a "cause-and-effect" relationship between a specific noise exposure and the amount of change in the distribution of hearing level. Perhaps "total population" is not the best descriptor, but we certainly do not see how it can be misinterpreted as the total population of the work force or of the United States population.

Mr. Botsford's comments do not concern the basic purpose and reasoning of our paper—as a matter of fact, they only emphasize the point we make, how difficult it is for the scientific community to separate damage risk criteria from the selection of enforceable, economically feasible and socially just exposure limits.

Subject Index